Fetal Medicine

Fetal Medicine

An Illustrated Textbook

Zarko Alfirevic

Emeritus Professor, University of Liverpool
Fetal Medicine Unit, Liverpool Women's Hospital
Liverpool, United Kingdom

Seshadri Suresh

Director of Mediscan Systems and Chief Functionary Voluntary Health Services
Chennai, India

Jonathan Hyett

Professor of Obstetrics and Gynaecology, Western Sydney University
Fetal Medicine Unit and Ingham Institute, Liverpool Hospital
Sydney, Australia

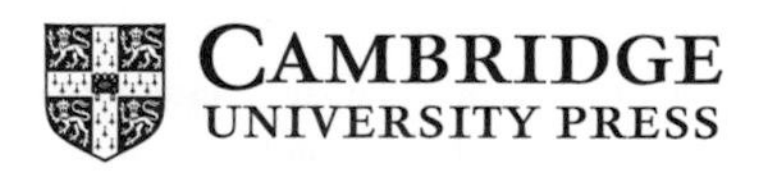

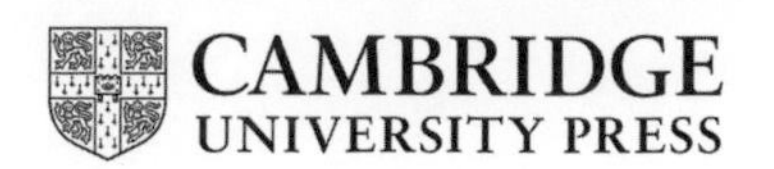

Shaftesbury Road, Cambridge CB2 8EA, United Kingdom

One Liberty Plaza, 20th Floor, New York, NY 10006, USA

477 Williamstown Road, Port Melbourne, VIC 3207, Australia

314–321, 3rd Floor, Plot 3, Splendor Forum, Jasola District Centre, New Delhi – 110025, India

103 Penang Road, #05–06/07, Visioncrest Commercial, Singapore 238467

Cambridge University Press is part of Cambridge University Press & Assessment, a department of the University of Cambridge.

We share the University's mission to contribute to society through the pursuit of education, learning and research at the highest international levels of excellence.

www.cambridge.org
Information on this title: www.cambridge.org/9781009015943

DOI: 10.1017/9781009030816

First published 2023

Printed in the United Kingdom by TJ Books Limited, Padstow Cornwall

A catalogue record for this publication is available from the British Library.

Library of Congress Cataloging-in-Publication Data
Names: Alfirevic, Zarko, editor. | Suresh, Seshadri, editor. | Hyett, Jonathan, editor.
Title: Fetal medicine : an illustrated textbook / edited by Zarko Alfirevic, Seshadri Suresh, Jonathan Hyett.
Other titles: Fetal medicine (Alfirevic)
Description: Cambridge, United Kingdom ; New York, NY : Cambridge University Press, 2022. | Includes bibliographical references and index.
Identifiers: LCCN 2022049376 (print) | LCCN 2022049377 (ebook) | ISBN 9781009015943 (paperback) | ISBN 9781009030816 (epub)
Subjects: MESH: Fetal Diseases | Congenital Abnormalities | Prenatal Diagnosis–methods | Fetal Therapies–methods | Perinatology–methods | Handbook
Classification: LCC RG626 (print) | LCC RG626 (ebook) | NLM WQ 39 | DDC 618.3/2–dc23/eng/20230119
LC record available at https://lccn.loc.gov/2022049376
LC ebook record available at https://lccn.loc.gov/2022049377

ISBN 978-1-009-01594-3 Paperback

Contents

Contributors

SIÂN BULLOUGH

Research Fellow, Fetal Medicine Unit
Liverpool Women's Hospital, Liverpool, United Kingdom
Chapter 14: Fetal Infections; Chapter 15: Drugs in Pregnancy and Teratogenesis

GLENN GARDENER

Director and Senior Staff Specialist
Maternal and Fetal Medicine, Mater Mother's Hospital, Brisbane, Queensland, Australia
Chapter 18: Fetal Surgery for Spina Bifida

SUJATHA JAGADEESH

Head of Department of Clinical Genetics Mediscan Systems, Chennai, India
Chapter 15: Drugs in Pregnancy and Teratogenesis

DAVOR JURKOVIC

Consultant Gynaecologist and Professor
at the University College London
Director Gynaecology Diagnostic Unit, University College Hospital, London, United Kingdom
Chapter 9: Abnormal Placenta

VICTORIA MCKAY

Consultant Clinical Geneticist and Clinical Lead at the Liverpool Centre for
Genomic Medicine
Liverpool Women's NHS Foundation Trust, United Kingdom
Chapter 19: Genetic Syndromes

RITU MOGRA

Senior Staff Specialist and Head of Department of Obstetric and Gynaecological Imaging
RPA Women and Babies, Royal Prince Alfred Hospital, Sydney, Australia
Chapter 12: Multiple Pregnancy

KATE NAVARATNAM

Consultant in Maternal Fetal Medicine
Fetal Medicine Unit, Liverpool Women's Hospital, Liverpool, United Kingdom
Chapter 16: Ultrasound Guided Invasive Diagnostic and Therapeutic Procedures; Chapter 20: Termination of Pregnancy for Fetal Abnormality

BORNA POLJAK

Research Fellow, Fetal Medicine Unit
Liverpool Women's Hospital, Liverpool, United Kingdom
Chapter 19: Genetic Syndromes

ANDREW SHARP

Senior Lecturer, Department of Women's and Children's Health, University of Liverpool, Liverpool, United Kingdom
Chapter 4: Small for Gestational Age (SGA) and Fetal Growth Restriction

BEENA SURESH

Consultant Geneticist, Mediscan Systems, Chennai, India
Chapter 19: Genetic Syndromes

INDRANI SURESH

Co-director, Mediscan Systems, Chennai, India
Chapter 3.2: Fetal Heart

Acknowledgments

Special thanks to Dr Lata Muralidharan, Head of Perinatal Pathology, Mediscan, for providing amazing images of various pathological specimens, and to Mrs Subbulakshmi Raghavan, Research coordinator, Mediscan, for her work with ultrasound images for the book.

CHAPTER 1

Fetal Anatomy

First Trimester Assessment

SUMMARY BOX

HEAD AND NECK

ANATOMY ASSESSMENT

- Head
  - Cranial bones, midline falx
  - Ventricles filled with choroid plexus – 'butterfly' sign (Fig. 1.1)
  - Intracranial translucency/posterior fossa
- Face
  - Eyes with lenses (Fig. 1.2)
  - Normal profile with nasal bone
  - Intact lips (Fig. 1.3)
- Neck
  - Normal appearance
  - Nuchal translucency (Fig. 1.4)

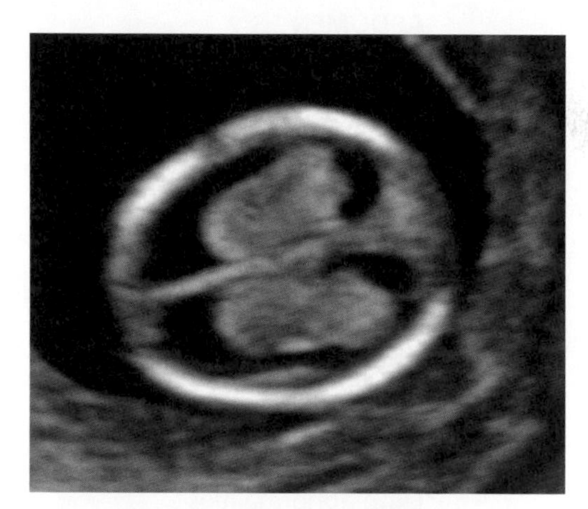

Fig. 1.1 Transverse view of the head. The appearance of the normal choroid plexus is called the 'butterfly sign'. Note that there is no space between the choroid plexus and the walls of the lateral ventricle.

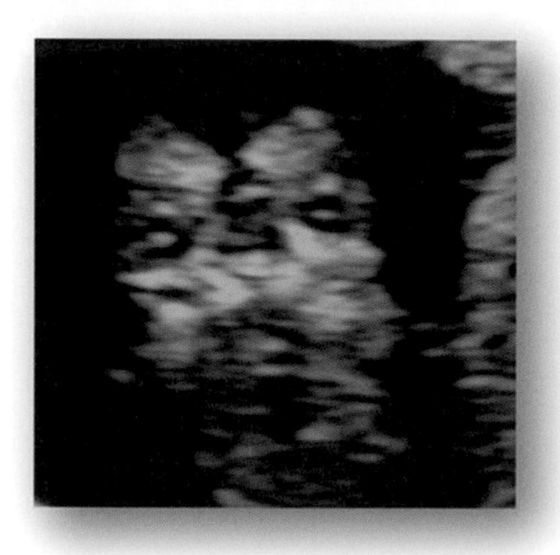

Fig. 1.2 Posterior coronal view of a normal face with large anterior fontanelle. The orbits are seen with the white dot indicating the lenses.

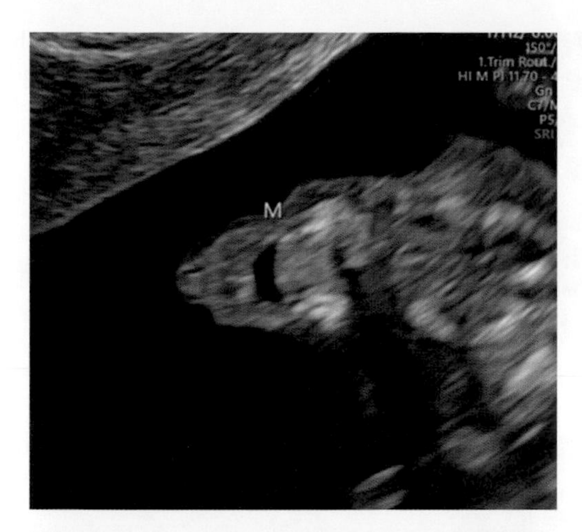

Fig. 1.3 Anterior coronal view of a normal fetal face with open mouth and intact lips.

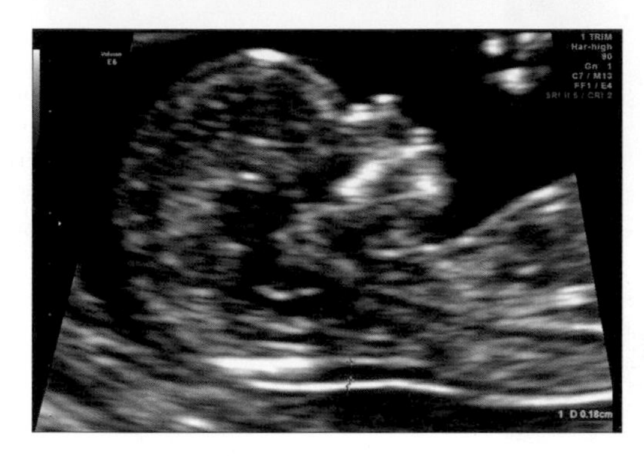

Fig. 1.4 Normal fetal profile with visible nasal bone and normal nuchal translucency (1.8 mm).

ABNORMAL SKULL

Acrania–Exencephaly–Anencephaly Sequence (Fig. 1.5)

Definitions and Characteristics

- Absent cranium – acrania
- Amorphous brain mass – exencephaly (Fig. 1.6)
- No recognisable brain tissue – anencephaly
- Commonly associated with neural tube abnormalities (craniorachischisis, spina bifida, iniencephaly) and facial, cardiac, renal and gastrointestinal malformations

Ultrasound Assessment

- Use transvaginal scan to exclude the presence of amniotic band sequence

Investigations

- Karyotyping may reveal an aneuploidy which would alter the risk for future pregnancy

Counselling and Management

- Offer termination of pregnancy
- Offer palliative care and discuss organ donation programme, if available
- Recurrence is ~3–4%
- Amniotic band sequence is sporadic with no increased risk for future pregnancies
- Advise folic acid supplementation (5 mg/day) in all future pregnancies

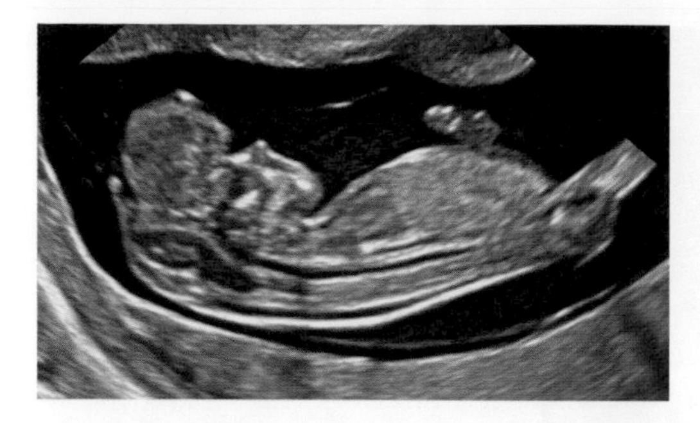

Fig. 1.5 Acrania–exencephaly–anencephaly sequence. Note the absent cranium and free-floating amorphous brain tissue. If first seen later in pregnancy, as the brain tissue is destroyed, this would present as a classic anencephaly.

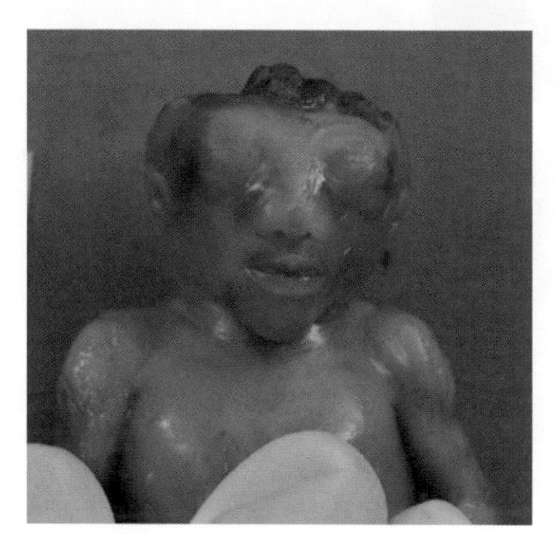

Fig. 1.6 Fetus with acrania. Only a small amount of amorphous brain tissue is still visible.

Skull Defects

Definitions and Characteristics

- Defects are most commonly occipital (85%) and may contain:
  - only meninges (meningocele) (Fig. 1.7)
  - brain tissue (encephalocele) (Figs. 1.8 and 1.9)
  - brain and part of the lateral ventricles (encephalocystocele)
- The clear distinction may not be accurate in the first trimester as contents of a defect may vary at later gestations

Ultrasound Assessment

- Look for *Meckel–Gruber syndrome* (occipital encephalocele with large cystic kidneys and polydactyly)
- Look for *amniotic band sequence* when defects are lateral or parietal

Investigations

- Offer invasive testing for karyotyping and microarray
- Exome sequencing can detect associated autosomal recessive ciliopathies including *Walker–Warburg syndrome* and *Joubert syndrome-related disorders*

Counselling and Management

Isolated Meningocele

- Good prognosis; >90% survival without sequelae

Encephalocele

- Counselling is complex and should involve neurosurgeons
- Sac size and the amount of brain tissue will determine prognosis
- Mortality approaches 30% despite appropriate treatment
- The long-term outcome of milder forms remains uncertain as most had termination of pregnancy

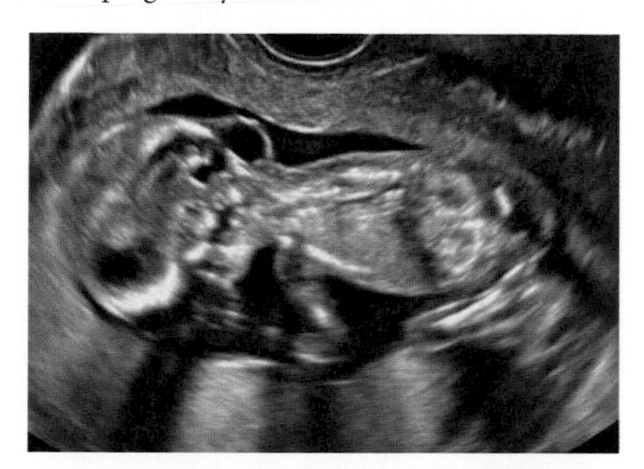

Fig. 1.7 Cystic swelling behind the occipital bone communicating with the posterior fossa through a small calvarial defect suggestive of occipital meningocele. This has to be differentiated from cystic hygroma or lymph cysts, wherein there will be no communication with intracranial structures.

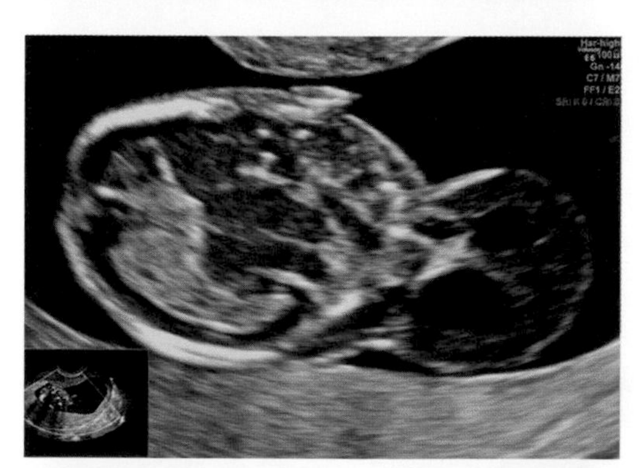

Fig. 1.8 Transverse view of an occipital encephalocele. Note the presence of the brain matter, calvarial defect and altered intracranial anatomy.

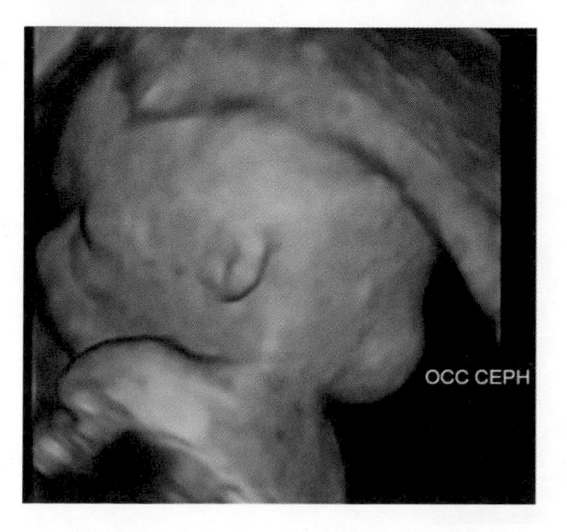

Fig. 1.9 3D view of an occipital encephalocele.

'BUTTERFLY SIGN' IS ABSENT

Definition and Characteristics

- 'Butterfly sign' describes the normal appearance of the choroid plexuses on transverse imaging of the fetal brain in the first trimester

Ultrasound Assessment

- Look for signs of *alobar holoprosencephaly* (single ventricle, fused thalami, absent falx) (Fig. 1.10)
- Less severe forms of *holoprosencephaly* are unlikely to be detectable in the first trimester
- Early *ventriculomegaly* presents as choroid plexus filling less than half of the ventricular space and not touching the medial and lateral ventricular walls (Fig. 1.11)
- Check for facial clefts and proboscis (a trunk-like nose)

Investigations

- Offer invasive testing

Counselling

- *Alobar holoprosencephaly* is usually lethal in early childhood; up to 80% of fetuses will have abnormal karyotype, mainly trisomy 13 (60%), but also trisomy 18, triploidy and deletions
- *Ventriculomegaly* in the first trimester is often associated with chromosomal and posterior fossa abnormalities, but can also be 'isolated' or transient, with good long-term prognosis

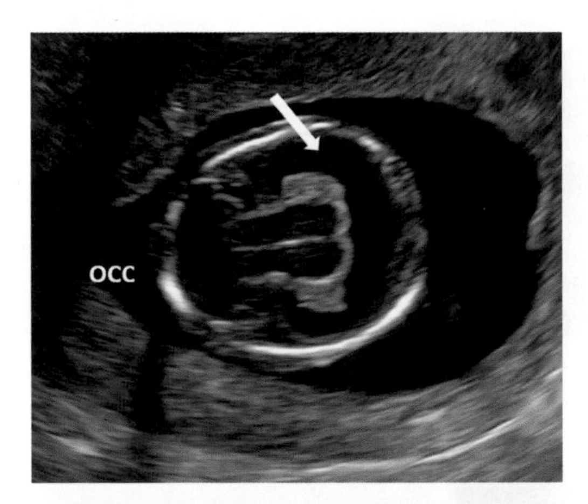

Fig. 1.10 Note the single ventricle (arrow) with absent midline falx and fused thalamus. The 'butterfly' sign is absent. Occ, Occiput.

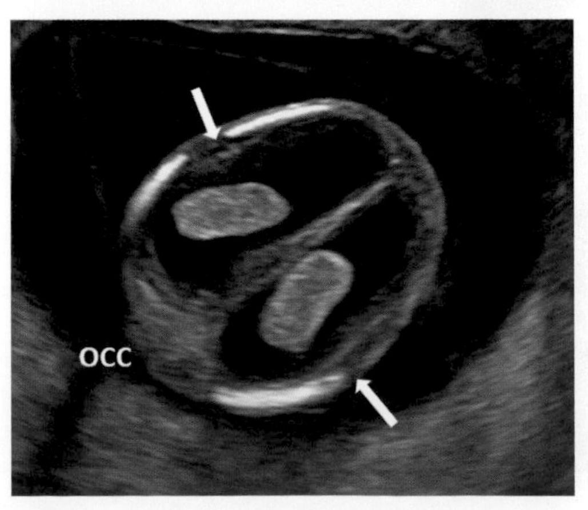

Fig. 1.11 Dilated lateral ventricles (arrows) are suspected in the first trimester when there is a visible space between the choroid plexus and the lateral wall of the lateral ventricles.
Occ, Occiput.

INTRACRANIAL TRANSLUCENCY IS ABSENT

Definition and Characteristics

- Intracranial translucency (IT) is the fourth ventricle which is seen in the mid-sagittal view of the head
- The IT is parallel to the nuchal translucency and appears between two echogenic borders – brainstem anteriorly and choroid plexus of fourth ventricle posteriorly (Fig. 1.12)
- Immediately below the fourth ventricle is a small translucent area representing the cerebromedullary cistern, which later forms the cisterna magna
- The IT increases from 1.5 mm at a CRL of 45 mm to 2.5 mm at a CRL of 84 mm

Ultrasound Assessment

- Absent or small IT in sagittal section (Fig. 1.13)
- In axial sections the choroid plexus appears to 'fill' the hemisphere and is often referred to as the 'dried up brain' (Fig. 1.14), or the 'crash' sign in the transverse plane (Fig. 1.15)
- Look for spinal defect – it may not be obvious even when using the transvaginal approach
- Absence of lemon and banana signs is not reassuring enough – these signs are not typically present before 14 weeks

Investigations

- Offer invasive testing

Counselling

- Absent IT as a sign of spina bifida or other pathology has a relatively high false-positive rate; therefore, a normal follow-up scan should be sufficiently reassuring

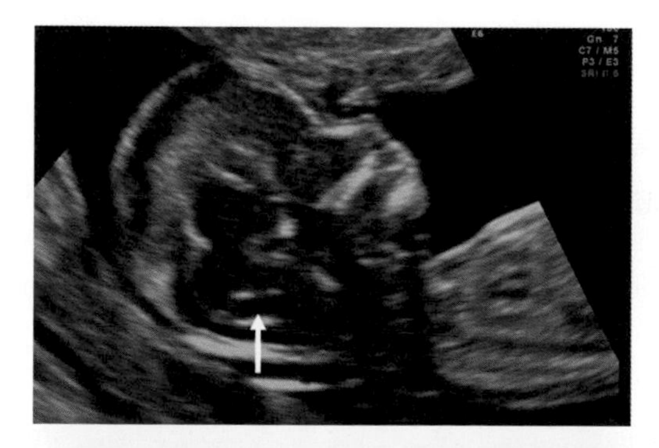

Fig. 1.12 Sagittal plane of the face with normal IT (arrow) which represents the fourth ventricle which lies between the brain stem (above) and the cisterna magna (below).

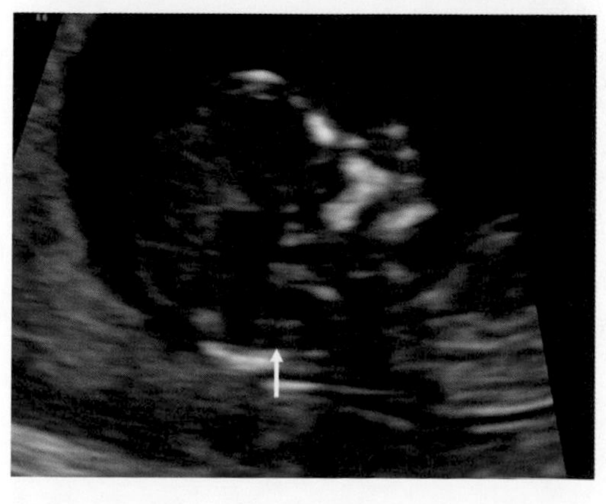

Fig. 1.13 Sagittal plane of the face in a fetus with an open neural tube defect. IT is absent due to the descent of the medulla oblongata through the foramen magnum and compression of the fourth ventricle (arrow).

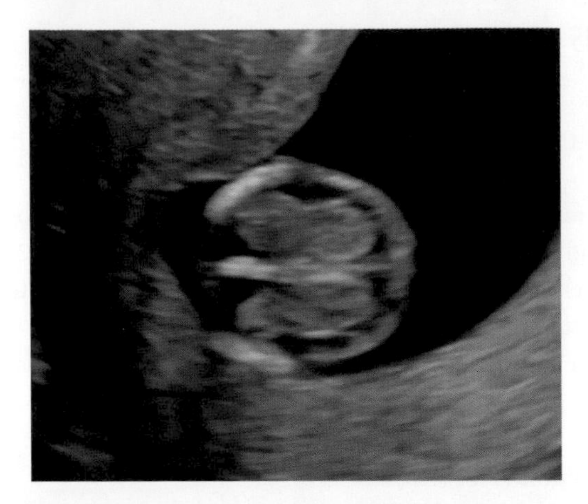

Fig. 1.14 Transverse section of the head in a fetus with spina bifida. The choroid plexus appears to fill up the entire hemisphere. This is referred to as the 'dried up brain'.

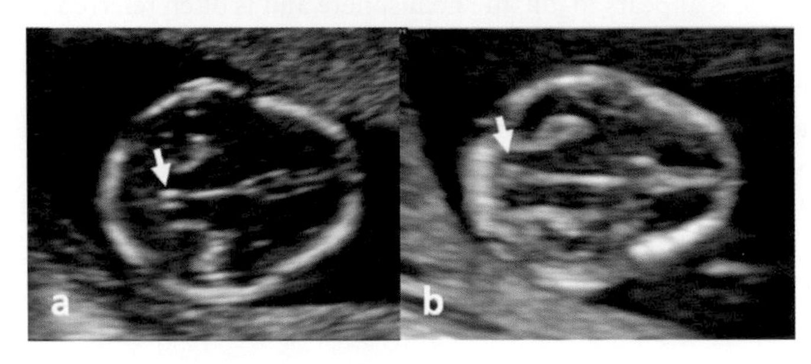

Fig. 1.15 (a) Transverse section of a normal fetal head, showing the thalami, cerebral peduncles and posterior fossa. The aqueduct is seen as a small slit (arrow) at a distance from the occiput. (b) Transverse section of the head in a fetus with spina bifida. The aqueduct is very close to the occiput (arrow) and is referred to as the 'crash sign'.

INTRACRANIAL TRANSLUCENCY IS ENLARGED

Definition and Characteristics

- 99th centile for IT ranges from 3.0 mm (CRL 45–54 mm) to 3.4 mm (CRL 75–84 mm)

Ultrasound Assessment

- Look for absent dividing septum between the IT (future fourth ventricle) and the cisterna magna
- There is a high chance of posterior fossa abnormalities (Dandy–Walker malformation, inferior vermian hypoplasia/Blake's pouch cyst) (Fig. 1.16)
- Arachnoid cysts may look similar

Investigations

- Offer invasive testing for aneuploidies and genetic syndromes (e.g. Walker–Warburg syndrome)

Counselling

- It is best to repeat a scan at 16–18 weeks to re-evaluate intracranial anatomy before discussing prognosis

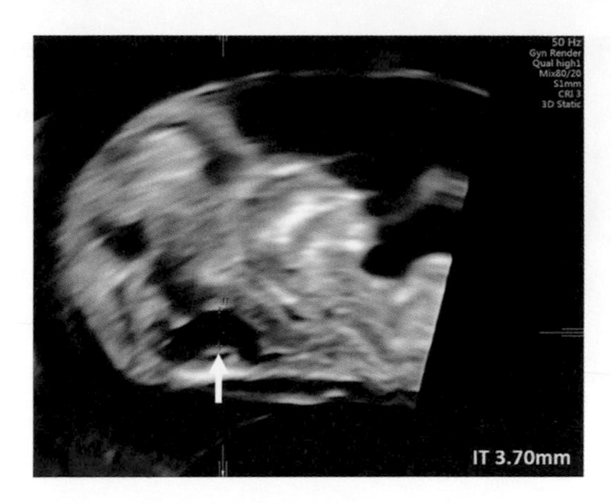

Fig. 1.16 Increased IT (arrow). A targeted scan at 16 weeks revealed a 'classic' Dandy–Walker malformation.

NASAL BONE IS 'ABSENT'

Definition and Characteristics

- The 'absence' describes lack of sonographic echogenicity, rather than absence of the bone/nose
- Prevalence in unselected population is 1–2% in the first trimester, <1% in the second trimester
- 65% of fetuses with trisomy 21 have an 'absent' nasal bone in the first trimester

Ultrasound Assessment

- Relies on comparison to overlying skin (Fig. 1.17)
- 'Absent' (unossified) nasal bone is less echogenic than skin and therefore only two dots are seen (Fig. 1.18)

Investigations

- If absent nasal bone has not been already included in the first trimester screening result, NIPT testing or karyotyping should be offered
- If absent nasal bone has been included in the first trimester screening and the result is low risk, the risk is not recalculated in the second trimester

Counselling

- When nuchal translucency and NIPT or karyotype are normal, interpret as a normal variant
- The couple can be informed that there is no risk of cosmetic problems after birth

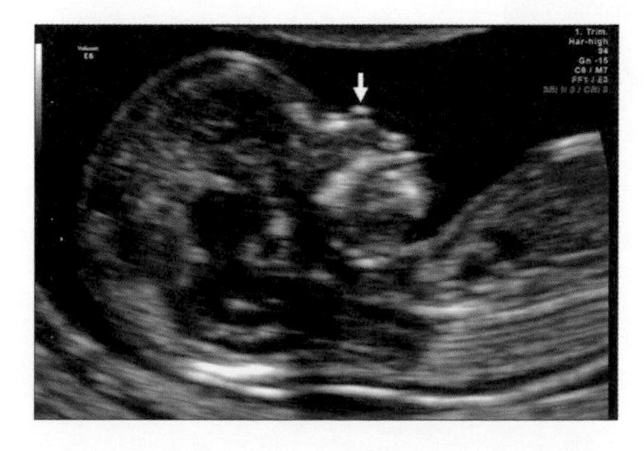

Fig. 1.17 Mid-sagittal view of the face showing an ossified nasal bone. Three 'dots' are visible – the brightest one is the nasal bone. Above the nasal bone is the skin; together they resemble = (equal sign). The third dot lying anteriorly is the tip of the nose (arrow). Note that the ultrasound beam is perpendicular to the nasal bone.

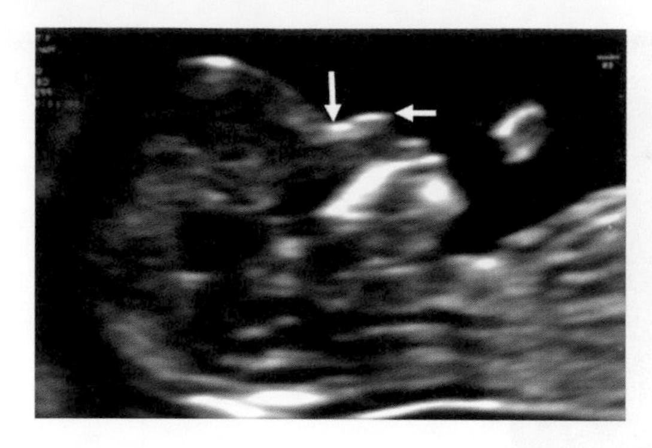

Fig. 1.18 Mid-sagittal view of the face showing 'absent' (unossified) nasal bone. Only two echogenic dots are seen, representing the skin and the tip of the nose (arrows).

MICROGNATHIA IS SUSPECTED

Definition and Characteristics

- Clinically significant facial abnormality should be suspected when the retronasal triangle is abnormal or the mandibular gap is absent

Ultrasound Assessment

- Visualise the retronasal triangle and mandibular gap on coronal section (Figs. 1.19 and 1.20)

Investigations

- Offer CVS when the retronasal triangle looks abnormal or mandibular gap is absent

Counselling

- As false positives are relatively common, detailed ultrasound assessment should be repeated around 16–18 weeks

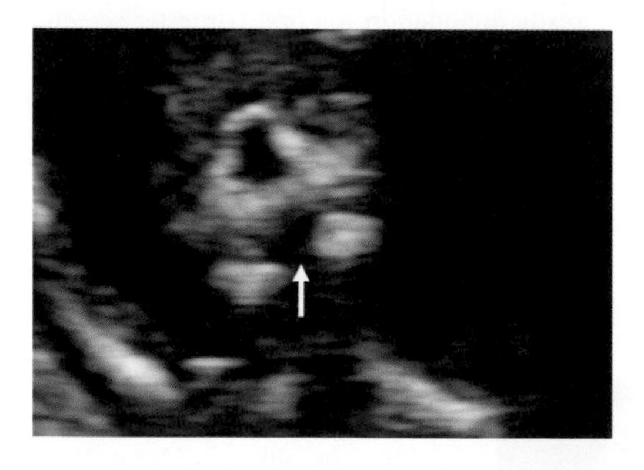

Fig. 1.19 Coronal view of the face with retronasal triangle and characteristic gap between mandibular bones (arrow). This mandibular gap is a normal finding. In cases of micrognathia the chin is still visible but this mandibular gap can be absent.

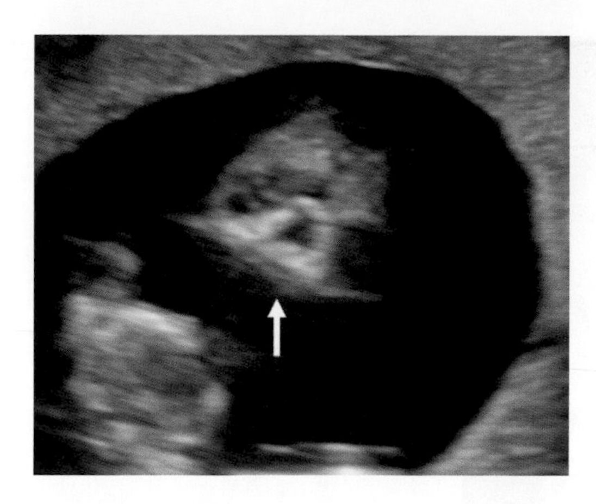

Fig. 1.20 In agnathia, no mandibular echogenicity is seen (arrow).

CLEFT LIP AND PALATE ARE SUSPECTED

Definition and Characteristics

- Cleft lip and palate are relatively common anomalies that are rarely suspected or detected during the first trimester scan
- The incidence of cleft lip and palate is around 1 in 1,250, although it is more common in some countries (e.g. 1 in 500 in Japan)

Ultrasound Assessment

- A cleft lip is recognised by lack of continuity of the upper lip in a coronal view (Fig. 1.21)
- Maxillary gap in the mid-sagittal view of the fetal face suggests that significant cleft palate is also present (Fig. 1.22)
- Assessment of the retronasal triangle may reveal its abnormal shape or defects in the base of the triangle when cleft palate is present (Fig. 1.23)

Investigations

- Offer CVS when facial clefts are detected

Counselling

- Detailed ultrasound assessment should be repeated around 16–18 weeks

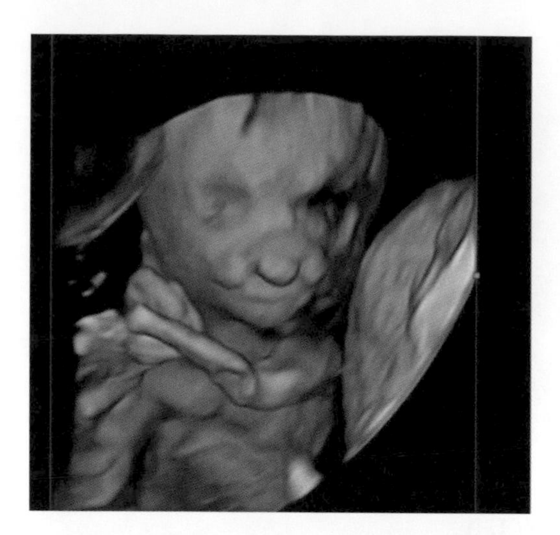

Fig. 1.21 3D picture of the face showing bilateral cleft lip.

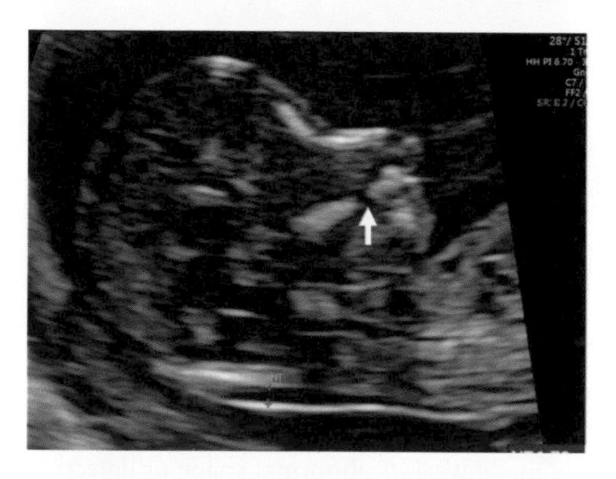

Fig. 1.22 Mid-sagittal view of the face showing a 'gap' in the maxilla which is indicative of cleft palate (arrow).

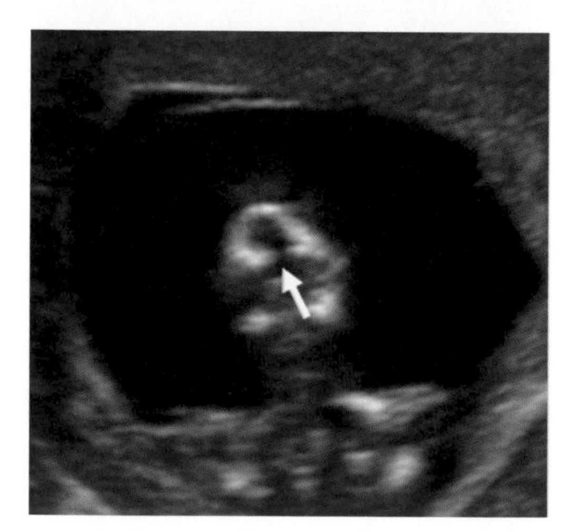

Fig. 1.23 Coronal view of the face of a fetus with cleft palate showing the retronasal triangle. The arrow points to the defect in the base of the triangle.

LARGE NUCHAL TRANSLUCENCY

Definition and Characteristics

- Nuchal translucency (NT) is the subcutaneous accumulation of fluid behind the fetal neck (Fig. 1.24)
- Typically identified during aneuploidy screening between 11^{+0} and 13^{+6} weeks of gestation (CRL 45–84 mm), it may also be identified before 11 weeks during pre-NIPT scans
- Increased NT before 11 weeks is usually defined as >2.2 mm, corresponding to the 95th centile at 10 weeks
- Raised NT before 11 weeks is best described as nuchal oedema to avoid confusion with 'classic' NT seen in a fetus with CRL > 45 mm after 11 weeks
- NT ≥ 3.5 mm between $11+^{0}$ and 13^{+6} weeks, corresponding to the 99th centile, is associated with chromosomal abnormalities, genetic syndromes and a wide range of structural defects commonly involving cardiac, skeletal and lymphatic systems

Ultrasound Assessment

- Identify correct sagittal plane and position callipers correctly
- Use colour Doppler to exclude nuchal cord (Fig. 1.25)
- If views are suboptimal, transvaginal scan is recommended to exclude the presence of generalised subcutaneous oedema, mild ascites and pleural/pericardial effusions

Investigations

- Offer chromosomal microarray analysis
- Large NT may also be an indication for exome sequencing – various cut-offs in terms of NT size have been proposed depending on local circumstances and availability of clinical geneticists to interpret variants of unknown significance

Counselling

- Normal NIPT test may provide false reassurance by missing atypical aneuploidies
- Structural abnormalities including hydrops may become apparent later in pregnancy (e.g. Noonan syndrome)
- If karyotype and 20 weeks scan are normal, long-term outcome is comparable to the general population
- Offer fetal echocardiography in the second trimester and a third trimester follow-up scan
- Nuchal oedema seen before 11 weeks will resolve in ~80% of cases when reviewed again between 11 and 13^{+6} weeks, but the risk of an adverse outcome (chromosomal abnormality, major structural defect or miscarriage) remains relatively high (~10%)

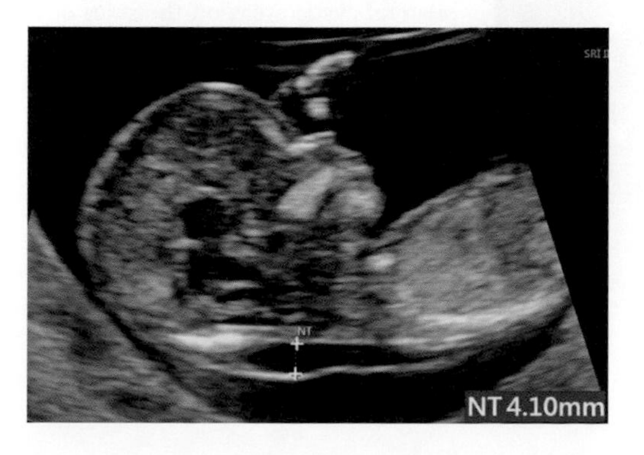

Fig. 1.24 Increased NT, no septa.

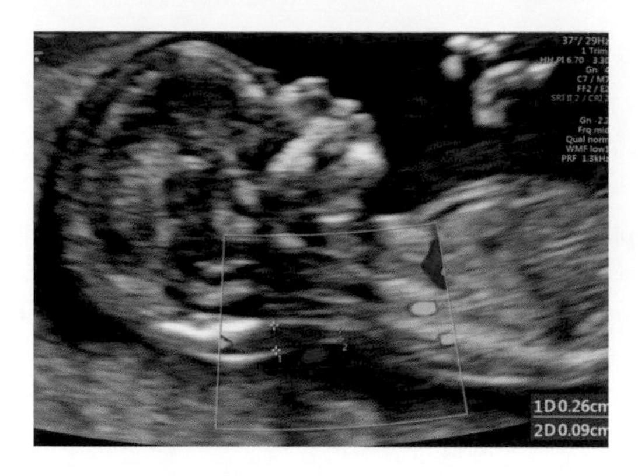

Fig. 1.25 NT with nuchal cord. Accurate measurement of the NT is compromised by the presence of nuchal cord. The measurements should be taken above and below the nuchal cord and the average used for risk calculation.

JUGULAR LYMPHATIC SACS

Definition and Characteristics

- Jugular lymphatic sacs (JLS) are accumulations of lymphatic fluid in the anterolateral region of the fetal neck
- Typically identified during anatomical survey of the neck in transverse section

Ultrasound Assessment

- Use both sagittal and transverse plane and colour Doppler to distinguish from increased NT, septated cystic hygroma or nuchal cord
- JLS will appear as spheroid echolucent 'cysts' in the anterolateral part of the neck (Fig. 1.26)
- The sacs do not cross the midline posteriorly

Investigations

- Offer invasive testing

Counselling

- If microarray and NT are normal, it is likely to be a normal variant
- If NT is increased but microarray analysis is normal, consider further testing for RASopathies (Noonan syndrome panel)

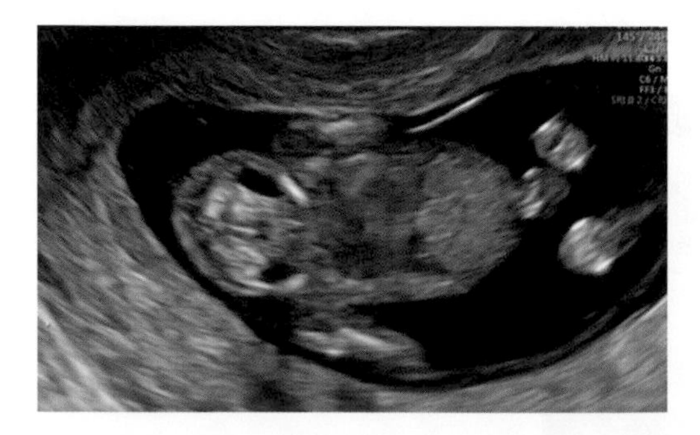

Fig. 1.26 Jugular lymphatic sacs are seen as small bilateral cystic areas on the sides of the neck.

CYSTIC HYGROMA

Definition and Characteristics

- Cystic hygroma have cystic areas by the side of the neck, while increased NT is strictly confined to the back of the neck (Figs. 1.27 and 1.28)
- The distinction between cystic hygroma and large NT is subjective – internal echoic structures are invariably present in both. Many experts will not attempt to make this distinction in the first trimester

Ultrasound Assessment

- Septation should be visible in the transverse plane
- Fetal echocardiography should be performed as early as possible

Investigations

- Offer microarray testing and, if available, testing for RASopathies (Noonan syndrome)

Counselling

- Very high risk (~50%) of chromosomal abnormalities
- Turner syndrome is the most common, but trisomies 21 and 18 and atypical chromosomal abnormalities are also represented
- Turner syndrome with large hygroma and generalised oedema has very low survival rate (<5%)
- Repeat fetal echocardiography in the second trimester and offer growth and wellbeing scans in the third trimester
- ~15–20% will have a good outcome with normal karyotype and normal paediatric follow-up

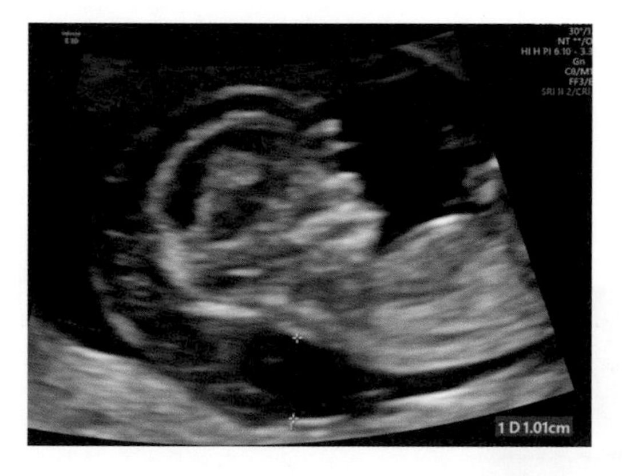

Fig. 1.27 Mid-sagittal view of the head and chest showing a large cystic hygroma. Generalised oedema is also present.

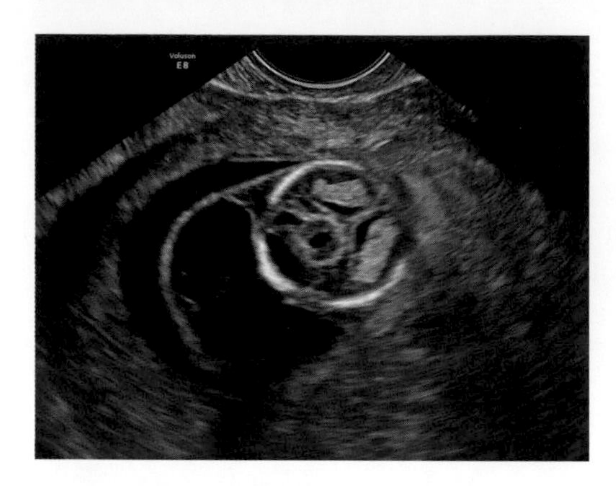

Fig. 1.28 Transverse view of the head with a septated cystic hygroma. Note that there is no communication with intracranial structures.

HEART

ANATOMY ASSESSMENT

Ultrasound Assessment

- Normal heart position with apex pointing to the left side of the chest (levocardia) (Fig. 1.29)
- Normal four-chamber view (Fig. 1.30)
- Normal three-vessel view/three vessels and trachea (3VV/3VT) view (Fig. 1.31)

Significant Heart Abnormality Should Be Suspected If

- Cardiac axis is abnormal
- NT is enlarged
- Tricuspid regurgitation is present (Figs. 1.32 and 1.33)
- Ductus venosus flow is abnormal (Figs 1.34 and 1.35)

Investigations

- If significant cardiac anomaly is suspected, CVS for chromosomal microarray testing should be offered

Counselling

- In most cases with normal microarray, the definitive diagnosis is best delayed until the second trimester

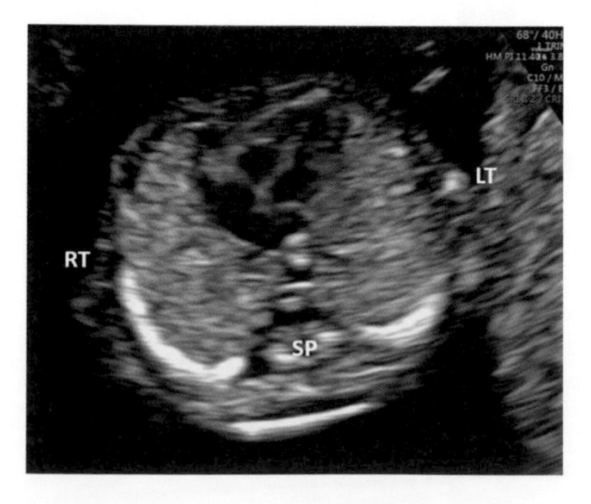

Fig. 1.29 Normal four-chamber view with the apex pointing to the left.

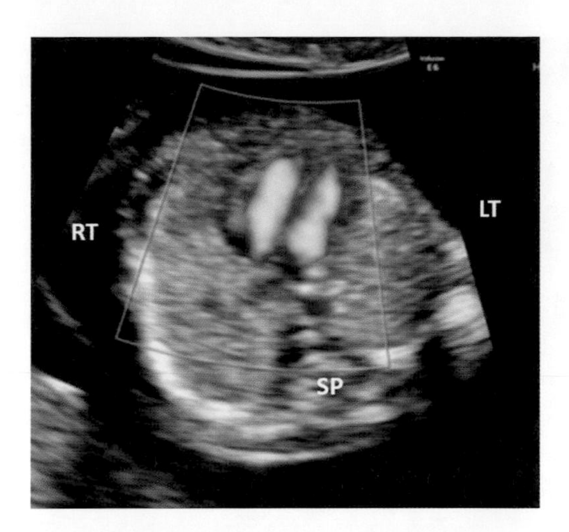

Fig. 1.30 Colour Doppler of the normal four-chamber view with blood flow reaching the apex of both ventricles.

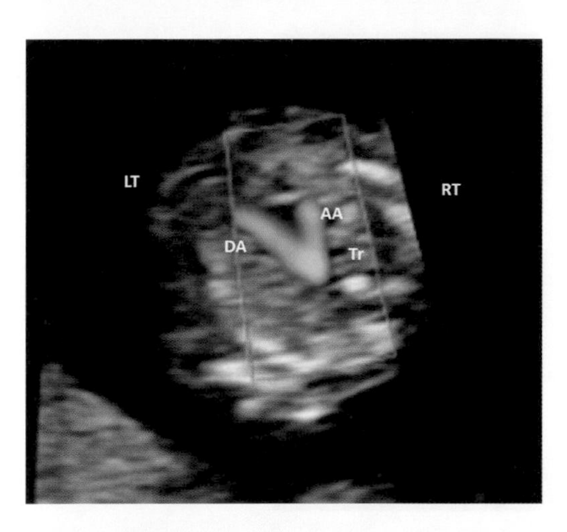

Fig. 1.31 Colour Doppler of the arches. Note that blood flow is towards the spine with both arches pointing to the left of the spine. AA, aortic arch; DA, ductal arch; Tr, trachea.

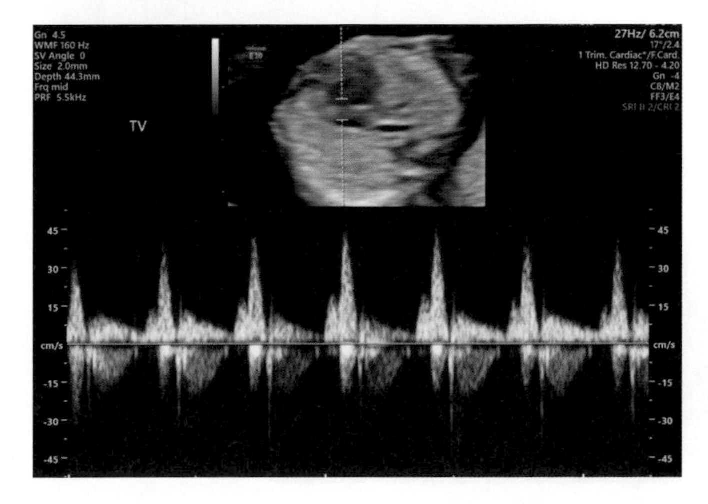

Fig. 1.32 Pulse wave Doppler showing normal flow across the tricuspid valve. Note that the sample volume is 3 mm and is placed across the whole tricuspid valve in an apical four-chamber view.

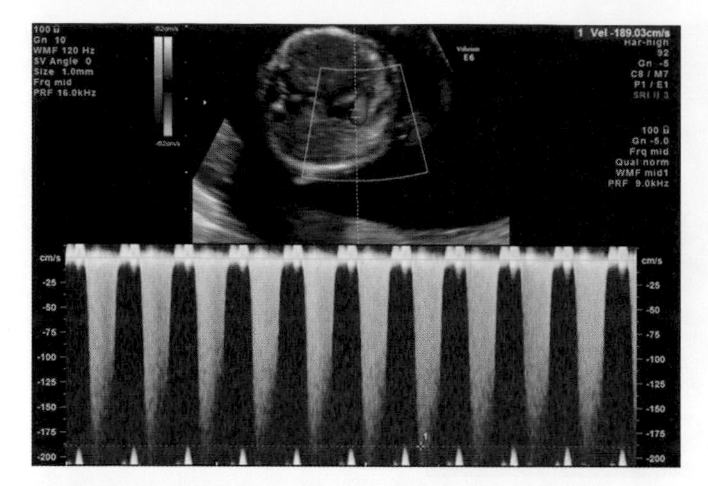

Fig. 1.33 Pulse wave Doppler showing tricuspid regurgitation. The regurgitant flow should reach at least 60 cm/s lasting at least two-thirds of the systole.

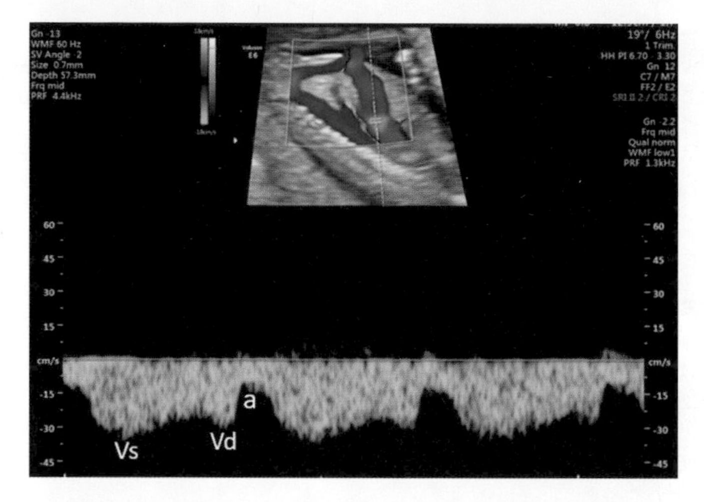

Fig. 1.34 Normal ductus venosus Doppler in the first trimester. The angle of the Doppler should be $<20^\circ$ in an adequately zoomed image with a sample volume of 0.5 mm placed at the colour aliasing point. In the typical 'M' waveform pattern the 'a' wave shows positive flow, which is normal. a, atrial systole; Vd, ventricular diastole; Vs, ventricular systole.

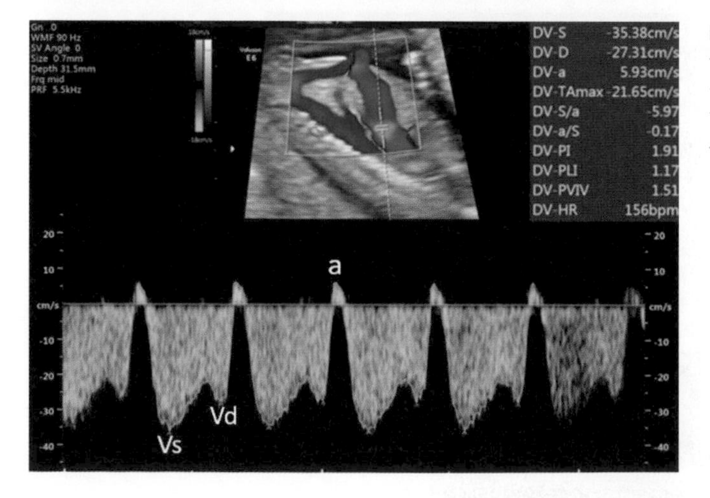

Fig. 1.35 Abnormal ductus venosus flow with reversal of the 'a' wave. a, atrial systole; Vd, ventricular diastole; Vs, ventricular systole.

ABNORMAL FOUR-CHAMBER VIEW

Table 1.1 Abnormal Four-Chamber View

Ultrasound presentation	Differential diagnosis
Single ventricle	Univentricular heart; hypoplastic left heart syndrome (HLHS), tricuspid atresia, mitral atresia, severe coarctation Large atrioventricular septal defect
Ventricular disproportion	
• Small left ventricle with unequal ventricular filling on colour Doppler (Figs. 1.36 and 1.37). Reversal of flow may be seen in the aortic arch (Fig. 1.38)	HLHS (Fig. 1.36), coarctation
• Hypoplastic, hypokinetic right ventricle	Pulmonary atresia
• Hypoplastic right ventricle, large left ventricle	Tricuspid atresia with ventricular septal defect
Single channel of blood entering both ventricles	Atrioventricular septal defect (Figs. 1.39 and 1.40)

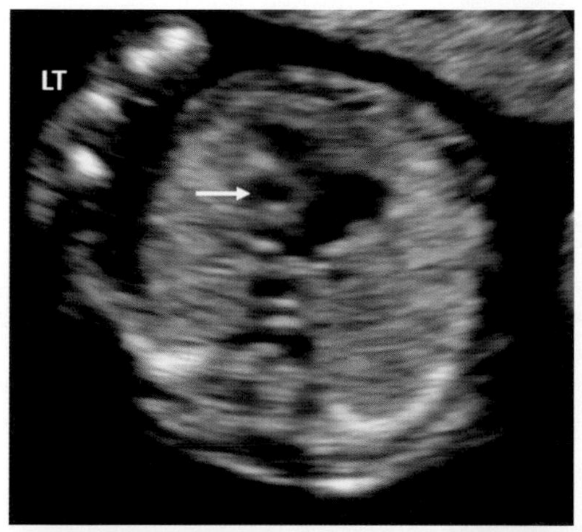

Fig. 1.36 Hypoplastic left heart syndrome (HLHS). Four-chamber view shows small left ventricle (arrow) and normal-sized right ventricle.

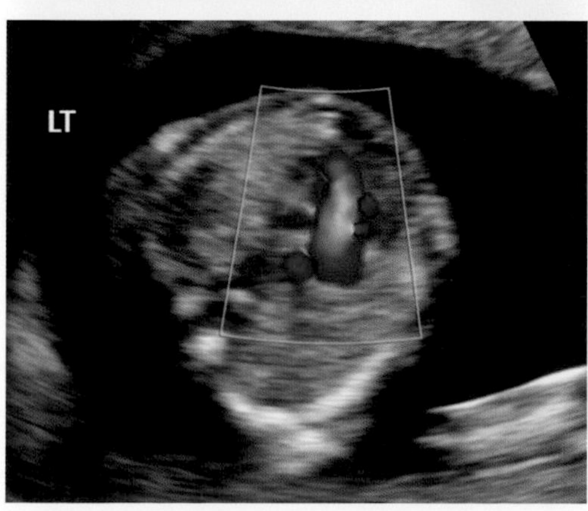

Fig. 1.37 Colour Doppler in HLHS shows single inflow filling on the right side and no filling on the left side.

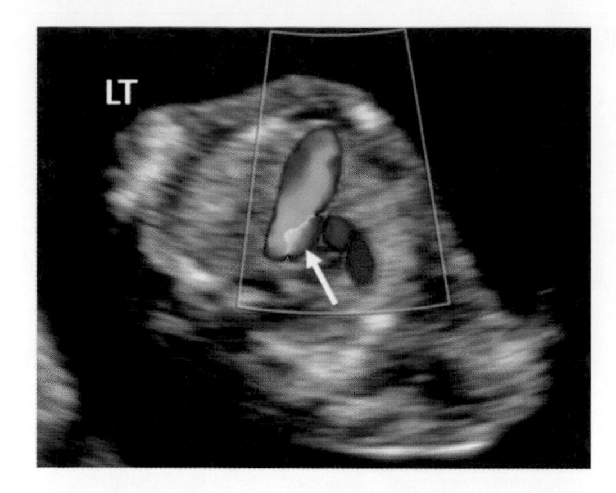

Fig. 1.38 Colour Doppler of the 3VT view in HLHS shows large pulmonary artery and reversal of flow in the aortic arch, shown in red (arrow).

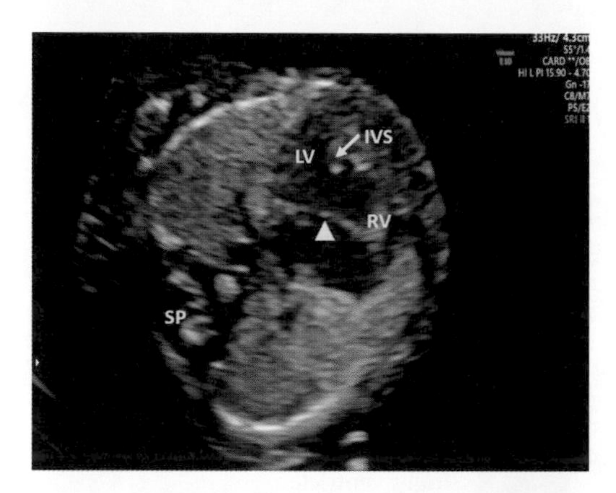

Fig. 1.39 Atrioventricular septal defect (AVSD). Note absence of crux and common AV valve (arrowhead). A small portion of the interventricular system is seen near the apex (arrow). LV, left ventricle; RV, right ventricle; SP, spine.

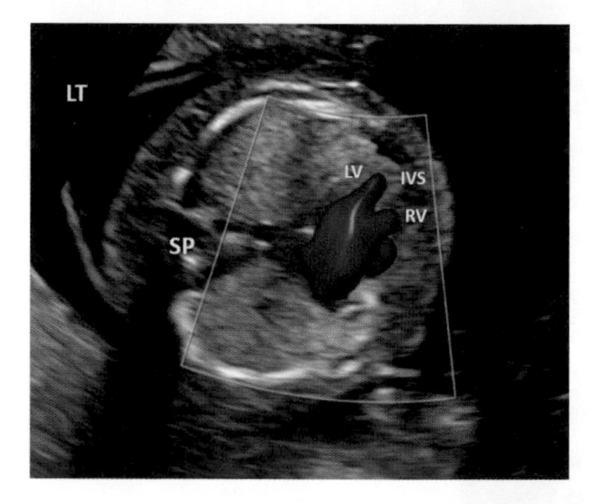

Fig. 1.40 Colour doppler in AVSD showing common atrioventricular flow. IVS, intraventricular septum; LV, left ventricle; RV, right ventricle; SP, spine.

ABNORMAL THREE-VESSEL VIEW

Table 1.2 Abnormal three-vessel view

Large pulmonary artery, small aortic arch with reversed colour flow	Hypoplastic left heart syndrome
Small aortic arch with antegrade flow	Coarctation
Reverse flow in pulmonary artery and ductus venosus	Pulmonary atresia with intact septum
Small pulmonary artery with antegrade flow	Tricuspid atresia with ventricular septal defect
Single great vessel	Transposition of great arteries (Figs. 1.41–1.44)

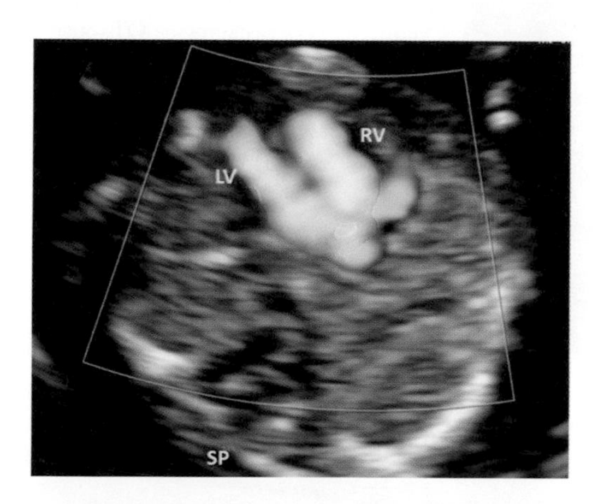

Fig. 1.41 Transposition of the great arteries (TGA). Colour Doppler in four-chamber view shows normal inflow into symmetrical ventricles. LV, left ventricle; RV, right ventricle; SP, spine.

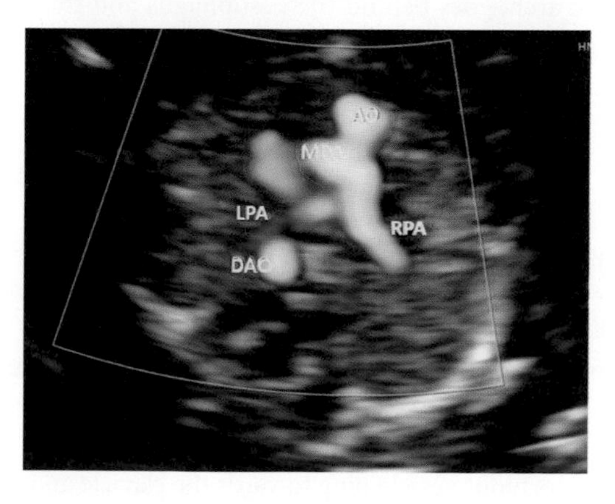

Fig. 1.42 Three-vessel view in TGA shows a cross section of the aorta anteriorly and the branching pulmonary artery posteriorly. In a normal fetus the anterior branching vessel is the pulmonary artery. AO, aorta; DAO, descending aorta; LPA, left pulmonary artery; MPA, main pulmonary artery; RPA, right pulmonary artery.

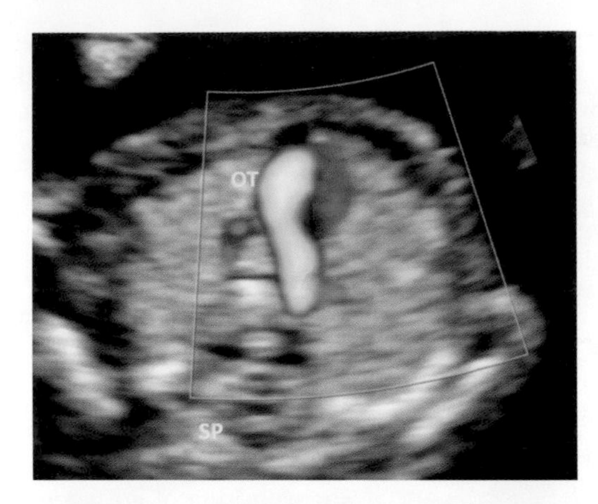

Fig. 1.43 Three-vessel trachea view in TGA shows a single outflow tract. The aorta is posterior and behind the PA and cannot be not seen at this level. OT, outflow tract; SP, spine.

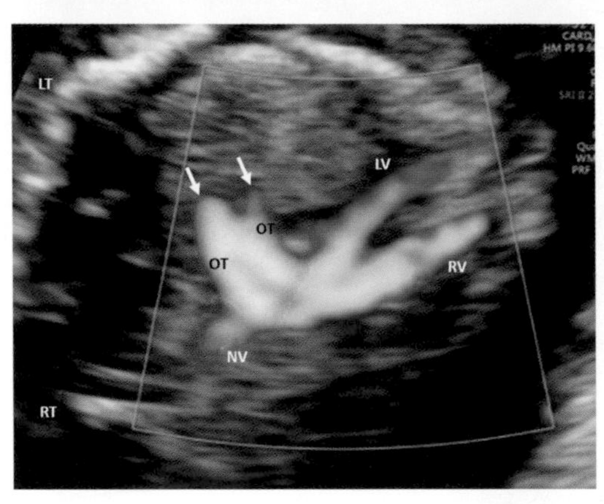

Fig. 1.44 Colour Doppler in sagittal view of TGA. Arrows show parallel outflow tracts (red colour) and ventricular blood flow (blue colour). LV, left ventricle; NV, neck vessel; OT, outflow tract; RV, right ventricle.

ABERRANT RIGHT SUBCLAVIAN ARTERY (ARSA)

Definition and Characteristics

- Arises most distally from the aortic arch, goes behind the oesophagus and trachea to the right upper arm (Fig. 1.45)
- The most common abnormality of the aortic arch

Ultrasound Assessment

- Measure NT
- Examine fetal heart in standard planes
- Exclude tricuspid regurgitation and abnormal ductus venosus
- Colour Doppler PRF set to 0.9–1.8 KHz
- Identify arches and aortic arch crossing trachea anterior and to the left of the spine (3VT view) (Fig. 1.46)
- Move the probe cranially to identify clavicles
- Normal subclavian artery is seen as a tortuous vessel going towards the clavicle and right arm
- Aberrant right subclavian artery is seen coursing behind the trachea

Counselling

- Isolated ARSA is not associated with an increased risk of aneuploidy
- Fetal karyotyping including 22q11 deletion is advisable, if the background risk is higher or additional markers are present

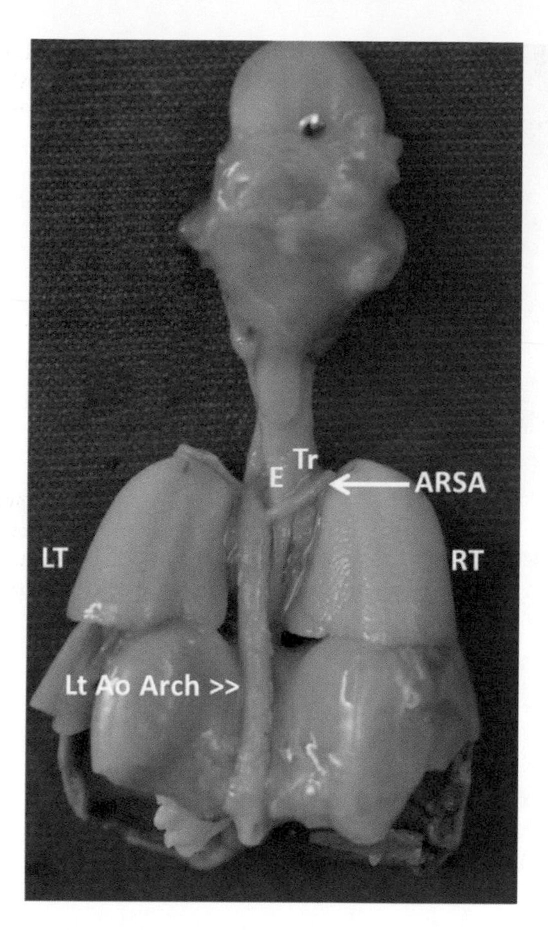

Fig. 1.45 Post mortem specimen viewed from the back showing the aberrant origin of the right subclavian artery (ARSA) from the aortic arch and traversing posterior to the oesophagus (E) and trachea (Tr).

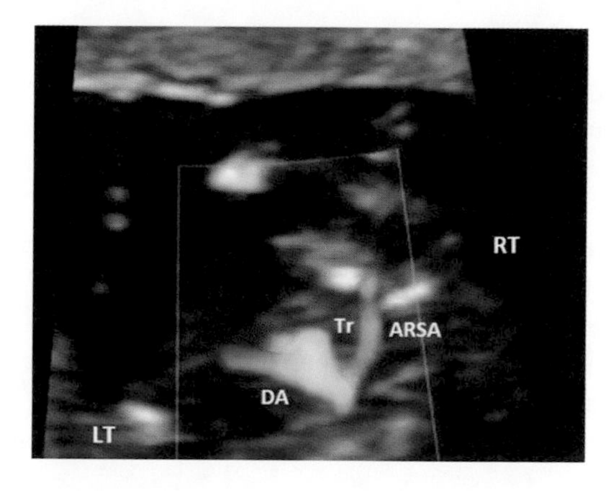

Fig. 1.46 Aberrant right subclavian artery (ARSA) seen in the 3VT view. DA, ductal arch; Tr, trachea.

CHEST

ANATOMY ASSESSMENT

- Homogeneous lung echogenicity should be seen on both sides without pleural effusions or cystic or solid masses (Fig. 1.47)
- Lungs are slightly more echogenic than cardiac muscles and fetal liver
- Diaphragmatic continuity with normal position of stomach and liver (Fig. 1.48)

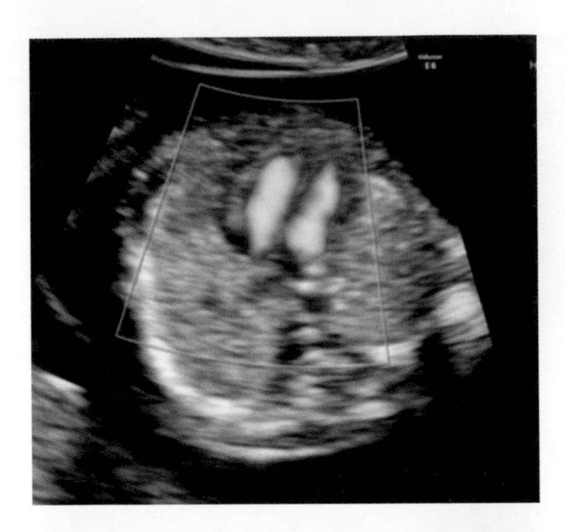

Fig. 1.47 Transverse section of the thorax at the four-chamber view with normal symmetrical lungs.

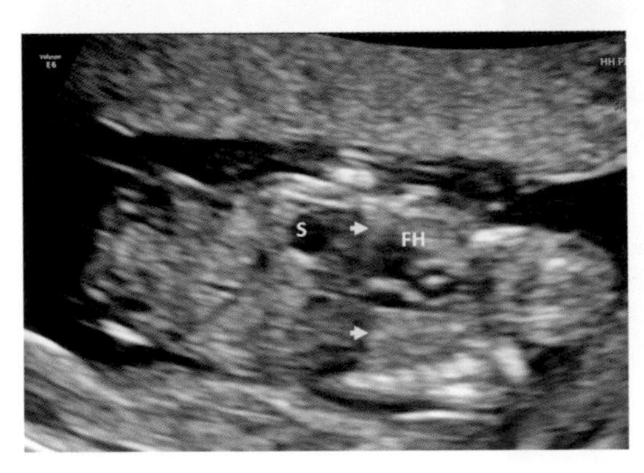

Fig. 1.48 Coronal view of the abdomen and thorax showing normal diaphragm (arrows). The stomach is seen below the diaphragm. FH, fetal heart; S, stomach.

MEDIASTINAL SHIFT

Ultrasound Assessment

- Mediastinal shift is diagnosed on a transverse four-chamber view plane by drawing an imaginary line connecting the spine and sternum, with the fetal heart lying on either side of the line
- Congenital diaphragmatic hernia (CDH) should be suspected in the presence of mediastinal shift, abnormal cardiac axis or herniated stomach (Figs. 1.49 and 1.50)
- Unilateral lung agenesis is also a (much rarer) possibility.
- In the sagittal sections of the abdomen an abnormal course of the ductus venosus and 'upturned' course of the superior mesenteric artery are pointers point to CDH (Fig. 1.51)
- In the coronal view the abdominal aorta is deviated

Investigations

- If CDH is suspected, offer invasive testing even if NT is normal; associated syndromes include trisomy 18, tetrasomy 12p (Pallister–Killian syndrome) and Cornelia de Lange syndrome

Counselling

- Definitive diagnosis of intrathoracic pathology, including diaphragmatic hernia, is best delayed until the second trimester

- Isolated unilateral lung agenesis may have a good outcome, but is more likely to be associated with congenital heart defects, including Scimitar syndrome (anomalous venous return from the right lung) with very high mortality rate

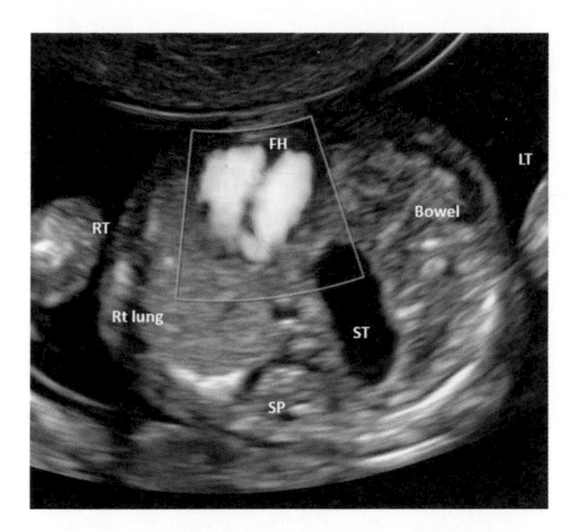

Fig. 1.49 Transverse section of the thorax showing left-sided diaphragmatic hernia. There is a mediastinal shift to the right. Stomach and small bowel are seen on the left side. FH, fetal heart; ST, stomach.

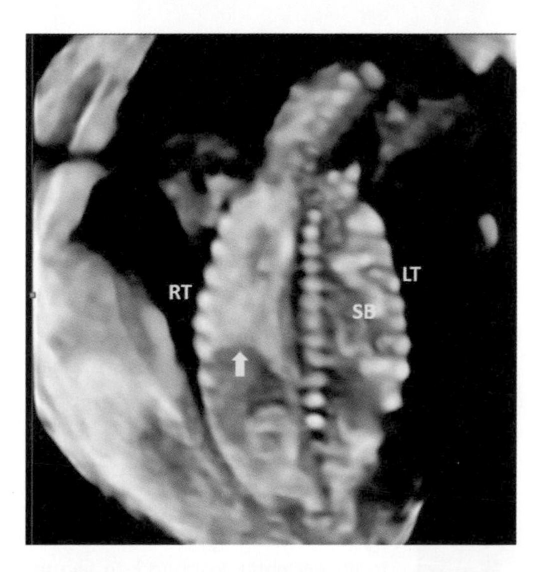

Fig. 1.50 Coronal 3D image of left diaphragmatic hernia with small bowel in the left hemithorax. The arrow points to the right hemidiaphragm. SB, small bowel.

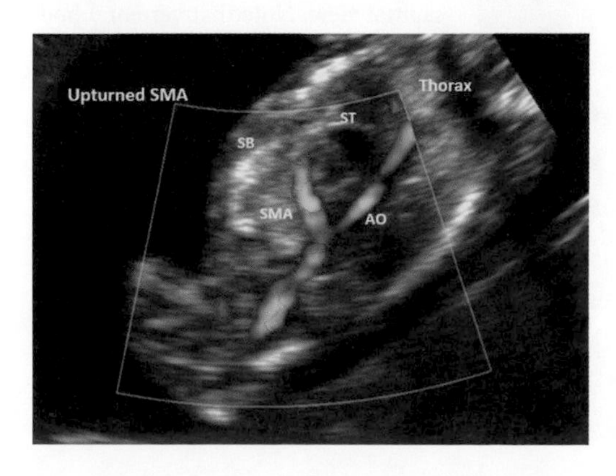

Fig. 1.51 Colour Doppler in a case of left-sided diaphragmatic hernia showing the upturned superior mesenteric artery. AO, aorta; SB, small bowel; SMA, superior mesenteric artery; ST, stomach.

PLEURAL EFFUSION

Definitions and Characteristics

- In pleural effusions an abnormal collection of fluid lies between the layers of pleura within the chest cavity
- Incidence of non-hydropic pleural effusions is around 1 in 10,000.
- Most isolated pleural effusions will present before 24 weeks, but rarely in the first trimester

Ultrasound Assessment

- Look for other evidence of hydrops (skin oedema, slight ascites)
- Pericardial effusion can be mistakenly described as pleural effusion – the fluid in pericardial effusion surrounds the heart and is, therefore, seen on the medial aspect of the lung
- Diagnosis should be confirmed on transvaginal scan
- Unilateral effusions are very rarely seen in the first trimester

Investigations

- Offer invasive testing (microarray)

Counselling

- Most babies with pleural effusions associated with hydrops and/or chromosomal anomalies are likely to die before 20 weeks (>80%).
- Non-hydropic unilateral effusions are likely to resolve spontaneously

SPINE

ANATOMY ASSESSMENT

- Normal vertebral alignment in longitudinal, coronal and transverse views (Figs. 1.52–1.54)
- Intact overlying skin
- Particular effort should be made to confirm normal appearance of the spine when
  - IT is absent
  - biparietal diameter is <5th centile

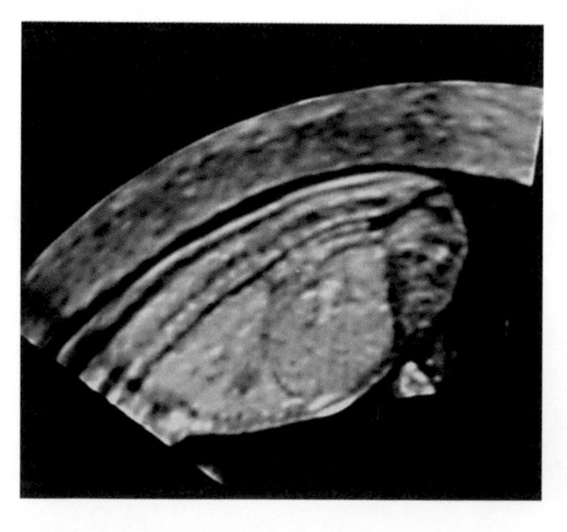

Fig. 1.52 Normal spine with intact skin posterior to the vertebrae from neck to sacrum in a mid-sagittal view. Note that vertebral bodies show ossification, but arches, which are still cartilaginous, are isoechoic or hypoechoic.

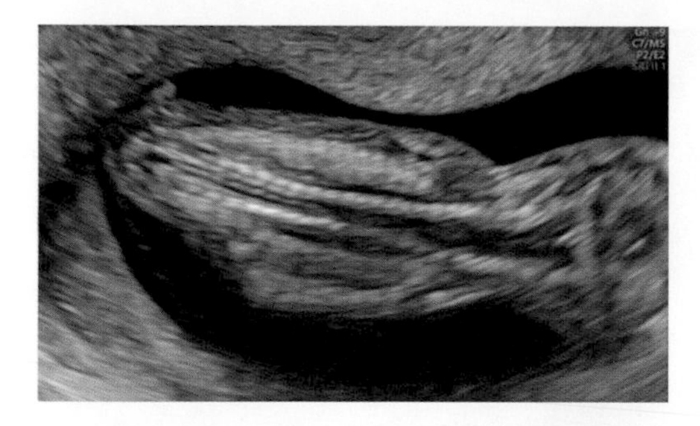

Fig. 1.53 Coronal view of the normal fetal spine at 13 weeks, showing normal cervical widening; the rest of the spine is parallel.

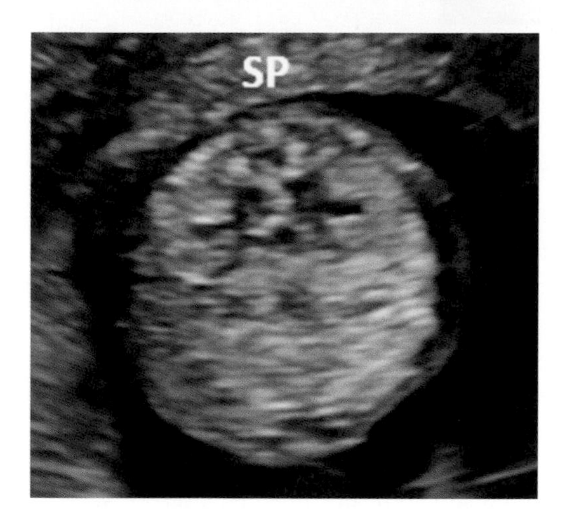

Fig. 1.54 Transverse view of the normal fetal lumbar spine of the same fetus (SP) showing the three ossification centres with intact overlying skin.

MENINGOMYELOCELE, MENINGOCELE

Ultrasound Assessment

- It is difficult to differentiate between meningocele and meningomyelocele as most first trimester defects are 'flat'
- Every effort should be made to determine whether the lesion is skin-covered (Fig. 1.55)

Investigations

- Offer invasive testing if spinal abnormality is detected

Counselling

- The outcome for open spina bifida is largely dependent on presence/absence of associated structural and chromosomal abnormalities, brain imaging later in pregnancy and the size and type of the lesion
- In apparently isolated meningocele, it is best to delay the definitive diagnosis until second trimester
- Even a large, thoracic skin-covered meningocele (limited dorsal myeloschisis) is associated with a very good long-term neurological outcome

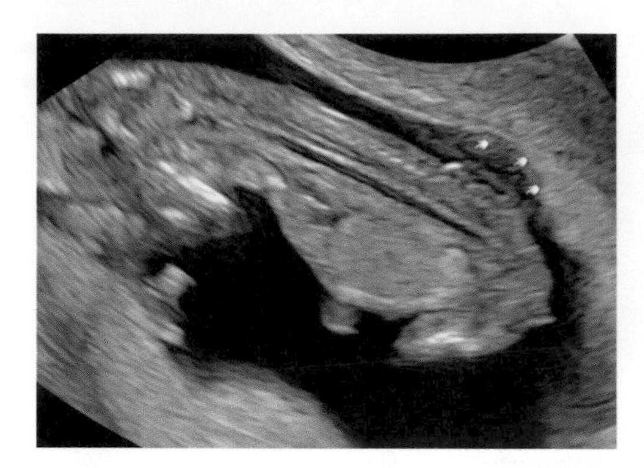

Fig. 1.55 Lumbosacral meningomyelocele. Note disruption of the skin line (small arrows) in the lumbosacral region.

ABDOMEN

ANATOMY ASSESSMENT

- A normal stomach filled with anechogenic gastric secretions is positioned in the left upper abdomen and is less echogenic than liver (on the right) (Fig. 1.56)
- The empty fetal stomach has no clinical significance in the first trimester as most fetuses don't swallow amniotic fluid before 14 weeks
- The gall bladder is almost always seen by 14 weeks' gestation, but non-visualisation in the first trimester has no clinical significance
- With normal situs, the inferior vena cava is anterior and to the right of the descending aorta
- Normal insertion of the umbilical cord should be documented after 12 weeks, together with the number of umbilical arteries
- Signs of gastrointestinal obstruction have been reported in the first trimester (e.g. double bubble); however, definitive diagnosis should be delayed until the second trimester

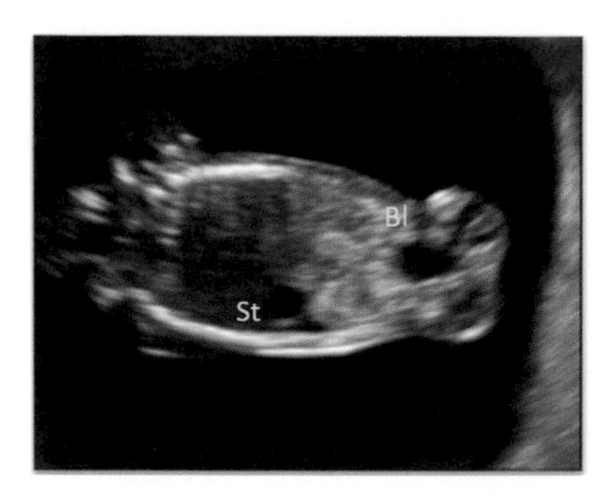

Fig. 1.56 Coronal view of fetal abdomen at 13 weeks, showing the stomach (St) and bladder (Bl).

EXOMPHALOS

Definition and Characteristics

- Exomphalos (*outside the navel* in Greek) and omphalocele (omphalos – umbilicus and cele – cavity) are synonyms
- Prevalence of exomphalos is around 1 in 5,000 births

- Small bowel herniation into a midline sac measuring <7 mm and seen before 13 weeks is likely to be a physiological midgut herniation

Ultrasound Assessment

- Abdominal defect is membrane-covered (Figs. 1.57 and 1.58).
- The umbilical cord arises from the dome of the sac
- Large defects can include liver and stomach as well as bowel
- Patent urachal cyst can be quite large and easily mistaken for an exomphalos

Investigation

- Invasive testing is indicated as exomphalos is associated with chromosomal abnormalities in 50% of cases (trisomy 18 is the most common)

Counselling

- Small, isolated exomphalos with normal NT and normal karyotype will often resolve spontaneously in the late second trimester
- If there is an isolated exomphalos with normal chromosomes, consider a possibility of Beckwith–Wiedemann syndrome; CVS material can be used for prenatal diagnosis by methylation analysis

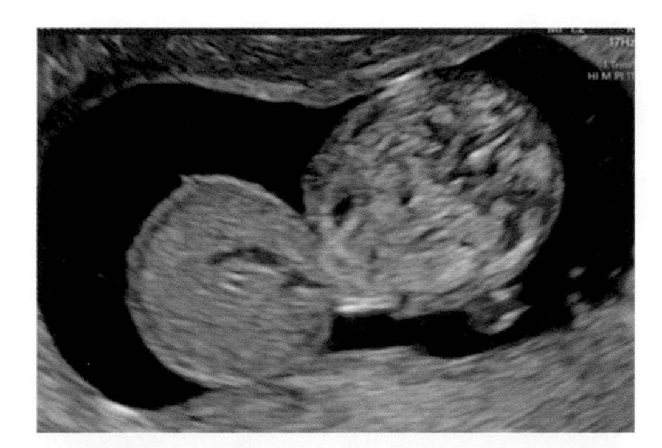

Fig. 1.57 Transverse view of the fetal abdomen showing a large anterior abdominal wall defect filled with liver. Note the covering membrane.

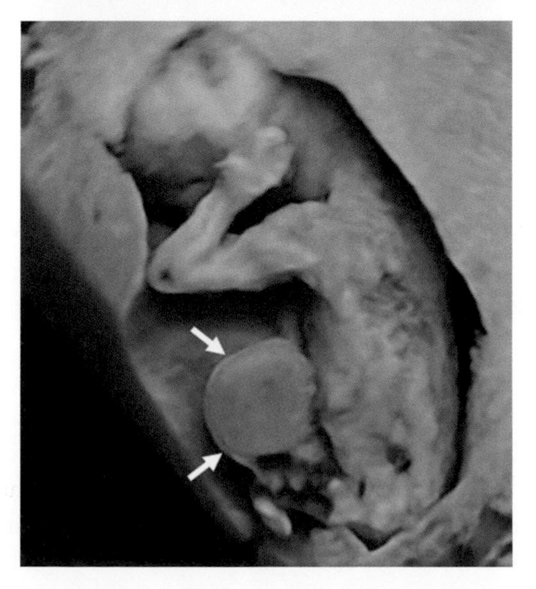

Fig. 1.58 3D image of the same fetus with exomphalos (arrows).

GASTROSCHISIS

Definition and Characteristics

- A full-thickness paraumbilical abdominal wall defect to the right of the umbilicus
- Prevalence of gastroschisis is rising, especially in young mothers where the prevalence has risen to 1 in 500

Ultrasound Assessment

- The defect has no covering membrane (Fig. 1.59)
- The defect is to the right of the normal cord insertion

Counselling

- Apparently isolated gastroschisis is rarely associated with chromosomal and structural abnormalities and is, therefore, not an indication for invasive testing in the first trimester

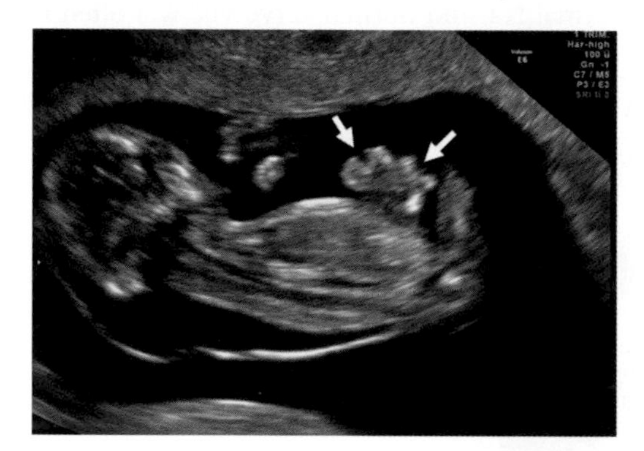

Fig. 1.59 Parasagittal longitudinal view of the fetus with an abdominal wall defect. Note the free-floating loops of bowel with no covering membrane (arrows).

ECTOPIA CORDIS, PENTALOGY OF CANTRELL OR BODY STALK ANOMALY?

Definitions and Characteristics

- The original description by Cantrell includes five parts (pentalogy):
  1. Deficiency of the anterior diaphragm
  2. Midline suprapubic abdominal wall defect
  3. Defect in the diaphragmatic pericardium
  4. Cardiac abnormalities
  5. Defect of the lower sternum
- In ectopia cordis the heart is either partly or completely protruding through the sternal defect
- Body stalk anomaly includes a large chest and abdominal wall defect with a very short or absent umbilical cord

Ultrasound Assessment

- A combination of ectopia cordis with supraumbilical omphalocele points to the pentalogy of Cantrell – a complete Cantrell pentalogy has been rarely reported (Fig. 1.60)
- In a body stalk anomaly, liver and bowel are often seen in the celomic cavity while an apparently intact amniotic sac contains the rest of the fetus. Umbilical cord is absent or

very short with a baby in very close proximity to the placenta. Some degree of kyphoscoliosis is almost always present (Fig. 1.61)
- Isolated ectopia cordis is very rare; therefore, the diagnosis should be confirmed in the second trimester

Counselling

- Body stalk anomaly is uniformly fatal, but fetal karyotype is usually normal
- Pentalogy of Cantrell and ectopia cordis have a very high mortality even if chromosomes are normal

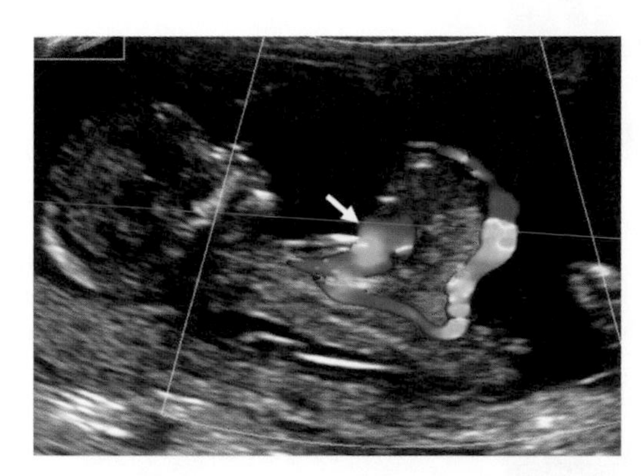

Fig. 1.60 Sagittal section of the fetus showing an abdominal wall defect with ectopia cordis (arrow).

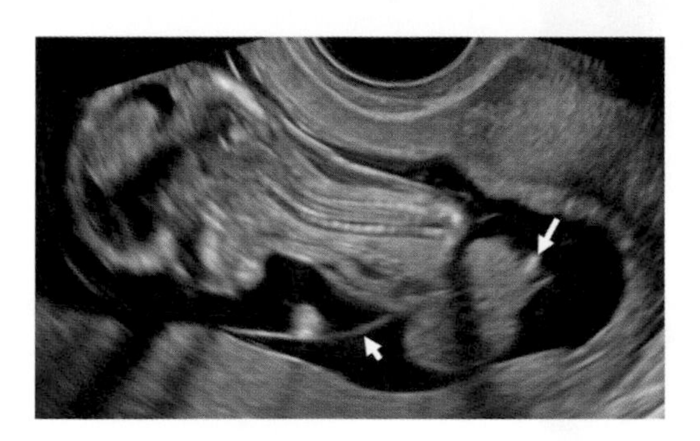

Fig. 1.61 Body stalk anomaly. The fetus is lying within the amniotic cavity, but the inferior abdominal wall defects (long arrow) is seen in the celomic cavity, which is beyond the amniotic membrane (short arrow). The umbilical cord is very short in body stalk anomaly.

GENITOURINARY SYSTEM

ANATOMY ASSESSMENT

- The fetal kidneys should be seen in a paraspinal location as bean-shaped, slightly echogenic structures with hypoechoic central renal pelvis
- In the first trimester kidneys are better visualised in the coronal plane (Fig. 1.62)
- Normal kidneys may appear hyperechoic
- Colour doppler helps to identify renal arteries and the location of the kidneys (Fig. 1.63)
- By 12 weeks' gestation, the fetal bladder should be visible as a median hypoechoic round structure in the lower abdomen and measures <7 mm in longitudinal diameter
- Colour Doppler can be used to confirm normal position of the bladder by identifying two umbilical arteries surrounding the bladder (Fig. 1.64)
- Absence of bladder filling may be indicative of renal agenesis

- Sex determination is 85% accurate and can be used in conjunction with cffDNA (cell-free fetal DNA) to ascertain the need for invasive prenatal diagnosis of X-linked conditions and management of congenital adrenal hyperplasia

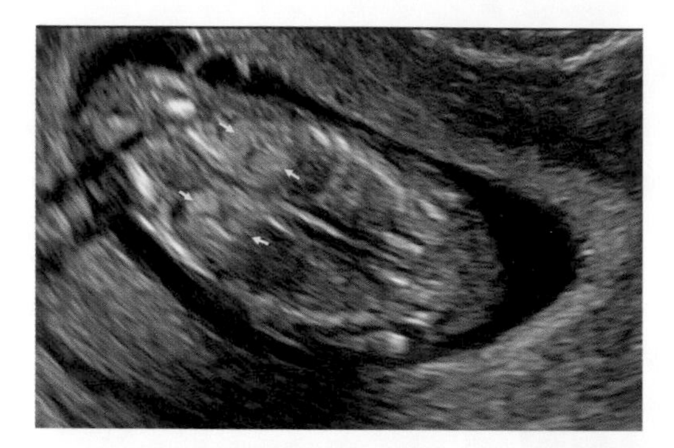

Fig. 1.62 Normal kidneys. Coronal view of the fetal abdomen showing normal kidneys, which are quite echogenic in the first trimester. Better visualisation can be achieved by increasing the dynamic range and by using 'chroma' colour.

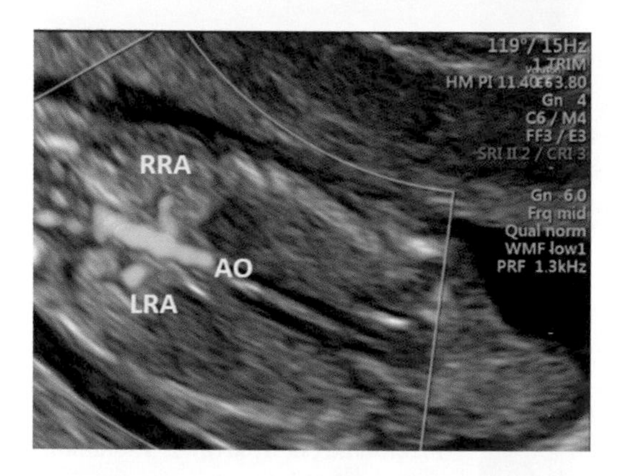

Fig. 1.63 Normal renal arteries. Coronal view of the fetal abdomen with colour Doppler showing both renal arteries. Ao, aorta; LRA, left renal artery; RRA, right renal artery.

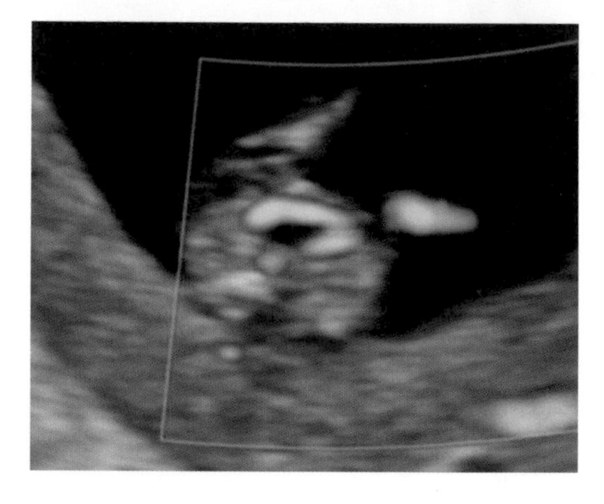

Fig. 1.64 Umbilical arteries. Colour Doppler of the lower abdomen showing a normal bladder surrounded by two umbilical arteries.

BLADDER IS LARGE (MEGACYSTIS)

Definition and Characteristics

- Usually defined as ≥7 mm in a longitudinal bladder diameter (LBD) (Fig. 1.65)
- Prevalence in the first trimester is around 1 in 1,500–2,000

- Around 40% of cases will be complex (chromosomal abnormalities, anorectal malformations or multiple anomalies)
- 40% will have a lower urinary tract obstruction (urethral atresia, stenosis or posterior urethral valve)
- 20% will resolve spontaneously

Ultrasound Assessment

- Measure NT
- Look for umbilical cord cysts
- A large urachal cyst can be easily mistaken for a megacystis/bladder extrophy when a communication between the bladder and an extra-abdominal cystic structure surrounded by umbilical arteries is visible

Investigations

- Offer invasive testing

Counselling

- Megacystis when NT is $>$95th centile:
  - high risk of complex pathology (chromosomal, anorectal or multiple abnormalities)
  - isolated posterior urethral valve is very unlikely
- Umbilical cord cyst is also present:
  - High risk of a urethral atresia in both female and male fetuses
- LBD < 12 mm with normal karyotype, normal NT and no cord cyst:
  - spontaneous resolution is likely
  - offer follow-up at 16, 20 and 28 weeks for reassurance
- LBD > 12 mm, normal karyotype and NT, no cord cyst, male fetus:
  - isolated posterior urethral valve is the most likely diagnosis
  - Survival is around 50% and 25–30% of survivors will develop end-stage renal disease requiring dialysis and renal transplant by the age of 5

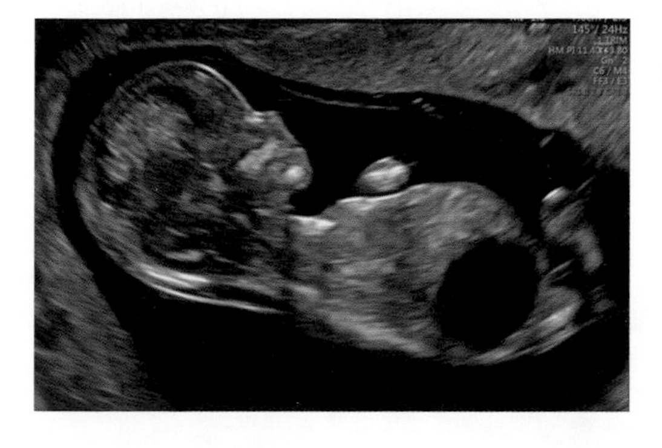

Fig. 1.65 Megacystis. Sagittal view of the fetus showing an abnormally large bladder.

SKELETAL SYSTEM

ANATOMY ASSESSMENT

- The presence of each bony segment of the upper and lower limbs and presence and normal orientation of the two hands and feet should be noted

LIMB ABNORMALITIES

Definition and Characteristics

- Limb abnormalities detected in the first trimester can be isolated, but are more likely caused by chromosomal abnormality or a genetic syndrome (Table 1.3)
- Terminal transverse defects are more common in the upper limbs; most of them are caused by a vascular injury or amniotic band sequence

Table 1.3 Limb abnormalities that can be detected in the first trimester

Talipes equinovarous or clubfeet	In most cases the foot is twisted downward and inward
Clinodactyly	Abnormally bent finger due to abnormal bone development of the small bones of that finger
Clenched hand	Adducted thumb; second and fifth finger overlapping third and fourth
Polydactyly	Extra digits (Fig. 1.66)
Syndactyly	Two or more digits fused together
Ectrodactyly	Split hand or foot deformity with a deep central cleft (Fig. 1.67)
Phocomelia	Hands or feet attached close to the trunk
Sirenomelia	Fused lower limbs (Figs. 1.68 and 1.69)

Ultrasound Assessment

- Use transvaginal ultrasound to look for other abnormalities
- Look for signs of amnion disruption

Investigation

- Offer karyotyping/microarray

Counselling

- The definitive diagnosis is best delayed until the second trimester

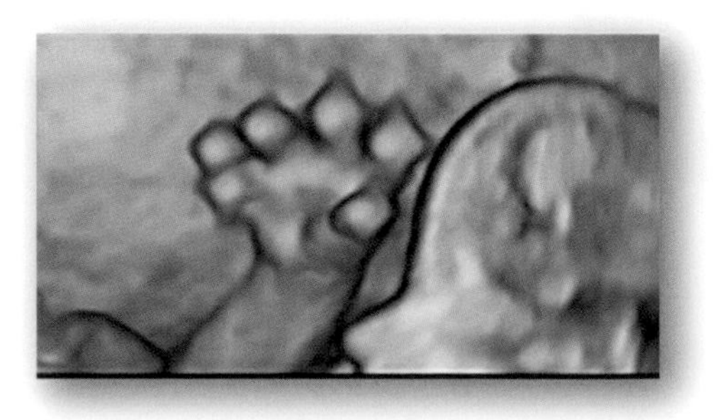

Fig. 1.66 Polydactyly. 3D image of a hand with post-axial polydactyly.

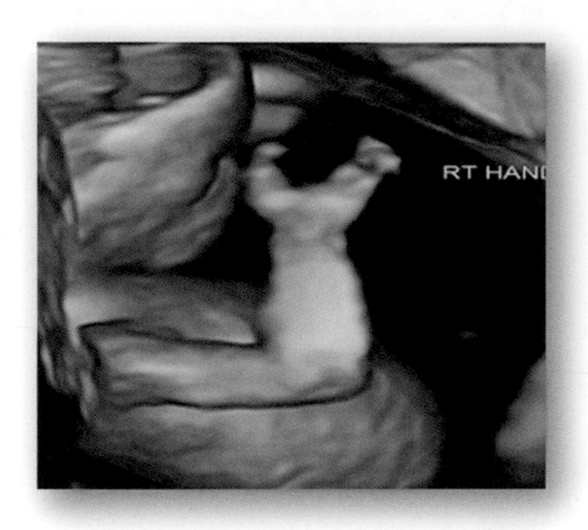

Fig. 1.67 Ectrodactyly. 3D image of a hand showing ectrodactyly (cleft hand).

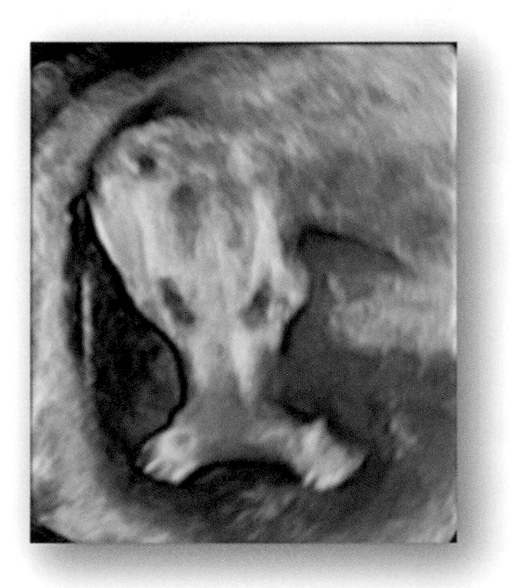

Fig. 1.68 3D image of fused lower limbs in sirenomelia (mermaid syndrome).

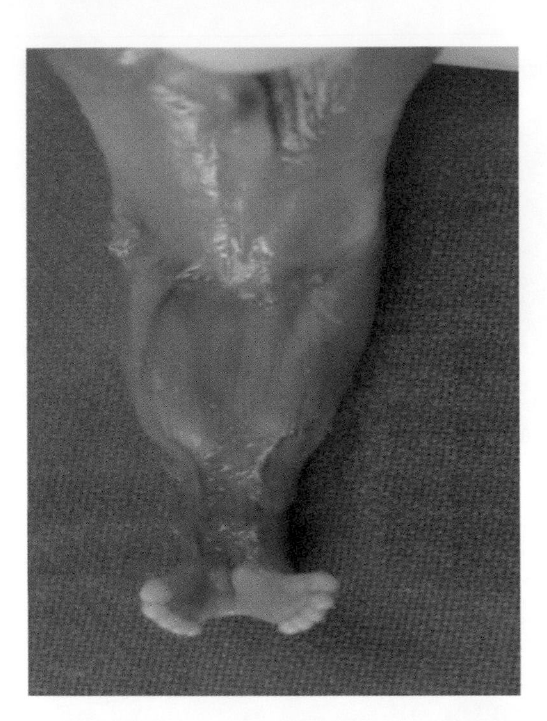

Fig. 1.69 Autopsy image of sirenomelia.

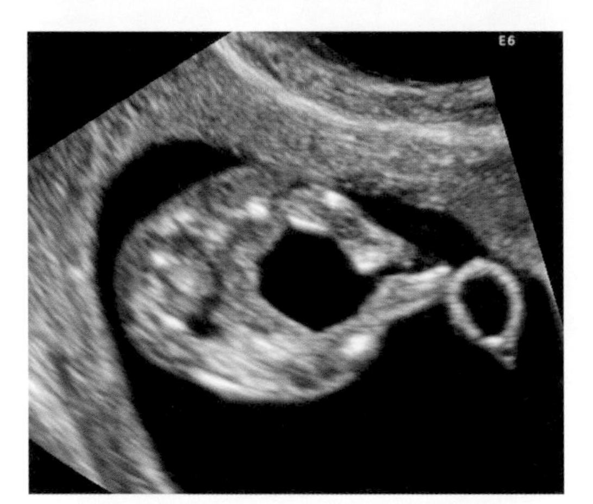

Fig. 1.70 2D image of both lower limbs showing short long bones in a fetus affected by achondrogenesis.

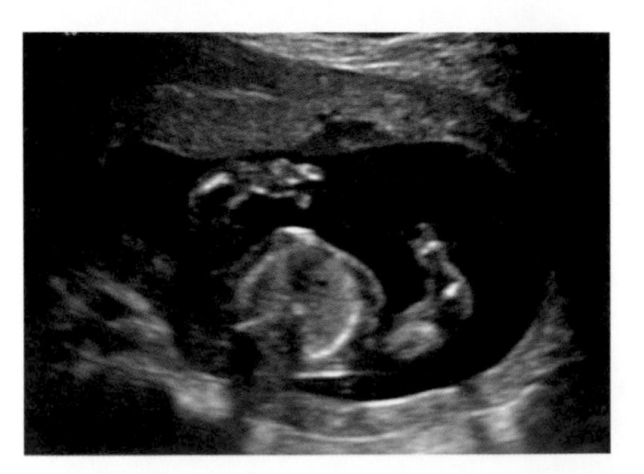

Fig. 1.71 2D image of the same fetus showing short upper limbs.

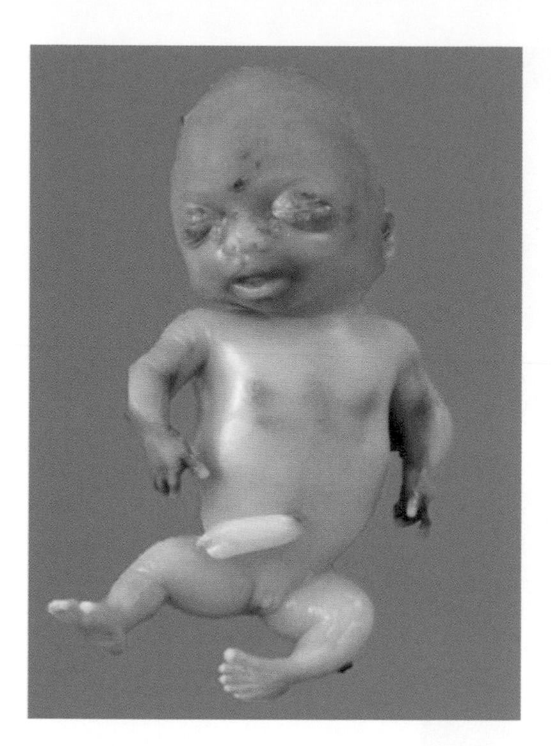

Fig. 1.72 Autopsy picture of the same fetus showing short limbs.

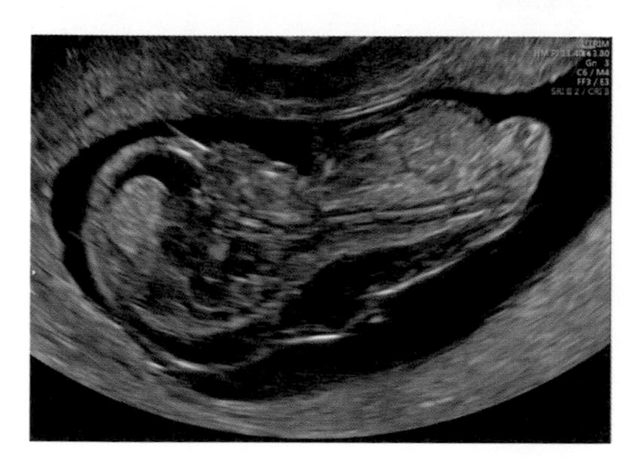

Fig. 1.73 Achondrogenesis at 13 weeks, showing significant oedema and poor mineralisation of the spine and skull.

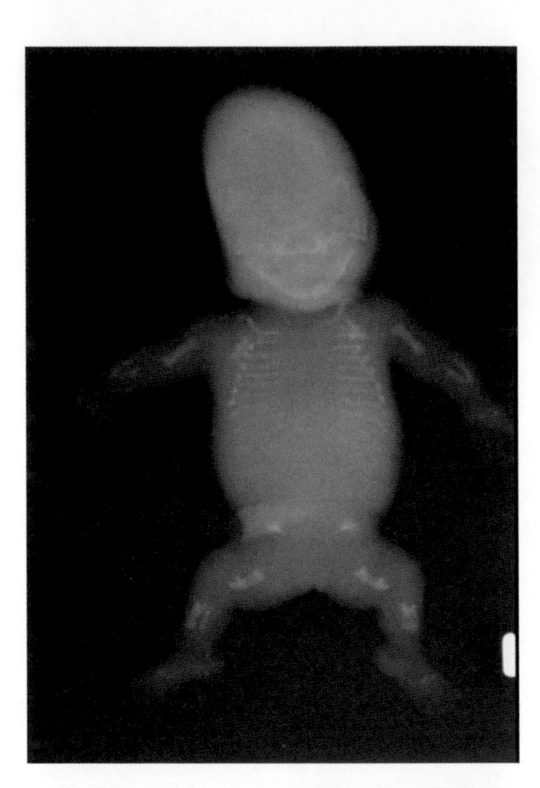

Fig. 1.74 X-ray of the same baby confirming poor ossification of the spine and skull.

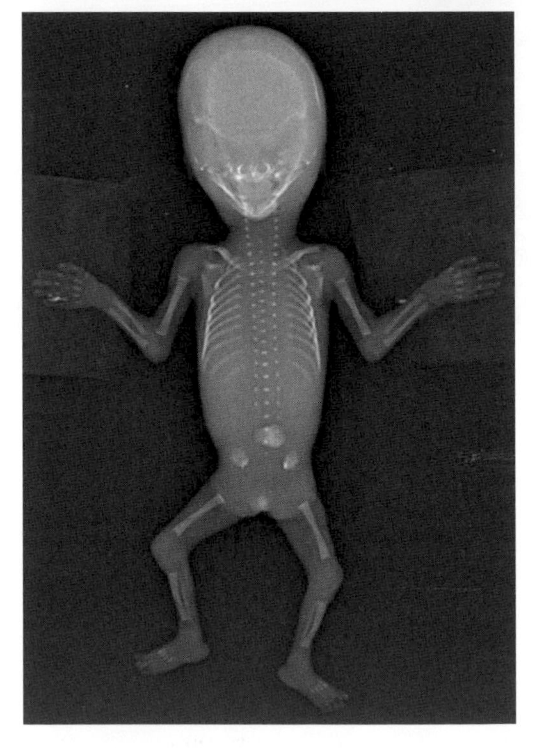

Fig. 1.75 Normal fetogram at 13 weeks. Note the distinct ossification of the spine and the normal long bones at this gestation.

SHORT FEMUR

Definition and Characteristics

- Femur length <5th centile

Ultrasound Assessment

- A combination of short femur (<5th centile) and increased NT should prompt a detailed skeletal survey including transvaginal scan using the same principles as in the second trimester assessment (Table 1.4)

Table 1.4 Differential diagnosis when a short femur (<5th centile) is seen in combination with increased NT in the first trimester

Additional phenotype	Differential diagnosis
Generalised oedema, hydrops	Achondrogenesis (Figs. 1.70–1.75), short rib polydactyly syndrome, Noonan syndrome
Poor skull ossification	Achondrogenesis, osteogenesis imperfecta, hypophosphatasia, boomerang dysplasia, Roberts syndrome
Small thorax	Achondrogenesis, Ellis-van Creveld syndrome, osteogenesis imperfecta, thantophoric dysplasia, campomelic dysplasia, hypophosphatasia, boomerang dysplasia, Jeune syndrome, short rib polydactyly syndrome
Polydactyly	Short rib polydactyly syndrome, Jeune syndrome, Ellis-van Creveld syndrome, acrocallosal syndrome
Oligodactyly	Roberts syndrome
Missing long bones	Boomerang dysplasia, Roberts syndrome, femoral facial syndrome
Hitchhiker's thumb/toe	Atelosteogenesis, diastrophic dysplasia
Talipes	Campomelic dysplasia, hypophosphatasia, atelosteogenesis, diastrophic dysplasia, Roberts syndrome
Cardiac anomaly	Ellis-van Creveld syndrome, Meckel–Gruber syndrome, Noonan syndrome
Posterior fossa cyst	Ellis-van Creveld, Meckel–Gruber syndromes

Investigations

- Short femur in combination with increased NT, or phenotype suggestive of skeletal dysplasia or genetic syndrome, is an indication for invasive testing

Counselling

- If skeletal dysplasia is suspected, a definitive diagnosis based on the first trimester ultrasound appearances is best avoided and should be delayed until the second trimester
- Increasingly, the definitive diagnosis can be made by targeted genetic testing (e.g. FGFR3 for suspected thanatophoric dysplasia)

HYDROPS

Definition and Characteristics

- Rather than using the umbrella term 'hydrops', it is more informative to be specific and describe a presenting phenotype more precisely; for example: pleural effusion, pericardial effusion, ascites, skin oedema, or a combination of these conditions (Fig. 1.76)
- Virtually all cases presenting in the first trimester are non-immune; immune hydrops due to feto-maternal blood group incompatibility occurs after 15 weeks
- Around 25% of cases presenting in the first trimester will have chromosomal abnormalities detected either by conventional karyotyping (20%) or microarray (additional 5%)
- Exome sequencing can identify pathogenic genetic variants in up to 30% of otherwise unexplained cases

Ultrasound Assessment

- Detailed structural survey
- Offer follow-up scan at 16 weeks to reassess anatomy with particular emphasis on fetal echocardiography and any changes in the amount of accumulated fluid

Investigations

- Offer invasive testing, including exome sequencing if available
- Maternal serology to exclude congenital viral infections (parvovirus B19, cytomegalovirus)

Counselling

- Significant, progressive hydrops has poor prognosis; termination of pregnancy should be considered
- Counselling for pathogenic genetic variants, if found, is complex and should involve clinical geneticists
- Unexplained cases should be followed regularly during pregnancy, even when the 20-weeks scan looks entirely normal as reappearance in the third trimester is relatively common (e.g. undiagnosed Noonan syndrome)
- In some cases of complete resolution in the second trimester, the definitive diagnosis has been established in early childhood (e.g. hereditary spherocytosis)

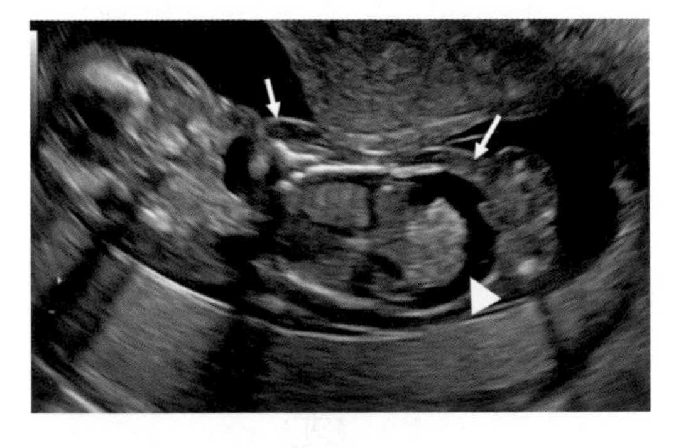

Fig. 1.76 Coronal section of fetus showing ascites (arrow head) and skin oedema (arrows).

PLACENTA AND UMBILICAL CORD

ANATOMY ASSESSMENT

- A three-vessel cord, cord insertion at the umbilicus and presence of cord cysts should be noted
- Evaluation of the placental size, thickness and localisation in the first trimester is of little clinical value

SINGLE UMBILICAL ARTERY

Definition and Characteristics

- Prevalence of single umbilical artery (SUA) is around 0.5%
- Aplasia/atrophy has been suggested as the underlying cause
- Laterality is of no clinical importance
- Around 80% will be 'isolated'

Ultrasound Assessment

- Use a transverse plane at the level of the fetal bladder
- Use colour Doppler mode to confirm the diagnosis (Fig. 1.77)
- Use the transvaginal approach to assess anatomy
- It is important to exclude renal agenesis
- Measure NT

Counselling

- If SUA appears to be isolated and NT is normal, invasive testing is not indicated
- Perinatal mortality is not increased
- Detailed structural survey should be arranged in the second and third trimesters because of an increased risk of gastrointestinal atresias/stenosis and heart defects
- If a third trimester scan (30–32 weeks) has confirmed that SUA is isolated, follow-up scans should be arranged to exclude fetal growth restriction
- If there is no evidence of fetal growth restriction, early delivery is not indicated

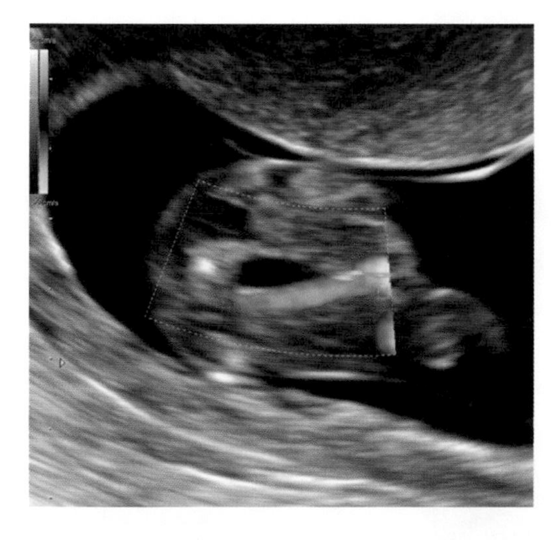

Fig. 1.77 Transverse section of fetal bladder. Colour Doppler shows an SUA.

UMBILICAL CYSTS

Definition and Characteristics

- Reported prevalence is higher (up to 3%) when transvaginal scans are used in the first trimester
- Differentiation between true cysts and 'pseudocysts' with no epithelial lining (*Wharton jelly cysts*) is of little clinical value

Ultrasound Assessment

- It is important not to describe the yolk sac (extra-amniotic cyst with echogenic borders) as an umbilical cyst
- Urachal cyst should be suspected when there is a communication between bladder and extra-abdominal cystic structure surrounded by umbilical arteries (Fig. 1.78)

Counselling

- Isolated umbilical cord cysts seen in the first trimester have no clinical significance, regardless of their size or location (Fig. 1.79)
- Even multiple umbilical cysts seen before 10 weeks are likely to disappear by 14 weeks
- Detailed anatomy scan should be arranged around 16 weeks
- In the absence of structural abnormalities, fetal karyotyping is not indicated
- Extra-abdominal urachal cysts can be quite large and should not be mistaken for exomphalos or bladder exstrophy. If karyotype is normal, the prognosis after surgery is very good

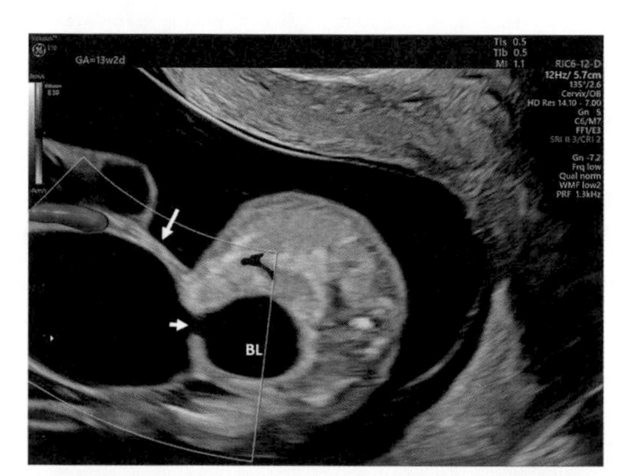

Fig. 1.78 Transverse section of the lower abdomen showing the bladder and a large urachal cyst in a fetus with trisomy 18. Note the communication (small arrow) between the bladder (BL) and a cyst (arrow).

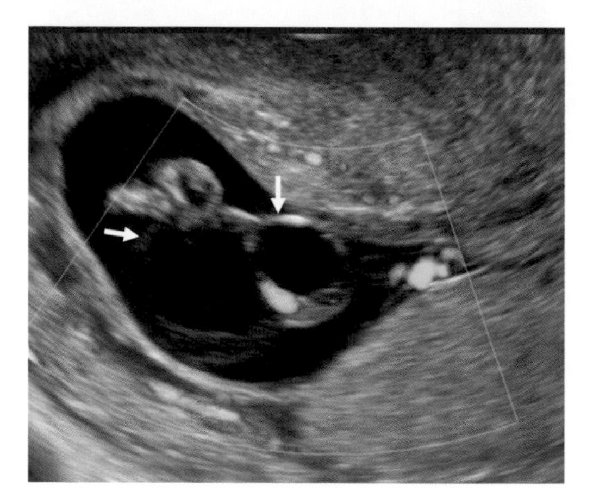

Fig. 1.79 Transverse section of the umbilical cord with two small umbilical cord cysts (arrows). If isolated, they have a good outcome.

SUGGESTED READING

PRIMARY RESEARCH

Bardi F, Bosschieter P, Verheij J, et al. Is there still a role for nuchal translucency measurement in the changing paradigm of first trimester screening? *Prenat Diagn* 2020;40(2):197–205.

Chaoui R, Benoit B, Mitkowska-Wozniak H, Heling KS, Nicolaides KH. Assessment of intracranial translucency (IT) in the detection of spina bifida at the 11–13-week scan. *Ultrasound Obstet Gynecol* 2009;34:249–252.

Shi Y, Zhang B, Kong F, Li X. Prenatal limb defects: epidemiologic characteristics and an epidemiologic analysis of risk factors. *Medicine (Baltimore)* 2018;97(29):e11471.

Sparks TN, Lianoglou BR, Adami RR, et al. Exome sequencing for prenatal diagnosis in nonimmune hydrops fetalis. *NEJM* 2020;383:1746–1756.

REVIEWS AND GUIDELINES

Abuhamad A, Chaoui R. *First Trimester Ultrasound Diagnosis of Fetal Abnormalities.* Wolters Kluwer, Philadelphia, 2018; 319–327.

Bakker M, Pace M, de Jong-Pleij E, et al. Prenasal thickness, prefrontal space ratio and other facial profile markers in first-trimester fetuses with aneuploidies, cleft palate, and micrognathia. *Fetal Diagn Ther* 2018;43(3):231–240.

Chaoui R, Orosz G, Heling KS, Sarut-Lopez A, Nicolaides KH. Maxillary gap at 11–13 weeks' gestation: marker of cleft lip and palate. *Ultrasound Obstet Gynecol* 2015;46(6):665–669.

de Mooij YM, Bekker MN, Spreeuwenberg MD, van Vugt JM. Jugular lymphatic sacs in first-trimester fetuses with normal nuchal translucency. *Ultrasound Obstet Gynecol* 2009;33(4):394–398.

Fantasia I, Stampalija T, Sirchia F et al. First-trimester absent nasal bone: is it a predictive factor for pathogenic CNVs in the low-risk population. *Prenat Diagn* 2020. doi: 10.1002/pd.5812.

Fontanella F, Duin L, van Scheltema PNA et al. Antenatal workup of early megacystis and selection of candidates for fetal therapy. *Fetal Diagn Ther* 2019;45:155–161.

Khalil A, Pajkrt E, Chitty LS. Early prenatal diagnosis of skeletal anomalies. *Prenat Diagn* 2011;31 (1):115–124.

Levy AT, Berghella V, Al-Kouatly HB. Outcome of 45,X fetuses with cystic hygroma: a systematic review. *Am J Med Genet A* 2020. doi: 10.1002/ajmg.a.61902.

Liao YM, Li SL, Luo GY, et al. Routine screening for fetal limb abnormalities in the first trimester. *Prenat Diagn* 2016;36(2):117–126.

Luo X, Zhai S, Shi N, et al. The risk factors and neonatal outcomes of isolated single umbilical artery in singleton pregnancy: a meta-analysis. *Sci Rep* 2017;7(1):7396.

Malone FD, Ball RH, Nyberg DA, et al. First-trimester septated cystic hygroma: prevalence, natural history, and pediatric outcome. *Obstet Gynecol* 2005;106(2):288–294.

Maruotti GM, Saccone G, D'Antonio F, et al. Diagnostic accuracy of intracranial translucency in detecting spina bifida: a systematic review and meta-analysis. *Prenat Diagn* 2016;36(11):991–996.

Morris RK, Quinlan-Jones E, Kilby MD, et al. Systematic review of accuracy of fetal urine analysis to predict poor postnatal renal function in cases of congenital urinary tract obstruction. *Prenat Diagn* 2007;27:900–911.

Nassr AA, Shazly SAM, Abdelmagied AM, et al. Effectiveness of vesicoamniotic shunt in fetuses with congenital lower urinary tract obstruction: an updated systematic review and meta-analysis. *Ultrasound Obstet Gynecol* 2017;49:696–703.

Quarello E, Lafouge A, Fries N, Salomon LJ, CFEF. Basic heart examination: feasibility study of first-trimester systematic simplified fetal echocardiography. *Ultrasound Obstet Gynecol* 2017;49(2): 224–230.

Ramkrishna J, Menezes M, Humnabadkar K, et al. Outcomes following the detection of fetal edema in early pregnancy prior to non-invasive prenatal testing. *Prenat Diagn* 2021;41(2):241–247.

Salomon LJ, Alfirevic Z, Bilardo CM, et al. ISUOG Practice Guidelines: performance of first-trimester fetal ultrasound scan. *Ultrasound Obstet Gynecol* 2013;41:102–113.

Sepulveda W, Wong AE, Viñals F, et al. Absent mandibular gap in the retronasal triangle view: a clue to the diagnosis of micrognathia in the first trimester. *Ultrasound Obstet Gynecol* 2012;39(2):152–156.

Sotiriadis A, Papatheodorou S, Makrydimas G. Neurodevelopmental outcome of fetuses with increased nuchal translucency and apparently normal prenatal and/or postnatal assessment: a systematic review. *Ultrasound Obstet Gynecol* 2012;39:10–19.

Syngelaki A, Hammami A, Bower S, et al. Diagnosis of fetal non-chromosomal abnormalities on routine ultrasound examination at 11–13 weeks' gestation. *Ultrasound Obstet Gynecol* 2019;54:468–476.

Tassin M, Benachi A. Diagnosis of abdominal wall defects in the first trimester. *Curr Opin Obstet Gynecol* 2014;26(2):104–109.

Volpe N, Dall'Asta A, Di Pasquo E, Frusca T, Ghi T. First-trimester fetal neurosonography: technique and diagnostic potential. *Ultrasound Obstet Gynecol* 2020. doi: 10.1002/uog.23149.

Wong L, Da Silva Costa F, Araujo Júnior E, Meagher S. Diagnosis of fetal multicystic dysplastic kidney in the first trimester of pregnancy by 2-D and 3-D ultrasonography. *J Obstet Gynaecol Can* 2019; 41(10):1397–1398.

CHAPTER 2

Screening for Common Chromosomal Abnormalities and Other Genetic Conditions

SUMMARY BOX

BACKGROUND INFORMATION

- Chromosomal abnormalities affect ~1% of all pregnancies that reach 11 weeks
- They are responsible for a significant proportion of miscarriages and are the commonest cause of structural and neurodevelopmental anomalies in infants
- A variety of screening tests can identify pregnancies at high risk of chromosomal abnormality. These screening tests have varying efficacy, advantages and disadvantages – the same screening tool will not necessarily suit all women
- The confirmatory diagnostic tests have varying constraints of performance and assess the genome at varying levels of resolution – choice of diagnostic test will vary according to clinical circumstance
- All pregnant women should be given the opportunity to opt into prenatal screening and/or prenatal diagnosis as early as possible in their pregnancy
- Appropriate resources for pre- and post-test counselling need to be available to allow informed consent for testing and to facilitate ongoing pregnancy management
- Newer forms of screening can potentially identify pregnancies at higher risk of chromosomal abnormalities other than common trisomies, including Turner syndrome and other sex chromosome aneuploidies, rare autosomal trisomies and microdeletions and/or duplications. The benefits and disadvantages of such extended forms of aneuploidy screening need to be carefully considered
- High-quality prescreening counselling is essential, but relevant information is often communicated to pregnant women by non-experts in busy antenatal clinics. Increasingly, women are getting information via social media and providers' promotional material, which is of variable quality. Using preformatted infographics provides higher consistency of information
- Fetal medicine specialists have to acknowledge that information regarding pros and cons of various screening options is difficult to communicate, even by experts
- Even when good-quality, accurate information is provided, it may be overshadowed by a large amount of other health and wellbeing information given to pregnant women in the first trimester

TEST ACCURACY STATISTICS

- **Sensitivity** = detection rate
- **Specificity** is easier to understand when described as **false-positive rate** (100 – specificity = false-positive rate)
- Sensitivity and specificity are important for decision making at the population level; however, both are not easily transferable to individuals' risk
- **Positive and negative predictive values** (PPV and NPV) are often described as being of more interest to clinicians and patients
- PPV in particular is often misunderstood and is, therefore, best avoided when counselling individual women
- The difficulty in using PPV for comparing different screening methods is illustrated in Table 2.1. Even more confusing is an example shown in Table 2.2, where two tests with vastly different detection rates (sensitivity) can have the same PPV rate

Table 2.1 Trisomy prevalence varies greatly with maternal age and these differences affect the NIPT performance results

	NIPT positive predictive value		
Maternal age	**Trisomy 21**	**Trisomy 18**	**Trisomy 13**
20	48%	14%	6%
30	61%	21%	10%
40	93%	69%	50%

PPV results are generated using the calculator available at: www.perinatalquality.org/Vendors/NSGC/NIPT.

Table 2.2 An example of how two screening tests applied to the same population of 50,100 women (50,000 unaffected and 100 with trisomy 21) would have the same PPV despite vastly different detection rates (sensitivity)

	Trisomy 21	
	Yes	No
NIPT+	100	100
NIPT−	0	49,900

- Detection rate (sensitivity) = 100%
- False-positive rate = 0.2% (specificity = 99.8%)
- PPV = 50%

(100 true positives/100 true positives + 100 false positives)

	Trisomy 21	
	Yes	No
NIPT+	50	50
NIPT−	50	49,950

- Detection rate (sensitivity) = 50%
- False-positive rate = 0.1% (specificity = 99.9%)
- PPV = 50%

(50 true positives/50 true positives + 50 false positives)

- In settings where individual women and their doctor have to decide which provider to use, *the cost, no call rate and support for test result interpretation* are far more important than test accuracy statistics. Information regarding diagnostic test accuracy of various tests can be easily manipulated in different ways and is, therefore, very hard to compare

ULTRASOUND IN THE CONTEXT OF GENETIC SCREENING

PRE-TEST ULTRASOUND

- Women who have consented to be screened should have a detailed ultrasound assessment after 11^{+0} weeks, not just a scan focusing on NT measurements
- For a twin pregnancy, chorionicity and accurate dating based on the larger twin should be noted; 'vanishing twin' should be excluded
- If a structural abnormality or NT $\geq$ 3.5 mm is found, women should be counselled accordingly and offered invasive testing for microarray. In this clinical scenario, combined screening or NIPT is *not appropriate* as negative results provides false reassurance
- If NT measurement is not possible after several attempts, the options, depending on availability, include:
  - NIPT
  - second trimester quadruple screening
  - invasive testing

POST-TEST ULTRASOUND

- All screen positive women should have a detailed scan looking for structural abnormalities that might have been missed on a pre-test scan.
- While a negative scan will not be sufficiently reassuring to avoid the need for invasive testing, the presence of structural abnormalities may alter management in terms of the type of genetic testing (e.g. microarray, exome) and follow-up

WHICH SCREENING TEST TO CHOOSE?

- For women with a viable pregnancy confirmed by ultrasound scan in the first trimester, the choices are between:
  - combined screening (nuchal translucency + maternal serum PAPP-A and free hCG)
  - non-invasive prenatal testing using cell-free fetal DNA (cfDNA) in maternal plasma
  - invasive testing
  - screening declined
- **Quadruple serum marker testing** (AFP, hCG, estriol and inhibin A) or a **triple test**, when inhibin A is not available, are screening options offered between 15 and 22 weeks to women who, for whatever reason, missed an opportunity to have the first trimester screening
- With wider availability of NIPT, various combinations of first and second trimester testing (e.g. **integrated, contingent, stepwise, sequential screening**) are now considered obsolete

HIGH RISK COMBINED FIRST TRIMESTER SCREENING

Risk Calculation

- Most commonly, the risk calculations are based on:
  - maternal characteristics (age, history of aneuploidy)
  - fetal characteristics (gestational age and **nuchal translucency**)
  - two serum markers (**PAPP-A** and free beta-**hCG**); values should be adjusted for gestation, ethnicity, smoking status, maternal weight and type of conception
- Each of these components has a considerable impact on the final result (Tables 2.3 and 2.4)

Table 2.3 Impact of maternal age on the trisomy 21 risk calculation* for a fetus with CRL of 56 mm with nuchal translucency of 2 mm and average PAPP-A and hCG (1 MoM)

	Age 30	Age 35	Age 40	Age 45
Trisomy 21 risk	1 in 5,000	1 in 2,500	1 in 769	1 in 189

* From FMF risk calculator: https://fetalmedicine.org/research/assess/trisomies.

Table 2.4 Impact of nuchal translucency measurements (NT) on the trisomy 21 risk calculation* for a 35-year-old mother with average PAPP-A and hCG (1 MoM) and a fetus with CRL of 56 mm

	NT = 2 mm	NT = 3 mm	NT = 3.5 mm
Trisomy 21 risk	1 in 2,500	1 in 111	1 in 70

* From FMF risk calculator: https://fetalmedicine.org/research/assess/trisomies.

- The choice of risk calculator is not trivial as there could be significant differences in the results, depending on the software used. For example, when the same maternal and fetal characteristics from Table 2.4 are entered in the software that uses the FMF Germany algorithm (https://hoehle.shinyapps.io/t21app/), the risk with NT of 3.5 mm rises from 1 in 70 to 1 in 7
- The cut-off for high risk may vary between health care providers. As an example, when the cut-off of 1 in 150 is used, the false screen positive rate at the population level is ~5%; that is, when 1,000 are screened, ~50 women will be offered invasive testing 'unnecessarily'
- Increasingly, women with so-called 'intermediate risk' on combined screening and a structurally normal fetus are being offered NIPT as a second screening test. This 'intermediate risk' window varies considerably between settings and depends largely on the affordability of NIPT. For example, intermediate risk defined as 1 in 50 to 1 in 1,000 will include ~15% of the screened population

Interpretation and Counselling

- While the distinction between a screen positive and screen negative result is predetermined at the population level (usually 1 in 150), for individual women the result is more often expressed as probability, risk, or chance – these terms are essentially synonymous
- Screen positive women who were found to have a structurally normal fetus, particularly those with NT <3 mm and no ultrasound markers associated with aneuploidy, can be offered NIPT instead of invasive testing
- Although ultrasound markers (absent nasal bone, reversed a-wave in ductus venosus, tricuspid regurgitation, ARSA) may be used to 'recalculate' the risk generated by the combined screening, we don't consider this to be good practice. Women who seek additional reassurance after combined screening should be advised to have invasive testing

- Screen positive women who consent for invasive testing should be made aware of the options available to them in terms of additional genetic testing (see the section on invasive testing in this chapter)
- When a high-risk woman, after detailed counselling, declines invasive testing, such a decision should be clearly documented, including the statement that significant chromosomal pathology may be present despite apparently normal ultrasound scans later in pregnancy
- When counselling goes beyond screen positive/negative and is based on an individual risk (chance) of having a fetus with an aneuploidy, great care must be taken to put the numbers in the clinical context, particularly when comparisons are made with the risks associated with invasive procedures
- It is, therefore, advisable to present the risk (chance) also as a percentage, to highlight that differences between risks in terms of clinical importance may be relatively small; that is, risks of 1 in 100, 1 in 200 and 1 in 300 correspond to 1%, 0.5% and 0.33%, respectively

NON-INVASIVE PRENATAL TESTING

METHODOLOGY

- Cell-free DNA detected in maternal plasma comes from trophoblast; fetal (placental) DNA fragments are shorter than maternal cfDNA
- NIPT is based on bioinformatic calculation of the relative contribution from each chromosome
- The main commercially available detection/quantification methods are (see also Table 2.5):
  - Massive parallel sequencing: this is genome-wide screening of the entire chromosome complement. It allows detection of sub-chromosomal copy number variants (CNVs) $\geq$7 Mb in size, as well as selected smaller microdeletions
  - Chromosomal-specific sequencing/microarray: in this method cfDNA fragments are amplified by PCR and quantified. Deviations in relative amount of fragments indicate an abnormality
  - Rolling circle amplification test: chromosomal-specific non-sequencing non-PCR method is based on counting and imaging fluorescently labelled DNA spheres
  - SNP-based analysis: cfDNA is amplified by PCR using specific SNP targets. A statistical algorithm is used to detect abnormalities in expected allele frequencies

Table 2.5 Key characteristics of different NIPT methods

	Massive parallel sequencing	Chromosome-specific sequencing/ microarray	SNP-based analysis	Rolling circle amplification test
Large providers	Verifi (Illumina), Iona, Nifty (BGI)	Harmony (Ariosa/Roche)	Panorama (Natera)	Vanadis (PerkinElmer)
Testing in addition to common trisomies	• Sex chromosome aneuploidies • Autosomal trisomies • Microdeletion syndromes (Prader–Willi, Angelman, DiGeorge, 1p36 deletion, Cri-du-chat), Jacobsen's, Wolf–Hirschorn	• Sex chromosome aneuploidies • DiGeorge	• Sex chromosome aneuploidies • Triploidy • Microdeletion syndromes (Prader–Willi, Angelman, DiGeorge, 1p36 deletion, Cri-du-chat)	
Sample failure rate on the first sample	0.1–3.8%	2.9–4.9%	2–8.1%	0.4–1.8%
Twins	• Monozygotic and dizygotic for common trisomies	• Monozygotic and dizygotic for common trisomies and fetal sex	• Monozygotic and dizygotic for common trisomies and fetal sex • Reports fetal fraction for each twin	• Monozygotic and dizygotic for common trisomies • Reports if there is a male fetus present

- Key questions that providers should be able to answer in order to make an informed choice regarding the most appropriate test are:
  - cost;
  - proportion of test results issued after five working days;
  - proportion of non-reportable results (no-calls), pathway for retesting ('redraws') and retest success rate; and
  - availability of post-test counselling/advice
- While detection rates (sensitivity) and false-positive rates (specificity) may be useful for decision-making at the population level, the differences in quoted figures between various NIPT providers are easily misinterpreted and are, therefore, not very helpful for individual

counselling. The confidence intervals around these estimates do overlap, 'head to head' comparisons between different NIPT tests on the same population are virtually non-existent, and the results will be influenced by the way the 'no calls' are handled – some providers include 'no calls' in their statistics, some don't

LOW FETAL FRACTION AND NON-REPORTABLE NIPT (NO CALL)

- The most common reasons for non-reportable results are:
  - low fetal fraction (FF)
  - insufficient cfDNA
  - borderline z score
  - altered maternal genomic profile (e.g. maternal lymphoma)

Fetal Fraction

- The average FF (ratio of fetal to maternal cfDNA) is ~10–15% between 10 and 20 weeks of gestation. However, there is no universally agreed method to estimate the fetal fraction – most of them compare relative sizes of DNA fragments and are rather imprecise
- Inadequate amount of fetal DNA or excessive maternal DNA (e.g. high BMI) will result in low fetal fraction, which makes the test less accurate and, therefore, 'not reportable'
- The actual 'FF cut-off' at which a result is withheld varies between different providers (laboratories), which is then reflected in different 'no-call' rates
- While reporting FF seems intuitively important, once a laboratory has estimated that a sample is reportable (i.e. above 'the detection threshold', which is externally regulated), the actual FF of a reported sample should not be used to influence clinical decision-making

Non-reportable Result (No-Calls)

- A relatively large proportion of samples (~1–5%) are no-calls
- No-call figures vary between providers and should be regarded as one of the key parameters when deciding which test to use
- It is important to ascertain whether a no-call is due to technical reasons (operator error, stuck pipette tips in automated protocols) or due to low FF
- The association of non-reportable NIPT due to low FF and higher risk of aneuploidy has been reported. One possible reason is that placentas in trisomy 18 and 13 are smaller and therefore have a lower FF
- The options following non-reportable results include:

Retest ('Redraw')

- Likely to be successful in at least 60–70% and even higher, if the reason for failure is 'technical', rather than low FF

Invasive Testing

- A better option for women with high BMI and very low FF (<2%)

NIPT TESTING FOR SINGLE-GENE DISORDERS

- It is now possible to use NIPT for single-gene disorders that are either inherited (e.g. cystic fibrosis, hemoglobinopathies and autosomal recessive deafness) or *de novo* mutations (e.g. Noonan syndrome, craniosynostosis syndrome and skeletal disorders)
- Single-gene testing may be clinically useful in women with family history or ultrasound markers suggestive of the disease; however, the value of offering these tests to general obstetric populations remains highly controversial
- As the prevalence of single-gene disorders in the general population is very low, PPVs are also likely to be very low, causing anxiety and unnecessary invasive testing

NIPT COUNSELLING

- For some women, first trimester combined screening may be a better choice than NIPT (Table 2.6)
- With adequate pre-test counselling a need for **confirmatory invasive testing** should have been already agreed and any confusion regarding the differences between screening and diagnostic testing avoided. However, anxiety following screen positive results is inevitable
- Requests for termination of pregnancy based on NIPT results should be declined, but handled sensitively and with compassion
- Most providers report the estimate of FF and the levels could be low (<4%). However, if the NIPT is reported, the FF fraction is judged to be above 'detection threshold' and the actual FF levels should not be used to influence the clinical decision-making
- In the event of a non-reportable result due to low FF, particularly at later gestations (>12 weeks), women should be advised to have invasive testing – any 'retesting' will have a high chance of repeated failure and further delays
- Fetal medicine specialists presented with a positive NIPT for microdeletions or single-gene disorders must ensure that the management options following confirmatory invasive testing, including provisions for late termination of pregnancy, are well understood. If at all possible, clinical geneticists should be *involved* in the decisions regarding invasive testing and follow-up plans in case of a positive result

Table 2.6 Contraindications for NIPT

NIPT is not appropriate test	NIPT is relatively contraindicated due to high no-call rate
• Maternal chromosomal abnormality (e.g. mosaic Turner)	• Obesity (BMI >35)
• Cancer (e.g. lymphoma)	• Low molecular weight heparin
• Bone marrow transplant	• Low PAPP-A
	• Consanguinity for SNP-based NIPT

SECOND TRIMESTER BIOCHEMISTRY SCREENING

- May be offered to women who missed out on the first trimester combined screening for whatever reason (late presentation, unable to measure nuchal translucency)
- Quadruple test includes: (1) alpha-fetoprotein (AFP); (2) unconjugated oestriol (uE_3); (3) human chorionic gonadotrophin (hCG) – total, intact or free beta subunit; and (4) inhibin-A
- The triple test may be offered in settings where inhibin-A is not available
- The gestational window for the test varies between providers, but can be done as early as 14^{+0} weeks up to 21^{+6} weeks
- The most common cut-off for screen positive test is 1 in 150
- Screen positive women are offered amniocentesis, although NIPT is a reasonable alternative if the ultrasound scan is normal

INVASIVE TESTING

- Some women may wish to avoid the uncertainty of a screen negative test and, therefore, choose a diagnostic rather than a screening test, accepting the relatively small risk of losing a healthy pregnancy (<1 in 200)
- The option of having CVS or amniocentesis on maternal request should be available to women, but access will depend on local circumstances and costs (funding)
- Women who consent for invasive testing should be informed of the options in terms of genetic testing and significant differences in terms of diagnostic potential, time needed to reach the diagnosis and cost (if relevant):
  - QF-PCR for trisomy 21, 18, and 13, Turner syndrome – usually four working days
  - Conventional karyotyping – 10–14 days
  - Microarray testing may detect deletions and duplications that would be missed by conventional karyotyping, but may not detect certain rearrangements (e.g. balanced translocations) – 7–10 days
- In most modern genetic laboratories, QF-PCR is considered to be diagnostic for amniocentesis
- When CVS samples are analysed with the QF-PCR method, there is a residual concern that confined placental mosaicism may be present. We therefore consider QF-PCR following CVS to be 'interim' reports and counsel women accordingly
- There is also a small possibility of a completely discrepant result (i.e. a QF-PCR indicating trisomy followed by a normal karyotype generated from the cell culture). Provided that laboratories are using the digest method for analysis, the risk of such a discrepant result is likely to be around 1 in 10,000, particularly for cases where three separate alleles (triallelic result) are clearly seen, indicating three different chromosomes
- Given the possibility, albeit extremely rare, of a false-positive QF-PCR result, the decision whether to proceed with termination of pregnancy based on QF-PCR result must be individualised, with the risks carefully explained and clearly documented. Appropriate pre- and post-test counselling is, therefore, essential. If there is any ambiguity with the result and its interpretation, this must be resolved with laboratory scientists before counselling takes place

SCREENING TEST DECLINED

- Most women who decline aneuploidy screen are still keen to have ultrasound scans performed to a high standard at the optimal time. It is, therefore, important to ascertain and discuss what is the local policy regarding the 11^{+0} to 13^{+6} week 'nuchal translucency scan' for women who decline aneuploidy screening
- Women who decline aneuploidy screening should not be denied the first trimester scan, which should be performed to ISUOG standards

SECOND TRIMESTER ULTRASOUND MARKERS

- Many 'soft' ultrasound markers seen in otherwise structurally normal fetuses at the second trimester scan have been linked with common aneuploidies, and more recently with pathological CNVs
- We consider the following to be clinically important when found after 18 weeks:
  - mild ventriculomegaly (≥10 mm)
  - absent or hypoplastic nasal bone
  - increased nuchal fold (≥6 mm)
  - aberrant right subclavian artery (ARSA)
  - short femur (<third centile)
- Renal pelvic dilatation and echogenic bowel, while not clinically important in the context of genetic testing, are associated with increased risk of specific structural abnormalities, fetal infection and cystic fibrosis (see the relevant chapters for more information)
- When short femur is found, it is important to note that previous low-risk aneuploidy screening does not provide adequate reassurance. While the risk for trisomy 21 may not be significantly increased, the possibility of skeletal dysplasia and/or pathological CNVs must be considered
- In some centres invasive testing may be offered for fetuses with isolated intracardiac echogenic foci, choroid plexus cysts or single umbilical artery. However, there are no good-quality data that show clinically important increased risks for women who were adequately screened in the first trimester

SCREEN NEGATIVE WOMEN WITHOUT ULTRASOUND MARKERS AT 20 WEEKS' SCAN

- For women who had low-risk combined test and/or NIPT, the risk of chromosomal abnormalities is further reduced after normal 20 weeks' scan, but we do not recommend recalculation of an already low risk

SCREEN NEGATIVE WOMEN WITH A SINGLE ULTRASOUND MARKER AT 20 WEEKS' SCAN

- The risk of aneuploidies and/or pathological CNVs in this group is likely to be in excess of 1%
- For women who already had a low-risk combined test and/or NIPT, amniocentesis should be offered for:

Ultrasound marker	Increased risk
Ventriculomegaly	Trisomy 21, pathological CNVs
Increased nuchal fold	Trisomy 21
Absent nasal bone	Trisomy 21
ARSA	DiGeorge syndrome
Short femur	Pathological CNVs

SCREEN NEGATIVE WOMEN WITH TWO OR MORE ULTRASOUND MARKERS AT 20 WEEKS' SCAN

- Amniocentesis should be offered
- The combined risk could be as high as 10% (~5% aneuploidies; ~5% pathological CNVs)

WOMEN WITH ULTRASOUND MARKERS AT 20 WEEKS' SCAN WHO DECLINED FIRST TRIMESTER SCREENING

- This is a difficult scenario that requires detailed counselling regarding the reasons for declining
- If a woman declined screening for Down syndrome she should be counselled that other clinically important genetic conditions can be present

MULTIPLE PREGNANCY

NIPT

- NIPT screening performance for twins is comparable to singleton pregnancies, particularly for trisomy 21
- As a general rule, if ultrasound identifies intrauterine death of one twin **(vanishing twin)**, then NIPT is best avoided as there is a higher risk of false-positive result
- If a woman with a vanishing twin prefers a reassurance of negative NIPT and accepts the risk of a false-positive result that may lead to an 'unnecessary' invasive test, NIPT remains a valid option in this scenario

SERUM BIOCHEMISTRY

- Serum biochemistry testing is less reliable in twins because the biochemical results from an unaffected twin may mask an affected twin
- Although serum marker calculations cannot be simply derived from singleton pregnancies, combined screening performance (NT, PAPP-A, hCG) in monochorionic twins is comparable to singleton pregnancies

HIGHER-ORDER MULTIPLES

- For higher-order multiple pregnancies, nuchal translucency measurement in combination with maternal age is the only method that can be used to screen for common aneuploidies

SUGGESTED READING

PRIMARY RESEARCH

Hu T, Tian T, Zhang Z, et al. Prenatal chromosomal microarray analysis in 2466 fetuses with ultrasonographic soft markers: a prospective cohort study. *Am J Obstet Gynecol* 2021;224:516.e1–516.e16.

REVIEWS AND GUIDELINES

Agathokleous M, Chaveeva P, Poon LC, Kosinski P, Nicolaides KH. Meta-analysis of second-trimester markers for trisomy 21. *Ultrasound Obstet Gynecol* 2013;41(3):247–261.

Kagan KO, Sonek J, Wagner P, Hoopmann M. Principles of first trimester screening in the age of non-invasive prenatal diagnosis: screening for chromosomal abnormalities. *Arch Gynecol Obstet* 2017;296(4):645–651.

Salomon LJ, Alfirevic Z, Bilardo CM, et al. ISUOG Practice Guidelines: performance of first-trimester fetal ultrasound scan. *Ultrasound Obstet Gynecol* 2013;41(3):102–113.

Yaron Y. The implications of non-invasive prenatal testing failures: a review of an under-discussed phenomenon. *Prenat Diagn* 2016;36(5):391–396.

CHAPTER 3

Fetal Anatomy

Second and Third Trimester Assessment

SUMMARY BOX

CHAPTER 3.1

Head and Neck

SUMMARY BOX

ANATOMY ASSESSMENT

- Transverse section at the level of the cavum septum pellucidum and posterior horns of the lateral ventricle posteriorly enables the assessment of:
  - cranial bones
  - cavum septum pellucidum and anterior horns of lateral ventricle ('anterior complex') (Fig. 3.1.1)
  - posterior horns of lateral ventricles and choroid plexus ('posterior complex') (Fig. 3.1.2)
  - third ventricle (Fig. 3.1.3)
  - cerebral parenchyma
  - sylvian fissure

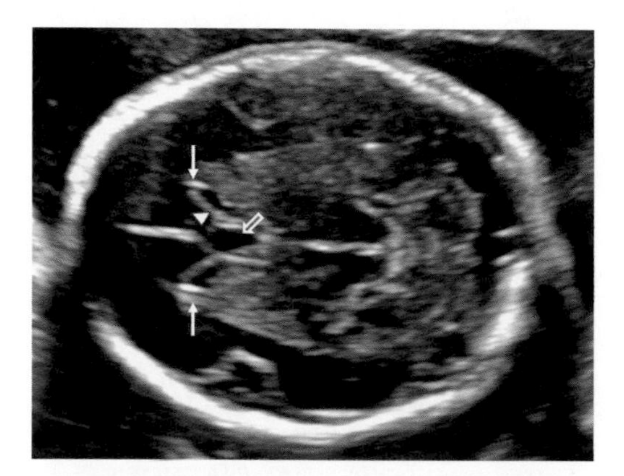

Fig. 3.1.1 Transverse view of the head showing the anterior echo complex. The interhemispheric fissure is seen as a bright line between the two frontal horns (arrows). The complex includes the cavum septum pellucidum (open arrow) and the genu of the corpus callosum (arrowhead).

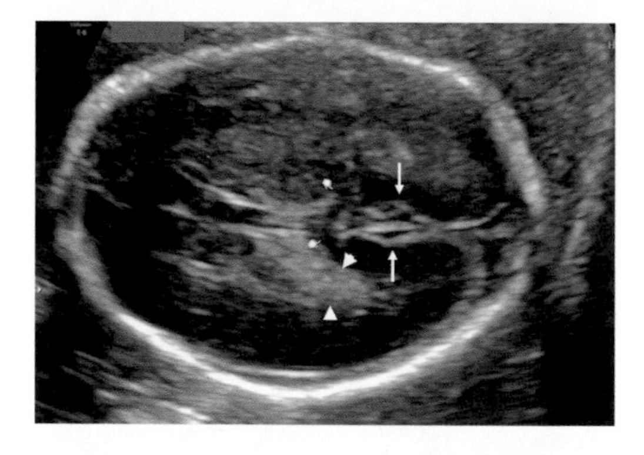

Fig. 3.1.2 Transverse view of the head showing the posterior echo complex with the choroid plexus (arrowheads). The complex includes the parieto-occipital sulci on either side of the midline (arrows) and the splenium of the corpus callosum (finger arrows).

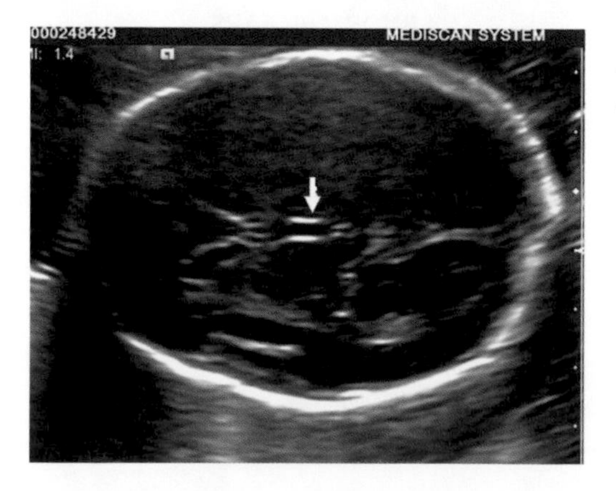

Fig. 3.1.3 Transverse view of the head showing the normal third ventricle as a small slit in the midline (arrow).

- The suboccipito-bregmatic section at the level of the cavum septum pellucidum anteriorly and cerebellum posteriorly enables the assessment of:
  - thalami and the midbrain
  - cerebellum and cerebellar vermis
  - cisterna magna and fourth ventricle (Fig. 3.1.4)
  - nuchal skin fold thickness can be measured in this plane

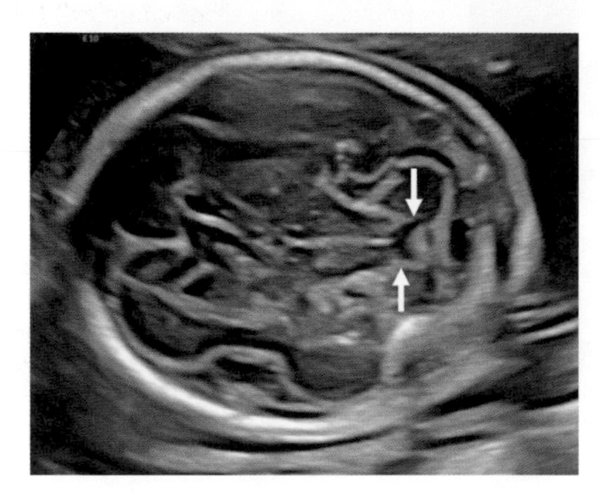

Fig. 3.1.4 Transverse view of the trans-cerebellar plane showing normally formed fourth ventricle (arrows). Note the width is larger than the antero-posterior (AP) diameter. The fourth ventricle index, calculated as the width (laterolateral diameter) divided by the AP diameter, in this case is normal (>1).

- Coronal views and sagittal sections enable the assessment of:
  - corpus callosum (Fig. 3.1.5)
  - brain stem, vermis, and tentorium

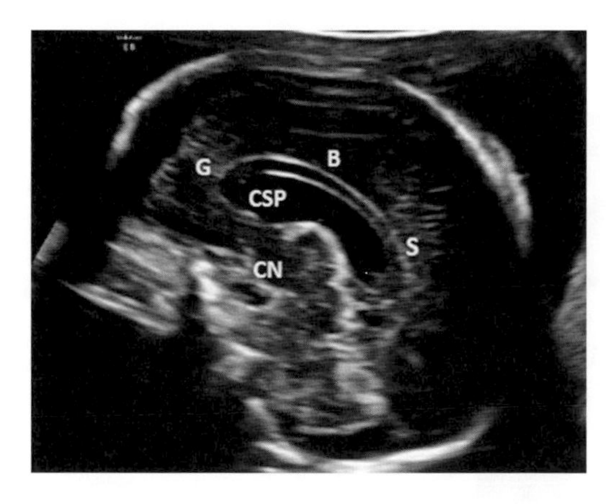

Fig. 3.1.5 Midline sagittal view of the head showing the normal corpus callosum. B, body; S, splenium; CN, caudate nucleus; CSP, cavum septum pellucidum; G, genu.

- Face and orbits:
  - interocular, binocular and orbital distances (Fig. 3.1.6)

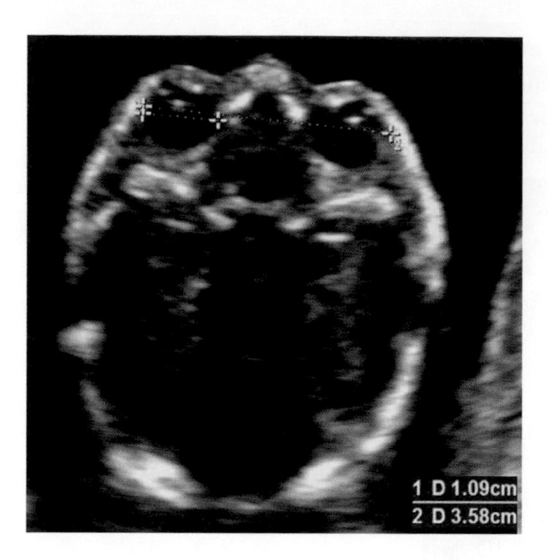

Fig. 3.1.6 Transverse section of the orbits. Note the two small echogenic dots representing the lenses. The orbital diameter (1) and binocular distance (2) measurements are shown.

- Ears:
  - best examined in the parasagittal view and 3D scan
  - mostly examined in detail only during phenotyping of suspected syndromic pathology
- Neck:
  - axial section
  - thyroid gland (Fig. 3.1.7)

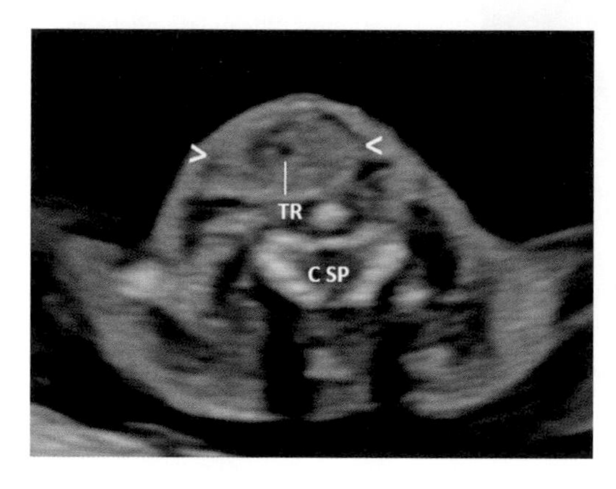

Fig. 3.1.7 Transverse section of the fetal neck showing the normal thyroid gland (>,<). CSP, transverse section of the cervical spine; TR, trachea.

ABNORMAL SKULL

ANENCEPHALY

Ultrasound Assessment

- Absent cranial vault (Fig. 3.1.8)
- Absent hemispheres, or minimal recognisable tissue above orbits and cranial floor
- It is important to exclude spinal defects or amniotic bands

Investigations

- Karyotyping may reveal aneuploidy, which would alter the advice about the risks for future pregnancy

Counselling and Management

- Lethal; therefore, offer termination of the pregnancy
- Palliative care can be discussed as an alternative
- Discuss possible organ donation
- Discuss relevant maternal risks of ongoing pregnancy, including polyhydramnios and its complications and post-term pregnancy
- Risk of recurrence is ~3–4%
- The recurrence risk can be reduced significantly with periconceptual folic acid (5 mg/day) in all future pregnancies
- Early ultrasound assessment ($11–13^{+6}$ weeks) should be arranged in all future pregnancies

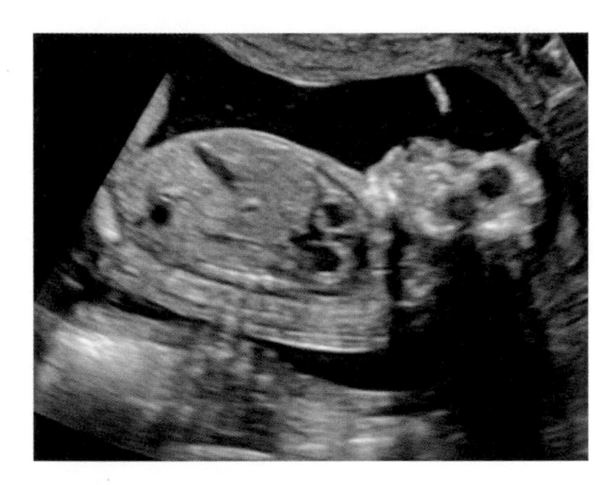

Fig. 3.1.8 Anencephaly: longitudinal section of the fetus showing absence of cranial vault. No brain parenchymal tissue is seen above the prominent orbits.

BONY DEFECTS IN CRANIUM

Ultrasound Assessment

- Skull defects are occipital in ~85% and frontal or ethmoidal in ~15% of cases
- Herniated meninges with or without brain tissue may be present (Fig. 3.1.9)
- Disruption of intracranial anatomy is often seen
- ~30% will have other structural anomalies, such as Meckel–Gruber syndrome (occipital encephalocele with large cystic kidneys and polydactyly)

Investigations

- Offer invasive testing (microarray)
- Consider exome sequencing when multiple anomalies are present
- MRI provides additional assessment of herniated tissue and brain parenchyma

Counselling and Management

- Isolated meningoceles have a good prognosis; survival without long-term sequelae is >90%
- Encephaloceles have a mortality risk of ~30% and neurodevelopmental morbidity of ~80%

- The long-term outcome is dependent on neurosurgical facilities and the size of the herniated defect

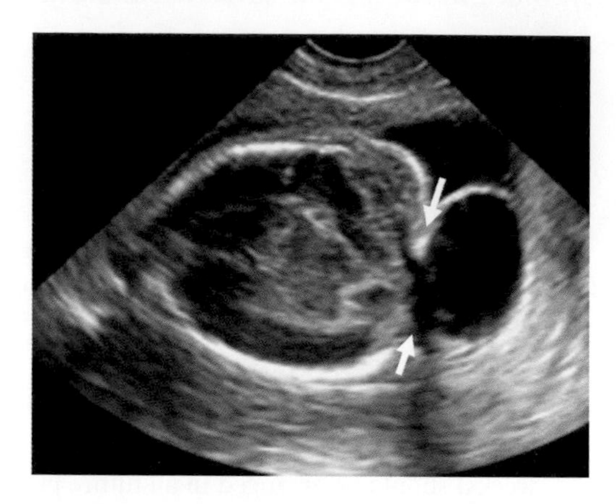

Fig. 3.1.9 Occipital meningocele. Transverse section of the fetal head showing a bony defect in the calvarium (arrows) with a cystic swelling that communicates with the intracranial structures.

ABNORMAL SKULL SHAPE

Definition and Characteristics

- Normal skull shape is oval, which can be confirmed by measuring the ratio of biparietal diameter (BPD) to occipitofrontal diameter (OFD)
- The cephalic index (BPD/OFD $\times$ 100) in the second trimester should be between 75 and 85

Ultrasound Assessment

- **Dolichocephaly:** low BPD/OFD ratio. Most commonly normal variant associated with breech presentation (Fig. 3.1.10)
- **Brachycephaly:** high BPD/OFD ratio. There is a weak association with trisomy 21 and small frontal lobes. May be associated with craniosynostosis of coronal and lambdoid sutures (Fig. 3.1.11)
- **Strawberry-shaped skull** (trigonocephaly). This is associated with trisomy 18, some skeletal dysplasias (thanatophoric dysplasia) and craniosynostosis of the median frontal (metopic) suture. Microdeletions on chromosomal microarray and genetic associations (exome) are found in ~30% of cases (Fig. 3.1.12)
- **Lemon-shaped skull** (scalloping of frontal bones). Look for other features of neural tube defects (spina bifida and encephalocele) and other CNS anomalies (Fig. 3.1.13)
- **Cloverleaf-shaped skull** is associated with craniosynostosis and a number of underlying genetic conditions, including *FGFR3* abnormalities (thanatophoric dysplasia type II), *FGFR2* abnormalities (severe Apert and Crouzon syndromes) and Carpenter syndrome (for more details on phenotypes, see Chapter 19) (Fig. 3.1.14)

Counselling and Management

- Detailed anatomy assessment, including full skeletal survey, is always needed
- Microarray and exome testing are indicated in the presence of other suspicious phenotypic features

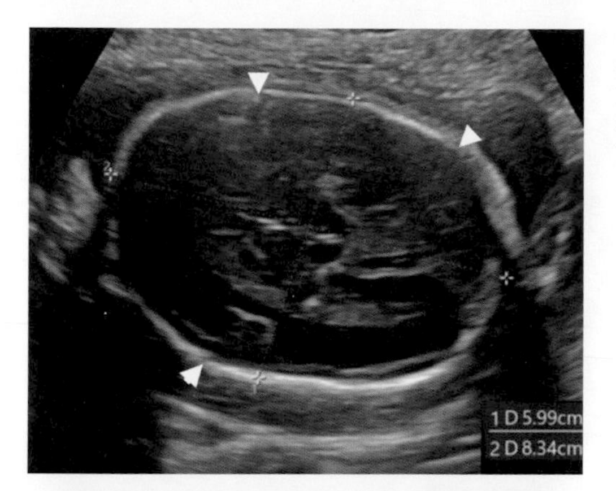

Fig. 3.1.10 Dolichocephaly in a normal breech presentation. The cephalic index is 72. Note the presence of the normal "gap" of the parietal and lambdoid sutures (arrowheads).

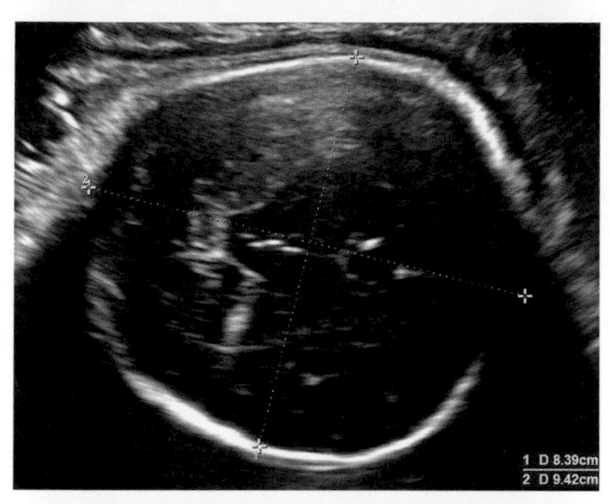

Fig. 3.1.11 Brachycephaly in a case of craniosynostosis. The cephalic index is 89. Note the absence of the normal "gaps" of the parietal and lambdoid sutures that are clearly seen in Fig. 3.1.10.

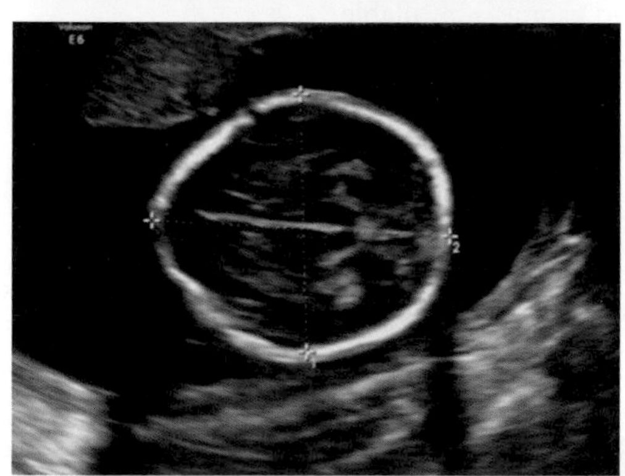

Fig. 3.1.12 Strawberry skull in trisomy 18. Note the pointed frontal end and a flattened occiput.

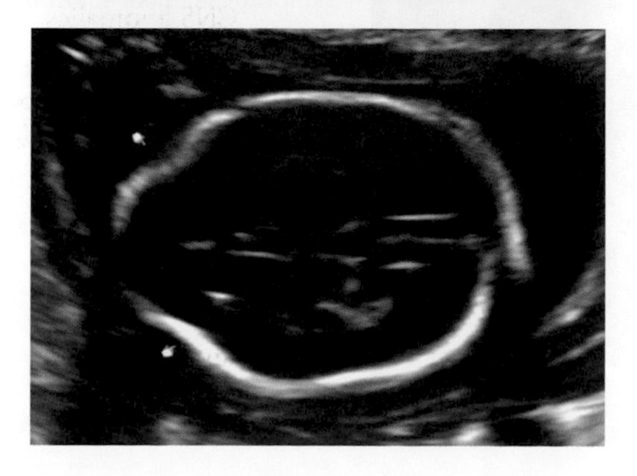

Fig. 3.1.13 Lemon-shaped skull in open spina bifida. The frontal bones appear scalloped (finger arrows).

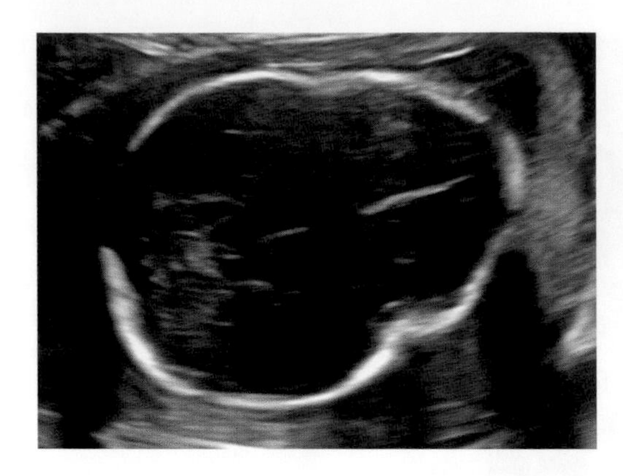

Fig. 3.1.14 Cloverleaf skull in a case of thanatophoric dysplasia. A similar appearance may also be seen in craniosynostosis.

ABNORMAL SKULL MINERALISATION

Ultrasound Assessment

- Demineralisation can be complete or partial
- Improved visualisation of intracranial structures is striking (Fig. 3.1.15a)
- Check the width of the median frontal (metopic) suture using a 3D scan (Fig. 3.1.15b)
- A full skeletal survey is essential to look for phenotypic features of skeletal dysplasias

Investigations

- Offer chromosomal microarray and exome, if available
- Skeletal panel/exome sequencing should be discussed with the clinical geneticist, as testing will be informed by the presence/absence of certain phenotypic features

Counselling and Management

- Significant risk of skeletal dysplasia, including osteogenesis imperfecta, achondrogenesis, Crouzon syndrome, Pfeiffer syndrome, Apert syndrome
- >80% chance of syndromic association

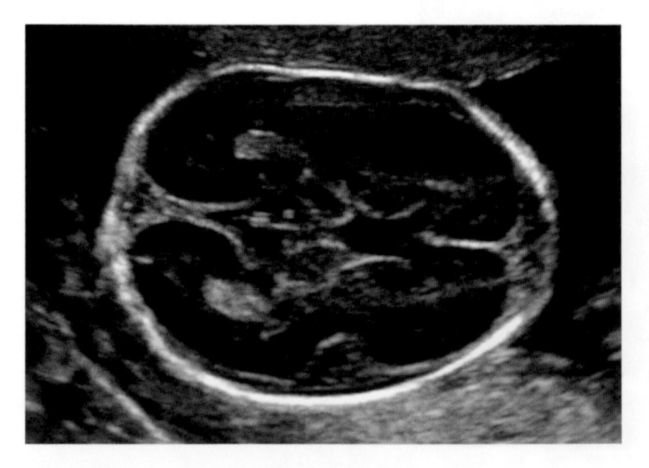

Fig. 3.1.15a Transverse section of the skull showing poor mineralisation of the cranial bones in a case of osteogenesis imperfecta. There is a flattening of the anterior portion of the skull. The contents of the near hemisphere are seen clearly.

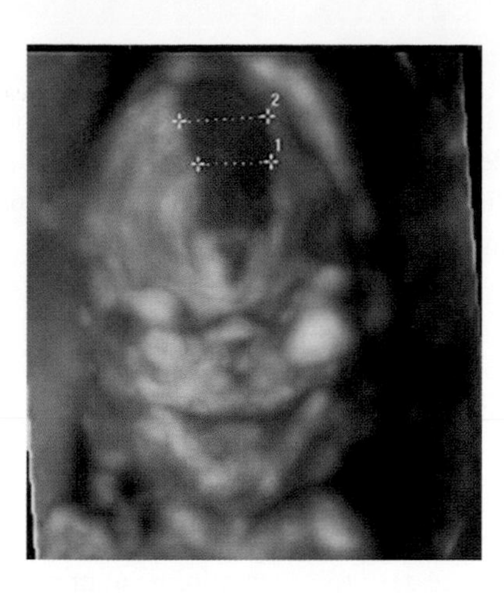

Fig. 3.1.15b 3D image of the fetal face showing a widened metopic suture (callipers) in the same baby with osteogenesis imperfecta.

ABNORMAL MIDLINE DIVISION OF THE CEREBRAL HEMISPHERES

Definition and Characteristics

- A range of midline anomalies caused by incomplete cleavage of the forebrain is collectively recognised as holoprosencephaly (Fig. 3.1.16)

Ultrasound Assessment

- Unable to identify falx
- Look for single 'anterior' ventricle and fused thalami
- Check for other midline defects – there is particularly high prevalence of midline facial clefts and proboscis (a trunk-like nose)

Alobar Holoprosencephaly

- Falx and interhemispheric fissure are absent anteriorly, but visible posteriorly
- There is a partial segmentation of the ventricles and cerebral hemispheres posteriorly (Fig. 3.1.17)

Semilobar Holoprosencephaly

- The falx is visible anteriorly and posteriorly as the fusion is typically confined to the inferior portion of the frontal lobes
- The cavum septum pellucidum is absent, but the corpus callosum may be normal or only partially present
- The third ventricle is usually visible (Fig. 3.1.18)

Lobar Holoprosencephaly

- Isolated small or absent cavum septum pellucidum with evidence of fused frontal horns
- MRI may show pituitary hypoplasia and optic nerve hypoplasia

Septo-optic Dysplasia

- Definitive antenatal diagnosis is usually not possible even when scans and MRI are combined
- Septo-optic dysplasia should be suspected when there is absence of the cavum septum pellucidum, fused or continuous frontal horns and optic nerve hypoplasia (Fig. 3.1.19)

Investigations

- Karyotyping should be offered as there is a strong association with trisomy 13 but also with trisomy 18, triploidy and some microdeletions
- Exome sequencing, if available, may be useful as there is high prevalence of autosomal dominant and autosomal recessive conditions

Counselling

- Alobar and severe semilobar holoprosencephaly are likely lethal
- Lobar is associated with significant rates of moderate or severe neurodevelopmental delay
- Septo-optic dysplasia is associated mainly with visual and endocrine disturbances, but there are reported cases of neurodevelopmental delay
- Interaction of several genetic events may be necessary to cause midline abnormalities, highlighting the complexity of inheritance. Clinical geneticists should, therefore, be involved in antenatal testing and subsequent counselling

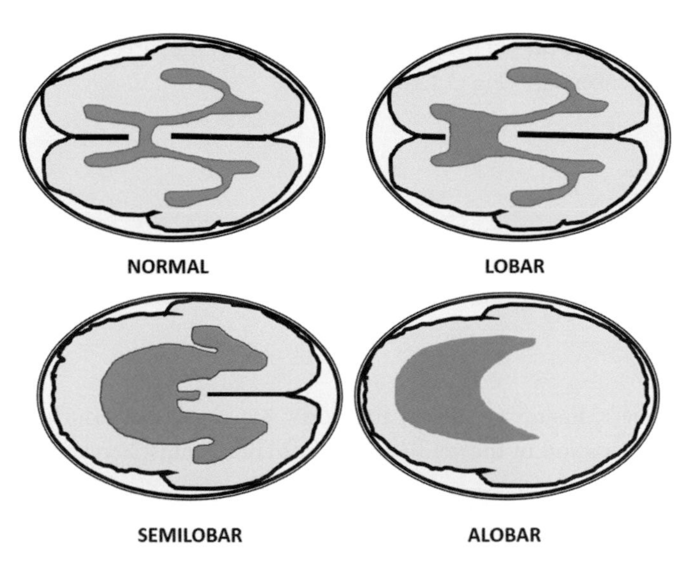

Fig. 3.1.16 Schematic drawing showing four types of holoprosencephaly.

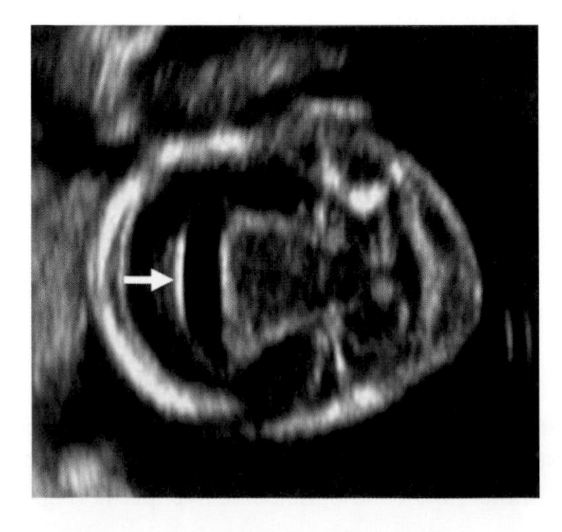

Fig. 3.1.17 Alobar holoprosencephaly. Transverse section of the head showing absence of the midline falx and a single ventricle (arrow).

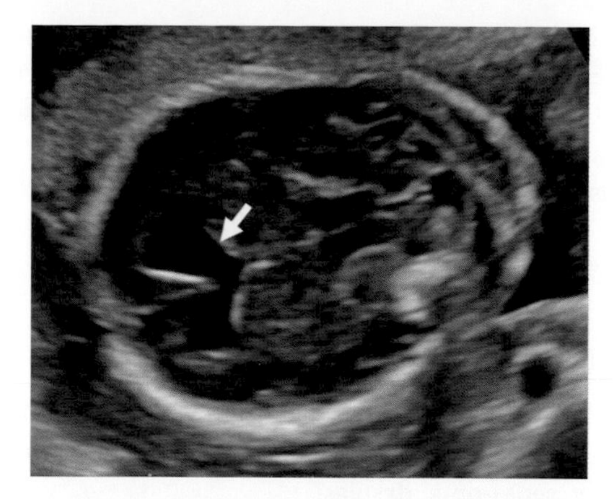

Fig. 3.1.18 Semilobar holoprosencephaly. Transverse section of the head showing part of the falx seen anteriorly and posteriorly, indicating partial cleavage of the frontal lobes. Fusion of the lateral ventricles is seen (arrow).

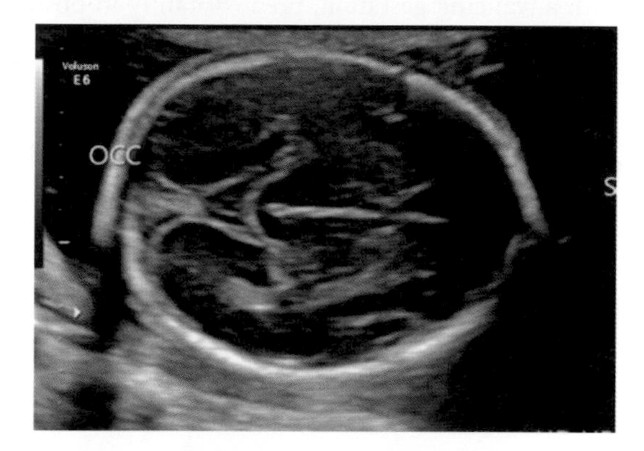

Fig. 3.1.19a Suspected septo-optic dysplasia. Transverse view of the head in a 22-week fetus showing absent cavum septum pellucidum. Occ, occiput.

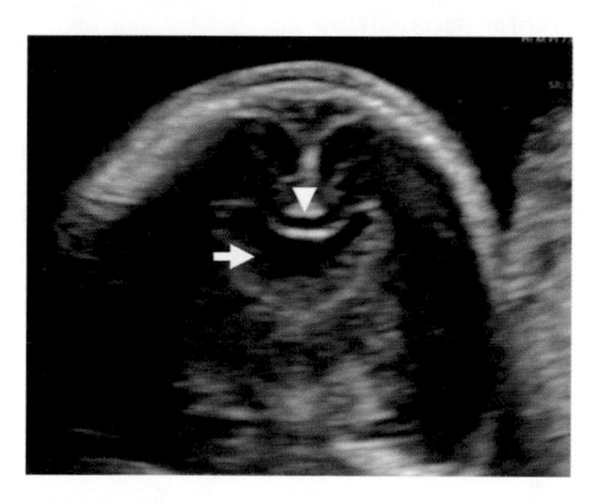

Fig. 3.1.19b Coronal view of the same case of suspected septo-optic dysplasia showing fused frontal horns (arrow). The corpus callosum is present (arrowhead).

ABNORMAL CAVUM SEPTUM PELLUCIDUM INCLUDING AGENESIS OF CORPUS CALLOSUM

Definition and Characteristics

- The corpus callosum (CC) runs beneath the cerebral hemisphere and has four distinctive parts: rostrum and genu anteriorly, body in the middle and splenium posteriorly
- Its development should be complete by 20 weeks. Maldevelopment can result in a CC that is totally or partially absent, or hypoplastic

- The septa pellucida are two thin leaves that hang from the anterior part of CC to the superior aspect of the fornix. They form part of the medial wall of the lateral ventricles
- The cavum septum pellucidum (CSP) is a cavity between the two leaves of the septum pellucidum, which separate the lateral ventricles
- The posterior extension of CSP is called cavum vergae and may be visible in ~80% of normal third trimester fetuses
- CSP will completely close in ~95% of children 5 months after birth

Absent CSP: Possible Agenesis of Corpus Callosum (ACC)

- Absence of the cavum septum pellucidum is strongly suggestive of ACC, but it is not diagnostic. This is because the septum pellucidum (and the cavum between two leaflets) can be absent with CC present (e.g. septo-optic dysplasia)
- Ventriculomegaly is common with advancing gestation, predominantly in posterior horns that look like a teardrop (colpocephaly) (Fig. 3.1.20a)
- The normal course of the pericallosal artery cannot be identified (Fig. 3.1.20b,c)

CSP Is Short or Thin: Possible Partial ACC

- Abnormal CC will be short (<18 mm) and/or very thin (<2 mm)
- Partial ACC usually involves loss of posterior parts – body and splenium
- If partial agenesis is suspected, look for arachnoid cysts, posterior fossa abnormalities and other structural anomalies

Investigations

- MRI to evaluate the development of cerebral parenchyma
- Exome testing is indicated, if available, as corpus callosum and septum pellucidum abnormalities are associated with >200 genetic syndromes

Counselling

- Isolated ACC has ~30% risk of moderate/severe neurodevelopmental delay and ~30% recurrence risk
- When associated with other CNS pathologies, the risk of neurodevelopmental delay is >50%

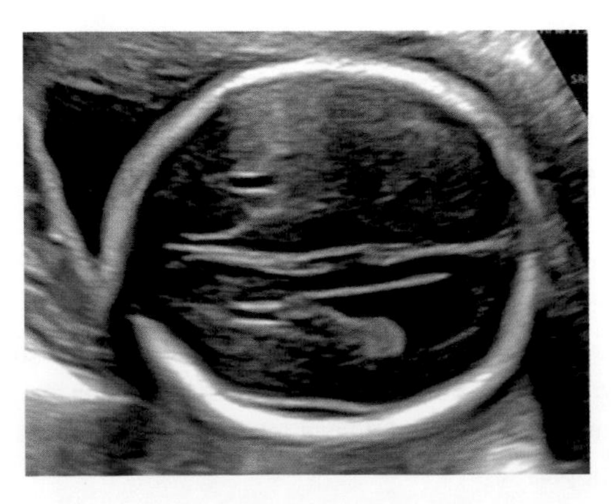

Fig. 3.1.20a Colpocephaly. Transverse section of the fetal head with agenesis of the corpus callosum showing a dilated occipital horn of the lateral ventricle. The "pinched" frontal horn gives an appearance of a "tear drop" shape of the lateral ventricle.

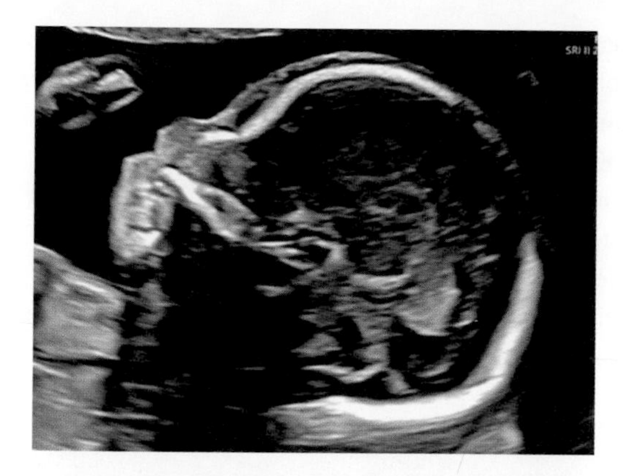

Fig. 3.1.20b Mid-sagittal view of the head of the same case showing absence of the corpus callosum.

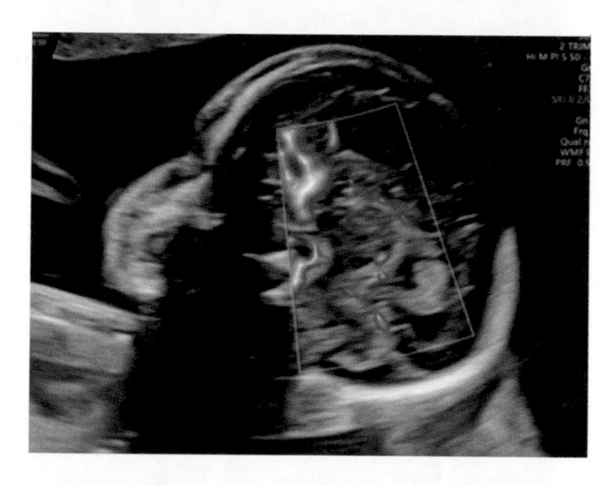

Fig. 3.1.20c Colour Doppler of the same case showing absence of the pericallosal artery.

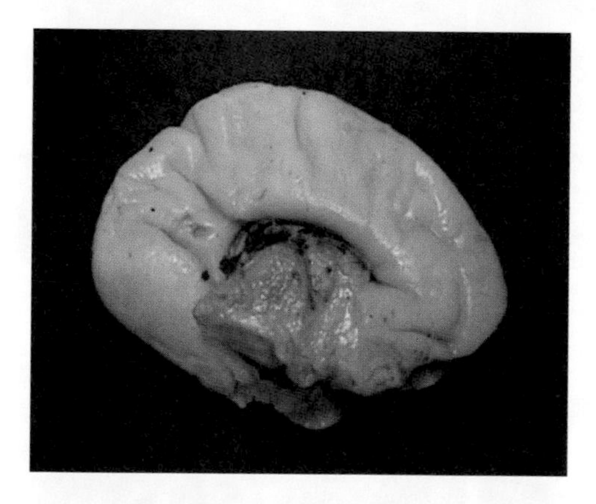

Fig. 3.1.20d Post mortem specimen of cerebral hemisphere showing absent corpus callosum.

CORTICAL MALFORMATIONS INCLUDING ABNORMAL SYLVIAN FISSURE

Definitions and Characteristics

Lissencephaly: Type 1 has 'smooth' brain with lack of gyri and sulci (neuronal undermigration). Sylvian fissure development (Fig 3.1.21) is delayed or incomplete (Fig 3.1.22). This type is a feature of Miller–Dieker syndrome.

Type 2 shows anarchic overmigration causing excessive number of cortical gyri that are abnormally formed and small (polymicrogyria). The result is bumpy cortical surface, hence the term cobblestone lissencephaly, seen in Walker–Warburg syndrome (see Chapter 19).

Hemimegaloencephaly: 'Overgrowth' of one hemisphere with ventriculomegaly, disruption of midline and abnormalities of sulcation and gyration (e.g. Proteus syndrome).

Schizencephaly: A cleft between the ventricle and the subarachnoid space, most commonly through the parietal lobe (Fig. 3.1.23). This is a migrational anomaly commonly associated with other CNS abnormalities.

Investigations

- MRI is essential to assess gyration and look for evidence of periventricular heterotopias and any other intracranial abnormalities (tumours, haemorrhage)
- Chromosomal microarray and exome sequencing, if available

Counselling and Management

- Prognosis is generally poor, but counselling is complex and should be multidisciplinary, involving clinical geneticists and neonatologists

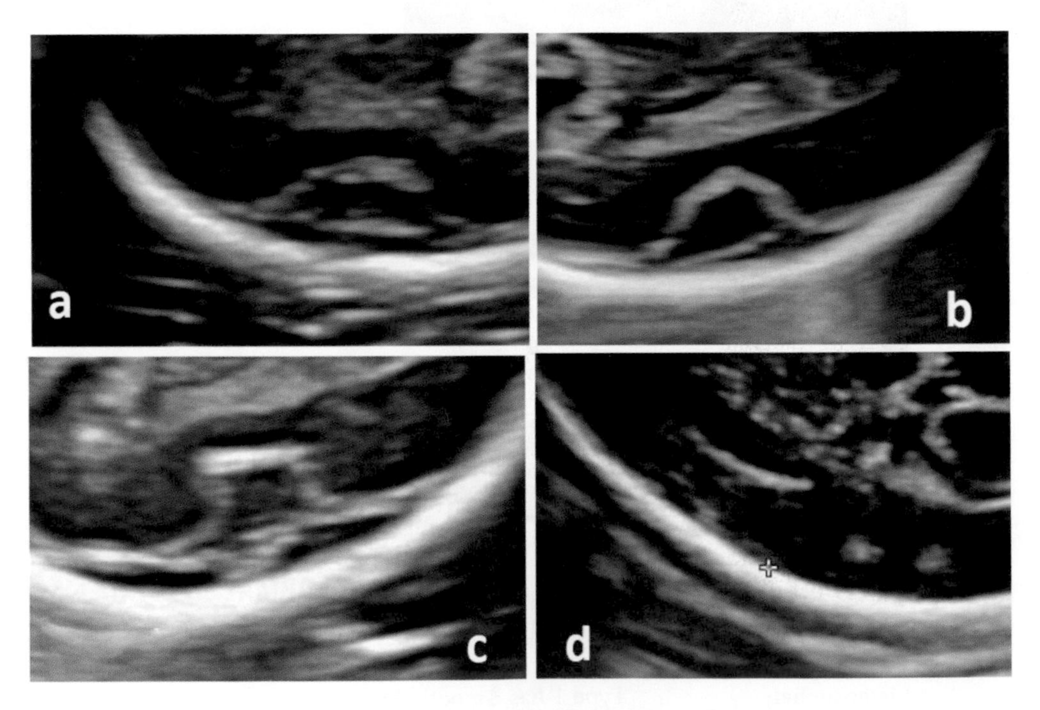

Fig. 3.1.21 Normal pattern of Sylvian fissure at different gestations. Note the variation in shape and narrowing of the sulcus with advancing gestational age (a = 22 weeks; b = 24 weeks; c = 28 weeks; d = 32 weeks).

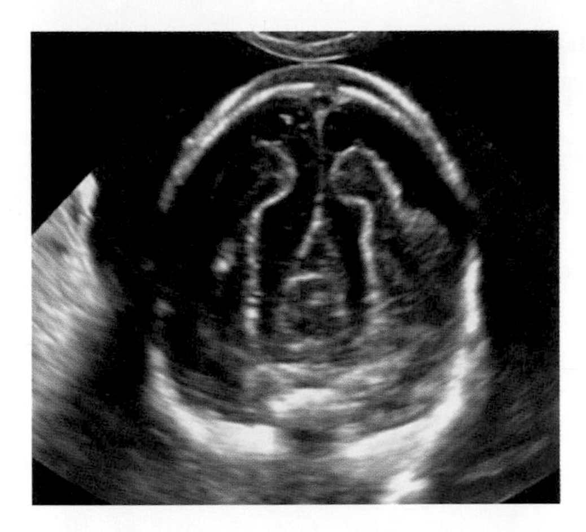

Fig. 3.1.22a Coronal view of the fetal head at 23 weeks in a fetus with lissencephaly. Note the smooth contour of the cerebral hemispheres and increased subarachnoid space.

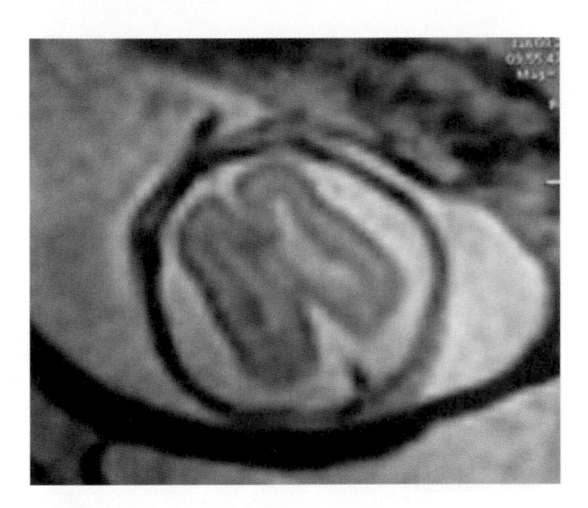

Fig. 3.1.22b MRI of the same fetus confirming the smooth contour of the cerebral hemispheres and increased subarachnoid space.

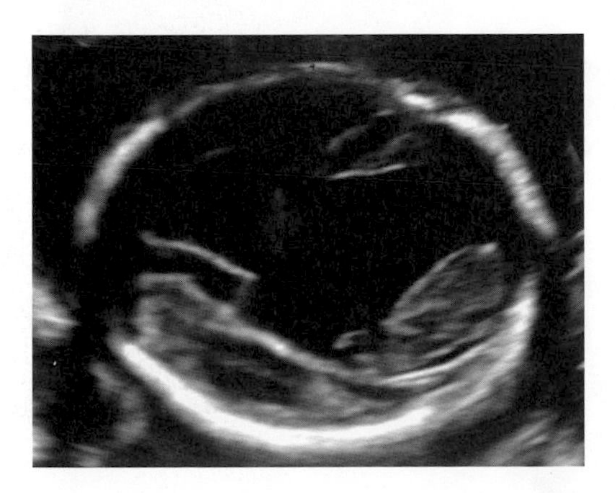

Fig. 3.1.23 Schizencephaly. Transverse view of the fetal head showing a full-thickness cleft of the hemisphere.

ABNORMAL HEAD CIRCUMFERENCE

LARGE HEAD CIRCUMFERENCE

- Secondary to hydrocephalus, large tumours or arachnoid cysts
- Benign (idiopathic), such as familial megalencephaly (Fig 3.1.24)

- Unilateral megalencephaly – isolated or syndromic
- Gigantism (Sotos, Weaver, Bannayan–Riley–Ruvalcaba syndrome)
- Achondroplasia

SMALL HEAD CIRCUMFERENCE

- Infection (Zika, rubella, chickenpox, toxoplasmosis, cytomegalovirus)
- Trisomies
- Fetal growth restriction – placental
- Primary microcephaly (autosomal recessive) (Fig. 3.1.25)
- Syndromes (Bloom, Cornelia de Lange, Roberts, Silver–Russel, Smith–Lemli–Opitz, Seckel)
- Craniosynostosis
- Fetal alcohol syndrome

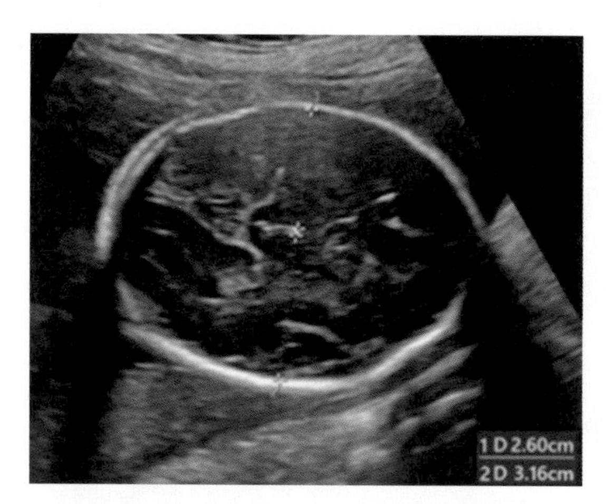

Fig. 3.1.24a Hemimegalencephaly. Transverse view of the head showing asymmetrical enlargement of the lower hemisphere.

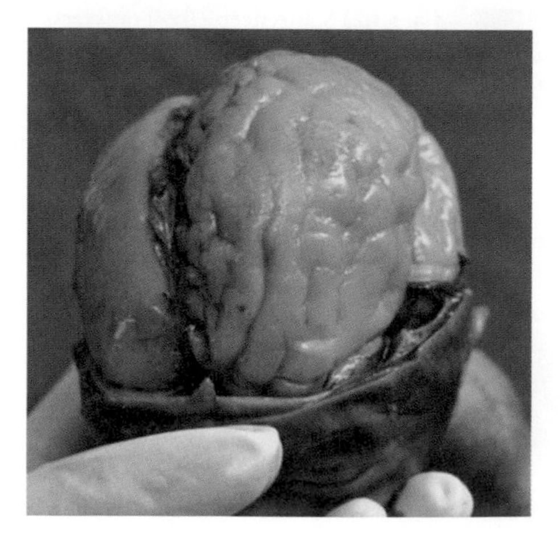

Fig. 3.1.24b Post mortem specimen of the same case showing asymmetrical enlargement of the right cerebral hemisphere.

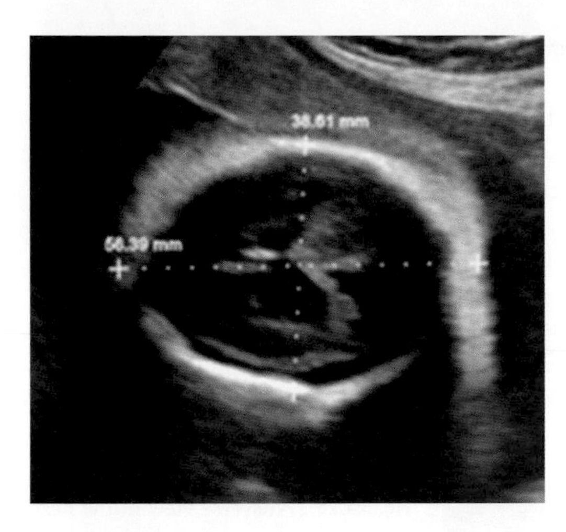

Fig. 3.1.25 22-week fetus with head measurements at –4 SD below the mean. This was a case of recurrent primary microcephaly.

VENTRICULOMEGALY

Description and Characteristics

- Enlargement of the intracerebral ventricle(s):
  - Ventriculomegaly can be subgrouped according to the degree of dilatation:
    - mild (ventricular diameter 10–12 mm)
    - moderate (12.1–15 mm)
    - severe (>15 mm)
  - Third ventricle (>3 mm)
  - Fourth ventricle (>5 mm)

Ultrasound Assessment

- Increased transverse diameter of the atrium of the lateral ventricle when measured in a transverse plane adjacent to the posterior aspect of the choroid plexus (Figs. 3.1.26–3.1.28)
- Check if unilateral or bilateral – coronal section may be useful to examine the side closer to the ultrasound probe
- The third ventricle should be examined – look for increased midline space between the thalami that communicates with lateral ventricles via the foramen of Monro (Fig. 3.1.28)
- Fourth ventricle – look for increased triangular space in front of the cerebellar vermis
- If presentation is cephalic, transvaginal scan should be used to complete full neurosonographic examination and exclude other structural anomalies (e.g. ACC, abnormal Sylvian fissure, delayed cortical maturation and signs of haemorrhage)
- Serial scans every 2–4 weeks are important to establish if ventriculomegaly is static, progressively decreasing or increasing

Investigations

- Chromosomal microarray (*L1CAM* mutation in X-linked hydrocephalus); exome sequencing
- Maternal serology (or amnio PCR) to exclude fetal infection (CMV, toxoplasmosis, Zika)

- If cerebral haemorrhage is suspected, look for maternal antiplatelet antibodies or *COL4A1* gene mutation
- MRI is mostly done in the third trimester to evaluate cerebral parenchyma and exclude neuronal migration pathology. In experienced centres MRI can be done as early as 20 weeks to exclude other intracranial pathologies not visible on ultrasound

Counselling

- Prognosis depends on the progression and degree of dilatation
- Isolated, non-progressive mild ventriculomegaly: >95% normal outcome
- Moderate ventriculomegaly: ~10% risk of neurodevelopmental delay
- Severe ventriculomegaly: ~50% risk of neurodevelopmental delay

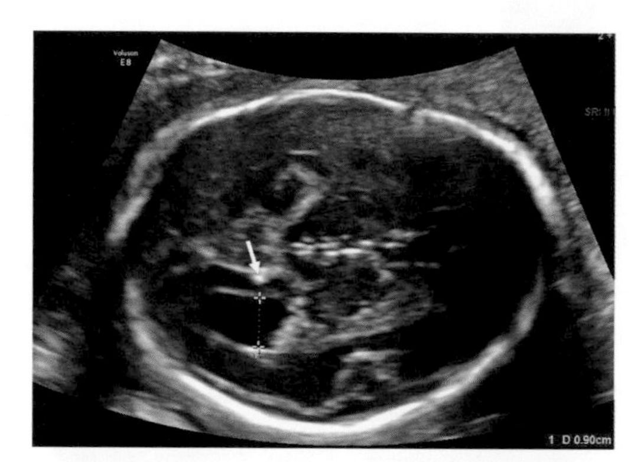

Fig. 3.1.26 Transverse view of the head showing correct measurement of the lateral ventricle. The callipers are placed perpendicular to the walls of the ventricle at the level of the parieto-occipital sulcus (arrow).

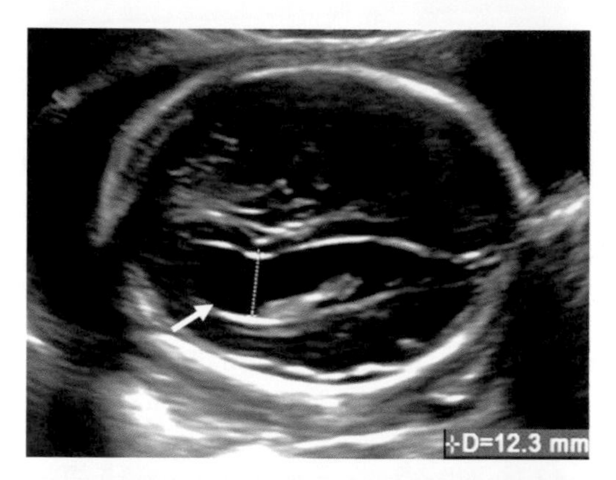

Fig. 3.1.27 Transverse view of the head showing mild ventriculomegaly (arrow).

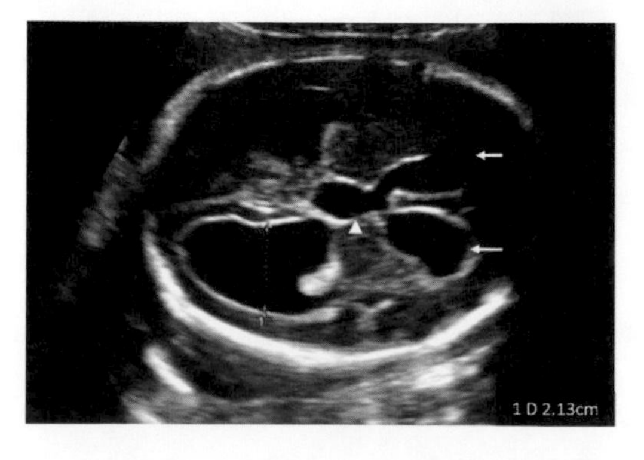

Fig. 3.1.28 Transverse view of the head showing severe ventriculomegaly. The frontal horns are dilated (arrow) and the third ventricle is also dilated (arrowhead).

INTERHEMISPHERIC CYSTS

- These are located in the interhemispheric fissure of the cerebral region, above the tentorium cerebelli

ARACHNOID CYSTS

- By definition, these cysts are extra-axial (external to brain parenchyma)
- Usually simple, unilocular and avascular midline cyst, and not communicating with lateral ventricles (Fig 3.1.29)
- They can also be located at the surface of the brain at the level of the Sylvian fissure, sella turcica, the anterior cranial fossa or the middle cranial fossa
- Relatively common in fetuses with agenesis of the corpus callosum

VEIN OF GALEN ANEURYSM

- Usually isolated and easily detectable due to high-velocity colour Doppler signal caused by arteriovenous shunting within a 'cyst' (Fig. 3.1.30)
- Shunting may cause progressive heart failure and hydrops due to the overload of the right heart
- Pressure effect and cerebral vascular steal may cause ventriculomegaly, cerebral infarcts, and leukomalacia

CAVUM VERGAE CYST

- Cavum vergae is best described as a posterior extension of the cavum septum pellucidum (Fig. 3.1.31)
- When cavum vergae is large (>1 cm) and has convex outer margin, it can be described as a 'cyst'

CAVUM VELI INTERPOSITI CYST

- Normal cistern of vellum interpositum is filled with cerebrospinal fluid and situated below the splenium of corpus callosum
- Vellum may appear to be dilated, which is a normal anatomical variant called cavum
- If cavum is >1 cm it is sometimes described as a cyst (Fig. 3.1.32)

DILATED SUPRAPINEAL RECESS

- Diverticulum (recess) of the posterior wall of the third ventricle may be dilated (Fig. 3.1.33)
- When recess is dilated it is likely that there is an obstruction below the third ventricle, leading to the obstructive ventriculomegaly

Investigations

- TORCH screen
- Microarray +/– exome
- MRI to look at neuronal migration, grey matter heterotopia and abnormal sulcation
- If haemorrhage is suspected, look for maternal antiplatelet antibodies or *COL4A1* gene mutation

Counselling and Management

- Most isolated arachnoid cysts and cavum veli interpositi cysts, even if quite large, are benign and should not have any impact on the obstetric management. Neonatal follow-up should be arranged
- Although most cavum vergae cysts are normal variants, some consider it a marker of possible impaired neurodevelopment; therefore, it seems prudent to arrange adequate paediatric follow-up
- Large vein of Galen aneurysms causing heart failure and cerebral findings have poor prognosis, and termination of pregnancy should be offered. Smaller aneurysms can be successfully embolised in the neonatal period, but still have variable long-term neurological outcomes

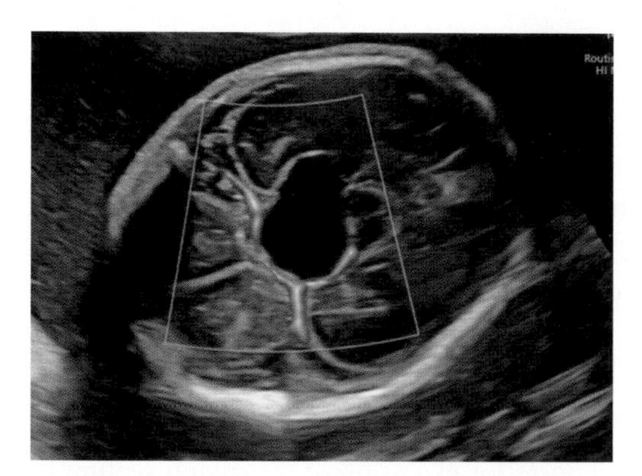

Fig. 3.1.29a Transverse view of the head showing a midline arachnoid cyst. Colour Doppler shows no flow within.

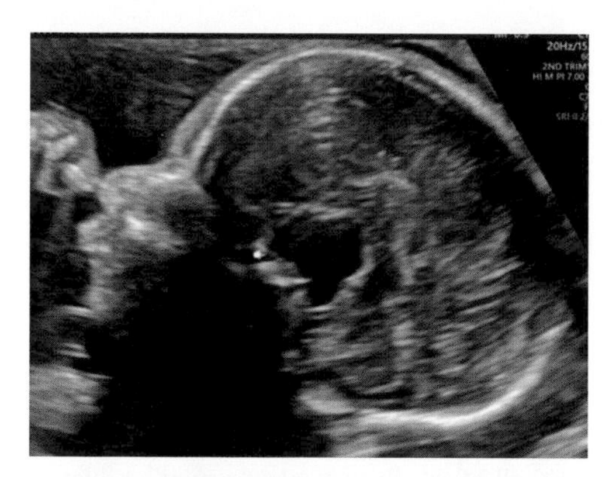

Fig. 3.1.29b Sagittal view of the same case. The cyst appears to be situated just above the sella turcica (finger arrow).

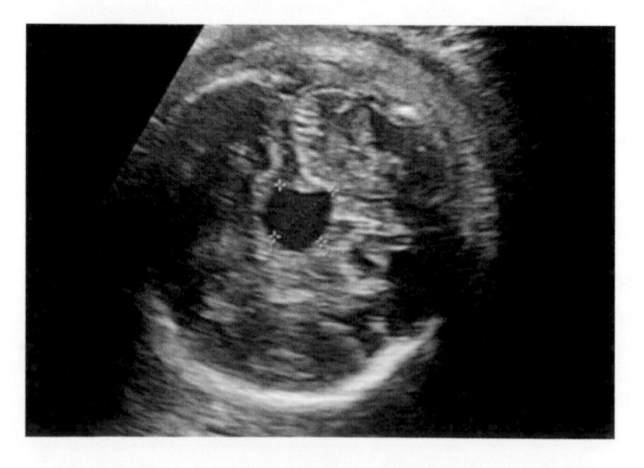

Fig. 3.1.30a Vein of Galen malformation. B-mode coronal view of the fetal head showing a midline cystic structure which was pulsating in real time. Fine echoes were swirling inside the cyst, suggesting a vascular lesion.

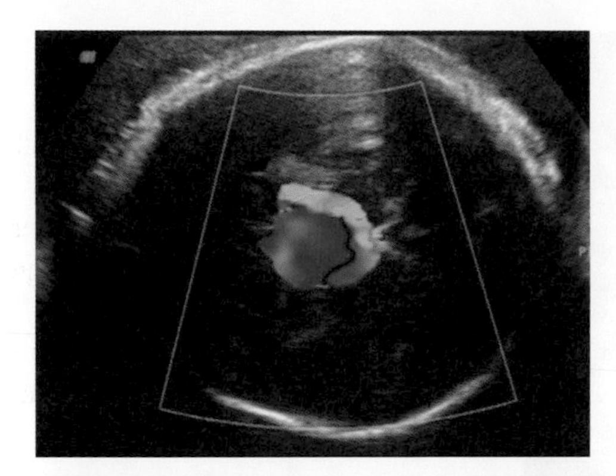

Fig. 3.1.30b Colour Doppler of the same case showing blood flow within the lesion which confirms the diagnosis of vein of Galen malformation.

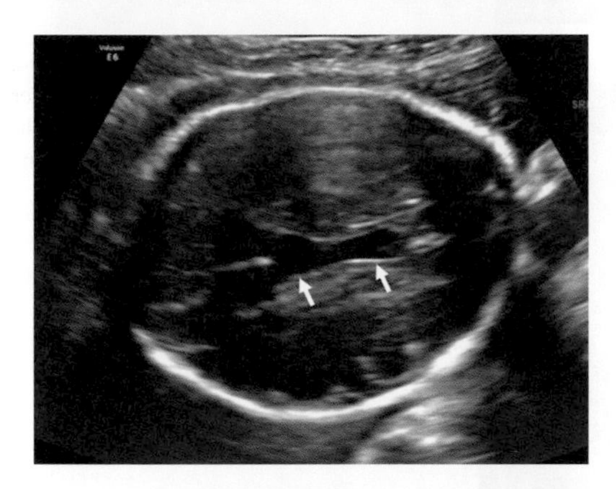

Fig. 3.1.31 Transverse view of the head showing a prominent cavum vergae (arrows).

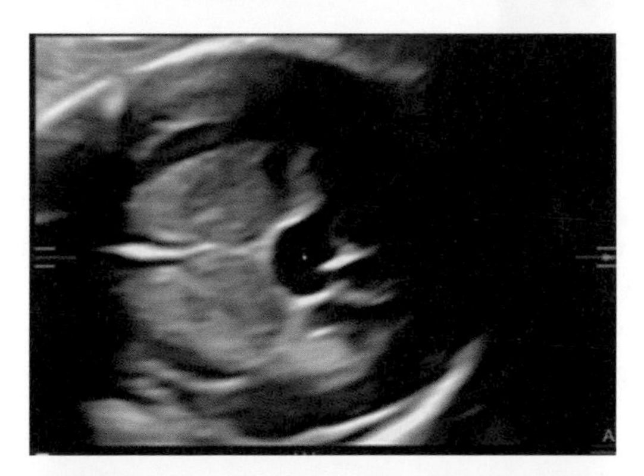

Fig. 3.1.32a Transverse view of the head showing a midline avascular cystic lesion. The origin of the cyst will be easier to ascertain in sagittal sections.

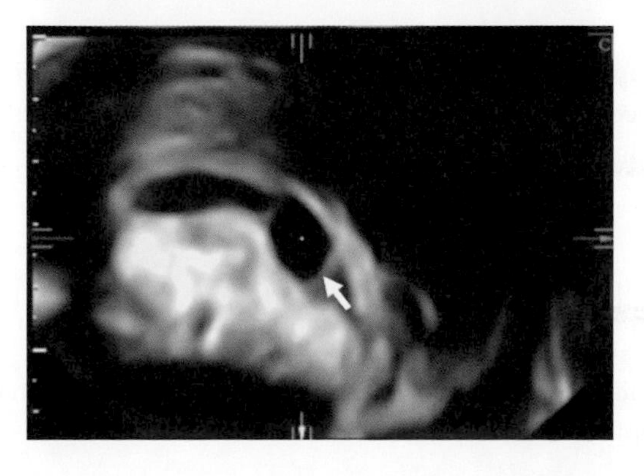

Fig. 3.1.32b Sagittal view of the same fetus showing that the cyst is located below the splenium of corpus callosum; this is typical of a cavum veli interpositi cyst (arrow).

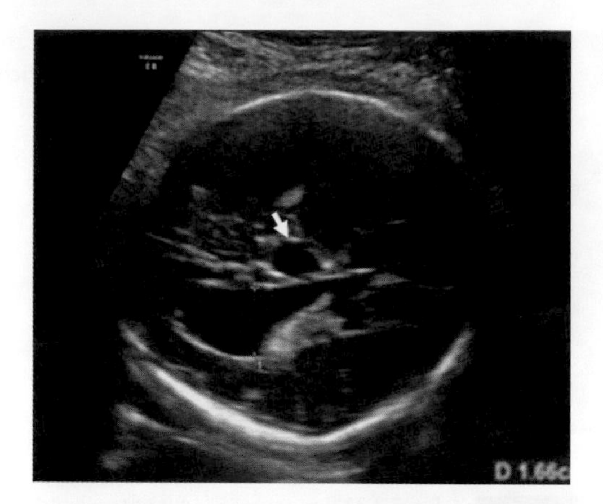

Fig. 3.1.33a Transverse view showing a small midline cyst (arrow) and mild ventriculomegaly.

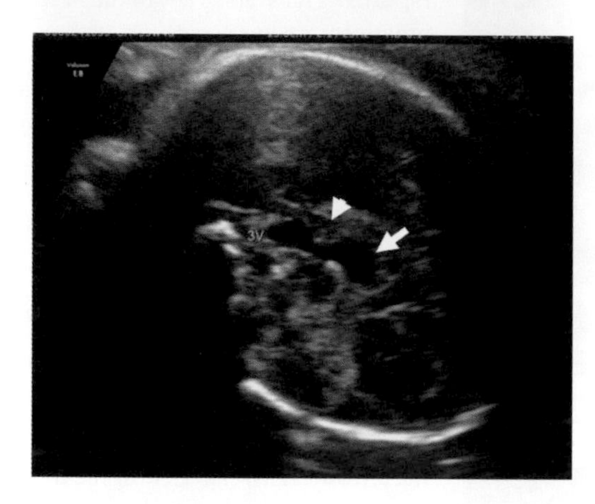

Fig. 3.1.33b Sagittal view shows that the cyst is communicating with the third ventricle (arrowhead). This is a typical finding in a dilated suprapineal recess (arrow).

INTRAPARENCHYMAL CYSTS

PORENCEPHALIC CYSTS

- One or more cystic areas, most commonly caused by an ischaemic event/focal necrosis
- Typically they arise from fissures or midline
- They tend to communicate with ventricles or subarachnoid space
- May be unilateral or bilateral (Fig. 3.1.34)

SUBEPENDYMAL PSEUDOCYSTS

- These cysts are commonly found in the thalamic region
- They are of varying size and shape (uni-/multilocular, uni-/bilateral) (Fig. 3.1.35)
- When other abnormalities are seen on a scan, the underlying pathology includes haemorrhage, infarctions, infection and abnormal karyotype

Investigations

- TORCH screen
- Chromosomal microarray and exome, if available
- MRI to exclude haemorrhage and cerebellar involvement and to look for neuronal migration, grey matter heterotopia and abnormal sulcation

- If haemorrhage is suspected, maternal antiplatelet antibodies or *COL4A1* gene mutation should be checked

Counselling and Management

- Porencephalic cysts diagnosed antenatally have poor prognosis and termination of pregnancy should be offered
- When subependymal cysts are isolated, they tend to regress spontaneously and their prognosis is good
- In association with other abnormalities these cysts have poor long-term neurological outcome

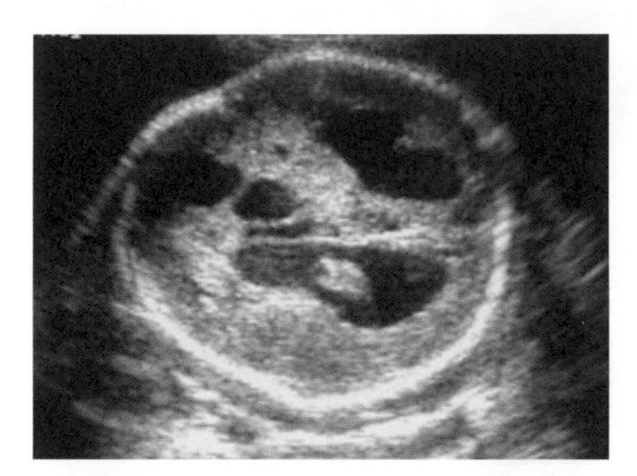

Fig. 3.1.34 Porencephalic cysts: transverse view of the head showing multiple cystic lesions in the parenchyma. The cysts were found to be communicating with the subarachnoid space.

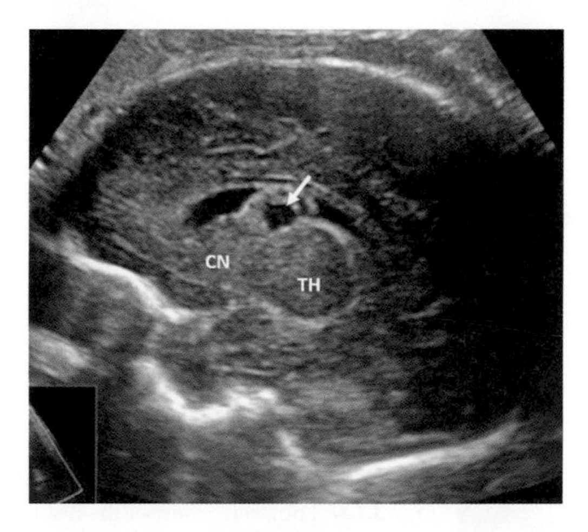

Fig. 3.1.35 Mid-sagittal view of the head showing a small subependymal pseudocyst (arrow) located in the thalamic region (TH), above the caudate nucleus (CN).

CHOROID PLEXUS CYSTS

Definition and Characteristics

- Single or multiple cysts within the choroid plexus of the lateral ventricles
- May be unilateral or bilateral

Ultrasound Assessment

- Document size/laterality/complexity of cystic lesions (Fig. 3.1.36)
- Look for structural anomalies and markers associated with trisomy 18

Investigations

- Review findings of combined first trimester screening
- If features of possible trisomy 18 are seen, offer karyotype – otherwise not indicated

Counselling

- If there are no other structural anomalies, then reassure
- ~95% will disappear before 36 weeks
- Even if they persist in the neonatal period, they are not clinically significant

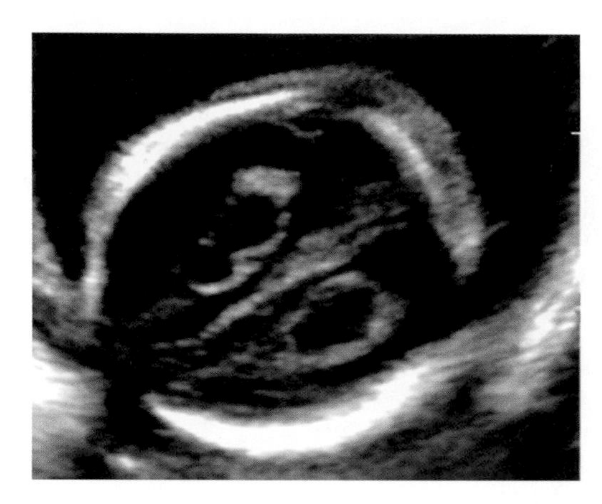

Fig. 3.1.36 Transverse view of the head showing bilateral multiple choroid plexus cysts.

BRAIN TUMOURS

- Classic presentation is an intracranial mass that may be associated with macrocephaly and ventriculomegaly
- The most common tumours are:
  - teratomas (Fig. 3.1.37)
  - astrocytomas
  - tuberous sclerosis
  - craniopharyngiomas
  - primitive neuroectodermal tumours
- The prognosis is generally poor

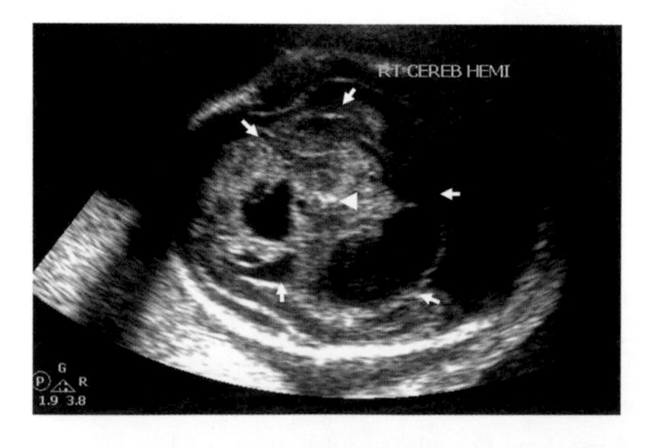

Fig. 3.1.37 Transverse view of the head showing a large intracranial teratoma (arrows) with solid and cystic areas. Small calcifications are also visible in the tumour (arrowhead).

ENLARGED POSTERIOR FOSSA

- The posterior fossa includes the cerebellar hemispheres, vermis, cerebral peduncles, the fourth ventricle, brain stem (pons and bulb), cisterna magna and the tentorium
- Biometry includes cerebellar diameter, measurement of cisterna magna (Fig. 3.1.38) and increasingly assessment of the angle between the brain stem and the vermis (Fig. 3.1.39)
- Most common causes of posterior fossa enlargement during the second trimester are:
  - Dandy–Walker malformation
  - Blake's pouch cyst
  - megacysterna magna
  - arachnoid cysts
  - dural sinus thrombosis (this pathology is included here because, although supratentorial, it is often mistakenly diagnosed as a posterior fossa pathology)

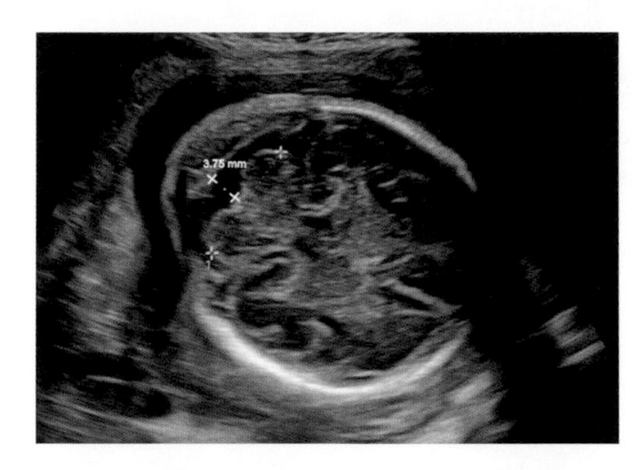

Fig. 3.1.38 Transverse view of the posterior fossa showing a normal size cisterna magna and normally formed cerebellum.

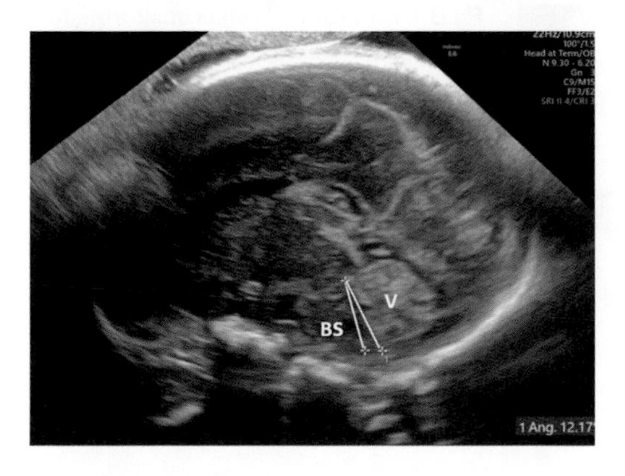

Fig. 3.1.39 Mid-sagittal view of a normal fetus showing a normal (narrow) brain stem–vermian (BV) angle $<45°$. BS, brain stem; V, vermis.

DANDY–WALKER MALFORMATION

Description and Characteristics

- A spectrum of anomalies that are best described separately because the nomenclature and definitions vary between neurosonographers, MRI experts and paediatric neurosurgeons, and often include so-called Dandy–Walker variants
- 'Classic' presentation includes:
  - significantly enlarged cisterna magna (>10 mm)
  - aplastic or hypoplastic vermis rotated upwards
  - cystic dilatation of the fourth ventricle extending posteriorly

- Cerebellar hemispheres should be displaced, but may have normal size and morphology
- Elevation of tentorium is always present
- Unfortunately, over- and misdiagnosis remain common, particularly before 18 weeks

Ultrasound Assessment

- Use coronal and sagittal planes as well as transverse plane for analysis (Fig. 3.1.40):
  - Are the cerebellar hemispheres normal size and echogenicity?
  - Is the trans-cerebellar diameter normal?
  - Is the cerebellar vermis present? Is it rotated? Is it dysplastic?
  - Is the fourth ventricle enlarged?
  - Is the cisterna magna enlarged?
- The diagnosis *should not be made* if the vermis looks normal, particularly if only rotated upwards, and if the tentorium is not elevated

Investigations

- Chromosomal microarray and exome sequencing, if available
- MRI is essential for additional assessment of brain stem and demonstration of parenchymal anomalies

Counselling and Management

- When ultrasound diagnosis is confirmed by MRI, even without associated genetic and other structural abnormalities, the prognosis is poor and termination of pregnancy should be offered
- Long term, problems related to hydrocephalus are the most common cause of death

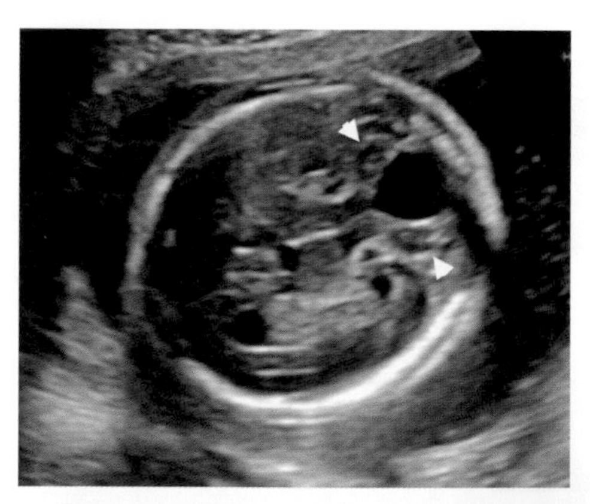

Fig. 3.1.40a Dandy–Walker malformation. Transverse view of the head showing a large posterior fossa cyst. The two cerebellar hemispheres are hypoplastic (arrowheads) and separated from each other. Vermis is absent.

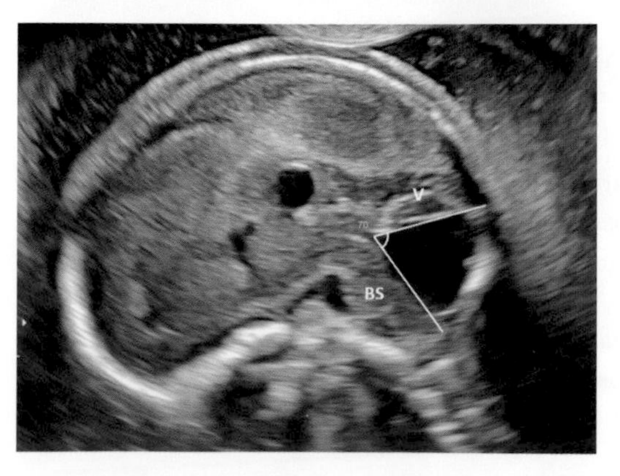

Fig. 3.1.40b Sagittal view of the same fetus with increased brain stem–vermian (BV) angle of 70° (see Fig. 3.1.39 for comparison).

BLAKE'S POUCH CYST

Definition and Characteristics

- Blake's pouch is a transient posterior fossa structure that normally regresses by 12 weeks
- The Blake's pouch cyst will form if a connection between the fourth ventricle and cisterna magna (foramen Magendie) fails to fenestrate
- ~50% of cysts will resolve by 26 weeks (delayed fenestration)

Ultrasound Assessment

- Often seen before 20 weeks when a presumed transverse plane is, in fact, semi-coronal
- Vermis is rotated, but normal in anatomy and size
- The BV angle is normal (<45°) (Fig. 3.1.41)
- Cisterna magna is normal (<10 mm)

Counselling and Management

- If isolated, Blake's pouch cyst should be considered a normal variant with good long-term prognosis

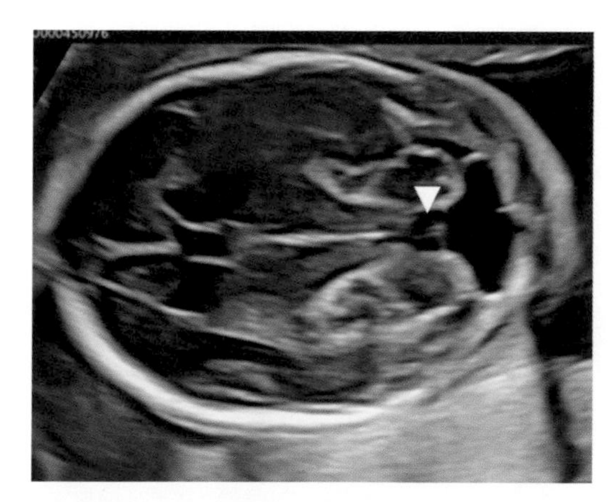

Fig. 3.1.41a Blake's pouch cyst in a trans-cerebellar plane at 22 weeks. There is a dilated fourth ventricle (arrowhead) ballooning into the cisterna magna.

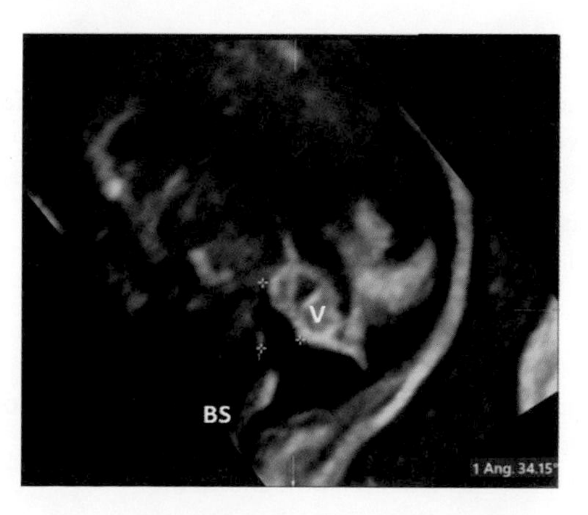

Fig. 3.1.41b Sagittal view of the same fetus showing a normal vermis and the normal BV angle <45°.

MEGA CISTERNA MAGNA

Definition and Characteristics

- Strictly speaking, cisterna magna is the space between the inferior vermis and posterior rim of the foramen ovale (normally 3–8 mm)
- The fetal mega cisterna magna measures >10 mm in transverse cerebral plane with normal vermis and no ventriculomegaly

Ultrasound Assessment

- The space between the internal surface of the cerebellar vermis and the internal edge of the occipital bone should be measured (Fig. 3.1.42)

Investigations

- Karyotype
- MRI is essential to confirm that the vermis is normal and there are no brain abnormalities

Counselling

- If truly isolated, the outcome is favourable

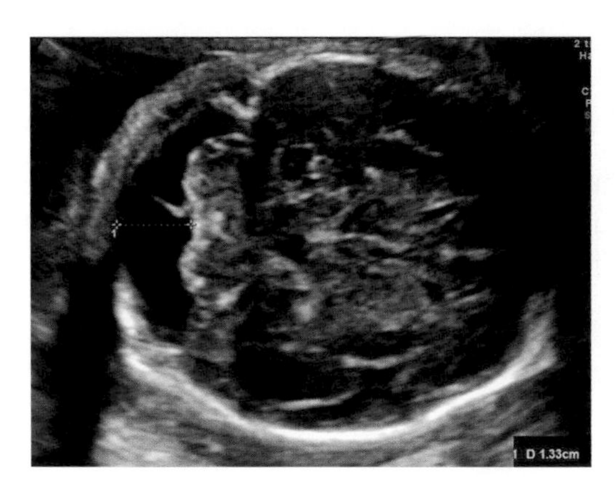

Fig. 3.1.42 Transverse view of the posterior fossa showing a mega cisterna magna of 13 mm. The normal measurement is <10 mm.

DURAL SINUS THROMBOSIS

Definition and Characteristics

- Cerebral veins drain into dural venous sinuses that anastomose posteriorly at the confluence of sinuses (torcular herophili)
- This area (torcular), which is in close proximity to the posterior aspect of the tentorium, is a focal point for venous thrombosis
- Occlusion by a large thrombus will result in a dural lake that can be very large

Ultrasound Assessment

- Large 'cisterna magna' is in fact dural lake that sits above the tentorium, with normal cerebellum and vermis below it (Fig. 3.1.43)
- Visualisation of a clot within a dural lake is virtually pathognomonic

Investigations

- Karyotype is not indicated
- MRI may be done to confirm the diagnosis

Counselling and Management

- There is no antenatal treatment
- Perinatal mortality ~10%
- Termination of pregnancy is not indicated as the majority of cases will either reduce in size or completely resolve during pregnancy
- Long-term outcome for survivors is generally very good

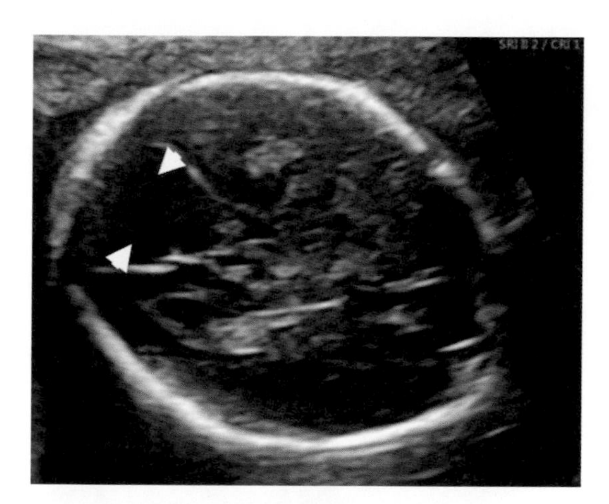

Fig. 3.1.43a Dural sinus thrombosis: transverse view of the head showing a large hypoechoic area with fine internal echoes (arrowheads). Colour Doppler did not reveal any vascularity.

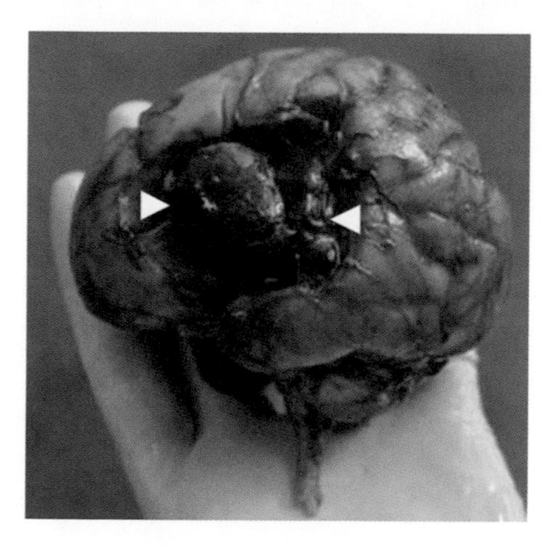

Fig. 3.1.43b Autopsy specimen of the same case showing a large clot (arrowheads) between the two occipital lobes.

ABNORMAL CEREBELLUM

RHOMBOENCEPHALOSYNAPSIS

Definition and Characteristics

- Complete absence of cerebellar vermis

Ultrasound Assessment

- Cerebellar hemispheres appear fused (Fig. 3.1.44)
- The fourth ventricle index is <1 ('keyhole')
- Ventriculomegaly is common (~50%)

Investigations

- MRI to confirm the diagnosis

Counselling and Management

- Rarely, if ever, truly isolated
- Prognosis is generally poor; termination of pregnancy should be offered

VERMIAN HYPOPLASIA

Definition and Characteristics

- Partial absence of the inferior part of the vermis
- Often described as a Dandy–Walker variant

Ultrasound Assessment

- Diagnosis should not be made before 18–20 weeks
- Some part of the vermis is visible
- Cerebellar hemispheres and the fourth ventricle look normal

Investigations

- Chromosomal microarray and exome, if available
- MRI

Counselling and Management

- If postnatal MRI confirms that the hypoplasia is isolated, normal neurodevelopment should be expected
- If isolated, long-term neurodevelopment is generally good

JOUBERT SYNDROME

See Chapter 19.

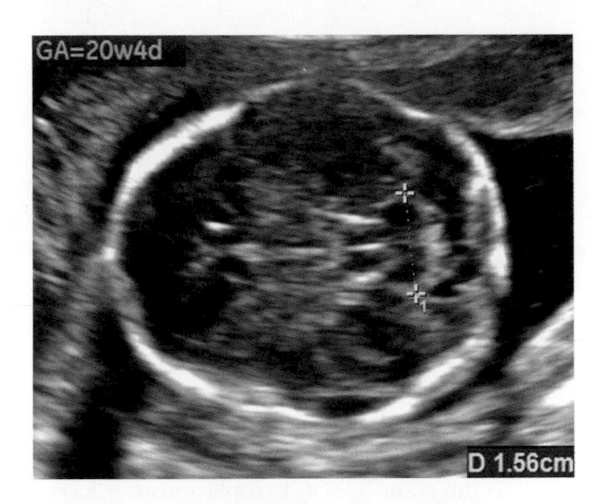

Fig. 3.1.44a Rhombencephalosynapsis: transverse view of the posterior fossa in a 20-week fetus showing a small fused cerebellum (between callipers) and absent vermis.

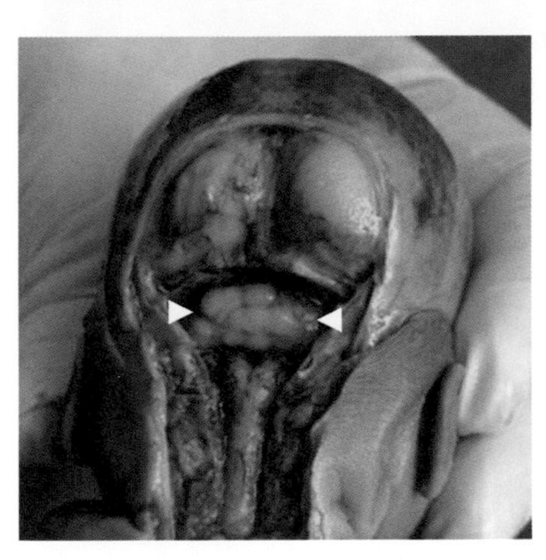

Fig. 3.1.44b Autopsy picture of the same case showing the fused cerebellum and the absence of vermis (arrowheads).

COMMON ABNORMAL CRANIAL ULTRASOUND FINDINGS WITH DIFFERENTIAL DIAGNOSIS

Ultrasound finding	Differential diagnosis
Head circumference >95th centile	• Secondary to hydrocephalus, large tumours or arachnoid cysts • Benign (idiopathic) familial megalencephaly • Unilateral megalencephaly • Gigantism (Sotos, Weaver, Bannayan–Riley–Ruvalcaba syndrome) • Achondroplasia
Head circumference <5th centile	• Infection (Zika, rubella, chickenpox, toxoplasmosis, CMV) • Trisomies • Fetal growth restriction – placental causes

(*cont.*)

Ultrasound finding	Differential diagnosis
	• Syndromes (Bloom, Cornelia de Lange, Roberts, Silver–Russel, Smith–Lemli–Opitz, Seckel) • Craniosynostosis • Fetal alcohol syndrome
Ventriculomegaly	• Normal variant • Abnormal karyotype • Aqueductal stenosis • Structural abnormality (agenesis of corpus callosum, spina bifida, heterotopias) • Infection (CMV, toxoplasmosis, Zika)
Cerebellum <5th centile	• Joubert syndrome • Rombencephalosynapsis • Vermian hypoplasia
Enlarged cisterna magna >10 mm	• Mega cisterna magna – normal variant • Blake's pouch • Dandy–Walker • Arachnoid cyst • Dural sinus thrombosis (supratentorial)
Absent cavum septum pellucidum	• Agenesis of corpus callosum • Holoprosencephaly • Septo-optic dysplasia • Hydrocephalus • Porencephaly • Schizencephaly • Dandy–Walker
Abnormal cavum septum pellucidum (length < width)	• Partial agenesis of corpus callosum
Abnormal fourth ventricle index	• Joubert syndrome and related disorders • Rhombencephalosynapsis • Cobblestone lissencephaly
Interhemispheric cysts	• Arachnoid cyst • Vein of Galen aneurysm • Cavum vergae cyst • Cavum veli interpositi cyst (true cyst of the roof of the third ventricle) • Dilated suprapineal recess
Intraparenchymal cysts	• Porencephalic cysts • Subependymal cysts
Extraparenchymal cysts	• Arachnoid cysts

(cont.)

Ultrasound finding	Differential diagnosis
Brain tumours	• Teratomas • Astrocytoma • Tuberous sclerosis • Craniopharyngioma • Primitive neuroectodermal tumour
Cortical malformations including abnormal Sylvian fissure	• Lissencephaly • Schizencephaly • Polymicrogyria • Pachygyria • Miller–Dieker • Tubulinopathies (tubulin-related cortical dysgenesis)

CLEFT LIP AND PALATE

Definition and Characteristics

- A cleft lip may be unilateral (75%), bilateral or midline (rare)
- A cleft lip may extend through the alveolar ridge into the hard palate (cleft lip and palate)
- Cleft palate can occur in the absence of cleft lip, and may include the hard and/or soft palate

Ultrasound Assessment

- The upper lip is assessed in coronal plane; the detection rate for cleft lip is ~90%
- The alveolar ridge and hard palate are assessed in a transverse plane; the detection rate for isolated cleft palate is ~30%
- Identify whether the cleft is unilateral or bilateral (Figs. 3.1.45 and 3.1.46)
- Exclude other structural anomalies

Investigations

- Karyotype is indicated because of association with a variety of aneuploidies and microdeletions
- Exome sequencing may be of value as a large number of autosomal dominant, autosomal recessive and X-linked conditions are associated with facial clefts
- Enquire about possible exposure to teratogens (e.g. exposure to valproate)
- MRI may be of value when midline clefts are found, as associated subtle midline brain defects (e.g. septo-optic dysplasia) are easily missed by ultrasound alone

Counselling

- With normal microarray/exome there is still ~10% residual risk of underlying genetic condition with neurodevelopmental sequelae
- The functional approach to repair with delayed cosmetic lip repair is the most common
- There is an ongoing need for speech and occupational therapy and specialist dentistry
- Repair of a complex cleft may require several surgical admissions through to teenage years

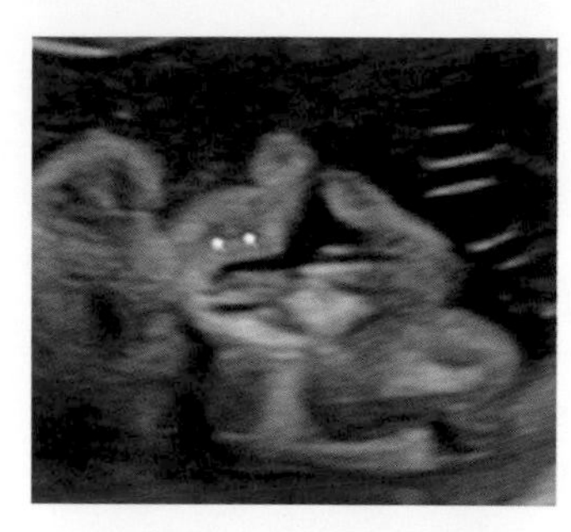

Fig. 3.1.45a Transverse view of the mouth showing unilateral cleft lip.

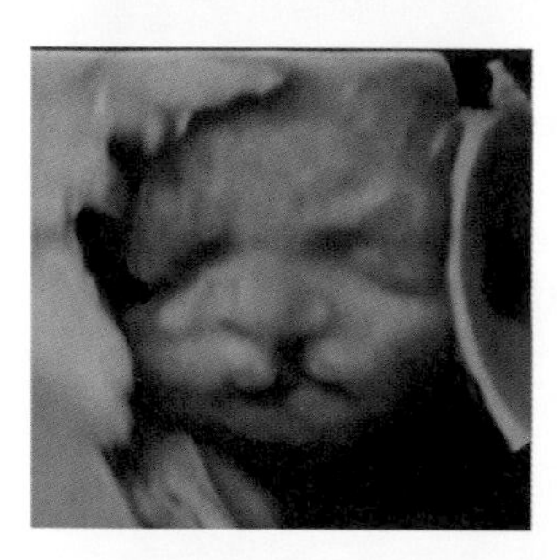

Fig. 3.1.45b 3D surface rendering of the face of the same fetus showing the cleft lip.

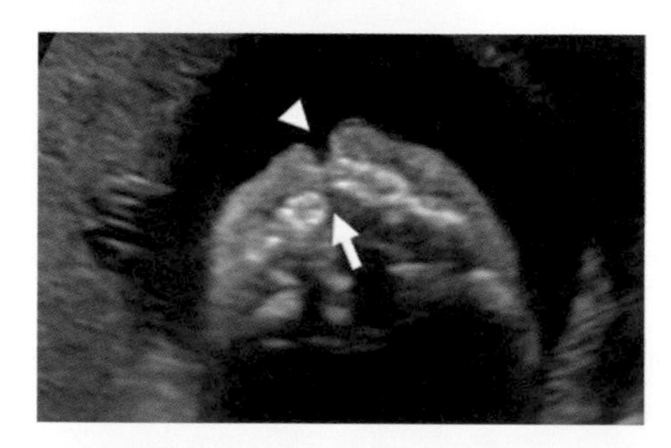

Fig. 3.1.45c 2D transverse view of the mouth showing a cleft in the hard palate (arrow). Cleft lip is also seen (arrowhead).

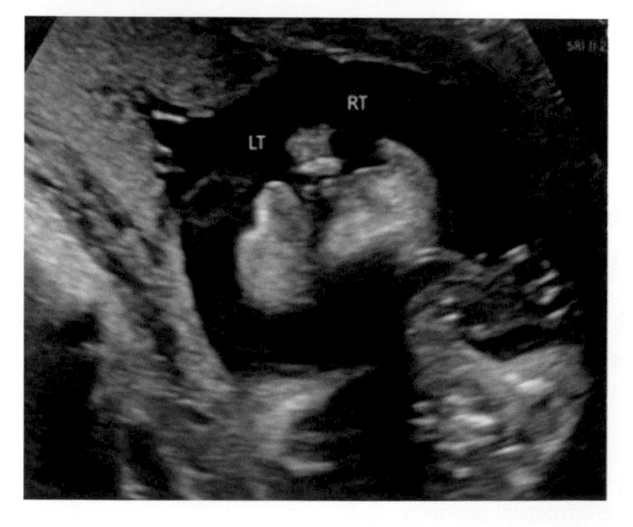

Fig. 3.1.46a Transverse view of the mouth showing bilateral cleft lip.

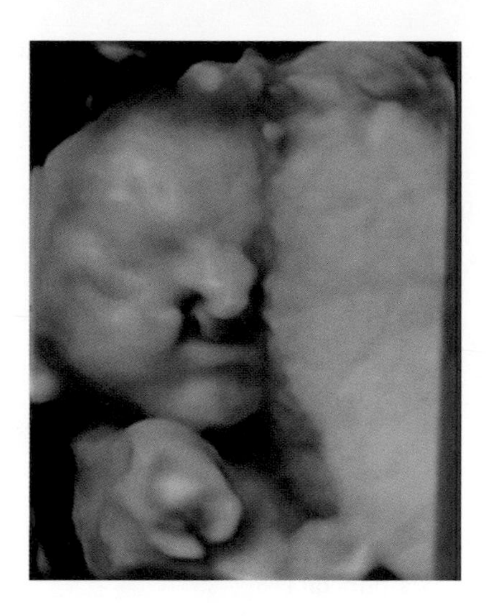

Fig. 3.1.46b 3D surface rendering of the face of the same fetus showing bilateral cleft lip.

ABNORMAL EYES

MICROPHTHALMIA OR ANOPHTHALMIA

- Only identified by recognising the small size or absence of the eyeball within the orbit (Fig 3.1.47)
- May be unilateral or bilateral
- High prevalence of genetic syndromes (e.g. Aicardi, Goldenhar)

ORBITS DISPLACED LATERALLY (HYPERTELORISM)

- Strong association with midline brain defects (e.g. frontal encephalocele, agenesis of corpus callosum) and many syndromes (e.g. frontonasal dysplasia, craniosynostosis)

Investigations

- Chromosomal microarray and exome sequencing, if available
- MRI to exclude subtle midline abnormalities

Counselling

- True hypertelorism is rarely isolated
- The prognosis will depend on the underlying pathology

REDUCED INTRA-ORBITAL DIAMETER (HYPOTELORISM)

- Normally associated with severe CNS anomalies such as holoprosencephaly
- Single median eye (cyclopia) is almost always associated with alobar form of holoprosencephaly

CATARACTS

Definition and Characteristics

- Mainly idiopathic
- No underlying pathology or risk factors can be found in ~90% of unilateral and ~40% of bilateral cases

Ultrasound Assessment

- 'Cloudy' lenses, either unilateral or bilateral (Fig. 3.1.48)

Counselling

- ~10% are associated with syndromes including cerebro-oculo-facio-skeletal, Neu–Laxova, pseudo-TORCH, and X-linked chondrodysplasia punctata
- ~30% are caused by an infection (CMV, toxoplasmosis, rubella)

DACROCYSTOCELE

Definition and Characteristics

- Also described as mucocele of the nasolacrimal duct
- Related to obstruction or delayed opening of the nasolacrimal duct; mainly in the third trimester

Ultrasound Assessment

- Appearance of three or four orbits (Fig. 3.1.49)
- ~25% bilateral
- Need to differentiate from frontal encephalocele and dermoid cysts

Counselling

- Karyotyping not indicated
- Most will resolve in the neonatal period

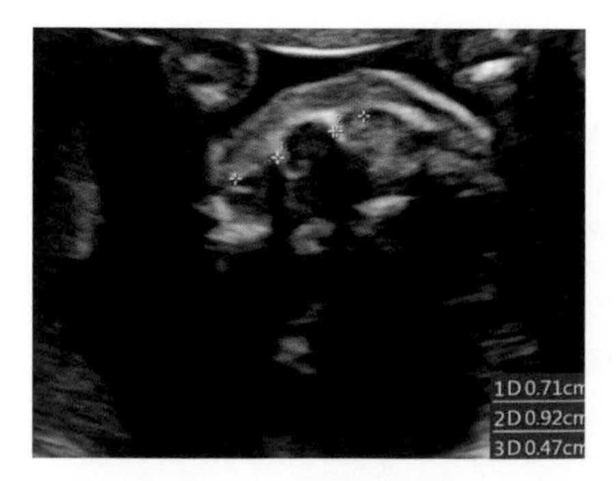

Fig. 3.1.47a Transverse section of the orbits showing severe microphthalmia. The orbital diameters are very small and the eyeballs are not seen.

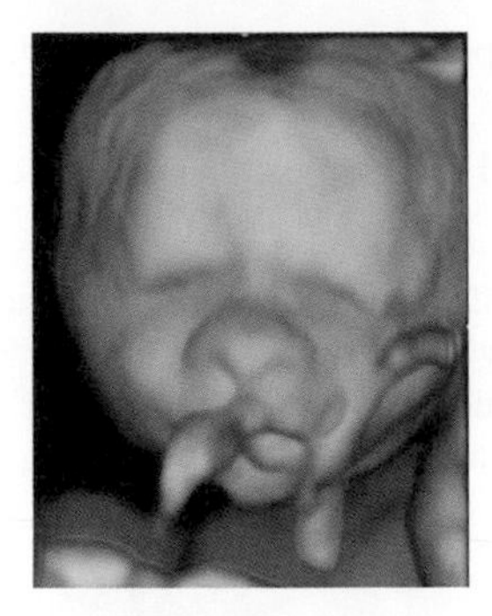

Fig. 3.1.47b 3D view of the same fetus showing "slit like" palpebral fissures. The fetus had multiple abnormalities including bilateral diaphragmatic hernia and horseshoe kidney. The nearest OMIM (Online Mendelian Inheritance in Man) match was Microphthalmia, syndromic.

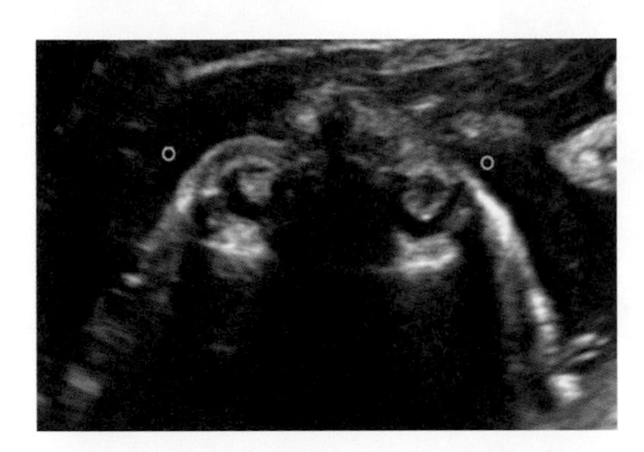

Fig. 3.1.48 Transverse view of the orbits showing bilateral cataracts. They are seen as echogenic structures inside the eyeball. The fetus also had microcephaly and duodenal obstruction. The family declined genetic counselling and further testing.

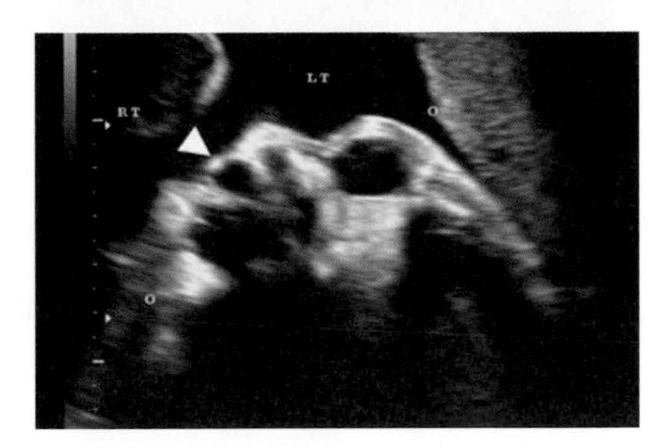

Fig. 3.1.49 Dacrocystocele: transverse view of the orbits showing a small cystic lesion (arrowhead) near the inner canthus of the eye on the left side.

ABNORMAL EARS

MICROTIA/ANOTIA

- Small or absent ear(s) (Fig. 3.1.50)
- Most commonly syndromic (branchial arch syndromes):
  - unilateral: Goldenhar syndrome
  - bilateral: Treacher Collins syndrome
- Exclude teratogen exposure (alcohol, retinoic acid)
- Usually sporadic if karyotype is normal

LOW-SET EARS

- Various biometric charts have been proposed for 2D/3D and MRI scans, but diagnostic accuracy is low

- Otocephaly is the extreme form (severe mandibular hypoplasia with anteromedial malposition of the ears)
- Antenatal diagnosis of isolated low-set ears is best avoided as false positives are too common

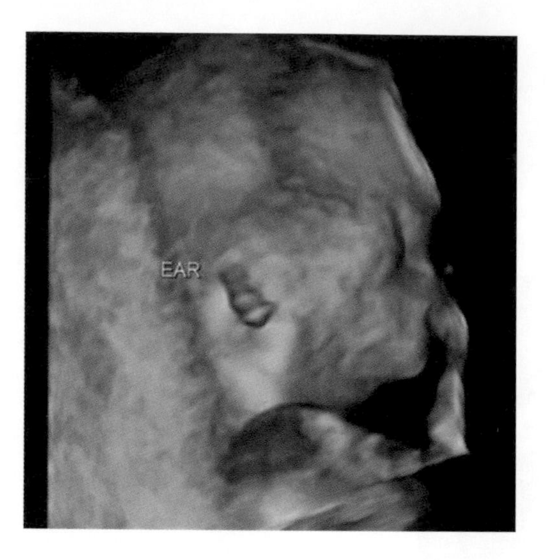

Fig. 3.1.50 3D image of the fetal face showing an abnormally formed earlobe (microtia). The fetus also had micrognathia. The family declined genetic counselling and further testing.

ABNORMAL PROFILE

MICROGNATHIA

Definition and Characteristics

- Small mandible and a receding chin
- Antenatal diagnosis is mainly subjective
- Biometry is available (inferior facial angle, jaw index), but the diagnostic accuracy of these measurements is limited
- May be present in numerous, mainly skeletal, syndromes, neuromuscular disorders and chromosomal abnormalities

Ultrasound Assessment

- Assess alignment of the lower jaw with the nose and upper jaw in profile view (Fig. 3.1.51)
- Confirm in coronal view
- Exclude cleft palate and glossoptosis (posterior displacement of the tongue, seen in Pierre–Robin sequence)

Investigations

- Karyotype, looking for trisomy 18, triploidy and microdeletions
- Exome/single gene disorder: Treacher Collins, Pierre–Robin sequence
- Exclude teratogen exposure (misoprostol, methotrexate)

Counselling

- Risk of false positives – repeat assessment in the third trimester
- Risk of respiratory compromise at birth – EXIT procedure may be indicated in severe cases

- High risk of associated structural anomalies/comorbidities
- Value of surgical intervention in childhood will depend on the associated pathologies and should be discussed with the local experts

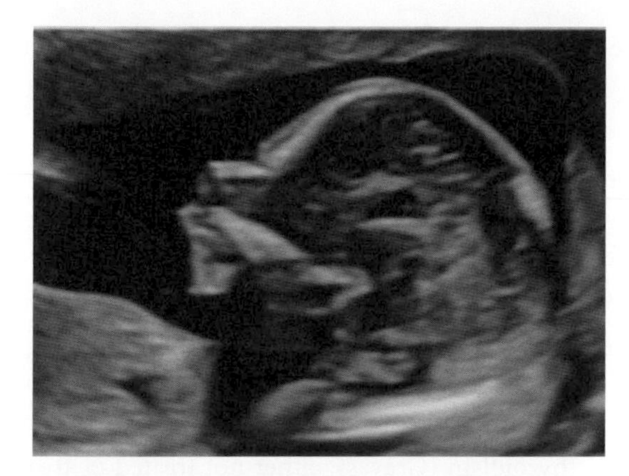

Fig. 3.1.51a Profile view showing the receding chin – micrognathia.

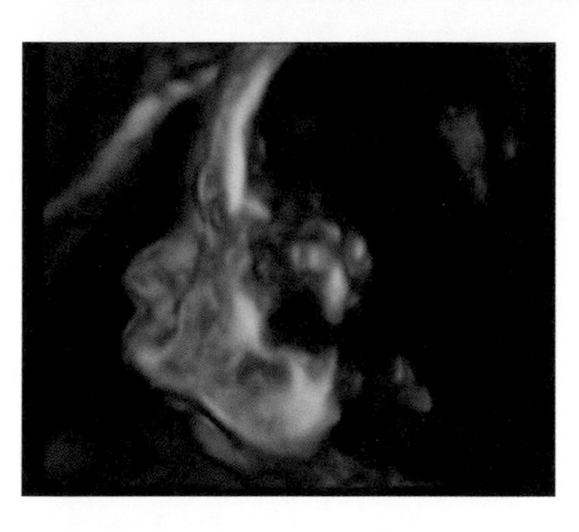

Fig. 3.1.51b 3D view of the same fetus with micrognathia.

PRENASAL OEDEMA

- Increased prenasal thickness (>4 mm at 20 weeks; >6 mm at 30 weeks) (Fig. 3.1.52)
- Relatively common in Down syndrome fetuses
- When prenasal thickness–nasal bone length ratio is >0.8, NIPT or karyotyping should be offered, if not already done

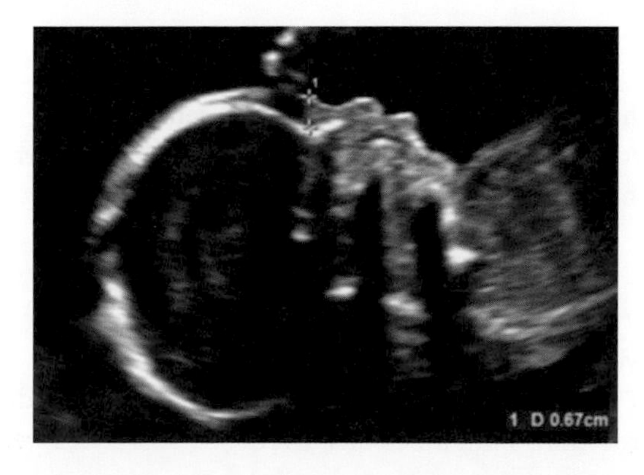

Fig. 3.1.52 Sagittal view of the face in a 20-week fetus showing prenasal oedema (marked by callipers). Karyotyping showed Down syndrome.

NECK MASSES

FETAL GOITRE

Definition and Characteristics

- Homogeneous mass of variable size in the anterior part of the fetal neck (Fig 3.1.53)

Hypothyroid Goitre

- More common cause of fetal goitre
- Usually caused by too aggressive treatment of maternal hyperthyroidism
- ~20% are caused by errors of fetal thyroid hormone synthesis (mother is euthyroid)
- May be caused by thyroid gland agenesis or hypoplasia

Hyperthyroid Goitre

- Rare cause of fetal goitre
- Usually caused by maternal hyperthyroidism (Graves); either not treated or treatment dose is too low

Ultrasound Assessment

- Not very helpful in accurately distinguishing between hypo- and hyperthyroidism (Fig 3.1.53)
- Colour Doppler patterns vary, although peripheral vascular pattern is more common in hypothyroid goitre
- Look for polyhydramnios and significant increase in size
- It is important to look for persistent hyperextension of the fetal neck
- Hypothyroid goitre may be associated with fetal growth restriction and bradycardia

Investigations

- Karyotyping is not indicated
- If the type of goitre cannot be ascertained from maternal history/investigations, both fetal blood and amniotic fluid can be tested
- If goitre is hypothyroid, fetal TSH will be high (>0.5 microIU/mL in amniotic fluid; >10 mU/L in fetal blood)

Counselling and Management

Fetal Hypothyroidism

- Reduce maternal medication
- Intra-amniotic injection of levothyroxine (180 µg/kg of estimated fetal weight)
- If no decrease in goitre size and/or colour Doppler vascularity within 1 week, serial injections every 1–2 weeks may be needed

Fetal Hyperthyroidism

- Adjust maternal antithyroid treatment
- If no fetal response within 1–2 weeks, recheck fetal thyroid hormone levels
- If persistent neck hyperflexion is present, it may cause problems in labour and during neonatal resuscitation – EXIT procedure should be considered

TUMOURS

- Teratomas are the most common
- Other tumours detectable by ultrasound include encephalomyelocele, lymphangiomas, sarcoma, haemangioma and neuroblastoma

Ultrasound Assessment

- Definitive diagnosis by ultrasound is rarely possible
- MRI provides clinically important additional information, including involvement of adjacent structures

Counselling and Management

- The long-term outcome will depend on the type of tumour, size, location and involvement of adjacent structures
- If persistent neck hyperflexion is present, it may cause problems in labour and during neonatal resuscitation – EXIT procedure should be considered

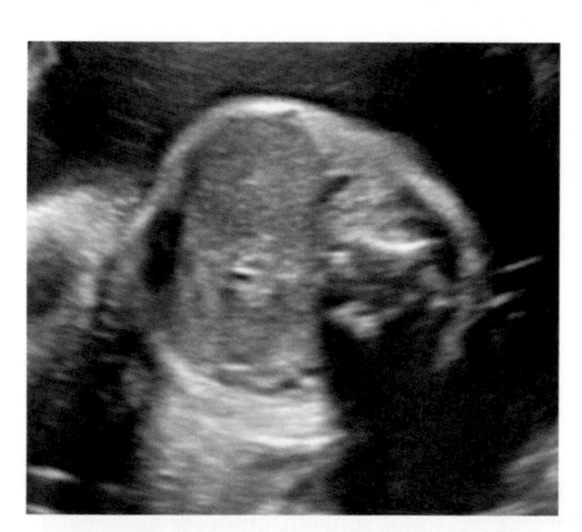

Fig. 3.1.53a Transverse view of the neck showing a large goitre. Fetus was hypothyroid with fetal TSH measuring 100 mIU/L (normal range 0.35–4.5 mIU/L).

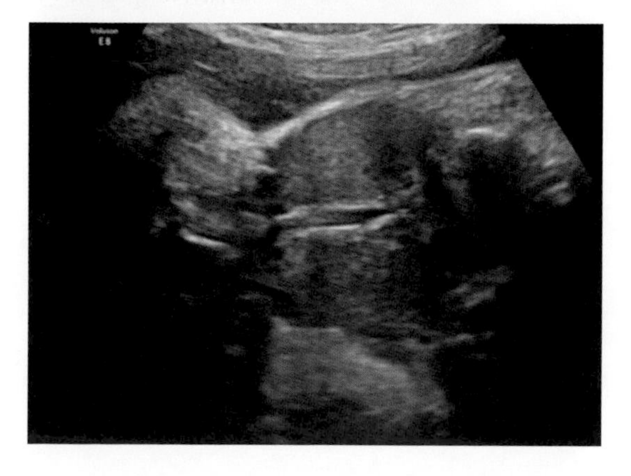

Fig. 3.1.53b Coronal view of the neck of the same fetus showing enlarged lobes of the thyroid. The parallel echogenic lines in the midline represent the trachea.

SUGGESTED READING

PRIMARY RESEARCH

Griffiths PD, Brackley K, Bradburn M, et al. Anatomical subgroup analysis of the MERIDIAN cohort: ventriculomegaly. *Ultrasound Obstet Gynecol* 2017;50(6):736–744.

Haratz KK, Shulevitz SL, Leibovitz Z, et al. Fourth ventricle index: sonographic marker for severe fetal vermian dysgenesis/agenesis. *Ultrasound Obstet Gynecol* 2019;53(3):390–395.

Maduram A, Farid N, Rakow-Penner R, et al. Fetal ultrasound and magnetic resonance imaging findings in suspected septo-optic dysplasia: a diagnostic dilemma. *J Ultrasound Med* 2020;39(8):1601–1614.

Paladini D. Fetal micrognathia: almost always an ominous finding. *Ultrasound Obstet Gynecol* 2010;35(4):377–384.

Pasquier L, Marcorelles P, Loget P, et al. Rhombencephalosynapsis and related anomalies: a neuropathological study of 40 fetal cases. *Acta Neuropathol* 2009;117(2):185–200.

Viñals F, Correa F, Gonçalves-Pereira PM. Anterior and posterior complexes: a step towards improving neurosonographic screening of midline and cortical anomalies. *Ultrasound Obstet Gynecol* 2015;46(5):585–594.

Vos FI, De Jong-Pleij EA, Bakker M, et al. Nasal bone length, prenasal thickness, prenasal thickness-to-nasal bone length ratio and prefrontal space ratio in second- and third-trimester fetuses with Down syndrome. *Ultrasound Obstet Gynecol* 2015;45(2):211–216.

REVIEWS AND GUIDELINES

Burns NS, Iyer RS, Robinson AJ, Chapman T. Diagnostic imaging of fetal and pediatric orbital abnormalities. *Am J Roentgenol* 2013;201(6):W797–W808.

Paladini D, Malinger G, Birnbaum R, et al. ISUOG Practice Guidelines (updated): sonographic examination of the fetal central nervous system. Part 2: performance of targeted neurosonography. *Ultrasound Obstet Gynecol* 2021;57(4):661–671.

Sacco A, Pannu D, Ushakov F, Dyet L, Pandya P. Fetal dural sinus thrombosis: a systematic review. *Prenat Diagn* 2021;41(2):248–257.

CHAPTER 3.2

Fetal Heart

SUMMARY BOX

ANATOMY ASSESSMENT

- Cardiac anomalies ~ 8 in 1000 births; 25% will need surgery or other procedures in the first year of life
- Detailed fetal echocardiography is usually carried out between 18 and 22 weeks, though it can be done earlier if needed
- Optimal views are obtained when cardiac apex is directed towards the anterior abdominal wall (Fig. 3.2.1)
- Optimal machine presets include focus, zoom, transducer frequency, gain, sample gate and pulse repetition frequency (Figs. 3.2.2–3.2.4)
- Fetal cardiac examination involves several key planes:
  - Upper abdomen to assess situs and arrangement of abdominal vessels (aorta and IVC) (Fig. 3.2.5)
  - Four chamber view to assess position, axis, size, symmetry and squeeze (mnemonic PASSS), atria, septum primum, foramen ovale, ventricles with interventricular septum and two pulmonary veins entering atrium. In this plane it is possible to assess the rhythm (Fig. 3.2.6)
  - Five chamber view (Fig. 3.2.7)
  - Three vessel view (Fig. 3.2.8)
  - Three vessel trachea view (Fig. 3.2.9)
  - Left outflow tract (Fig. 3.2.10)
  - Right outflow tract (Fig. 3.2.11)
  - Sagittal views of the systemic veins and arches (Fig. 3.2.12)

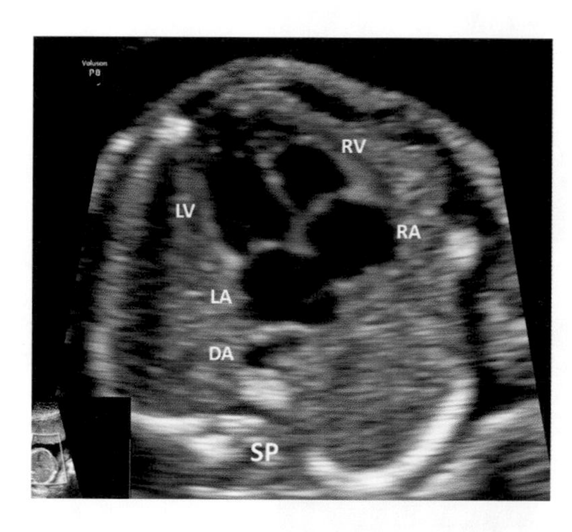

Fig. 3.2.1 Optimal depth, zoom and gain are important to obtain good, interpretable images of the heart. Optimal zoom should include spine, lungs and heart. DA, descending aorta; LA, left atrium; LV, left ventricle; RA, right atrium; RV, right ventricle; SP, spine.

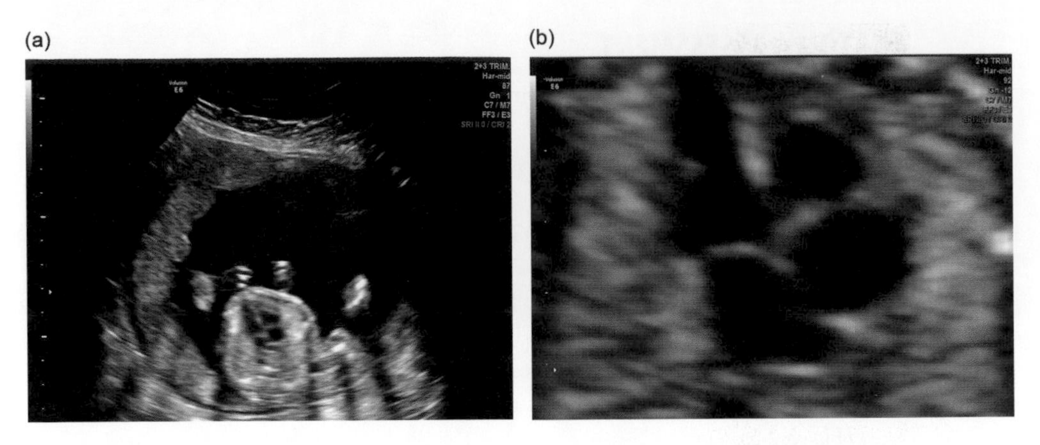

Fig. 3.2.2 (a) The heart appears too small. The depth and the sector angle should be reduced. Both of these settings will increase the frame rate. (b) Zoom should be reduced to include spine and lungs.

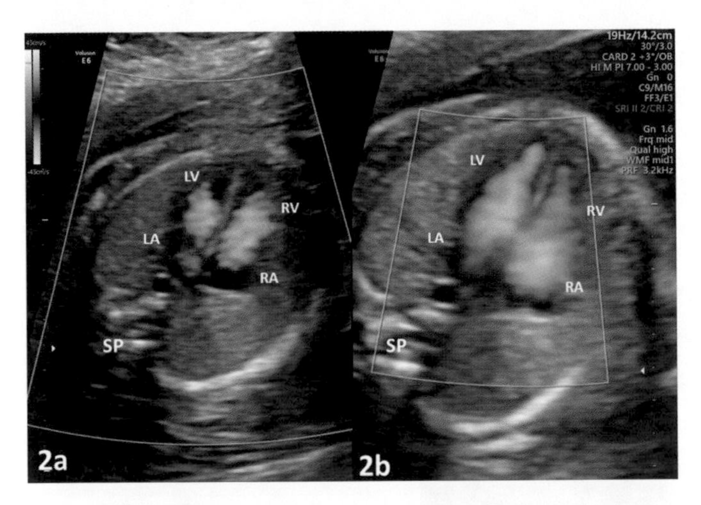

Fig. 3.2.3 Colour Doppler with a large colour box which results in a slower frame rate (left). Optimal colour Doppler box filling the region of interest (right). LA, left atrium; LV, left ventricle; RA, right atrium; RV, right ventricle; SP, spine.

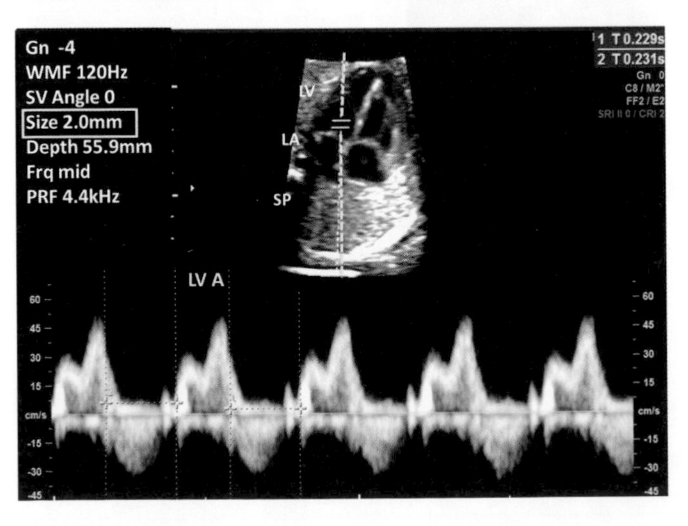

Fig. 3.2.4 Pulsed Doppler of the mitral valve. The sample gate of 2.0 mm is placed in the left ventricle close to the mitral valve.

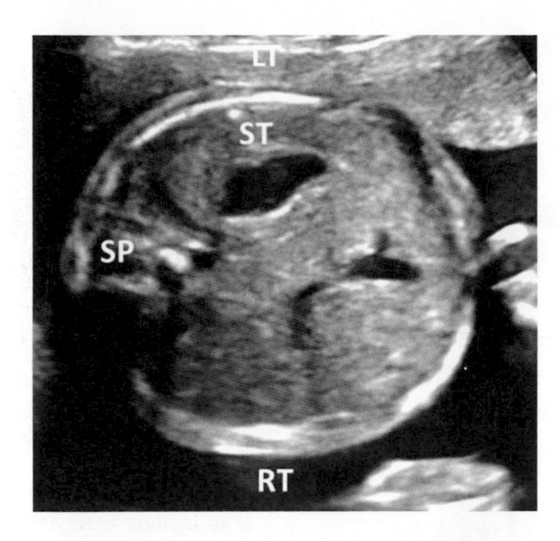

Fig. 3.2.5 Transverse section of the upper abdomen with the stomach (ST) on the left side of the fetus.

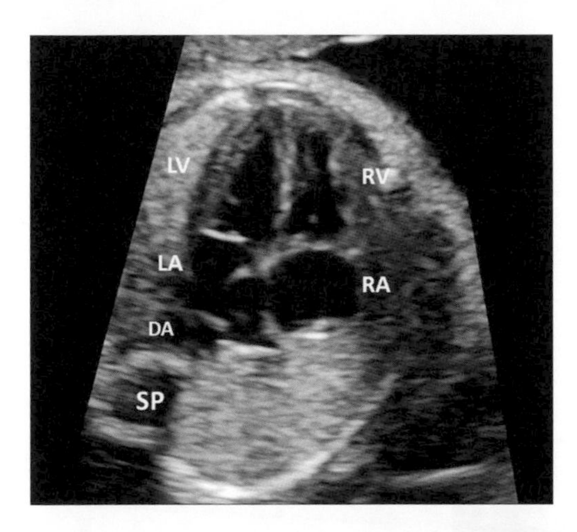

Fig. 3.2.6 Transverse section of thorax showing an apical four chamber view. The apex of the heart is on the same side as the stomach (left side) – situs solitus.

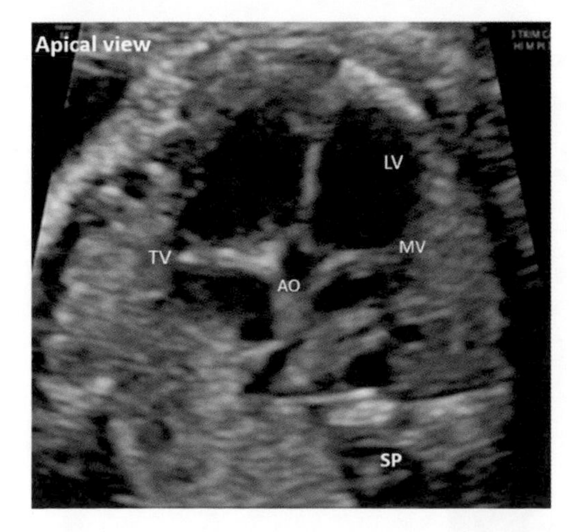

Fig. 3.2.7 Five chamber view of the heart. AO, aorta; LV, left ventricle; MV, mitral valve; TV, tricuspid valve; SP, spine.

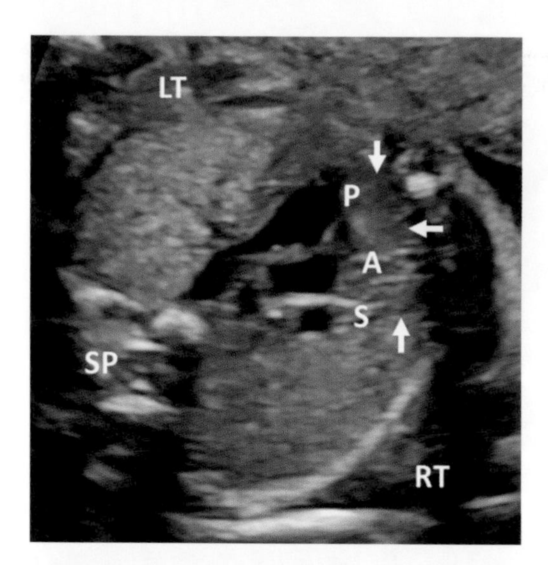

Fig. 3.2.8 Three vessel view. Transverse section of the upper thorax showing pulmonary artery (P), aorta (A) and superior vena cava (S). The thymus is seen in the anterior mediastinum (arrows).

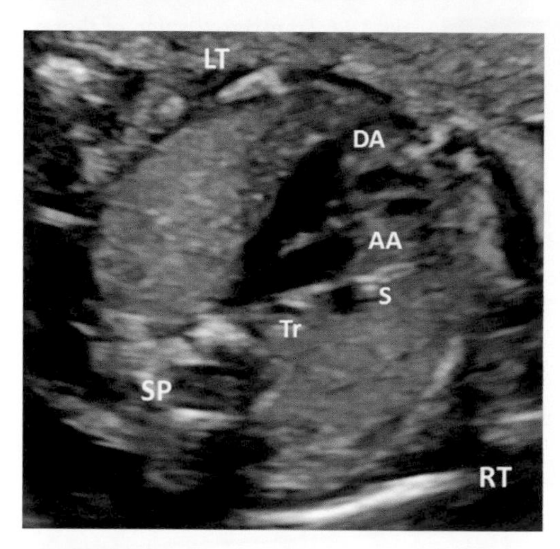

Fig. 3.2.9 Three vessel trachea view (3VT view) showing the arches. AA, aortic arch; DA, ductal arch; LT, left; RT, right; SP, spine.

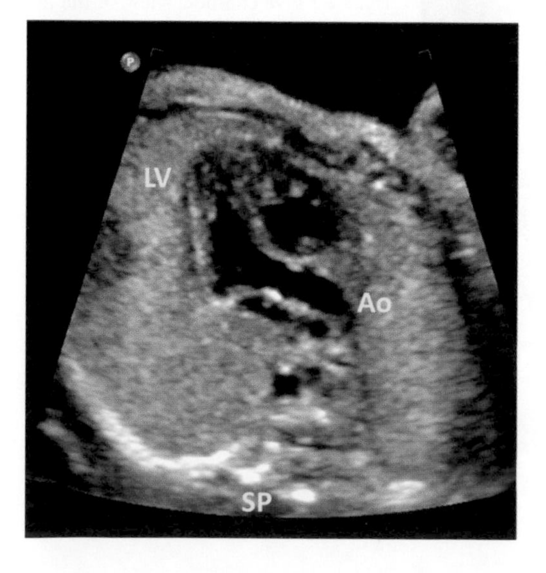

Fig. 3.2.10 Left ventricular outflow tract view (LVOT). AO, aorta; LV, left ventricle; SP, spine.

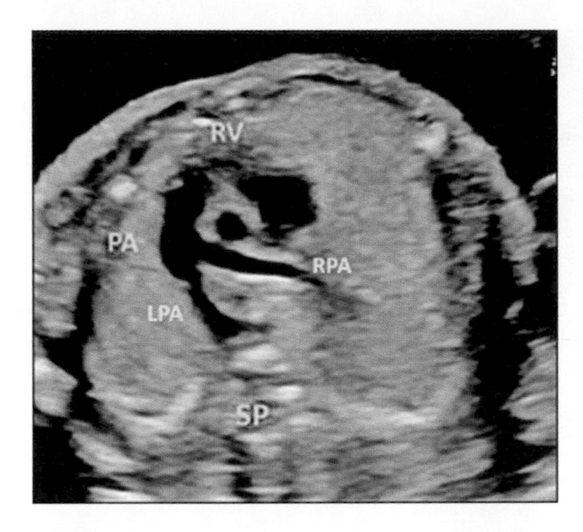

Fig. 3.2.11 Short-axis view showing the right ventricular outflow tract (RVOT). The pulmonary artery is seen bifurcating into the right and left pulmonary artery (RPA, LPA). RV, right ventricle; PA, pulmonary artery; SP, spine

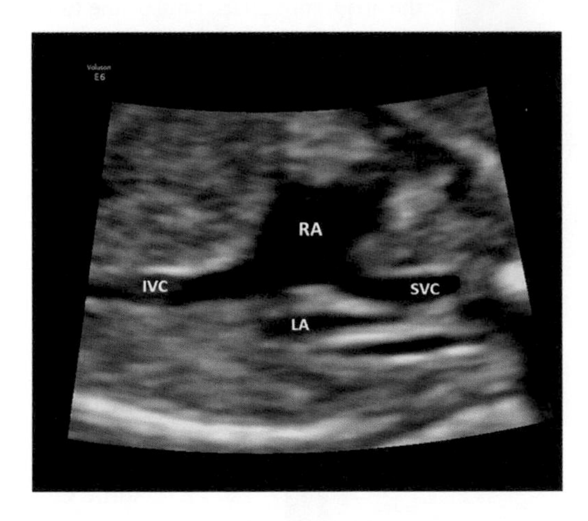

Fig. 3.2.12 Long-axis view of the thorax showing the inferior vena cava (IVC) and superior vena cava (SVC) draining into the right atrium (RA). LA, left atrium.

CARDIAC BIOMETRY

Cardiac biometry is performed only when an abnormal appearance of the cardiac chambers is suspected during a screening examination. The following measurements can be done:

- ventricular measurements (Figs. 3.2.13 and 3.2.14)
- annulus of great vessels (Fig. 3.2.15)
- ascending aorta and pulmonary artery (Fig. 3.2.16)
- arches (Fig. 3.2.17)

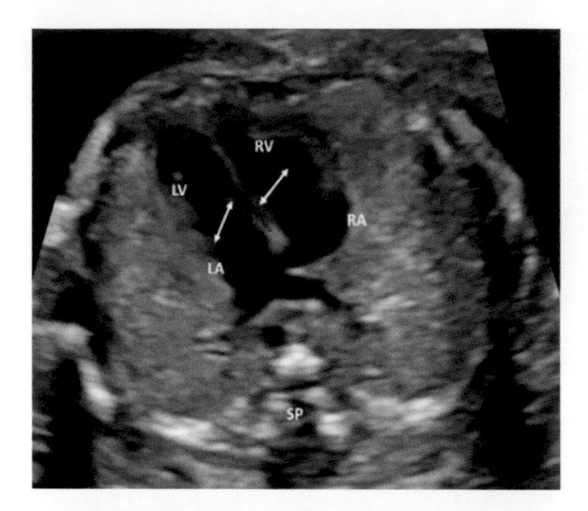

Fig. 3.2.13 Width of both ventricular cavities is measured in the apical four chamber view. Atrioventricular valve annulus is best measured with callipers placed from hinge point to hinge point of valve attachment. Valve attachment is best visualised in diastole. SP, spine.

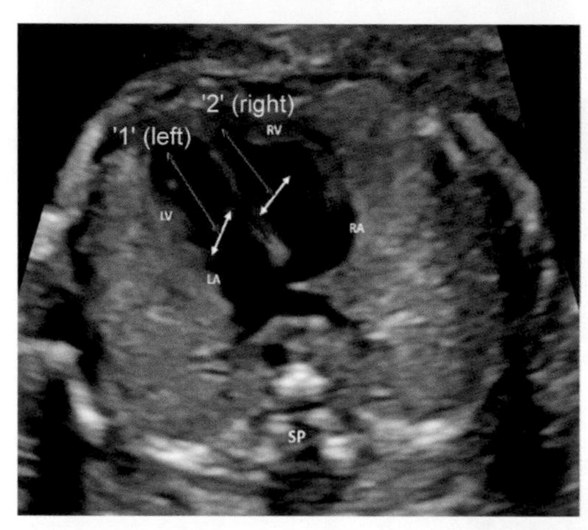

Fig. 3.2.14 Ventricular length is measured from the atrioventricular annular line to the ventricular apex; 1 = left ventricular length, 2 = right ventricular length.

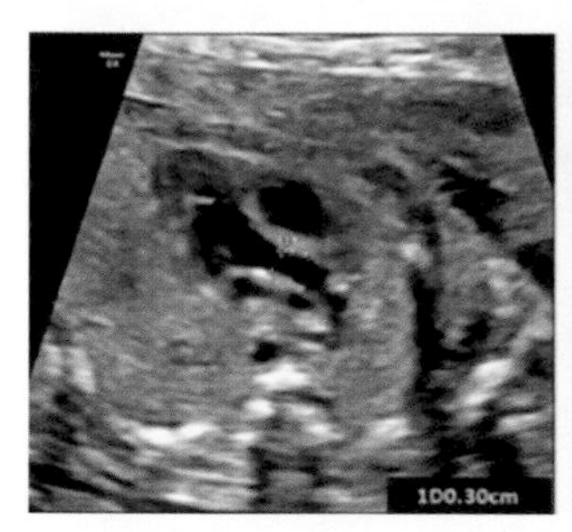

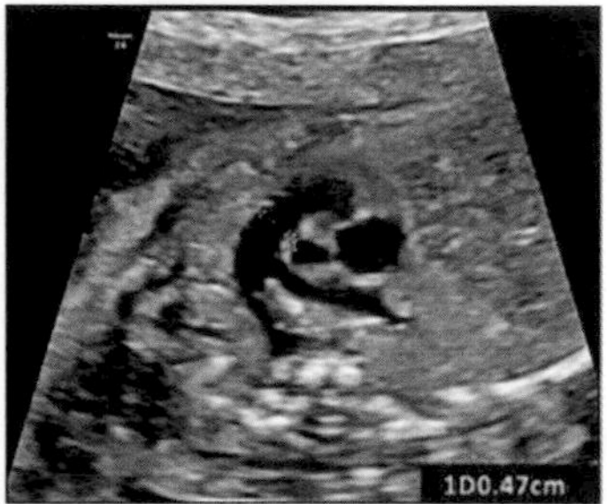

Fig. 3.2.15 Aortic valve annulus is measured with the valve in systole (left). The pulmonary artery annulus is measured with the valve in systole (right).

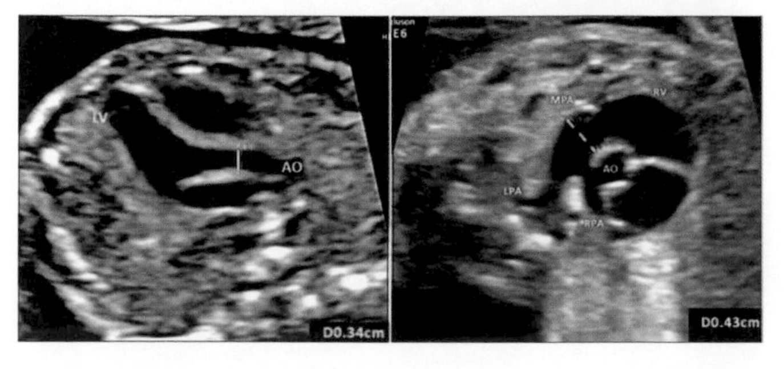

Fig. 3.2.16 The ascending aorta is measured beyond the valve before the arch (left). The main pulmonary artery is measured in the RVOT view between the valve and the bifurcation (right). AO, aorta; LPA, left pulmonary artery; LV, left ventricle; MPA, main pulmonary artery; RPA, right pulmonary artery.

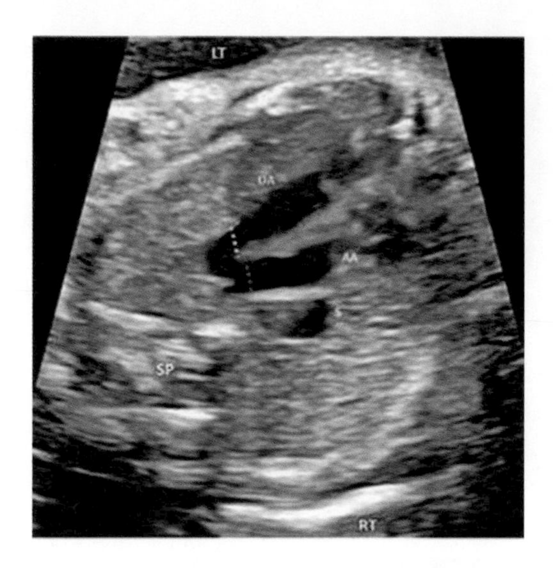

Fig. 3.2.17 The arches are measured before the confluence. AA, aortic arch; DA: ductal arch; LT, left; RT, right; S, superior vena cava; SP, spine.

CARDIAC RHYTHM ASSESSMENT

PULSED WAVE DOPPLER

The best sites to assess cardiac rhythm by pulsed Doppler are:

- the left ventricular outflow (Fig. 3.2.18)
- pulmonary vein and artery (Fig. 3.2.19)
- inferior vena cava and descending aorta (Fig. 3.2.20)
- superior vena cava and ascending aorta (Fig. 3.2.21)
- renal vein and artery (Fig. 3.2.22)

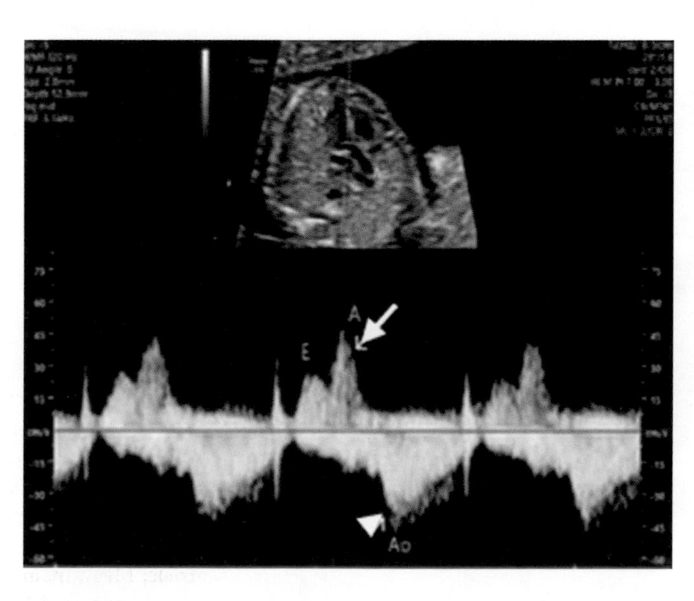

Fig. 3.2.18 Apical parasternal view with the Doppler sample gate placed before the aortic valve and near the mitral valve. Doppler signal of left ventricular outflow (Ao ejection) and inflow (mitral EA) are seen. Atrial systole (arrow) and ventricular systole (arrowhead) indicate normal 1:1 atrioventricular conduction.

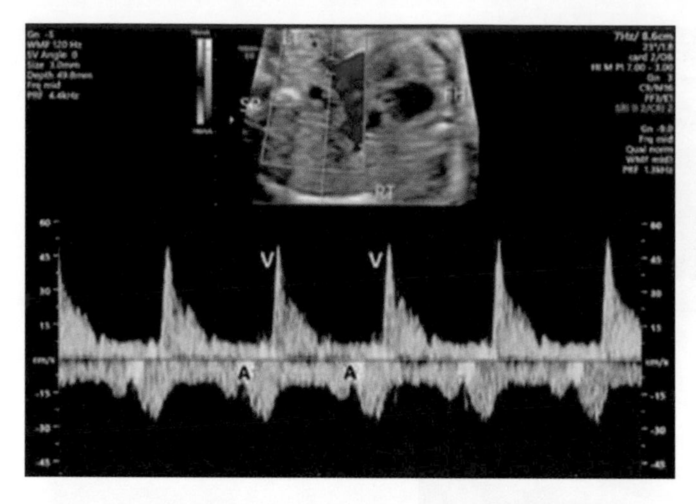

Fig. 3.2.19 Pulsed Doppler sample volume placed in the pulmonary vein. The adjacent pulmonary artery signal is also seen. The arterial signal represents ventricular events (V) and the venous signals represent the atrial events (A). There is 1:1 atrioventricular conduction.

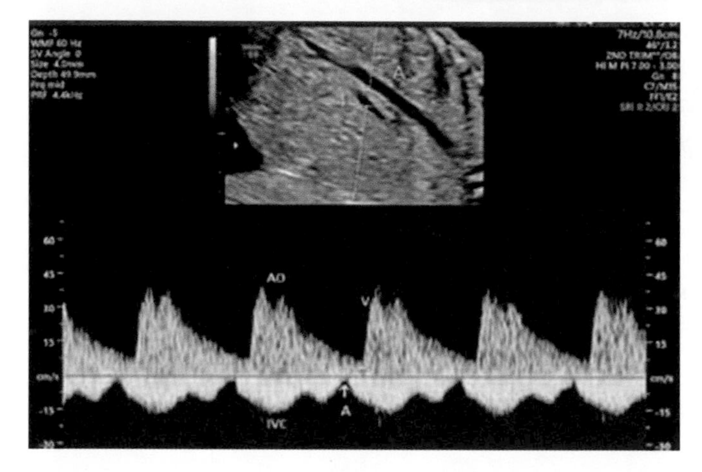

Fig. 3.2.20 Pulsed Doppler sample gate in the infrahepatic portion of the inferior vena cava (IVC) and descending aorta. A, atrial systole; V, ventricular systole. Note that the gate does not cover the full lumen of the aorta but is very close to the wall to ensure optimal aortic signals.

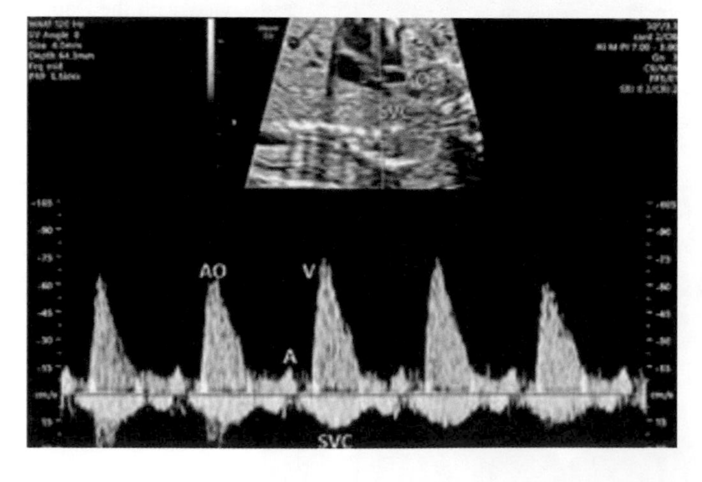

Fig. 3.2.21 Doppler sampling of superior vena cava (SVC) and ascending aorta (Ao). The atrial systole (A) is clearly seen as it is close to the heart. V, ventricular systole.

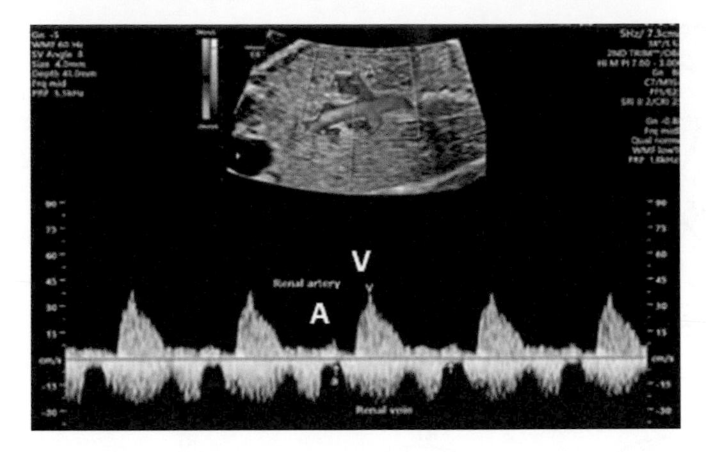

Fig. 3.2.22 Sampling of renal artery and renal vein by pulsed Doppler. Atrial systole (A) and ventricular systole (V) demonstrate normal conduction.

M-MODE

- M-Mode may be used to assess:
  - heart rate and rhythm abnormalities (Fig. 3.2.23)
  - biventricular cardiac function – ejection fraction and shortening fraction
  - excursion of valves
- For most fetal medicine specialists, fetal cardiac rhythm and function can be assessed better by pulsed wave Doppler

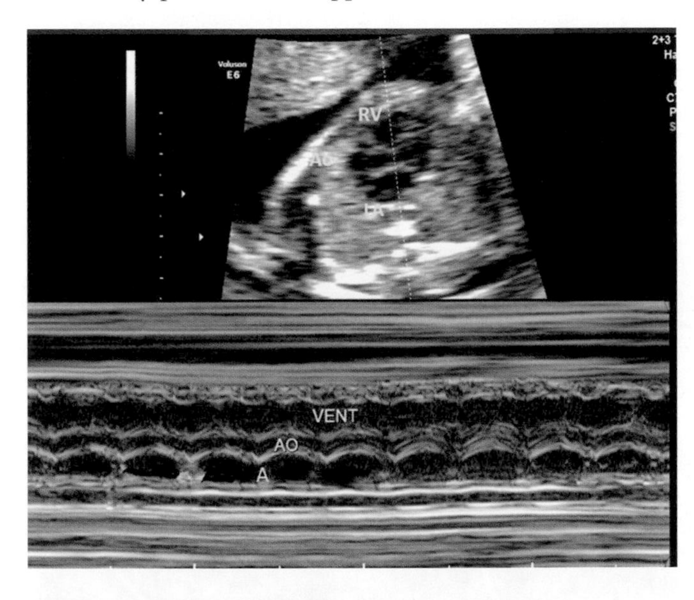

Fig. 3.2.23 M-mode tracing with the M-line passing through the right ventricle (RV) and left atrium (LA). A, atrium; Ao, aorta; VENT, ventricle.

SITUS ABNORMALITIES

- When situs is assessed, it is critically important to ensure that the probe is held **correctly** – that is, the marker on the ultrasound probe always corresponds with the left side of the screen. If there is any doubt, check with the little finger of the hand that is holding the probe

Cephalic Presentation: Transverse Planes

- In a cephalic presentation, using the fetal spine as the starting point, the **left side of the fetus is always clockwise (red arrow in** Fig. 3.2.24)
- In a normal situs, stomach and portal vein should always be clockwise from the fetal spine and apex of the heart should point clockwise (Fig. 3.2.24)

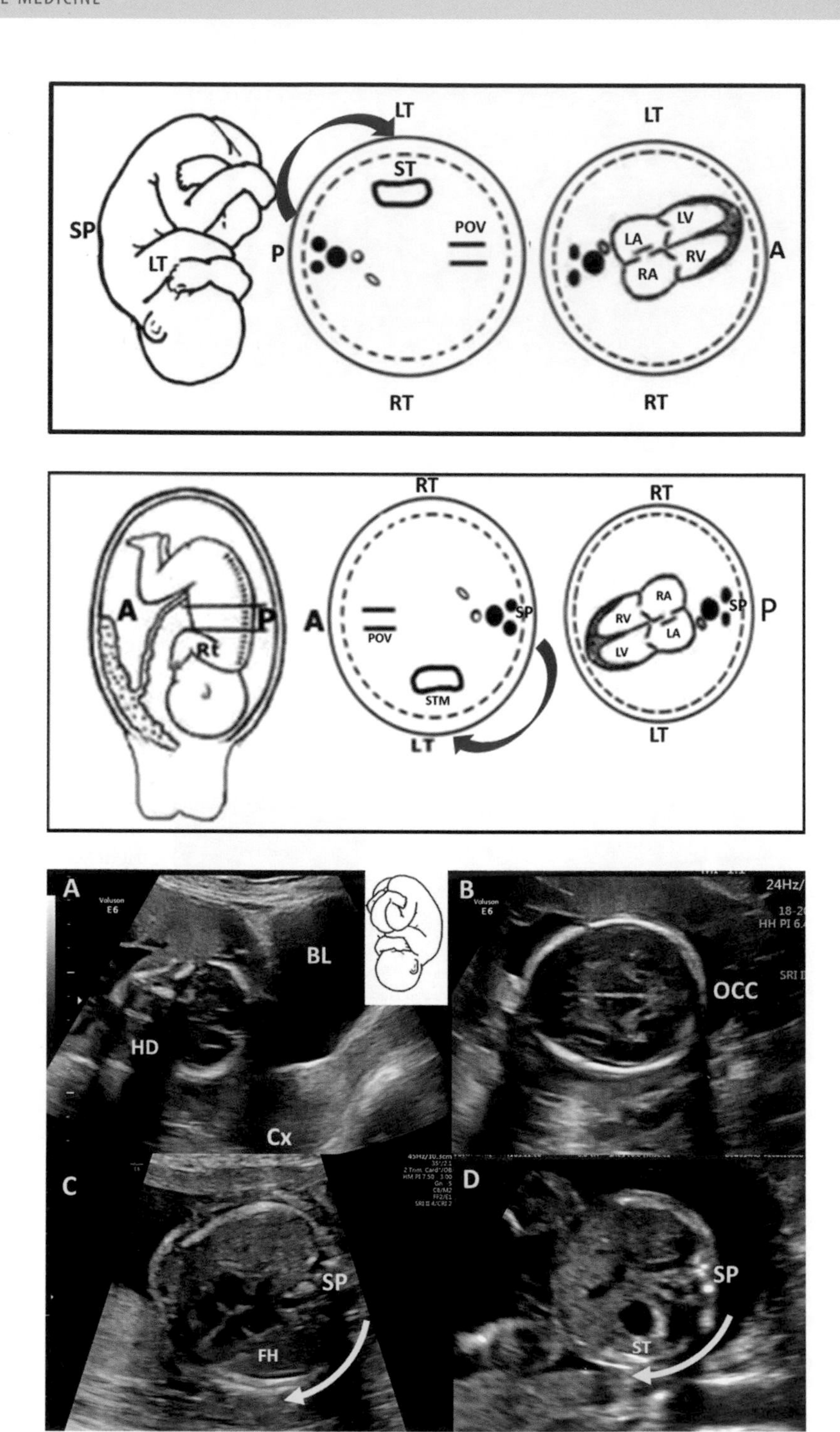

Fig. 3.2.24 The probe is held correctly – that is, the left edge of the screen corresponds to the left edge of the probe. *Cephalic presentation:* The stomach, portal vein and the apex of the heart all point clockwise; therefore, **the situs is NORMAL.**

Breech Presentation: Transverse Planes

- In a breech presentation, using the fetal spine as the starting point, the **left side of the fetus is always anticlockwise (black arrows in** Fig 3.2.25)

- The stomach and portal vein should always be anticlockwise from the fetal spine and apex of the heart should also point anticlockwise (Fig 3.2.25)

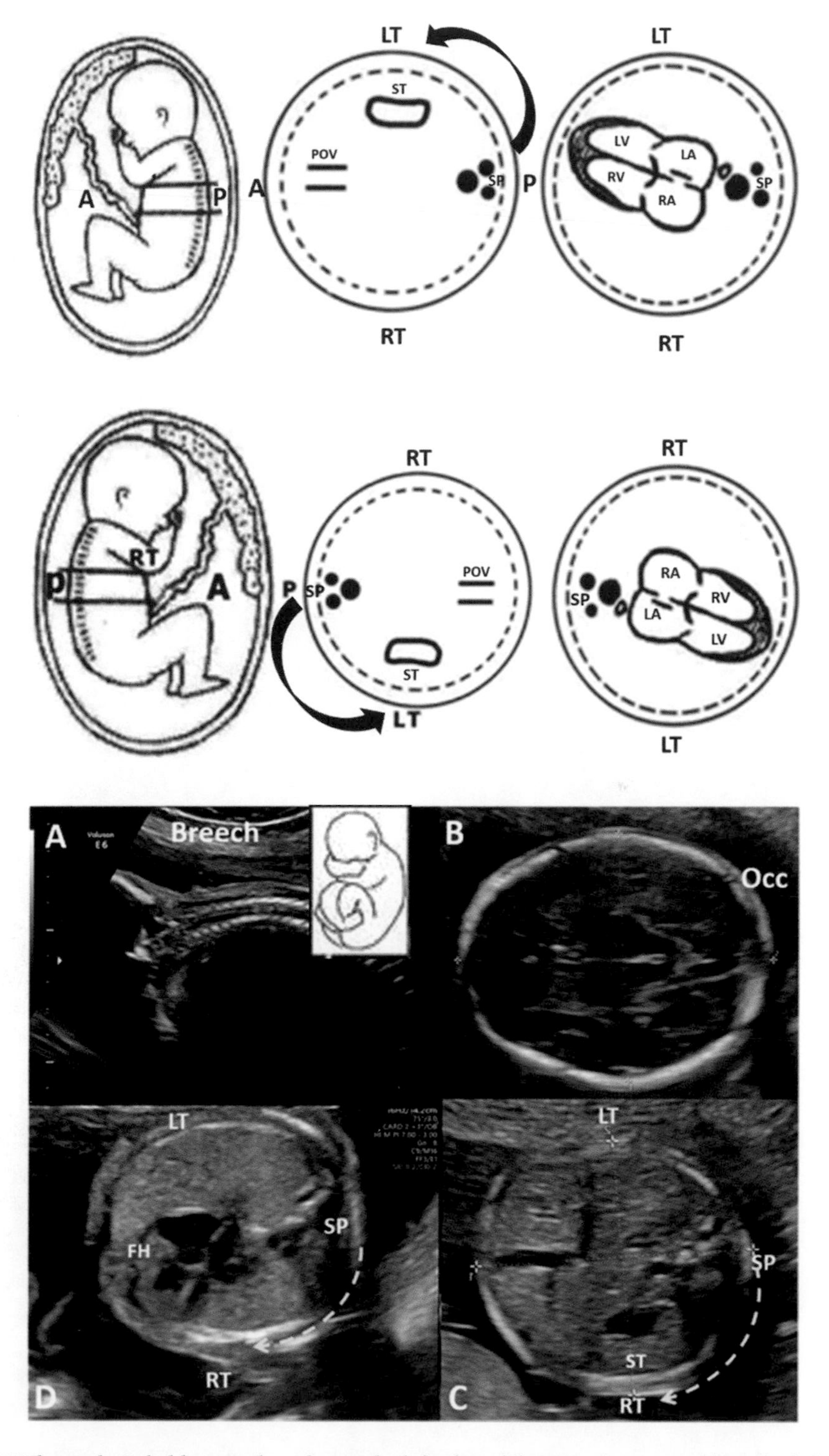

Fig. 3.2.25 The probe is held correctly – that is, the left edge of the screen corresponds to the left edge of the probe. **Breech presentation:** The stomach, portal vein and the apex of the heart all point anticlockwise; therefore, **the situs is NORMAL.**

SITUS INVERSUS TOTALIS

Definition and Characteristics

- Complete inversion (mirroring) of the normal anatomy
- Prevalence ~1 in 10,000 births
- Multiple gene mutations have been implicated, with autosomal recessive pattern of inheritance (e.g. primary ciliary dyskinesia)

Ultrasound Assessment

- In cephalic presentation, using the spine as a starting point, stomach and portal vein are in an anticlockwise direction (Fig. 3.2.26)
- In breech presentation, using the spine as a starting point, stomach and portal vein are in a clockwise direction. The apex of the heart and stomach are on the right side
- Look for transposition of the great arteries (TGA) as it will be present in ~3–5% of cases
- Look for right-sided aortic arch as it will be present in ~80% of cases

Investigations

- Chromosomal microarray and exome, if available

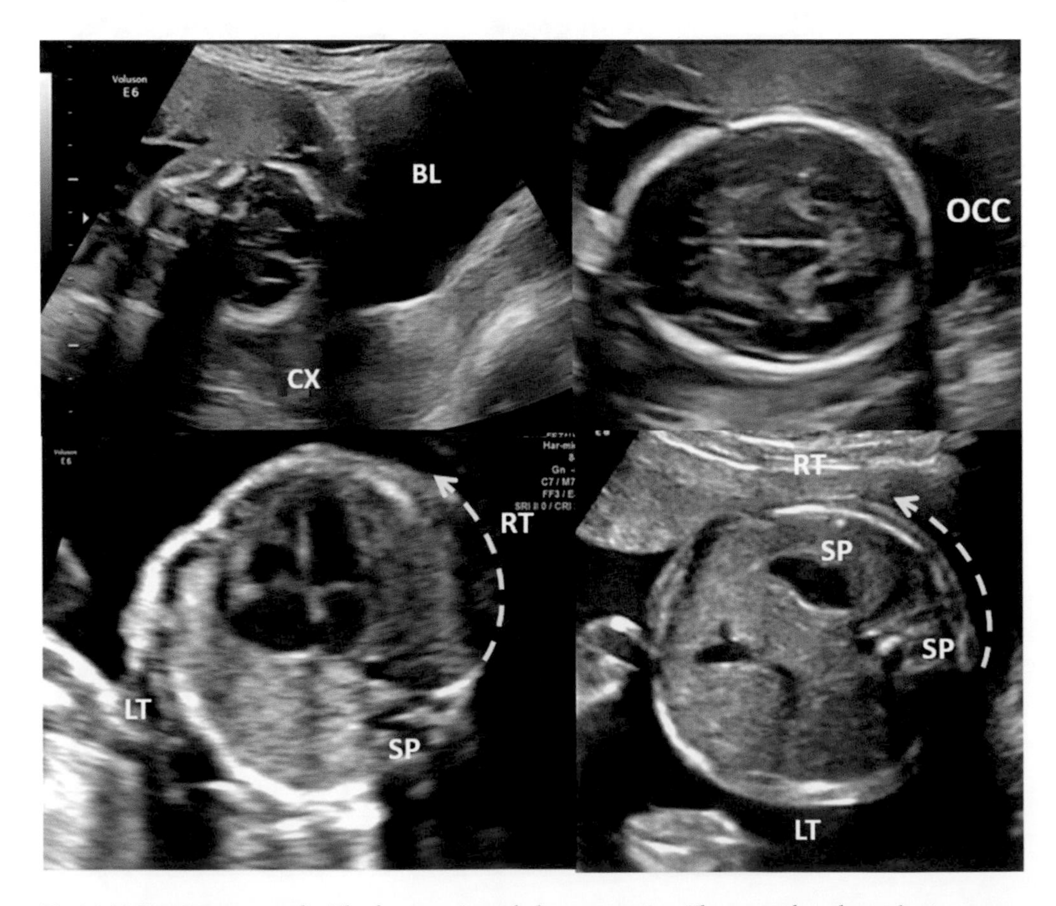

Fig. 3.2.26 Situs inversus totalis. The fetus was in cephalic presentation. The stomach and portal vein are seen in the anticlockwise direction using the spine as a starting point. The apex of the heart is pointing to the right.

Counselling

- If isolated, no major health issues are expected
- No significant benefit from delivery at a tertiary facility
- ~20% can have Kartagener syndrome, a rare autosomal recessive primary ciliary dyskinesia
- If there is associated Kartagener syndrome, neonatal respiratory distress may be present. Frequent bronchiectasis, respiratory infections and sinus and middle ear infections are common

HETEROTAXY

Definition and Characteristics

- Heterotaxy (isomerism) is suspected when there is an abnormal arrangement of the heart and viscera across the right and left axis but the situs is neither solitus nor inversus
- It is also called situs ambiguous, but this term should be avoided. Detailed description of the abdominal findings should be reported instead
- Other terms also used include cardiosplenic syndrome and right or left isomerism

Ultrasound Assessment

- The stomach and heart are on the opposite sides (Fig. 3.2.27)
- The stomach is seen on the right side posteriorly, close to the spine
- Look for IVC that is very close to the spine, or IVC that is not entering the atrium ('interrupted')
- Look for two vessels in front of the spine in the thoracic section (descending aorta and azygos/hemi-azygos vein)
- Look for complex cardiac abnormality, seen in >80% of cases (e.g. AVSD, DORV, interrupted IVC, persistent LSVC)

Investigations

- Chromosomal microarray (abnormal in ~3%), exome if available

Counselling

- Extracardiac anomalies include gut malrotation, polysplenia, and biliary atresia, which are difficult to diagnose antenatally, even in expert hands
- Children with left atrial isomerism, heart anomalies requiring biventricular repair, antenatal bradycardia or associated extracardiac anomalies have a poor long-term prognosis

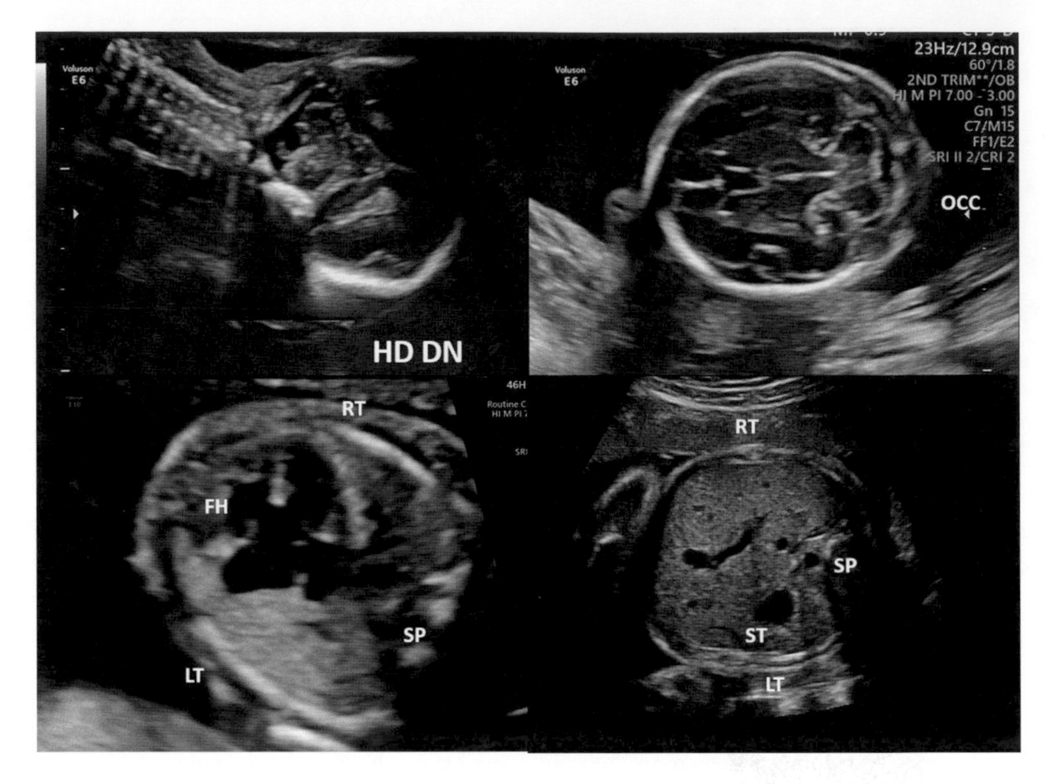

Fig. 3.2.27 The fetus with heterotaxy in cephalic presentation. The stomach is on the left side and the heart is on the right side. AVSD is also clearly visible.

ABNORMAL HEART AXIS

SHIFT TO THE LEFT

- Look for signs of *tetralogy of Fallot* (Fig. 3.2.28)
- Look for signs of *Ebstein's anomaly*
- Look for *common arterial trunk*
- Dilated right heart (right heart overload)

SHIFT TO THE RIGHT (MESOCARDIA)

- Can be a normal variant (Fig. 3.2.29)
- Look for corrected TGA (cTGA)
- Look for abnormalities of extracardiac space (e.g. CHAOS, kyphoscoliosis)

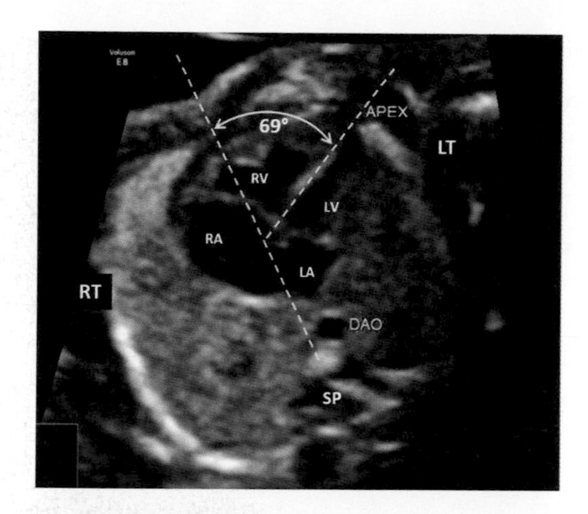

Fig. 3.2.28 Apical four chamber view in tetralogy of Fallot. There is left axis deviation. LV, left ventricle.

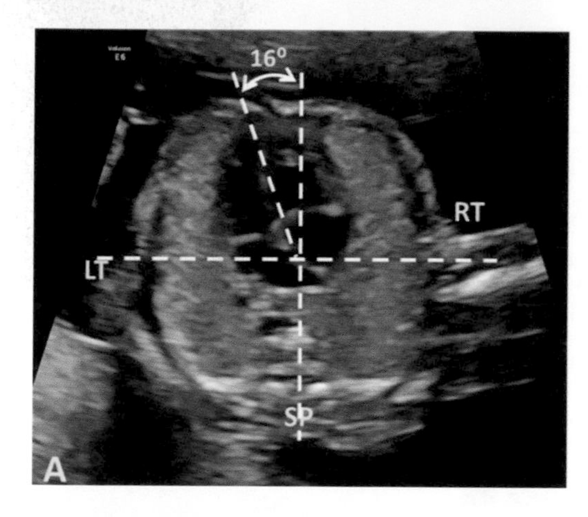

Fig. 3.2.29 Mesocardia. In this fetus no cause was found for the reduced axis. Reduced axis may also be seen in corrected transposition of great arteries.

ABNORMAL HEART SIZE

- Cardiothoracic ratio can be measured by the calliper or ellipse method. The ellipse method is preferred (Fig. 3.2.30)

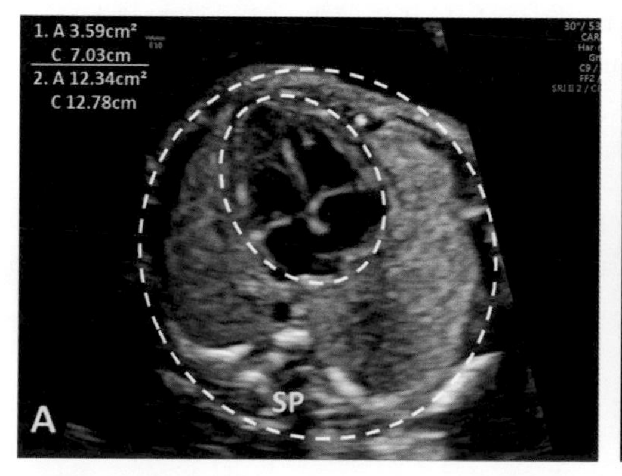

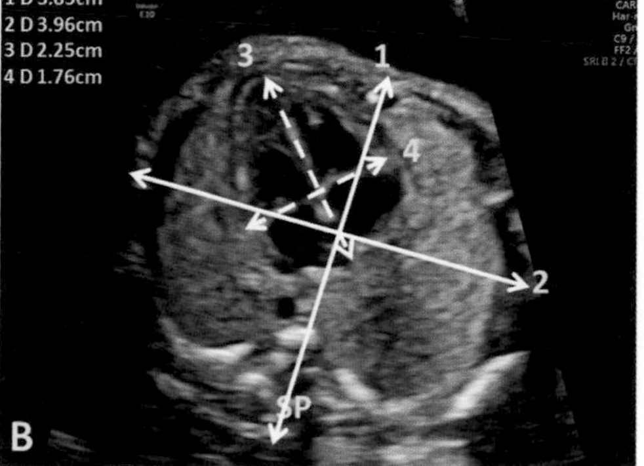

Fig. 3.2.30 (a) Measurement of area [A] and circumference [C] of fetal heart and thorax by the ellipse method. (b) Calliper method of measuring diameters of the fetal thorax [1,2] and heart [3,4] from which circumference can be calculated. Cardiac circumference/thoracic circumference >50% indicates cardiomegaly.

CARDIOMEGALY

- Cardiomegaly is usually diagnosed when the heart occupies more than 50% of the thorax
- Common causes include:
  - Ebstein's anomaly (Fig. 3.2.31)
  - cardiomyopathy (CMV, parvo)
  - fluid overload (fetal growth restriction, fetal anaemia, TTTS, chorioangioma, vein of Galen aneurysm)

INCREASED CARDIOTHORACIC RATIO WITHOUT CARDIOMEGALY

- Pulmonary hypoplasia secondary to bilateral renal agenesis or severe skeletal dysplasia
- Pulmonary agenesis
- Significant pericardial effusion

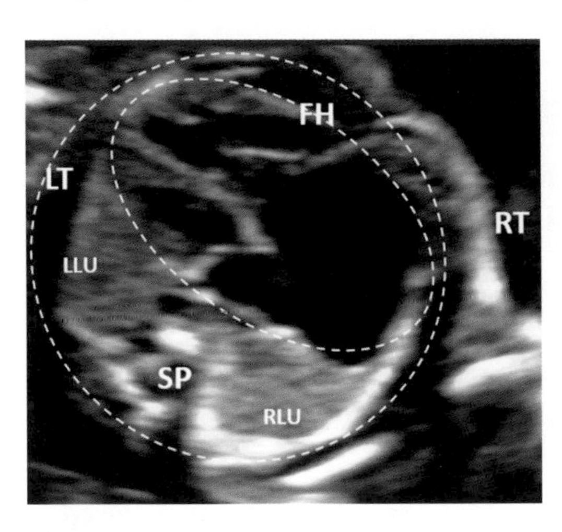

Fig. 3.2.31 Increased cardiothoracic circumference in Ebstein's anomaly. FH, fetal heart; LLU, left lung; RLU, right lung; SP, spine; LT, left; RT, right.

ABNORMAL ATRIA

REDUNDANT SEPTUM PRIMUM FLAP

- Aneurysmal flap valve extending to almost half of the left atrium (Fig. 3.2.32)
- Can be isolated or because of conditions that cause increased right atrial pressure

Counselling

- Benign if the rest of the anatomy is normal
- Associated anomalies include atrial septal defect, hypoplastic right heart, and Ebstein's anomaly

FLAP OF FORAMEN OVALE IN THE RIGHT ATRIUM

- Look for hypoplastic left heart

DILATED CORONARY SINUS

- Coronary sinus drains blood from the cardiac veins into the right atrium
- A large left atrial appendage may be mistaken for a coronary sinus (Fig. 3.2.33)
- Persistent left superior vena cava (PLSVC) is the common cause for a dilated coronary sinus due to increased volume flow through a coronary sinus (Fig. 3.2.34)
- Can be due to anomalous pulmonary venous connection
- Can be mistaken for AVSD (Fig. 3.2.35)

Counselling

- If isolated, the prognosis is good and does not require delivery in a tertiary unit

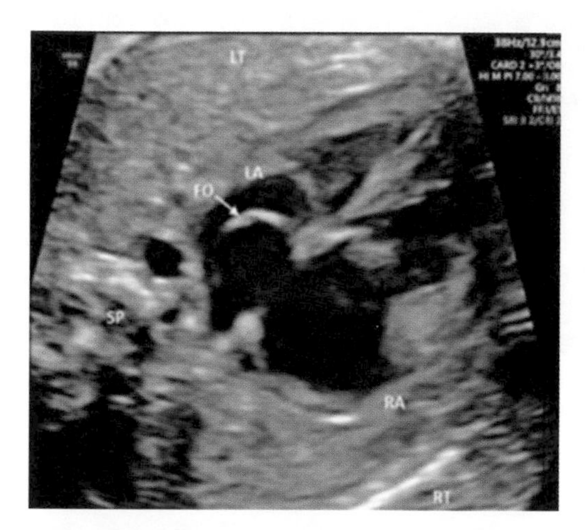

Fig. 3.2.32 Aneurysmal flap of foramen ovale (FO). Note the flap extending more than halfway into left atrium (LA). LT, left; RA, right atrium; RT, right; SP, spine.

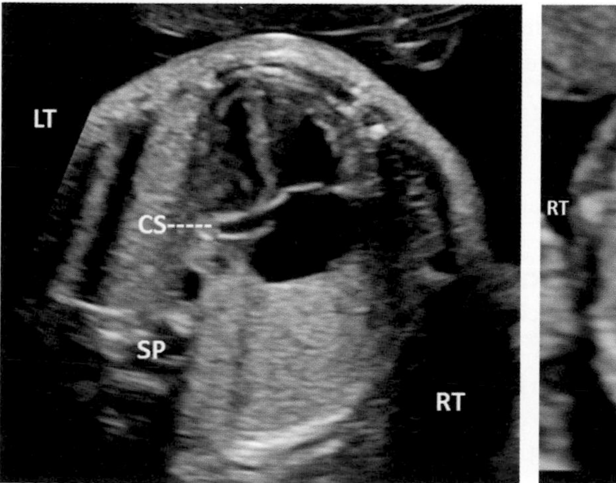

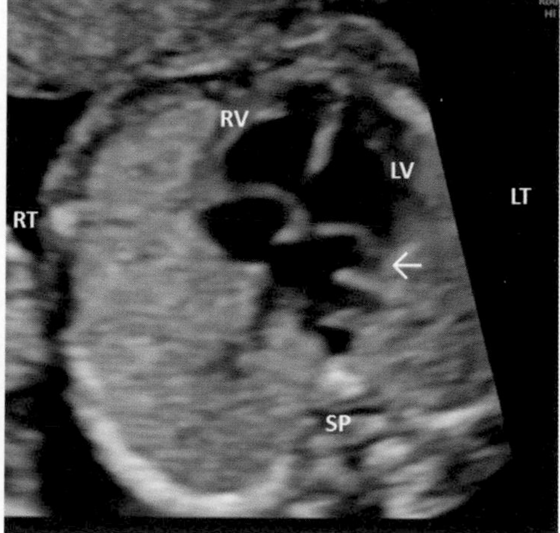

Fig. 3.2.33 Normal coronary sinus imaged in the four chamber view. Note that the left atrium is not seen. Left atrial appendage (arrow) can mimic a coronary sinus. CS, coronary sinus; SP, spine.

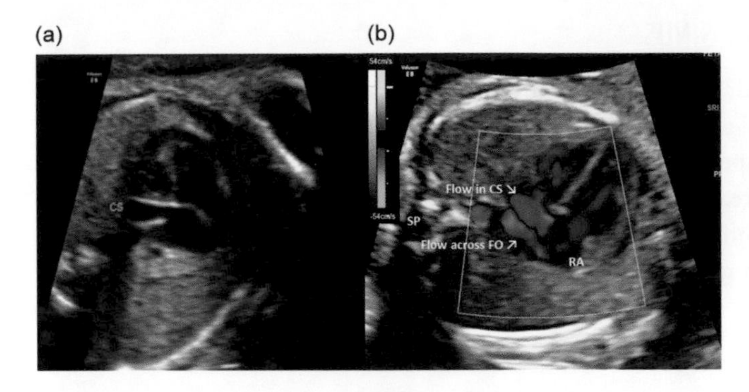

Fig. 3.2.34 (a) Dilated coronary sinus (CS) in a fetus with persistent LSVC. (b) Note the colour flow in the opposite direction – coronary sinus flow in blue and foramen ovale flow from right to left atrium in red.

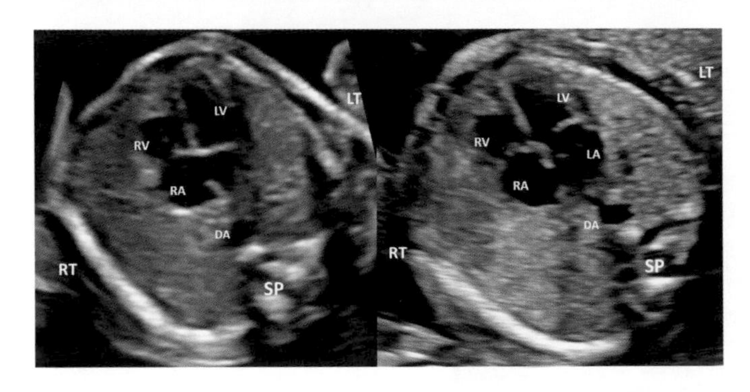

Fig. 3.2.35 (Left) Dilated coronary sinus may give an impression of an absent crux with loss of valve offset that can be mistakenly interpreted as AVSD. (Right) A slight angulation to ensure that the intraventricular septum is oblique will show intact crux and normal septum primum.

ABNORMAL VENTRICLES

VENTRICULAR SEPTAL DEFECTS

- Ventricular septal defects (VSD) can be located in:
  - perimembranous septum (inlet or outlet)
  - muscular septum (mid-muscular, apical, anterior or posterior)

Ultrasound Assessment

- In a true perimembranous septal defect, the aortic override is unlikely
- Muscular septal VSD may have tortuous course and be hidden by hypertrophied right ventricular muscle, hence they can be easily missed antenatally (Fig. 3.2.36)
- If true inlet VSD is present, an 'edge' or 'T' artefact can be seen even when colour Doppler crossing is not obvious (Fig. 3.2.37)
- When a septal defect extends to include subaortic VSD, the aortic override will be visible (e.g. tetralogy of Fallot)
- Colour Doppler is superior to B-mode in the diagnosis of muscular VSD

Investigations

- Amniocentesis for chromosomal microarray

Counselling

- Spontaneous closure after delivery:
  - VSD <3 mm ~85%
  - VSD ≥3 mm ~30%
- Muscular VSDs have a higher closure rate compared to perimembranous VSDs
- Postnatal echo for confirmation

ATRIOVENTRICULAR SEPTAL DEFECTS

Description and Characteristics

- A combination of a septum primum defect and inlet VSD with a common AV valve
- Incidence ~1 in 5,000 births
- If one parent has AVSD the recurrence is ~10–15%
- In a complete AVSD there is a common AV junction associated with deficient AV septation. There is a common AV valve
- Partial AVSD is diagnosed when there is an ostium primum septal defect and a common AV junction but separate AV valvular orifices and valves. There is loss of offset of the AV valves (Fig. 3.2.38)

Ultrasound Assessment

- Absent or abnormal crux in four chamber view
- Loss of valve offset
- Outflow tracts may be normal or anomalous
- LVOT appears elongated and shows a "goose neck" appearance
- Symmetrical size of the ventricles implies balanced AVSD (Fig. 3.2.39)
- Asymmetrical size of the ventricles implies unbalanced AVSD
- AV regurgitation, heart block and RVOT stenosis may be present.
- Exclude complex heart anomalies (tetralogy of Fallot, DORV, heterotaxy, coarctation)
- Look for signs of associated chromosomal abnormalities (trisomies 21, 18, 13) and syndromes (Holt–Oram, Ellis–van Creveld)
- A large isolated inlet VSD and partial AVSD should be considered in the differential diagnosis
- A dilated coronary sinus, if present, may mimic an AVSD

Investigations

- Amniocentesis for chromosomal microarray and DNA storage is recommended

Counselling

- Delivery in a tertiary centre with advanced paediatric cardiology should be arranged
- For non-syndromic, balanced AVSD, surgical correction is usually scheduled 6–12 weeks after birth with good long-term outcomes. In 5–10% of cases repeated surgery is needed for AV regurgitation
- Unbalanced AVSD requires multiple staged palliative surgeries with guarded prognosis. Complete heart block may develop, requiring permanent pacemaker

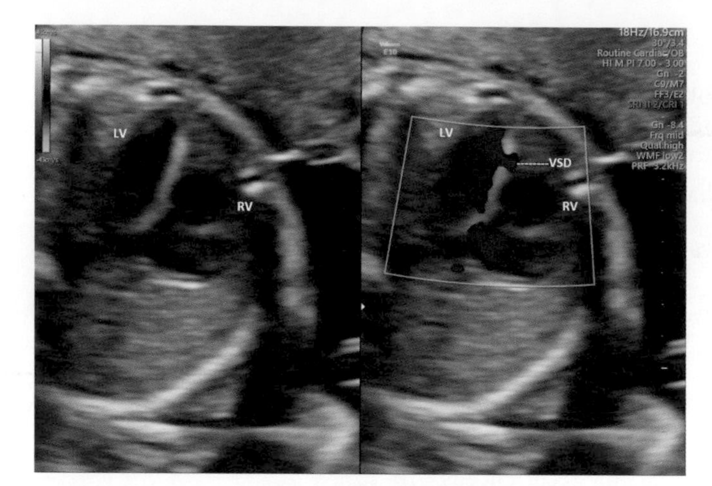

Fig. 3.2.36 Muscular VSD. On the left, B-mode shows an apparently normal septum. On the right, colour Doppler shows a mid-muscular VSD with flow from the right to the left ventricle. Such small VSDs are often missed during fetal cardiac screening.

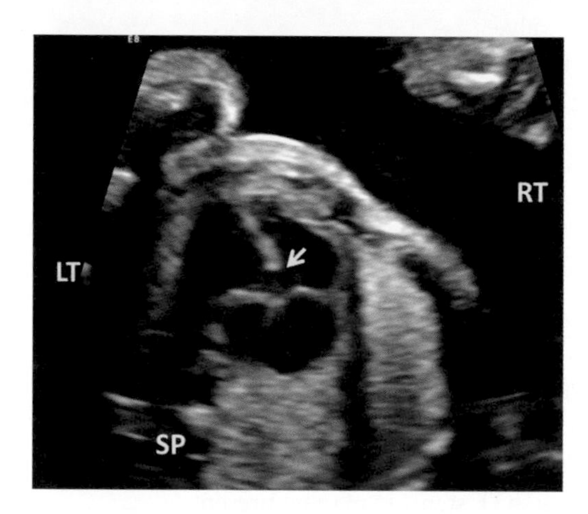

Fig. 3.2.37 Perimembranous inlet VSD (arrow). Note the echogenic tip of the septum. This helps to differentiate a true VSD from a false echo dropout in an apical four chamber view.

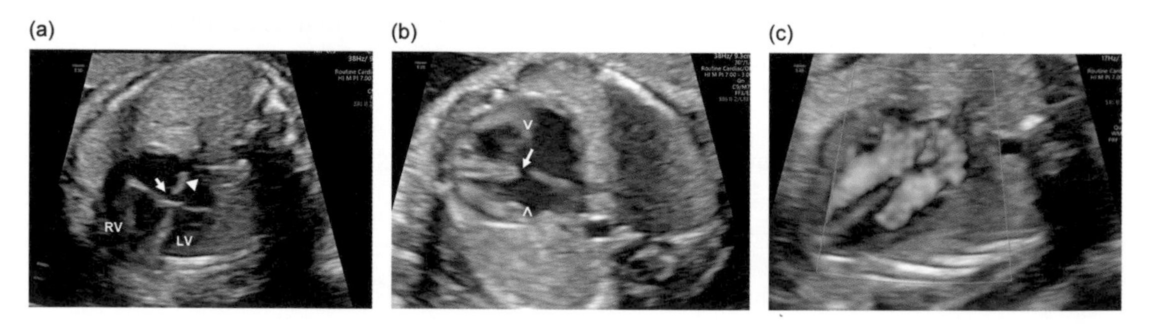

Fig. 3.2.38 Partial AVSD. (a) Basal four chamber view in systole showing a septum primum defect (arrow) and absence of the crux. The upper part of the septum primum is intact (arrowhead). The two AV valves are seen. (b) Lateral four chamber view confirms the septum primum defect (arrow) with two distinct AV orifices. (c) Colour Doppler shows two distinct inflows.

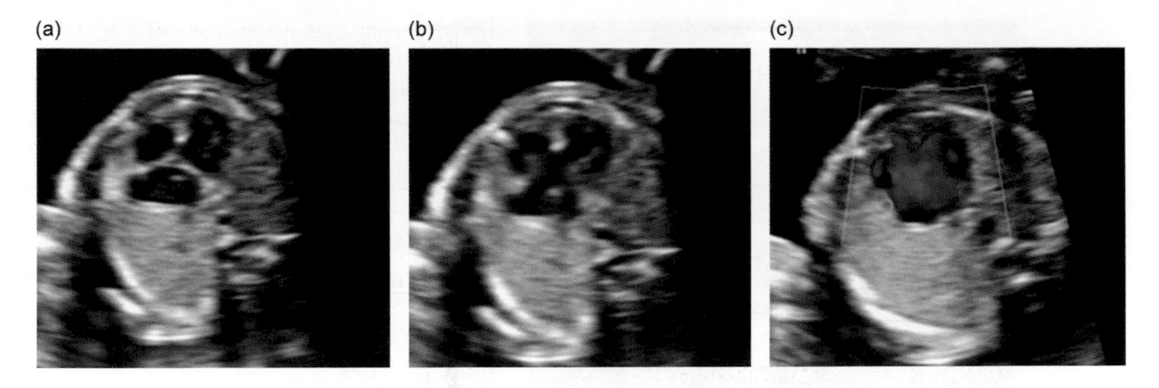

Fig. 3.2.39 Balanced AVSD. (a) Apical four chamber view in systole shows a closed common AV valve. (b) AV valve in diastole. (c) Colour Doppler in diastole has a 'H' shape indicating 'merging' of flows.

VENTRICULAR ASYMMETRY

Look for:

- hypoplastic left heart (Fig. 3.2.40)
- coarctation of aorta
- hypoplastic right heart
- Ebstein's anomaly

INTRACARDIAC ECHOGENIC FOCI

Definition and Characteristics

- Calcifications of the papillary muscle
- Prevalence ~5%

Ultrasound Assessment

- May be single or multiple (Fig. 3.2.41)
- May be seen in one or both ventricles
- Look for signs of aneuploidy

Investigations

- If isolated, karyotyping is not indicated

Counselling

- Most of them will disappear in the third trimester
- If isolated in an otherwise low-risk woman, the risk of aneuploidy is not increased

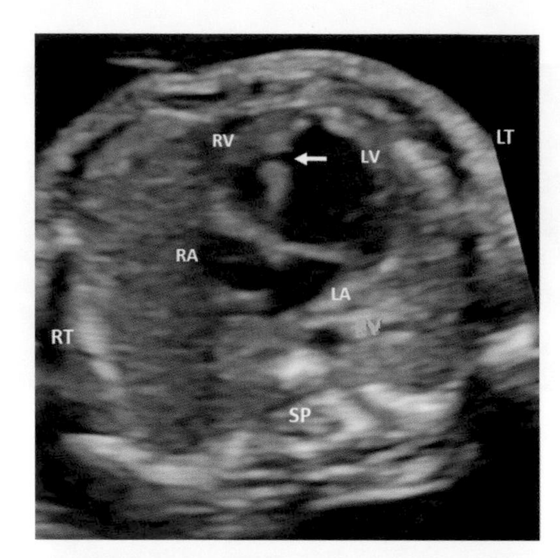

Fig. 3.2.40 Four chamber view showing ventricular asymmetry. The right ventricle is smaller (RV) as compared with the left ventricle (LV). There is a small muscular VSD seen near the apex. This was a case of hypoplastic right heart syndrome.

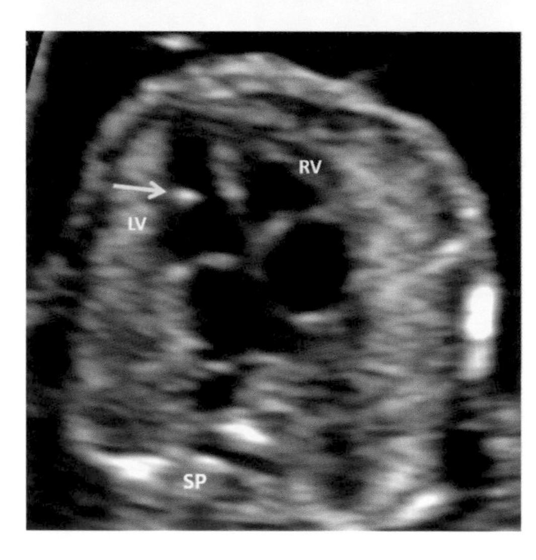

Fig. 3.2.41 Apical four chamber view showing an echogenic intracardiac focus (arrow) in the left ventricle (LV). The fetus was otherwise normal (RV, right ventricle; SP, spine).

RHABDOMYOMA

Definition and Characteristics

- A benign primary tumour of the heart composed of overgrown myocardial cells considered to be a hamartoma
- Incidence ~1 in 10,000 livebirths, more commonly reported in fetal series
- Often associated with tuberous sclerosis (~70%)

Ultrasound Assessment

- Hyperechogenic lesions of various sizes (Fig. 3.2.42)
- Avascular with smooth homogeneous appearance
- May be single or multiple
- Commonly attached to the septum or ventricles
- They can cause brady/tachyarrhythmia and hydrops
- Colour Doppler is helpful to assess the extent of flow obstruction (Fig. 3.2.43)

Differential Diagnosis

- Teratoma
- Fibroma
- Myxoma
- Haemangioma

Investigations

- Clinical examination of parents for hypopigmented macules, adenoma sebaceum in the face
- Genetic testing for tuberous sclerosis, with carrier testing for parents
- Fetal MRI may identify tubers, subependymal cysts in the brain or angiomyolipomas in the kidney

Counselling

- May remain static, regress or increase in size
- Large cardiac tumours may cause either inflow obstruction of the ventricle, outflow obstruction or both. In some cases, hydrops may develop
- Although cardiac tumours usually regress in the third trimester, or in the immediate neonatal period, tubers in the brain may increase
- Delivery should be in a unit with neonatal intensive care
- If there is no hydrops, delivery is planned for 38 weeks, earlier if hydrops is present
- If obstruction of inflow/outflow tract is suspected, prophylactic use of prostaglandins in the immediate neonatal period should be discussed with neonatologists/cardiologists
- If tumours are isolated and asymptomatic, prognosis is favourable

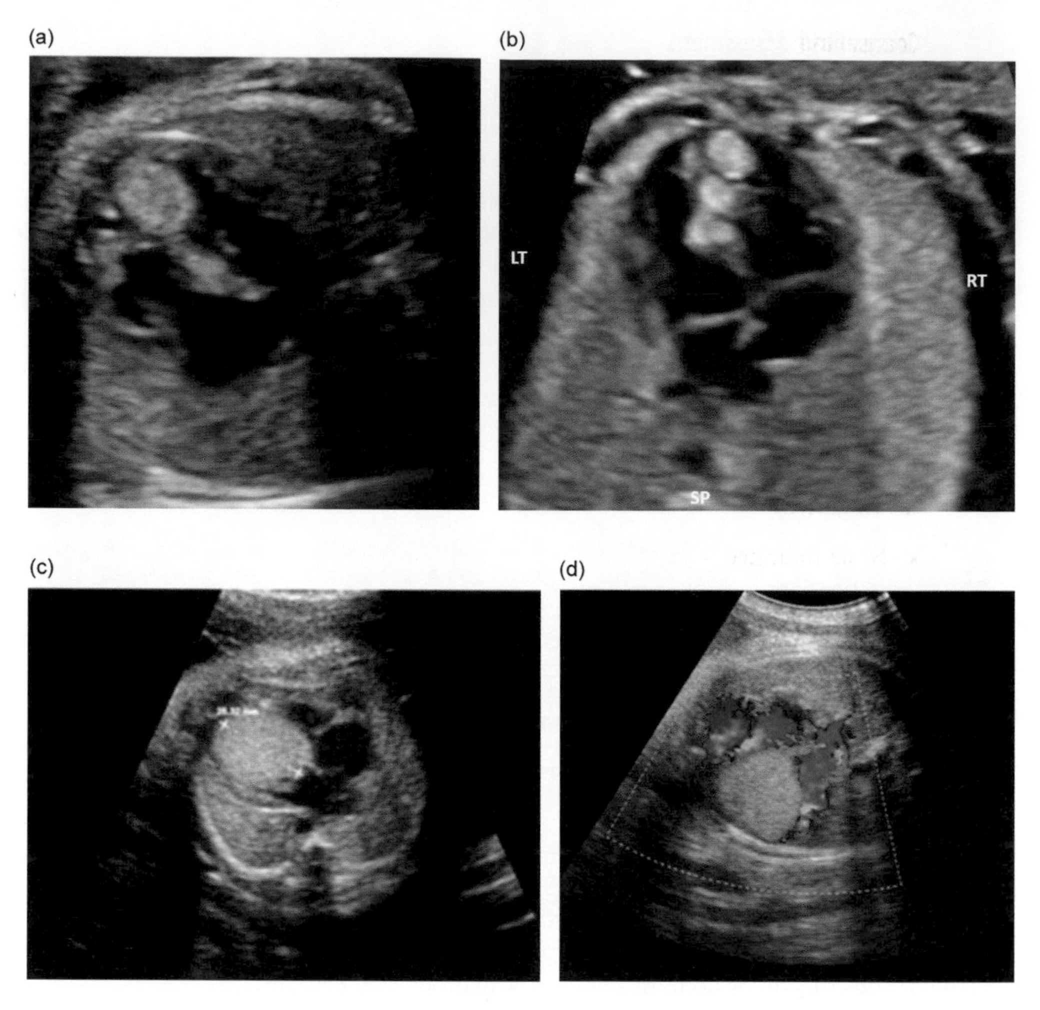

Fig. 3.2.42 Rhabdomyoma. (a) This tumour often presents as a solitary echogenic mass, but these tumours can be (b) multiple and (c) very large. (d) Colour Doppler helps to identify obstruction to flow. In this four chamber view there was no obstruction to flow despite large intraventricular rhabdomyoma.

ABNORMAL SYSTEMIC VEINS

PERSISTENT LEFT SUPERIOR VENA CAVA (SVC) DRAINING INTO CORONARY SINUS

Ultrasound Assessment

- SVC is usually seen as the fourth vessel in the three vessel trachea view (~90%)
- Drains into the coronary sinus, hence coronary sinus may be dilated
- Dilated coronary sinus may mimic an ASD or AVSD
- ~30% will have increased nuchal translucency in the first trimester
- Association of extra- and intracardiac anomalies in ~40–60%
- ~20% of isolated cases will develop coarctation of the aorta

Investigations

- Isolated persistent left SVC (PLSVC) does not require further testing
- Microarray if associated with other defects

Counselling

- Isolated PLSVC has a good outcome
- Serial scans to be done to look for development of coarctation of aorta
- Postnatal echo to be done in all cases

ABSENT RIGHT SVC WITH PERSISTENT LEFT SVC

Ultrasound Assessment

- In ~10% of PLSVC, the right SVC will be absent
- The left SVC will appear as an abnormal arrangement of the 3VT view (PLSVC, PA, Ao from left to right)
- Requires detailed examination to look for associated heterotaxia

Investigations

- None indicated

Counselling

- If heterotaxy is excluded, isolated LSVC has a favourable prognosis

INTERRUPTED INFERIOR VENA CAVA (IVC)

Ultrasound Assessment

- Diagnosed on longitudinal scans as a parallel vessel to the aorta in the suprarenal portion (azygous connection) (Fig. 3.2.43)
- "Piggy back" appearance of the parallel vessels on transverse scans of the upper abdomen (Fig. 3.2.44)
- Part of heterotaxy – hence situs/cardiac evaluation to be done

Investigations

- None indicated

Counselling

- As per heterotaxy

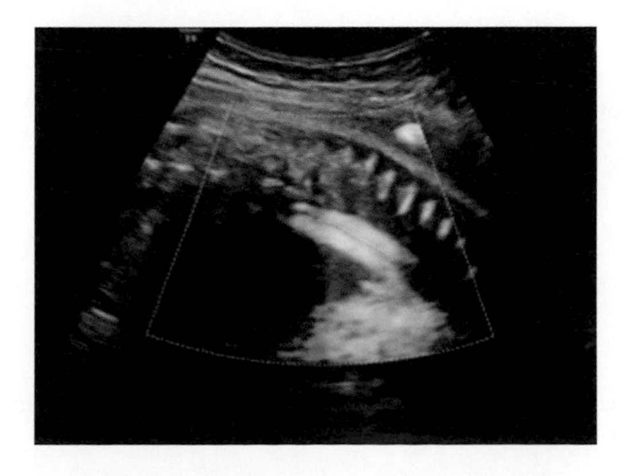

Fig. 3.2.43 Interrupted inferior vena cava (IVC). Sagittal section of the abdomen showing the abdominal aorta in red and the azygous vein in blue. The azygous vein runs parallel to the aorta as it goes through the diaphragm

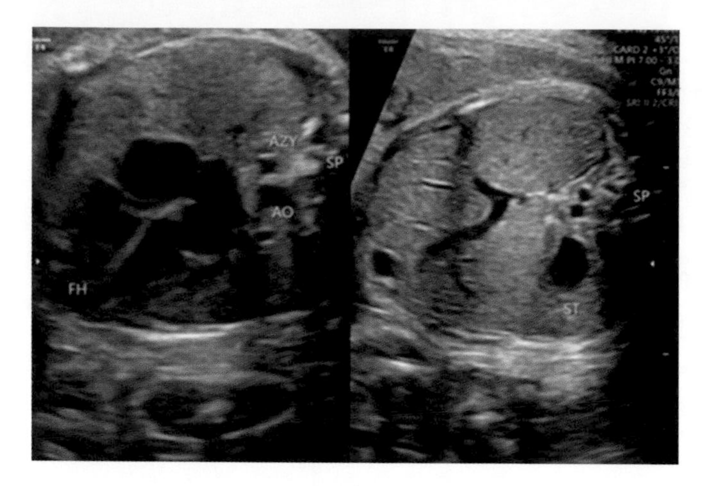

Fig. 3.2.44 Transverse sections of the abdomen and thorax showing cross sections of the aorta (AO) and azygous vein (AZY) side by side. In a normal fetus the IVC will be to the right of and anterior to the aorta.
SP, spine; ST, stomach.

ABNORMAL PULMONARY VEINS

TOTAL ANOMALOUS PULMONARY VENOUS CONNECTION (TAPVC)

Description and Characteristics

- Abnormal drainage of pulmonary veins into the right atrium and not into the left atrium
- Also known as total anomalous venous return or drainage
  - **Supracardiac TAPVC:** the pulmonary veins drain to the right atrium via the superior vena cava
  - **Cardiac TAPVC:** the pulmonary veins come together behind the heart and drain to the right atrium via the coronary sinus
  - **Infracardiac TAPVC:** the pulmonary veins drain into the right atrium via the hepatic vein and inferior vena cava
- Incidence is ~1 in 12,000
- Partial APVC is present when only one or two pulmonary veins are draining into the right atrium; partial APVC is very rarely diagnosed antenatally

Key Ultrasound Features

- Two inferior pulmonary veins cannot be seen draining into the left atrium
- In total APVC there is increased space behind the left atrium with a confluent vein behind the left atrium (Fig. 3.2.45)

Supracardiac TAPVC

- The fourth vessel in the 3VV view that is seen to the left of the pulmonary artery
- Coronary sinus is not dilated

Cardiac TAPVC

- Coronary sinus is dilated

Infracardiac TAPVC

- An abnormal vein descends below the diaphragm and joins the portal vein, hepatic vein or inferior vena cava

Investigations

- Invasive genetic testing (amniocentesis) is not indicated

Counselling

- Major but surgically correctable anomaly
- Delivery in a tertiary centre with advanced paediatric cardiology
- Balloon atrial septostomy is only attempted in an emergency when open heart surgery is not possible
- Urgent corrective surgery is needed if veins are obstructed, otherwise early corrective surgery is usually performed in the first 2–3 months of life
- There are good outcomes for supracardiac cardiac types
- The infracardiac type has higher morbidity and mortality

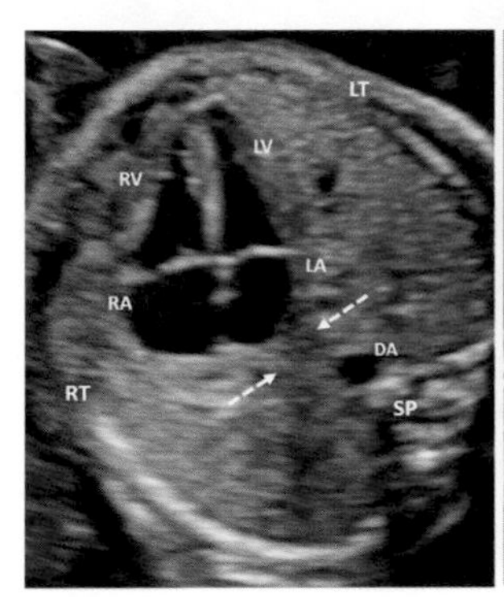

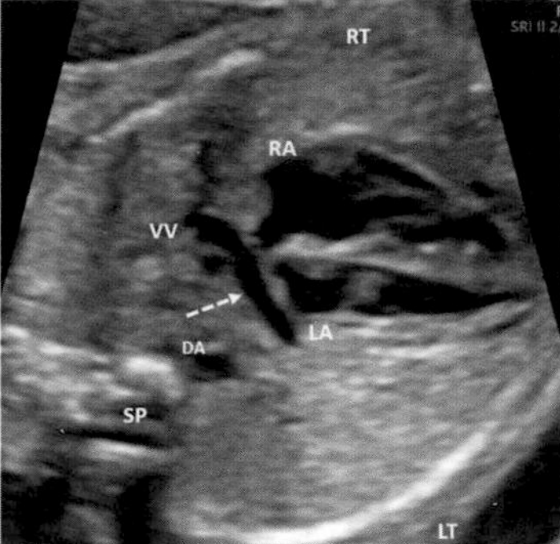

Fig. 3.2.45 Total anomalous pulmonary venous connection (TAPVC). Apical four chamber view on the left showing increased retroatrial space and a "bald" left atrium (arrow). The LA appears smaller than the RA. On the right, there is a confluent vertical vein behind the left atrium (arrow) with no connection to the left atrium. The vertical vein (VV) joins the superior vena cava

ABNORMAL THREE VESSEL VIEW

FOURTH VESSEL SEEN: CORONARY SINUS VISIBLE

- Persistent left superior vena cava draining into coronary sinus (Fig. 3.2.46)
- Serial scans to look for signs of aortic coarctation

Counselling

- Postnatal scan to rule out coarctation
- If there is no coarctation, this is considered as a normal variant

FOURTH VESSEL SEEN: CORONARY SINUS NOT VISIBLE

- Document pulmonary venous connections with left atrium
- If vertical vein and dilated SVC seen, look for signs of supracardiac TAPVC (Fig. 3.2.47)

Counselling

- If TAPVC is excluded, this can be considered as a normal variant

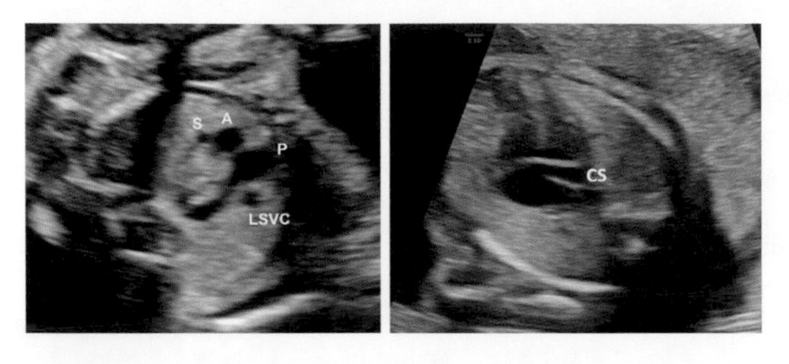

Fig. 3.2.46 Three vessel view with four vessels. Persistent left SVC lies adjacent to the left pulmonary artery (left). Four chamber view with a dilated coronary sinus (right). P, pulmonary artery, A, aorta, S, right superior vena cava, CS, coronary sinus.

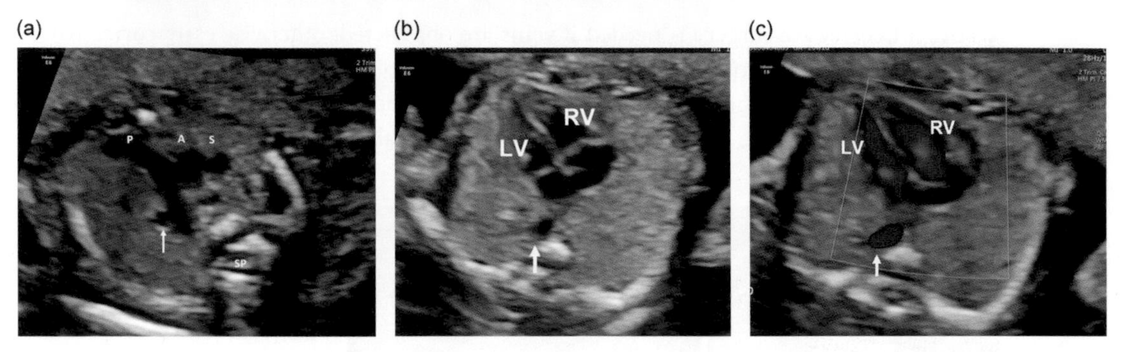

Fig. 3.2.47 Supracardiac total anomalous pulmonary connection. (a) Three vessel view includes the fourth vessel (arrow). (b) Four chamber view shows a 'bald' left atrium and a confluent vessel behind the left atrium. Note absence of a dilated coronary sinus. In (c) colour Doppler detected the inflows to both ventricles and the confluent vessel behind the left atrium. A, aorta; LV, left ventricle; P, pulmonary artery; RV, right ventricle; S, right superior vena cava.

ONLY TWO VESSELS SEEN

- Look for signs of a single outflow tract
- In hypoplastic left heart syndrome (HLHS), two vessels from left to right are the pulmonary artery and superior vena cava (Fig. 3.2.48)
- In hypoplastic right heart the two vessels from left to right are the aorta and SVC
- In severe tetralogy of Fallot with pulmonary atresia the two vessels that will be seen are the aorta and SVC

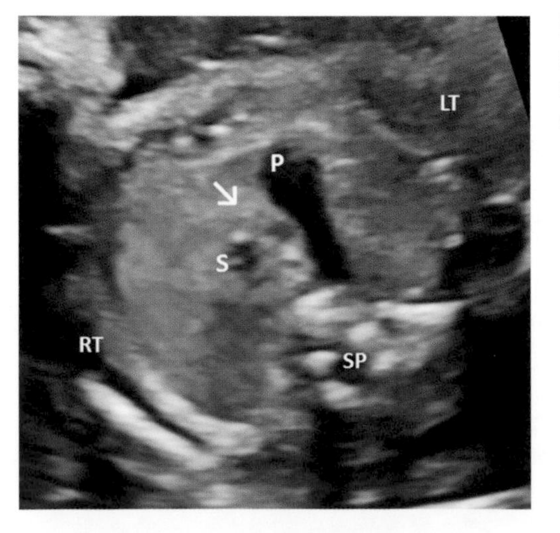

Fig. 3.2.48 Three vessel view showing two vessels in HLHS. Due to aortic atresia, only pulmonary artery (P) and right superior vena cava (S) are seen. Note the increased gap between P and S.

THREE VESSELS: ABNORMAL ARRANGEMENTS

- Absent right SVC with PLSVC
- There is a change in the normal order of three vessels from left to right: superior vena cava, pulmonary artery and aorta (Fig. 3.2.49)

Counselling

- This is considered a normal variant

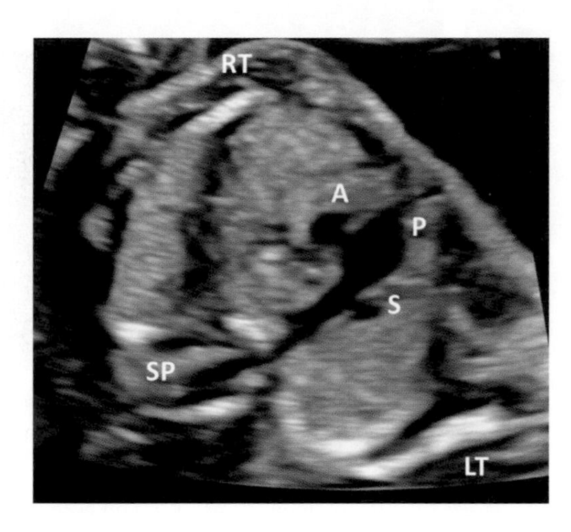

Fig. 3.2.49 Abnormal arrangement in absent right SVC with PLSVC. From left to right, instead of PAS, the order is SPA. A, aorta; P, pulmonary artery; S, Left SVC.

THREE VESSELS: ABNORMAL ALIGNMENTS AND ARRANGEMENT

- If the aorta is anterior to the pulmonary artery, TGA should be suspected (Fig. 3.2.50)
- The diagnosis is confirmed by imaging the origin of the aorta from the right ventricle and the pulmonary artery from the left ventricle

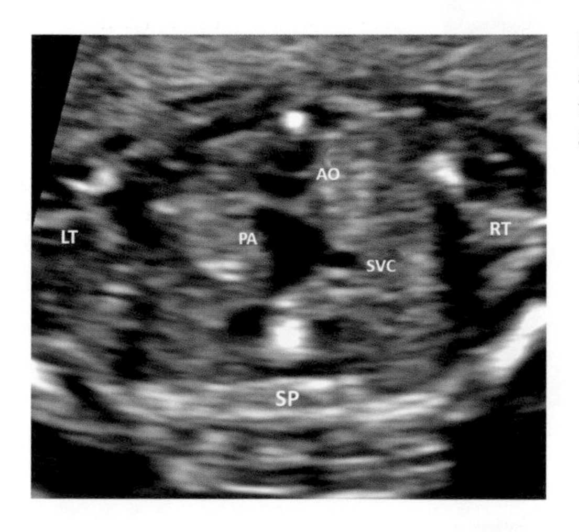

Fig. 3.2.50 Abnormality in alignment and arrangement in TGA. Aorta (AO) lies in front of the pulmonary artery (PA). LT, left; RT, right; SP, spine; SVC, superior vena cava.

THREE VESSELS: ABNORMAL SIZE

- In a normal fetus the pulmonary artery is slightly bigger than the aorta
- When the aorta looks bigger than the pulmonary artery, look for signs of tetralogy of Fallot (Fig. 3.2.51)
- When the superior vena cava looks bigger than the aorta, look for signs of supracardiac TAPVC (Fig. 3.2.52)

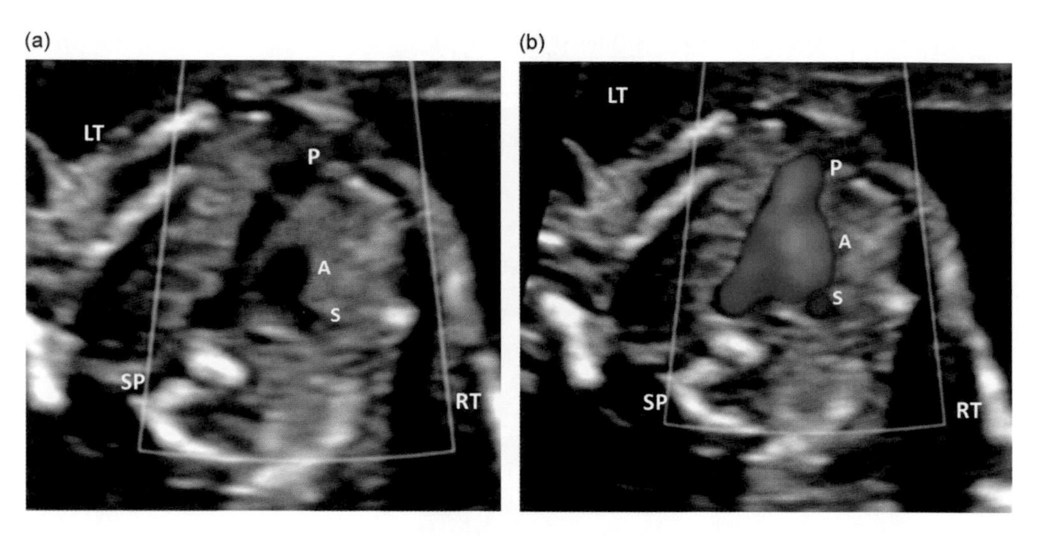

Fig. 3.2.51 Tetralogy of Fallot. The aorta (A) is larger than the pulmonary artery (P) on both (a) B-mode and (b) colour Doppler. LT, left; RT, right; S, superior vena cava; SP, spine.

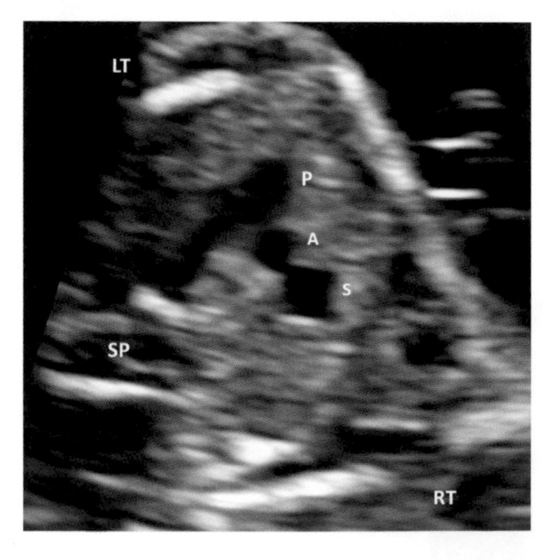

Fig. 3.2.52 Three vessel view showing the right SVC that is bigger than the aorta in TAPVC.

ABNORMAL THREE VESSEL TRACHEA VIEW

RIGHT AORTIC ARCH WITH LEFT DUCTUS

- The three vessel trachea view appears U-shaped instead of the normal V-shape (Fig. 3.2.53)
- The trachea is seen between two arches, forming a partial ring. This is more commonly seen if aberrant left subclavian artery is present
- Normal four chamber view and outflows
- If thymus is absent or small, suspect DiGeorge syndrome

Investigations

- Amniocentesis to exclude 22q11.2 deletion (DiGeorge syndrome)

Counselling

- Normal variant of a vascular anatomy
- Good long-term prognosis if isolated
- The right aortic arch (RAA) forms a vascular ring that may cause tracheal and oesophageal obstruction
- Surgical correction of the vascular ring is required in symptomatic cases
- Postnatal echocardiogram followed, if indicated, with MRI and CT

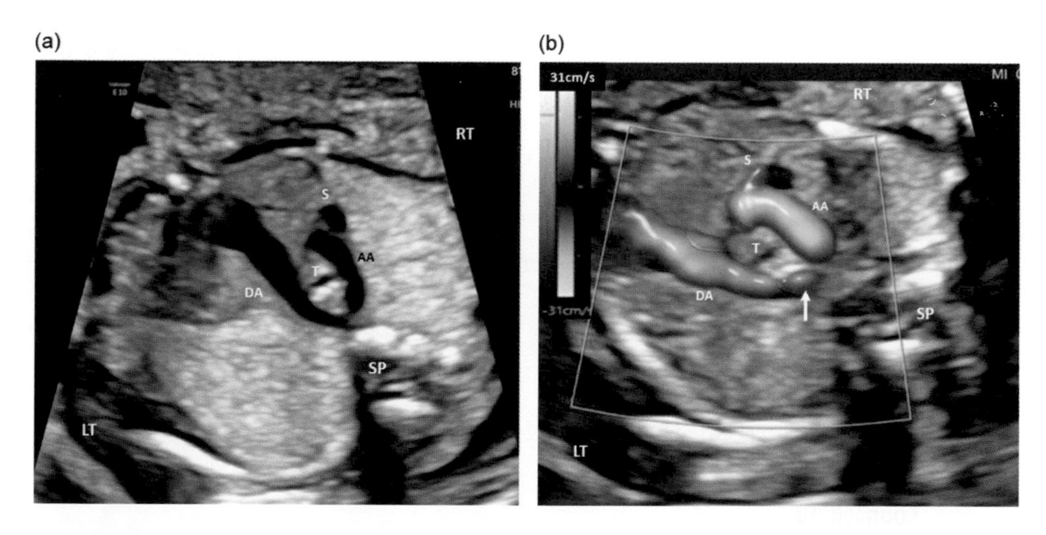

Fig. 3.2.53 Right aortic arch in 3VT view. (a) The trachea is seen between the aorta arch (AA) and ductus (DA). (b) The left ductus is seen behind the trachea (arrow). LT, left; RT, right; S, superior vena; SP, spine.

RIGHT AORTIC ARCH WITH RIGHT DUCTUS

- The 3VT view maintains the V-shape, but the apex of the V points towards the right instead of the left (Fig. 3.2.54)
- The trachea is positioned behind the right ductus
- Aberrant left subclavian artery may be present in ~10% and may form an incomplete vascular ring

Investigations

- Amniocentesis to exclude 22q11.2 deletion (DiGeorge syndrome)

Counselling

- If isolated, it is considered as a normal variant

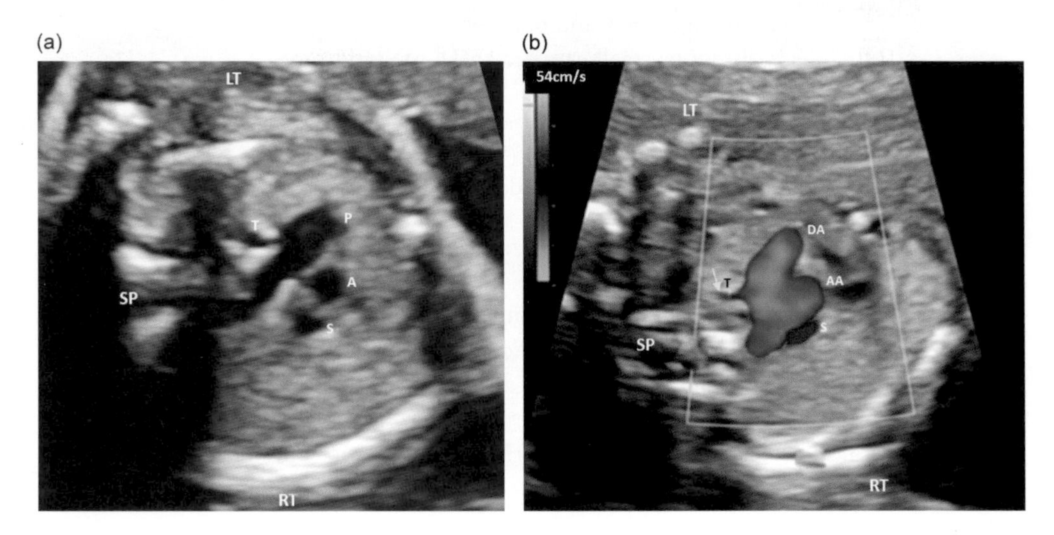

Fig. 3.2.54 Right arch, right ductus. (a) The 3VT looks normal. (b) Both the aortic and ductal arches form a V-shape, but the apex of the V is not pointing towards the left side as usual, it is pointing to the right. The arrow points to the trachea (T).

DOUBLE AORTIC ARCH

- Right and left aortic arch form a complete vascular ring, with the trachea within the circle (Fig. 3.2.55)

Investigations

- Amniocentesis to exclude 22q11.2 deletion (DiGeorge syndrome)

Counselling

- The vascular ring may compress the trachea/oesophagus and cause neonatal respiratory distress
- Children may present with wheezing/stridor or dysphagia and/or respiratory problems in childhood

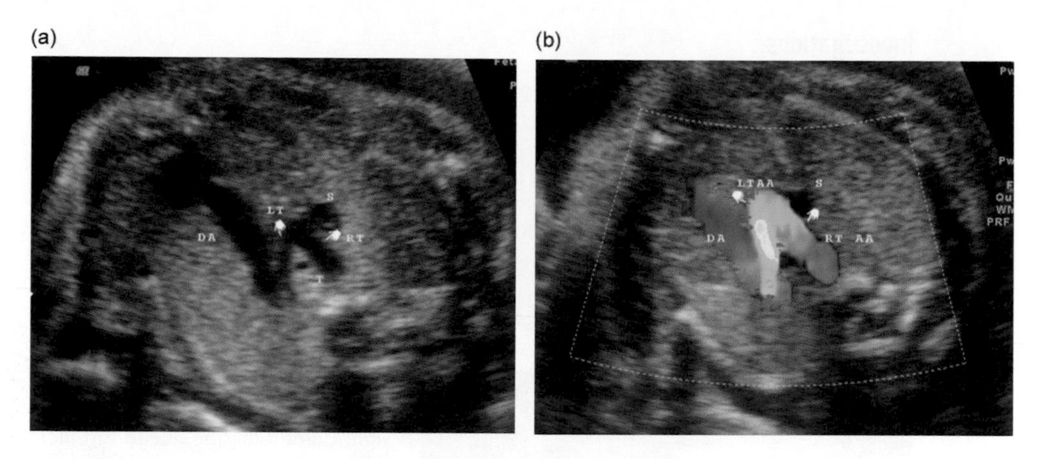

Fig. 3.2.55 Double aortic arch. (a) The trachea (T) is seen between the left and right aortic arch (RT and LT, finger arrows). (b) Colour Doppler shows left aortic arch (LTAA) joining the left ductus (DA). The right aortic arch is also seen.

MIDLINE DESCENDING AORTA

- This is a variation of the left aortic arch
- The confluence of the arches (V sign) is seen in the midline just in front of the vertebral body (Fig. 3.2.56)

Investigations

- None indicated

Counselling

- Normal variant

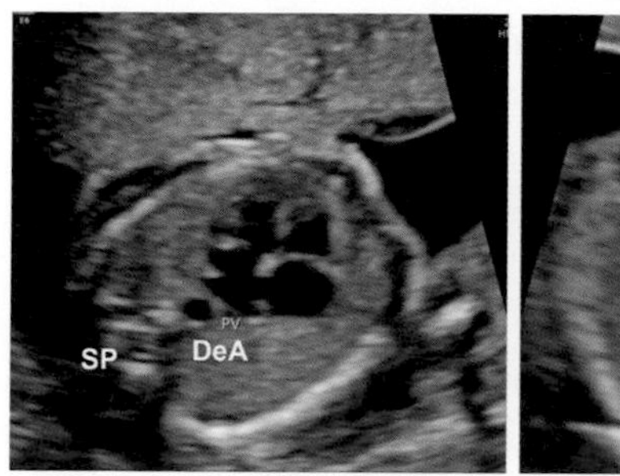

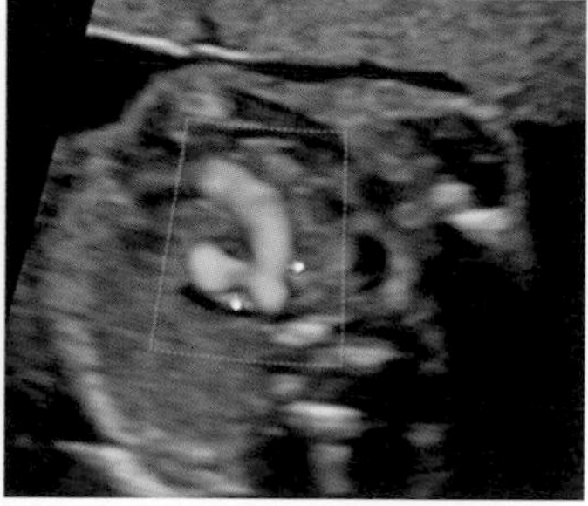

Fig. 3.2.56 Midline descending aorta. (Left) The four chamber view shows descending aorta that lies directly in front of the vertebral body, rather than to the left of the spine. (Right) Colour Doppler shows that the pulmonary artery has a skewed course to continue as the ductus to join the descending aorta. DeA, descending aorta; PV, pulmonary vein.

TORTUOUS DUCTUS

- The ductus courses parallel to the aortic arch
- The ductus joins the transverse arch, resulting in a π sign instead of V sign (Fig. 3.2.57)
- Aneurysm of the ductus arteriosus could be present

Investigations

- Amniocentesis to exclude 22q11.2 deletion (DiGeorge syndrome)

Counselling

- The majority diminish in size as the ductus closes
- Small risk of spontaneous rupture or thromboembolism
- Postnatal evaluation in a paediatric cardiac unit is advisable

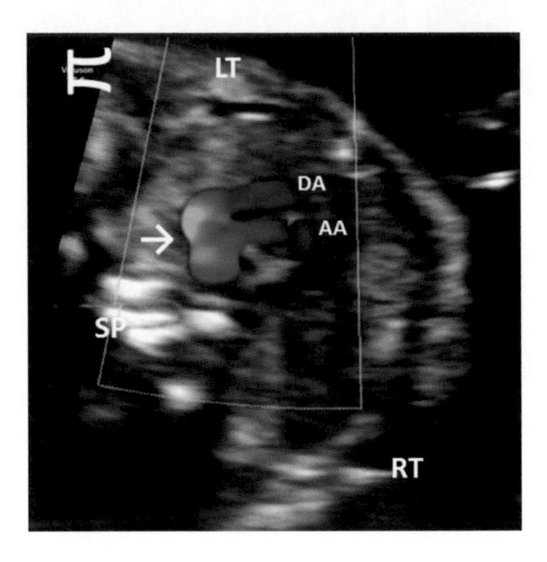

Fig. 3.2.57 Tortuous ductus arteriosus. Confluence of the arches (arrow) is seen as a π sign. Colour aliasing due to turbulent flow in a tortuous ductus arteriosus. AA, aortic arch; DA, ductal arch; LT, left; RT, right; SP, spine.

ABNORMAL CARDIAC RATE AND RHYTHM

Definition and Characteristics

- Arrhythmia (irregular heartbeats) is suspected while assessing heart rate by Doppler or observing the beating heart in real time during a routine examination (Table 3.2.1)
- When rhythm abnormality is suspected, atrial and ventricular rate have to be counted separately to assess AV conduction
- High risk for arrhythmias include:
  - women with anti-RO/SSA and anti-La/SSB autoantibodies since they cross the placenta and may cause conduction disturbances in the fetus
  - previous pregnancy with fetal heart block
  - fetuses with structural heart anomalies, especially those with AVSD, cTGA and heterotaxy
- Fetal bradycardia:
  - heart rate <100 bpm
  - sinus bradycardia – 1:1 conduction
  - complete heart block
- Fetal tachycardia >180 bpm:
  - Sinus tachycardia – fetal heart rate is 180–220 bpm. 1:1 conduction. Associated with maternal fever, infection, maternal beta mimetics or anxiety. If no cause is found, likely to be normal variant

  - Supraventricular tachycardia (SVT) – atrial rate is usually 220–240 bpm. Atrioventricular re-entry type is the most common
  - SVT may be intermittent or sustained. Risk of developing cardiac failure and hydrops
  - Atrial flutter may occur later in pregnancy. Atrial rates may be faster (>300 bpm). Atrioventricular conduction is mostly 2:1 AV conduction, although 1:1 conduction may be seen at slower rates

Ultrasound Assessment

- The following should be considered first if variations in the heart rate are seen:
  - Excessive probe pressure can cause bradycardia. Release of pressure will revert rate to normal
  - Fetal movements can cause variations in beat-to-beat variability. Hence, measurements must always be taken during fetal quiescence
  - Cord compression
  - Fetal hiccups
- Heart rate and rhythm can be assessed by M-mode and pulsed Doppler. Pulsed Doppler is the preferred method
- It is important to exclude structural heart anomalies, in particular heterotaxy and corrected transposition of great arteries

Pulsed Wave Doppler Assessment

- More precise assessment of rhythm is possible (Fig. 3.2.58)
- Mechanical events assessed by timing of blood flow
- Umbilical artery waveforms represent ventricular rate

M-Mode Assessment

- The cursor is placed across the right atrium and a ventricle (Fig. 3.2.59)
- Atrial rate and ventricular rate can be assessed (Fig. 3.2.60)
- Assessment of AV valves is difficult
- Timing of cardiac events is also difficult
- Ventricular and atrial rates are measured separately when abnormal rate or rhythm is suspected

Counselling

- If fetal heart rate is very low in combination with hydrops and valvular regurgitation, parents should be warned about the high risk of in utero demise. In such cases preterm delivery may be of benefit, but neonatologists and paediatric cardiologists should be consulted to carefully balance the benefits with risk of prematurity

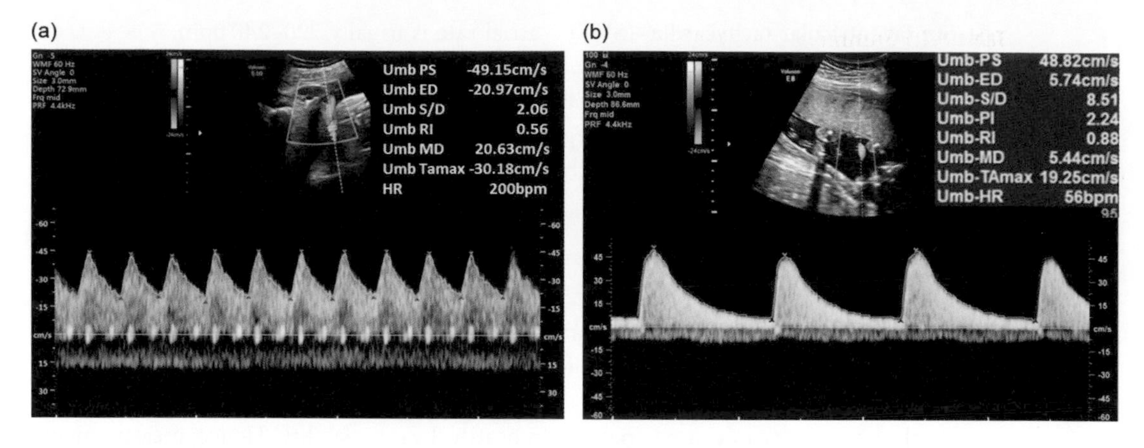

Fig. 3.2.58 Fetal supraventricular (a) tachycardia and (b) bradycardia.

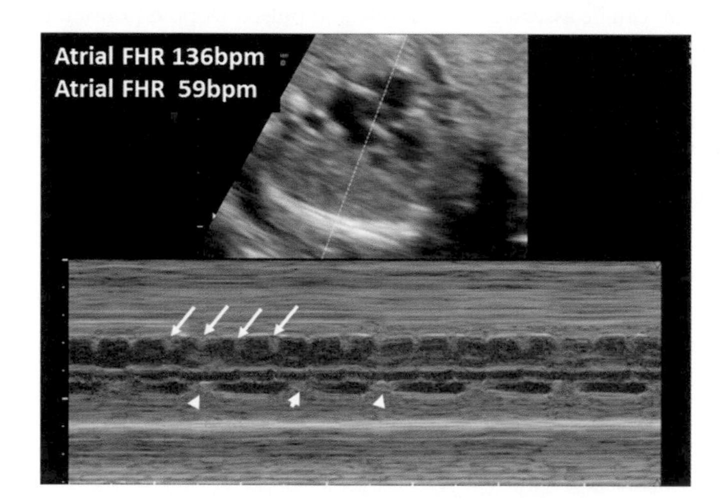

Fig. 3.2.59 M-mode tracing showing AV dissociation – complete heart block. Atrial rate is 136 bpm (arrows). Ventricular rate is 59 bpm (arrowheads).

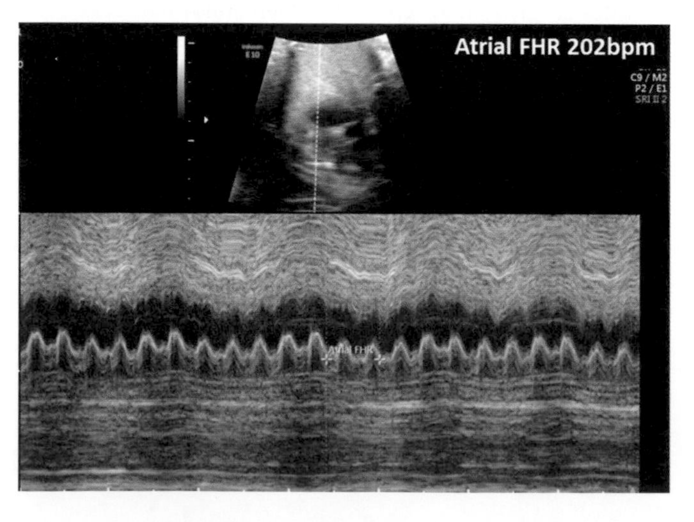

Fig. 3.2.60 M-mode tracing in a case of supra ventricular tachycardia. Heart rate is 202 bpm.

Table 3.2.1 Summary of arrhythmias

Fetal heart rate & pattern	Pulsed Doppler and M-mode	Type of arrhythmia
<60 bpm: Fixed and persistent pattern	• Complete AV dissociation • Normal atrial rate of 110–160 bpm with reduced ventricular rate	• Complete heart block
60–80 bpm	• Atrial bigeminy which is not conducted	• Non-conducted bigeminy or 2nd/3rd degree heart block • May be difficult to differentiate from 2:1 block
<110 bpm: Fixed pattern	Bradycardia with 1:1 conduction	• Sinus bradycardia

Management

- Check maternal autoantibodies (anti SSA-Ro and La).
- Maternal 12 lead ECG and family history of arrhythmia should be obtained.
- **Sinus bradycardia** is not associated with fetal distress and does not require treatment.
- **Blocked atrial ectopics** – bigeminy or trigeminy; no treatment is required.
- **Complete heart block** – there is no consensus on optimal treatment. Mainly dexamethasone (4–8 mg daily, tapered to 2 mg toward the end of pregnancy). Intravenous immunoglobulin therapy has also been tried, either alone or in combination with betamethasone.

Fetal heart rate & pattern	Pulsed Doppler and M-mode	Type of arrhythmia
100–160 bpm: Varying heart rates	• Atrial and ventricular rates equal • Every atrial contraction is followed by a ventricular contraction (1:1 conduction) with normal AV intervals	• Sinus rhythm

Management

- No action needed.

Fetal heart rate & pattern	Pulsed Doppler and M-mode	Type of arrhythmia
50–180 bpm: Irregular rhythm with 1:1 conduction	• 1:1 conduction. Atrial contractions appearing early.	• Premature atrial contractions or premature ventricular contractions
50–180 bpm with sudden drops in heart rate with difference between atrial and ventricular rates	• Some atrial contractions not followed by ventricular contractions	• Blocked atrial beats
	• Every 2 atrial beats are followed by a ventricular beat	• Blocked atrial bigeminy or ectopic atrial tachycardia

Management

- **Premature atrial contractions or blocked atrial beats** do not require active management before birth. Whilst most recover spontaneously some may convert to supraventricular tachycardia.

Fetal heart rate & pattern	Pulsed Doppler and M-mode	Type of arrhythmia
180 to 220 bpm with regular heart rate pattern: May be sustained or with intermittent normal rates	1:1 conduction with normal AV time intervals	• Persistent supraventricular tachycardia (SVT) • Permanent junctional reciprocating tachycardia

Management

- **Intermittent SVT** with no hydrops – expectant management with monitoring 2–3 times a week.
- **Sustained tachycardia** – digoxin, flecainide, Sotalol or amiodarone. Dose estimated as per fetal weight. Success rates 80–90%. Five per cent mortality in hydropic cases. Delivery should be in a tertiary unit with paediatric cardiac facilities.

COMMON ANTENATALLY DIAGNOSED CARDIAC ANOMALIES

HYPOPLASTIC LEFT HEART SYNDROME

Description and Characteristics

- Underdeveloped left heart structures (left ventricle, mitral valve, aorta and aortic arch)
- Valves may or may not be atretic
- Incidence ~2 in 10,000 births
- Inheritance – mainly sporadic, but in some families gene mutations have been implicated (*GJA1*, *NKX2*, *NOTCH1*, *HAND1*)
- 22q microdeletion rarely reported

Key Ultrasound Features

- Small left ventricle with no or minimal filling with colour Doppler (Fig. 3.2.61)
- Abnormal three vessel view:
  - small aorta (Fig. 3.2.62)
  - retrograde filling in the transverse arch (Fig. 3.2.63)

Differential Diagnosis

- Unbalanced AVSD
- Single ventricle with indeterminate morphology

Investigations

- Amniocentesis for chromosomal microarray and DNA storage is recommended

Counselling

- Late intrauterine death can occur due to restricted foramen ovale (Fig. 3.2.64)
- In utero transfer to tertiary centre with advanced paediatric cardiology
- Poor long-term prognosis
- Complex staged surgery is needed – mainly palliative
- Long-term neurological sequelae are likely

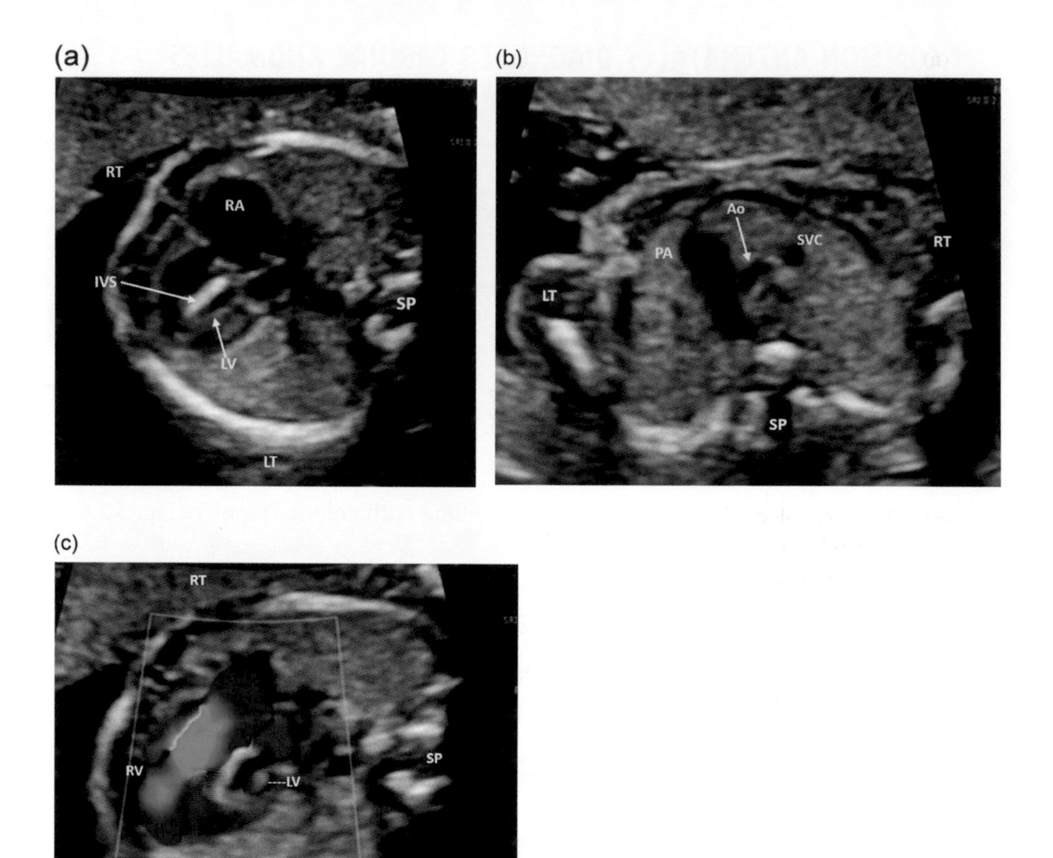

Fig. 3.2.61 (a) Four chamber view showing hypoplastic left ventricle with echogenic interventricular septum (IVS) due to endocardial fibroelastosis. (b) Three vessel view showing small aorta denoted by arrow. (c) Colour Doppler filling in right ventricle (RV) and no filling in left ventricle (LV). Note the apex forming right ventricle 'overhanging' left ventricle. Ao, aorta; IVS, interventricular septum; LT, left; LV, left ventricle; PA, pulmonary artery; RA, right atrium; RT, right; SP, spine; SVC, superior vena cava.

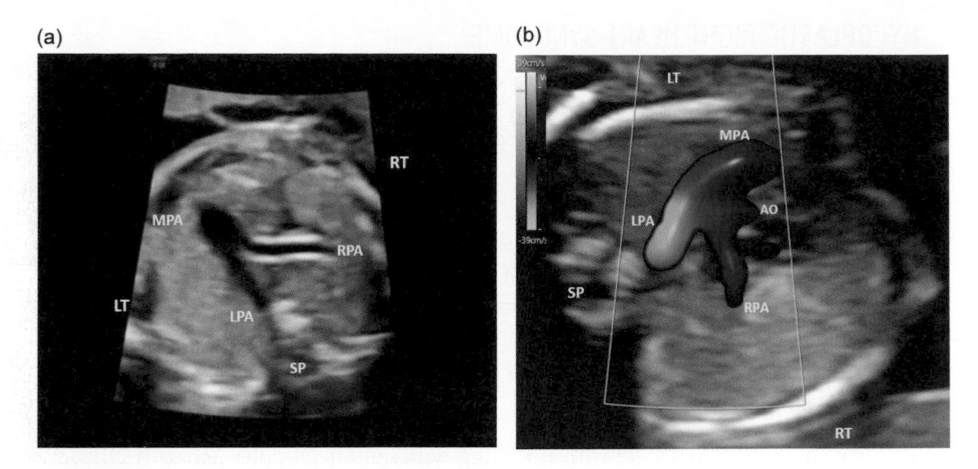

Fig. 3.2.62 Hypoplastic left heart syndrome. Pulmonary artery with branches in (a) B-mode and (b) in colour Doppler. The aorta, which is smaller, is not seen well in B-mode, but is visible in colour Doppler. The bright wall of the right pulmonary artery is due to specular reflection. LPA, left pulmonary artery; MPA, main pulmonary artery; RPA, right pulmonary artery

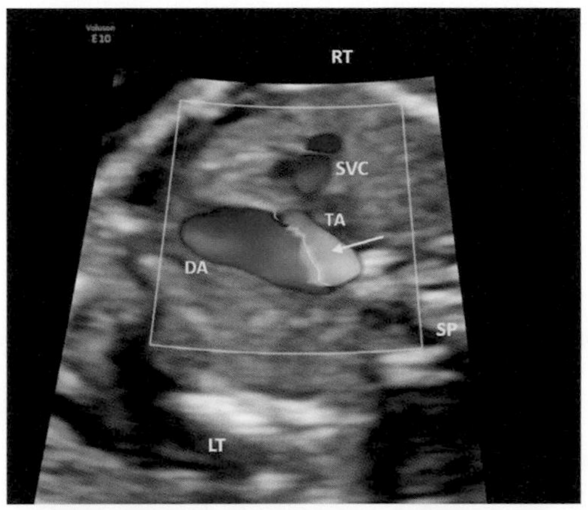

Fig. 3.2.63 Hypoplastic left heart syndrome. Retrograde colour Doppler flow in the transverse arch (arrow).

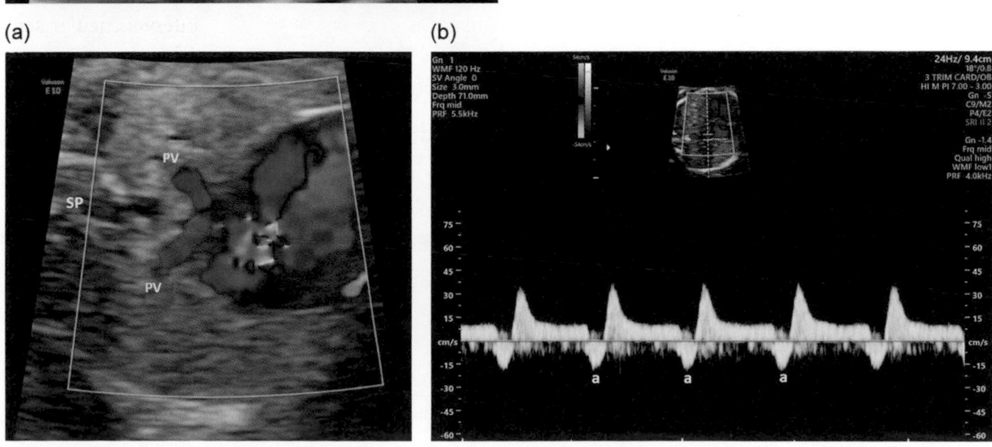

Fig. 3.2.64 Hypoplastic left heart syndrome. Colour Doppler showing pulmonary veins (PV) draining into the left atrium. Pulsed Doppler of the pulmonary vein showing flow reversal (a) in the pulmonary vein which is indicative of restrictive foramen ovale.

HYPOPLASTIC RIGHT HEART SYNDROME

Description and Characteristics

- Underdeveloped right heart structures (right ventricle, tricuspid valve, pulmonary artery). Valves may or may not be atretic
- Incidence ~1 in 15,000 births
- Familial cases are very rare
- 22q microdeletion may be present if pulmonary atresia is present

Key Ultrasound Features

Intact Ventricular Septum

- Very small right ventricle with no filling with colour Doppler across tricuspid valve (Fig 3.2.65)
- Abnormal 3VV and 3VT – small pulmonary artery (Fig 3.2.66)
- Retrograde flow in the ductus arteriosus (Fig 3.2.67)

With Ventricular Septal Defect

- Smaller right ventricle but outflow portion is formed
- Atretic tricuspid valve with no flow across it
- Small pulmonary artery in 3VV
- Flow through VSD into the right ventricle causes antegrade flow in the pulmonary artery

Differential Diagnosis

- Critical pulmonary stenosis with intact septum

Investigations

- Amniocentesis for chromosomal microarray and DNA storage is recommended

Counselling

- Delivery in tertiary centre with advanced paediatric cardiology should be arranged when pulmonary atresia/stenosis is suspected
- Staged palliative surgeries are needed after birth
- Arrhythmias and exercise intolerance are common – guarded long-term prognosis

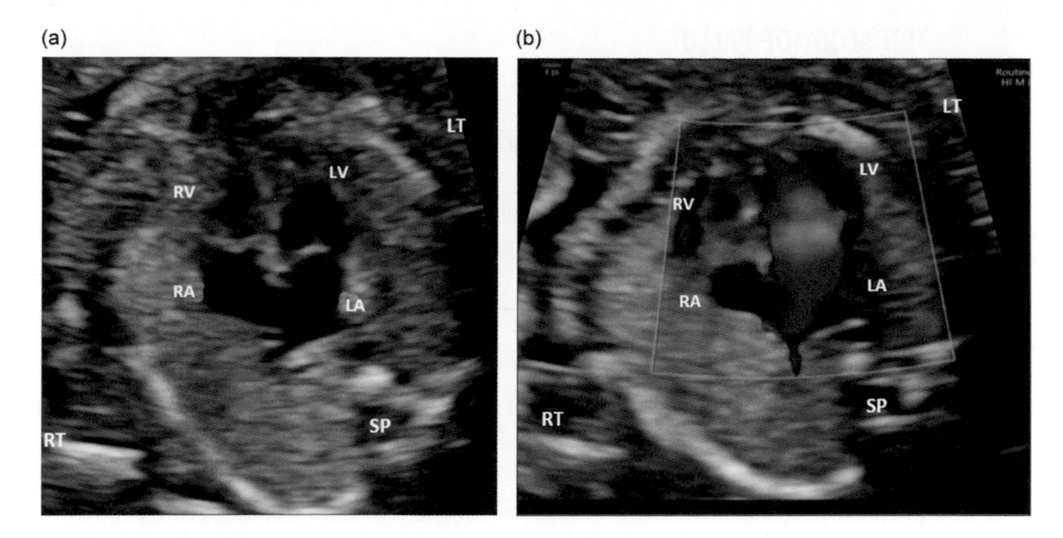

Fig. 3.2.65 Hypoplastic right heart syndrome. (a) Apical four chamber view showing hypoplastic right ventricle with intact septum. (b) No colour filling across the tricuspid valve. LA, left atrium; LT, left; LV, left ventricle; RA, right atrium; RT, right; RV, right ventricle; SP, spine.

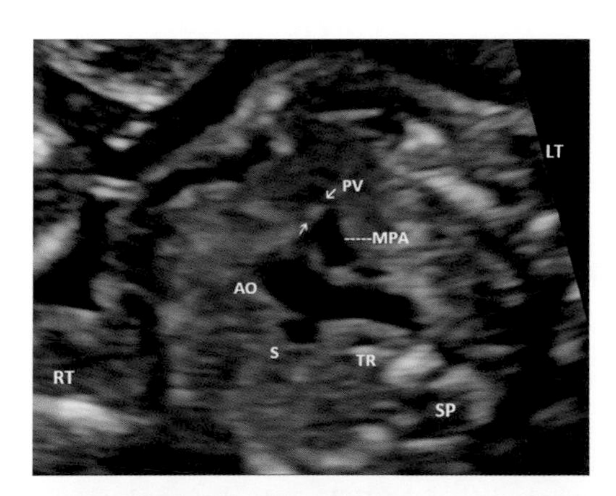

Fig. 3.2.66 Hypoplastic right heart syndrome. 3VT view in HRHS showing thickened pulmonary valve (arrows). The main pulmonary artery (MPA) is smaller than the aorta. LT, left; RT, right; S, superior vena cava; SP, spine; TR, trachea.

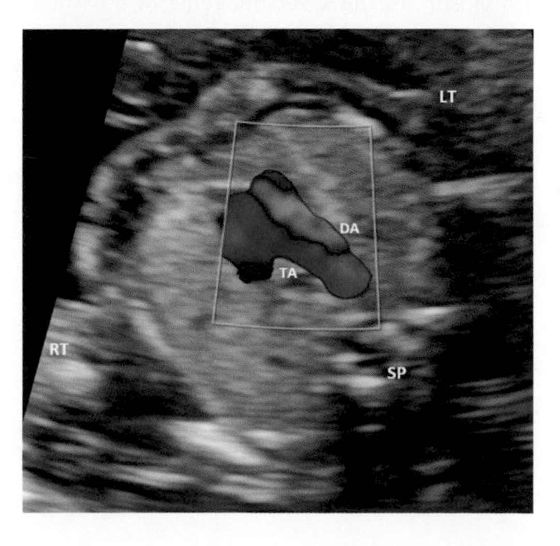

Fig. 3.2.67 Hypoplastic right heart syndrome. Transverse arch (TA) showing normal direction colour in blue. Reversed colour Doppler flow in the ductus arteriosus (DA) seen in red.

TETRALOGY OF FALLOT

Description and Characteristics

- Subaortic VSD, aortic overriding and pulmonary stenosis
- Incidence ~1 in 3,000 births
- Syndromic – 22q11 deletion; trisomies 21, 13, and 18; Noonan, Alagille syndromes
- Teratogen exposure – alcohol, anticonvulsants, retinoic acid
- Maternal illness – phenylketonuria, diabetes

Key Ultrasound Features

- Four chamber view is usually normal (Fig. 3.2.68). In some cases the cardiac axis is rotated to the left
- In the 3VV view the pulmonary artery is smaller than the aorta (Fig. 3.2.69)
- Malaligned subaortic VSD with dilated aortic root and overriding aorta in left ventricular outflow tract (LVOT) view. Aorta is committed to both ventricles (Figs. 3.2.70 and 3.2.71)
- High-velocity flow in the pulmonary artery due to pulmonary stenosis. Colour Doppler aliasing in right ventricular outflow tract (RVOT) view

Differential Diagnosis

- VSD with pulmonary atresia
- Double outlet right ventricle (DORV) with pulmonary stenosis
- Truncus arteriosus

Investigations

- Amniocentesis for chromosomal microarray and DNA storage is recommended

Counselling

- Delivery in a tertiary centre with advanced paediatric cardiology
- Major, surgically correctable heart defect
- The definitive repair is surgical, with closure of the VSD and relief of obstruction to pulmonary blood flow
- Type of corrective staged surgery depends on the severity of the pulmonary obstruction
- Pulmonary valve replacement may be needed in adolescence/adulthood

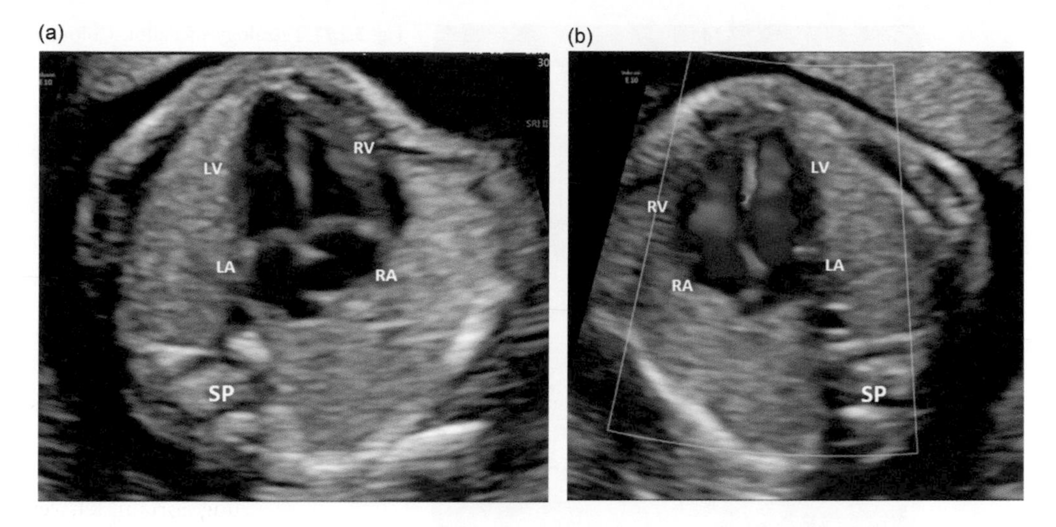

Fig. 3.2.68 Tetralogy of Fallot. The apical four chamber view appears normal on (a) B-mode and shows (b) normal inflow colour Doppler filling of both ventricles (LV, RV). LA, left atrium; RA, right atrium; SP, spine.

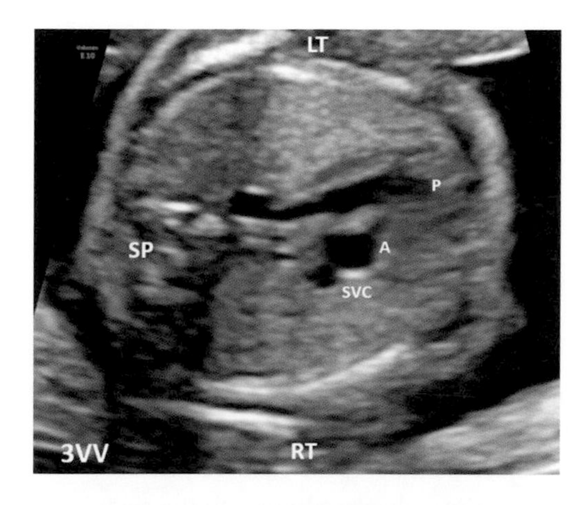

Fig. 3.2.69 Tetralogy of Fallot. Three vessel view in the same patient showing the pulmonary artery (P) which is smaller than the aorta (A). The superior vena cava (SVC) appears normal.

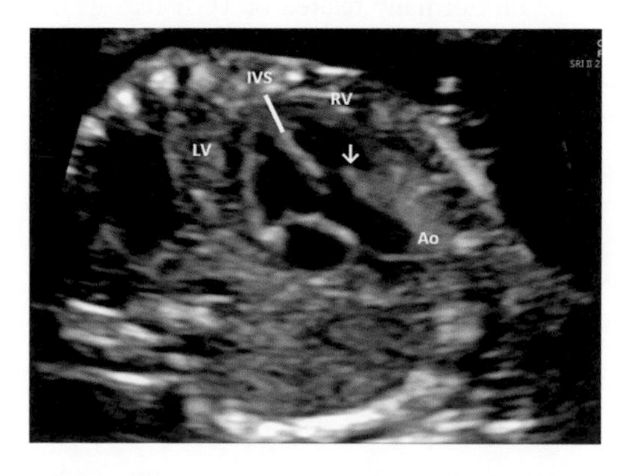

Fig. 3.2.70 Tetralogy of Fallot. LVOT view showing the aorta committed to both ventricles (LV, RV). Aortic override in systole showing the anterior aortic wall (arrow) not continuous with interventricular septum (IVS).

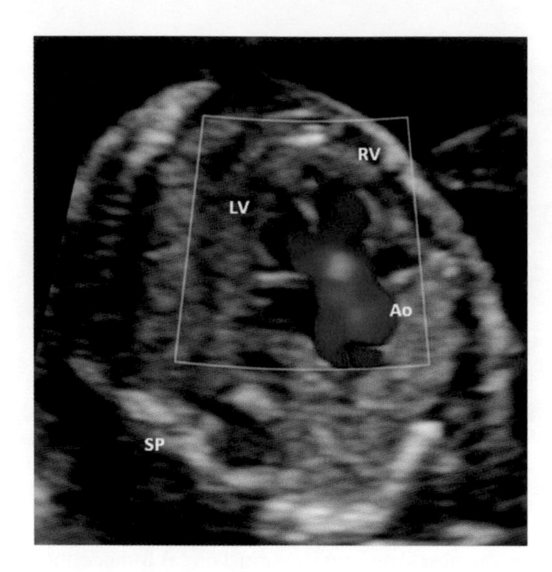

Fig. 3.2.71 Tetralogy of Fallot. Colour Doppler showing flow from both ventricles into the aorta (Ao). Ao, aorta; LV, left ventricle; RV, right ventricle; SP, spine

DOUBLE OUTLET RIGHT VENTRICLE

Description and Characteristics

- This is defined as a lesion where both great arteries arise exclusively or predominantly (at least 50%) from the right ventricle
- Virtually all cases have a VSD; the position and size are variable
- DORV with transposition-like arrangement of great vessels (TGA): both outflow tracts are parallel
- DORV with tetralogy of Fallot physiology: the great vessels are normally related
- Incidence ~1 in 20,000 births

Key Ultrasound Features

- The four chamber view can be normal or there can be ventricular disproportion with a larger right ventricle; VSD and straddling valves can be noted in this view (Figs. 3.2.72 and 3.2.73)
- Both outflow tracts arising from (or more than 50%) the right ventricle
- In the three vessel view, the aorta is anteriorly displaced more to the right
- Three vessel view is variable, depending on normally related or TGA-like arrangement of great vessels
- Parallel outflow tracts are seen (Fig. 3.2.74)

Differential Diagnosis

- Subaortic VSD
- Tetralogy of Fallot
- Transposition of great arteries with VSD

Investigations

- Amniocentesis for chromosomal microarray and DNA storage is recommended (22q11 deletion)

Counselling

- Delivery in a tertiary centre with advanced paediatric cardiology
- The surgical correction depends on the size and location of VSD and relationship of the great arteries
- Single-stage corrective surgery after birth when outflows are normally related
- Staged surgery will be needed if there are unbalanced chambers and outflow tract obstruction or great arteries are placed remote from VSD, leading to univentricular palliation (i.e. Fontan pathway)

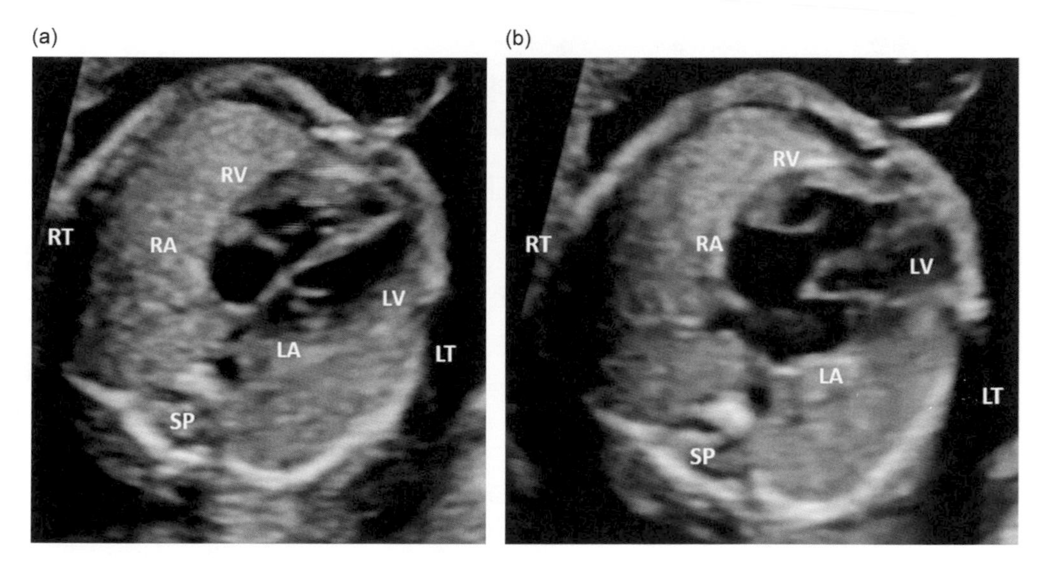

Fig. 3.2.72 Double outlet right ventricle. Apical four chamber view in (a) systole and (b) diastole. Note the chamber asymmetry with a larger right ventricle. LA, left atrium; LT, left; LV, left ventricle; RA, right atrium; RT, right; RV, right ventricle; SP, spine.

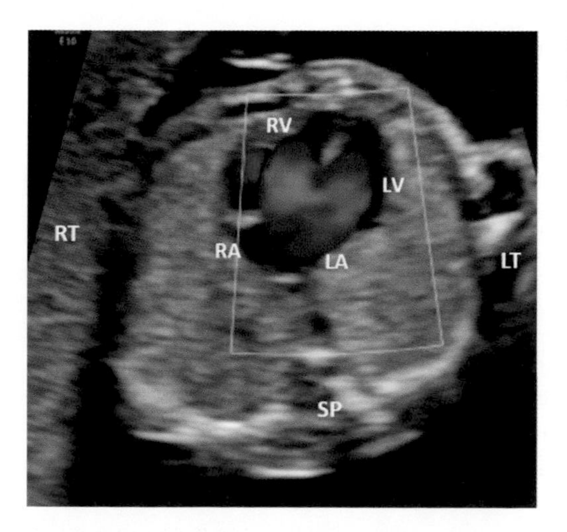

Fig. 3.2.73 Double outlet right ventricle: four chamber view with VSD shows normal filling of ventricles.

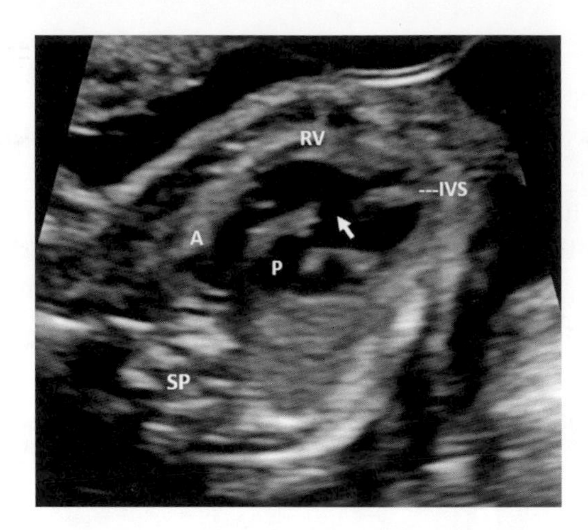

Fig. 3.2.74 Double outlet right ventricle. Parallel outflow tracts and a large muscular VSD are present (arrow). A, aorta; IVS, interventricular septum; P, pulmonary artery; RV, right ventricle; SP, spine.

TRANSPOSITION OF THE GREAT ARTERIES

Description and Characteristics

- Atrioventricular concordance with ventriculoarterial discordance
- Incidence ~1 in 3,500 births

Key Ultrasound Features

- Normal four chamber view
- Only two vessels in the 3VV view (aorta and SVC)
- In the 3VT view, the aorta and pulmonary artery are seen as a single line because the PA is parallel and posterior to the aorta – 'I' sign (Fig. 3.2.75)
- The outflow tracts are parallel (Fig. 3.2.76)

Differential Diagnosis

- Double outlet right ventricle
- Corrected transposition of great arteries

Investigations

- Amniocentesis for chromosomal microarray and DNA storage is recommended (22q11 deletion reported in some cases)

Counselling

- Delivery in a tertiary centre with advanced paediatric cardiology
- With intact septum and wide open foramen ovale, prostaglandin infusion will be needed
- Early major neonatal surgery (arterial switch) with good outcomes
- Later in life, further surgery or catheter intervention may be needed for outflow stenosis

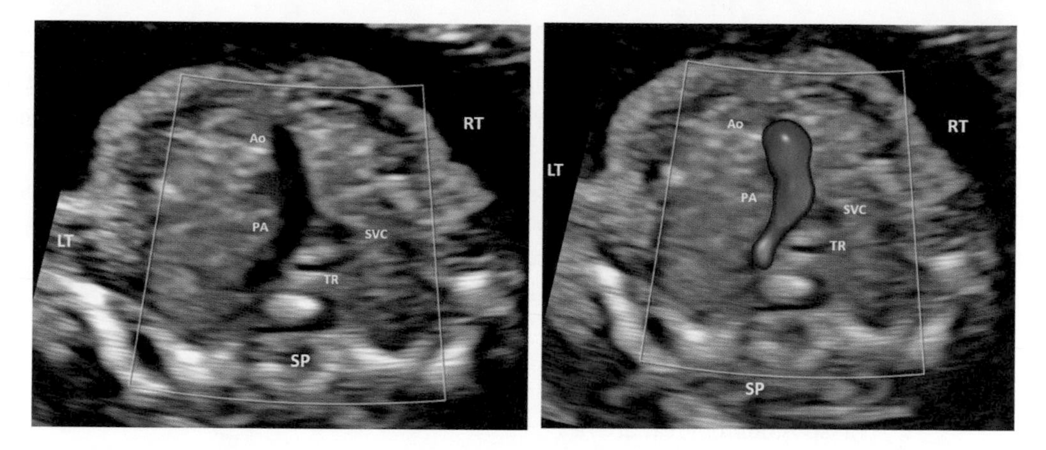

Fig. 3.2.75 Transposition of the great arteries. In the 3VT view, the aorta (Ao) and pulmonary artery (PA) are seen as a single line since the PA is parallel and posterior to the aorta. This is termed as the "I" sign. Superimposed colour Doppler flow demonstrates flow in the pulmonary artery. LT, left; RT, right; SP, spine; SVC, superior vena cava; TR, trachea.

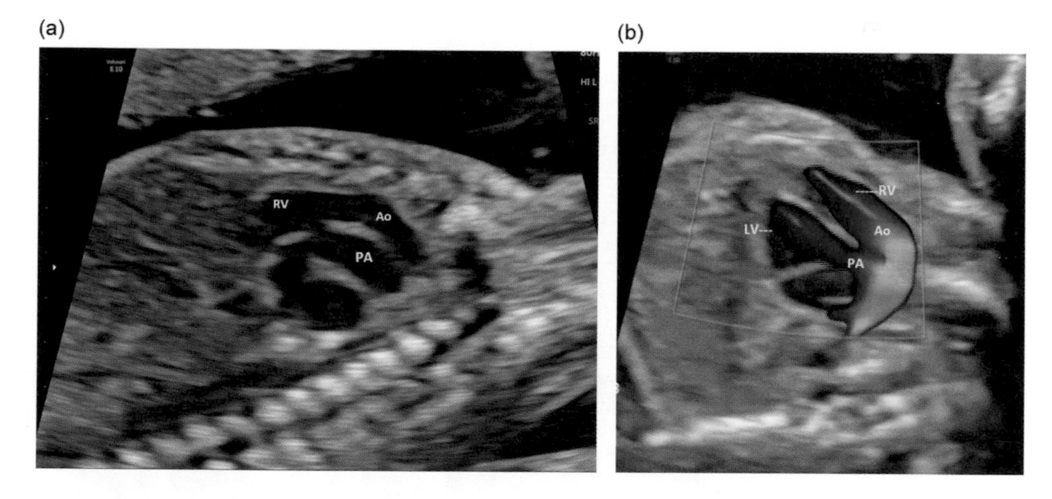

Fig. 3.2.76 Sagittal view in B-mode (a) and colour showing parallel outflow tracts (b). Ao, aorta; LV, left ventricle; PA, pulmonary artery; RV, right ventricle.

CORRECTED TRANSPOSITION OF THE GREAT ARTERIES

Description and Characteristics

- Atrioventricular and ventriculoarterial discordance
- Left atrium is connected to the right ventricle
- Right atrium is connected to the left ventricle
- Aorta arises from the right ventricle
- Pulmonary artery arises from the left ventricle (Fig. 3.2.77)
- Incidence ~1 in 33,000 births

Key Ultrasound Features

- In the four chamber view there is a reverse atrioventricular valve offset. The left-sided ventricle is morphologically the right ventricle with tricuspid valve and more apical septal hinge point
- The left-sided ventricle has coarse trabeculation and moderator band and the right-sided ventricle will be smooth (morphologically the left ventricle)
- In 3VV view only two vessels are seen
- The aorta is anterior and to the left of the pulmonary artery (Fig. 3.2.78)

Differential Diagnosis

- Transposition of great arteries

Investigations

- Amniocentesis for chromosomal microarray and DNA storage is recommended

Counselling

- Most newborns will have a stable haemodynamics and do not require immediate intervention
- Can be delivered in level II unit unless heart block is noted
- In the absence of other cardiac lesions, yearly follow-up is arranged
- Corrective surgery is complex and a double-switch operation is performed only in selected cases

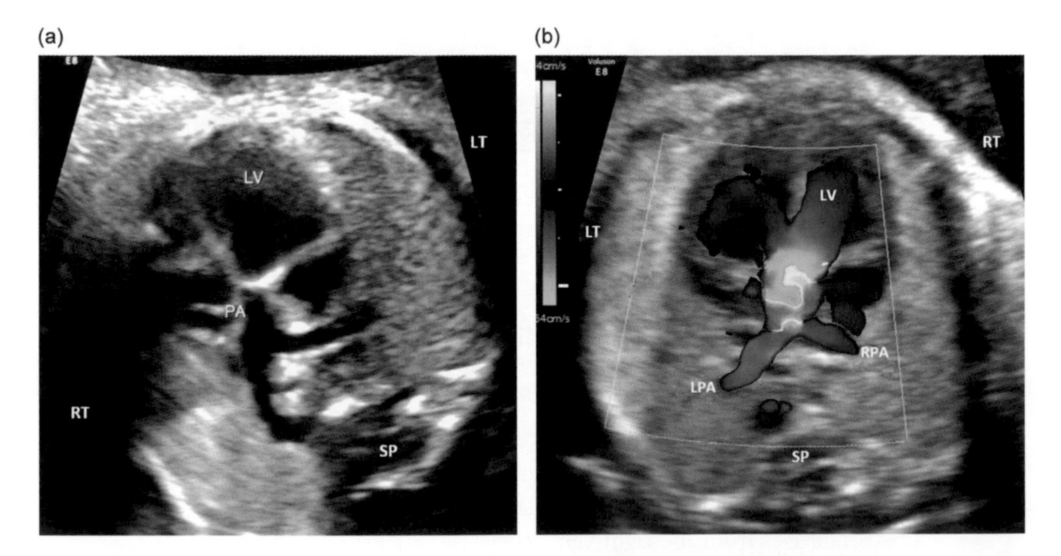

Fig. 3.2.77 Corrected transposition of the great arteries. (a) The pulmonary artery is seen arising from the left ventricle (LV). (b) Colour Doppler filling in systole showing the main pulmonary artery (identified by the branches) arising from the left ventricle. LPA, left pulmonary artery; LT, left; RPA, right pulmonary artery; RT, right; SP, spine.

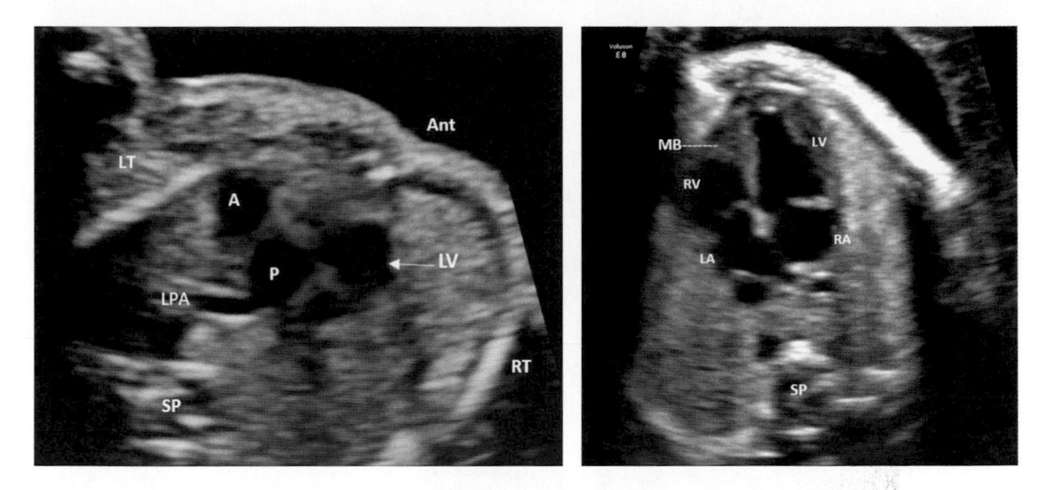

Fig. 3.2.78 Corrected transposition of the great arteries. Transverse section of the heart above the level of the four chamber view with the aorta (A) seen anterior and to the left of the pulmonary artery (P). The portion of the left ventricle is seen on the right side (LV). LPA, left pulmonary artery; LT, left; RT, right; SP, spine.

CRITICAL AORTIC STENOSIS

Description and Characteristics

- Narrowing at the level of the aortic valve leading to left ventricular outflow obstruction
- Incidence ~1 in 2,500 births

Key Ultrasound Features

- The four chamber view shows dilated, globular, non-contractile, echogenic left ventricle with no forward flow across the mitral valve and variable degree of mitral regurgitation (Figs. 3.2.79 and 3.2.80)
- The left ventricle becomes very hypoplastic in the later part of the pregnancy
- Thickened aortic valves with post-stenotic dilatation (Fig. 3.2.81)
- Colour Doppler aliasing across the aortic valve
- Retrograde flow in the aortic arch (Fig. 3.2.82)
- Pulsed wave peak systolic velocity at the aortic valve site may be elevated >100 cm/s or may be within normal range, reflecting reduced left ventricular function

Differential Diagnosis

- Cardiomyopathy

Investigations

- Amniocentesis for chromosomal microarray is recommended

Counselling

- Explain the evolving nature and need for postnatal intervention
- Mild stenosis can be delivered locally with postnatal echo and regular follow-up
- For severe (critical) stenosis, in selected cases there remains a potential to intervene before birth (in utero fetal aortic balloon valvuloplasty has been attempted to prevent progression to HLHS)
- Delivery should be in a tertiary centre with advanced paediatric cardiology as prostaglandin infusion is needed after birth with early intervention – either percutaneous balloon dilatation or surgical valvotomy
- If the left heart structure is not adequately developed then staged surgical procedure towards univentricular palliation will be required

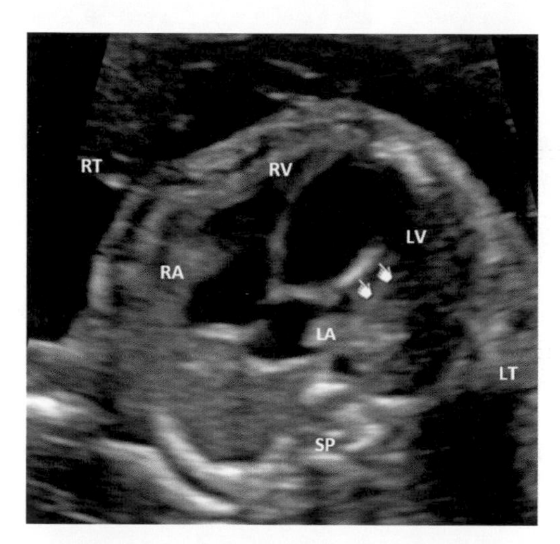

Fig. 3.2.79 Critical aortic stenosis. Apical four chamber view showing dilated globular left ventricle (LV). Echogenic papillary muscle is seen (arrows) indicative of endocardial fibroelastosis. LA, left atrium; LT, left; LV, left ventricle; RA, right atrium; RT, right; RV, right ventricle; SP, spine.

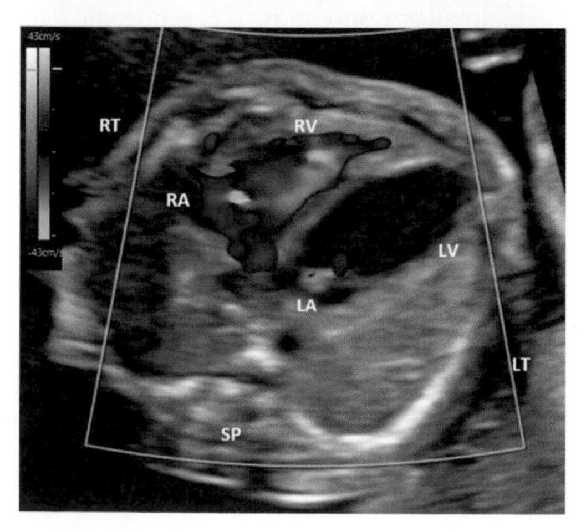

Fig. 3.2.80 Critical aortic stenosis. Absent colour Doppler filling of the left ventricle (LV). LA, left atrium; LT, left; RA, right atrium; RT, right; RV, right ventricle; SP, spine.

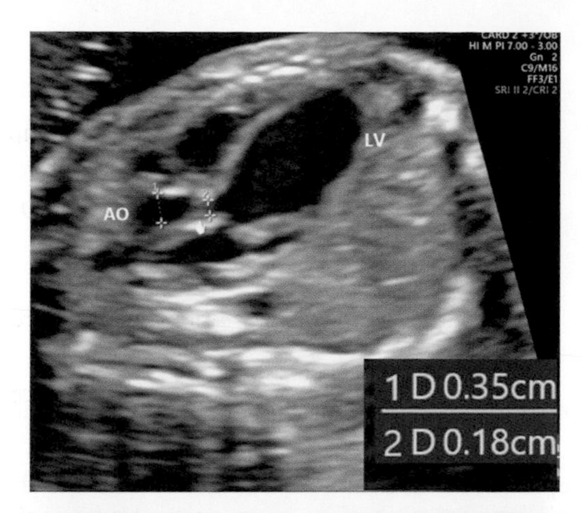

Fig. 3.2.81 Critical aortic stenosis. LVOT view shows a thickened aortic valve with post-stenotic dilatation.

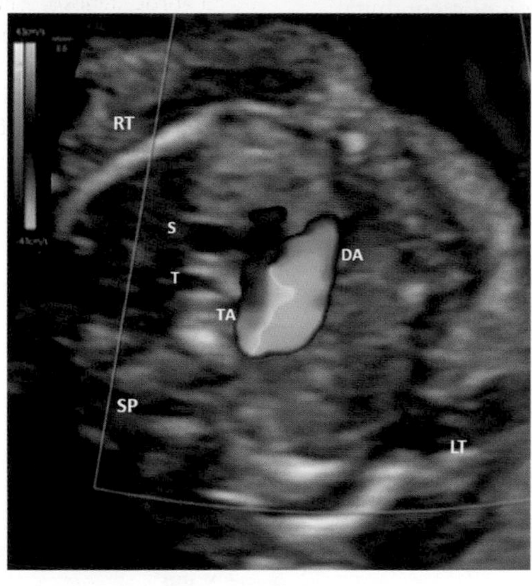

Fig. 3.2.82 In the 3VT view, the ductal arch (DA) shows normal flow but the aortic arch (TA) shows retrograde flow). LT, left; RT, right; S, superior vena cava; SP, spine; T, trachea.

COMMON ARTERIAL TRUNK

Description and Characteristics

- Also known as truncus arteriosus
- A single arterial trunk from which systemic, coronary and pulmonary branches originate
- Incidence ~1 in 10,000 births

Key Ultrasound Features

- The four chamber view is usually normal – in some cases the apex may be rotated to the left
- VSD with large overriding vessel in the LVOT view
- Single outflow tract (Figs. 3.2.83 and 3.2.84)
- Thickened dysplastic valve committed to both ventricles
- Single arch – two vessels in 3VV/3VT views (Fig. 3.2.85)
- No flow reversal in the single arch
- Usually absent ductus arteriosus

Differential Diagnosis

- Pulmonary atresia with VSD

Investigations

- Amniocentesis for chromosomal microarray is recommended (22q11 deletion)

Counselling

- Delivery in a tertiary centre with advanced paediatric cardiology
- Prostaglandin infusion is usually not indicated unless there is an interrupted aortic arch or duct-dependent circulation
- Surgical repair consists of VSD repair and connection of the right ventricle to the pulmonary circulation (i.e. insertion of a conduit)
- Replacement of the right ventricle to pulmonary artery conduit is usually required in childhood
- Poor prognosis with truncal valve regurgitation

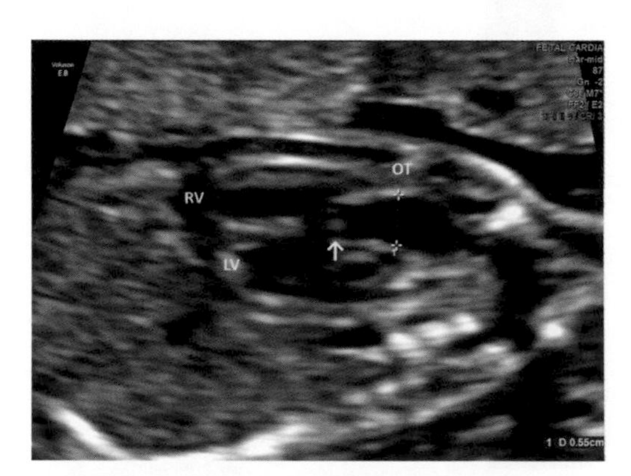

Fig. 3.2.83 Common arterial trunk (OT). Ventricular septal defect (arrow) with large overriding vessel in the left ventricular outflow tract view (LVOT). RV, right ventricle; LV left ventricle.

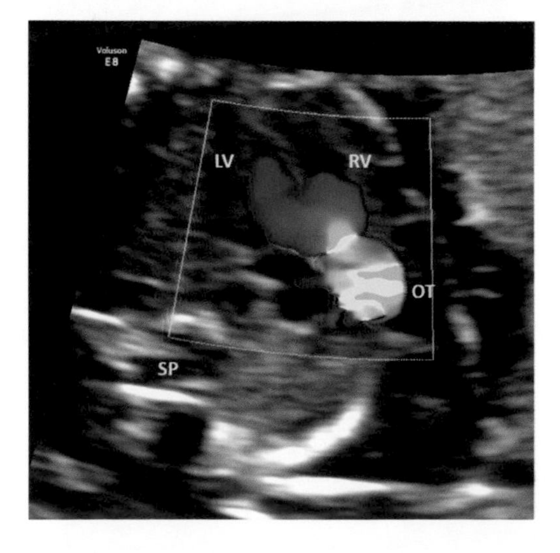

Fig. 3.2.84 Common arterial trunk (OT) with turbulent colour Doppler flow seen as aliasing. RV, right ventricle; LV, left ventricle; SP, spine.

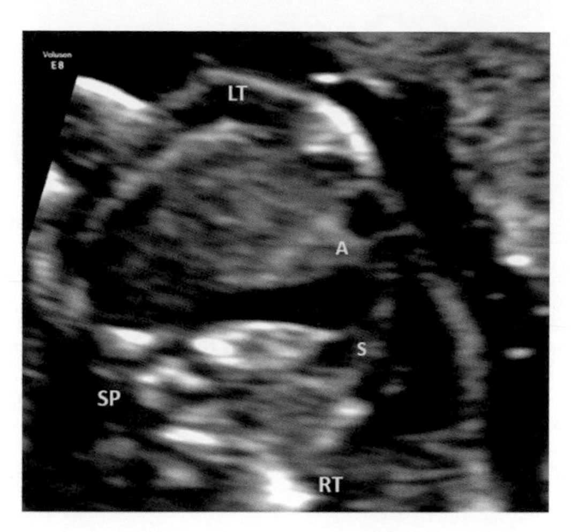

Fig. 3.2.85 Common arterial trunk. 3VT view showing two vessels. SVC (S) and left arch (A). Spine (SP), left (LT), right (RT).

SUGGESTED READING

REVIEWS AND GUIDELINES

Donofrio MT, Moon-Grady AJ, Hornberger LK, et al. Diagnosis and treatment of fetal cardiac disease: a scientific statement from the American Heart Association. *Circulation* 2014;129(21):2183–2242. Erratum in: *Circulation*. 2014;129(21):e512.

International Society of Ultrasound in Obstetrics and Gynecology, Carvalho JS, Allan LD, et al. ISUOG Practice Guidelines (updated): sonographic screening examination of the fetal heart. *Ultrasound Obstet Gynecol* 2013;41(3):348–359.

Suresh S, Indrani S, Shanthi C, Vijayalakshmi S. *Mediscan Manual of Fetal Echocardiography*. Avichal Publishing Company, New Delhi, 2021.

CHAPTER 3.3

Thoracic and Pulmonary Abnormalities

SUMMARY BOX

ANATOMY ASSESSMENT

- Both lungs should be routinely assessed in transverse section of the thorax at the level of the four chamber view (Fig. 3.3.1)
- The lungs should occupy approximately two-thirds of the chest
- The lungs have homogeneous echogenicity and are more echogenic than the liver
- Both left and right diaphragms should be clearly identified in the coronal and sagittal section (Fig. 3.3.2)
- In a transverse section of the upper part of the thorax, at the three vessel view, the thymus can be seen as a homogeneous mass in front of the aorta and pulmonary trunk (Fig. 3.3.3)
- Just above the three vessel view, the thymus is surrounded by two internal mammary arteries ('thybox view') (Fig. 3.3.4)

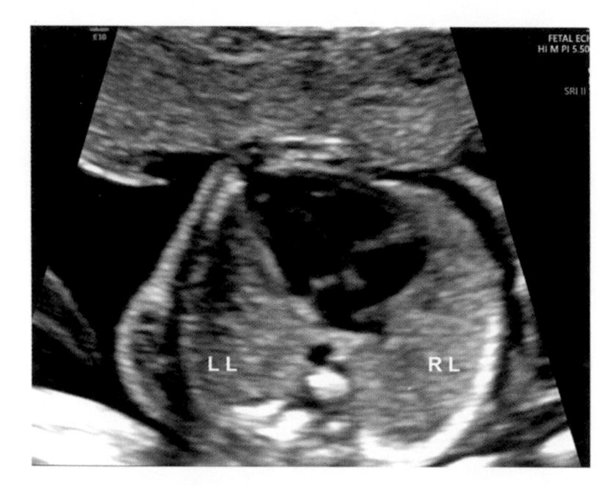

Fig. 3.3.1 Transverse view of the thorax at the level of the four chamber view showing both lungs. LL, left lung; RL, right lung.

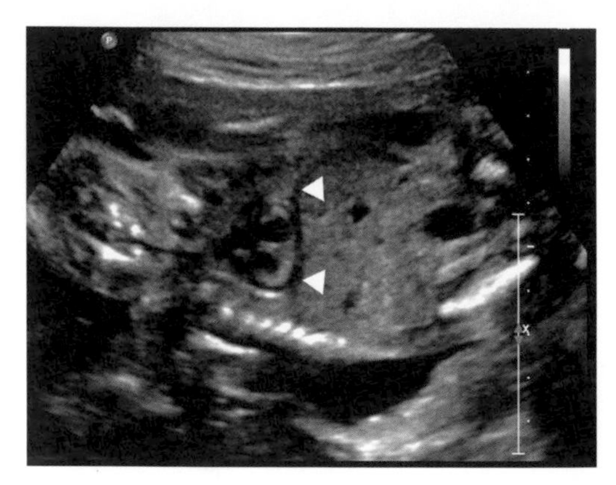

Fig. 3.3.2 Anterior coronal view of the fetus showing intact domes of the diaphragm (arrowheads).

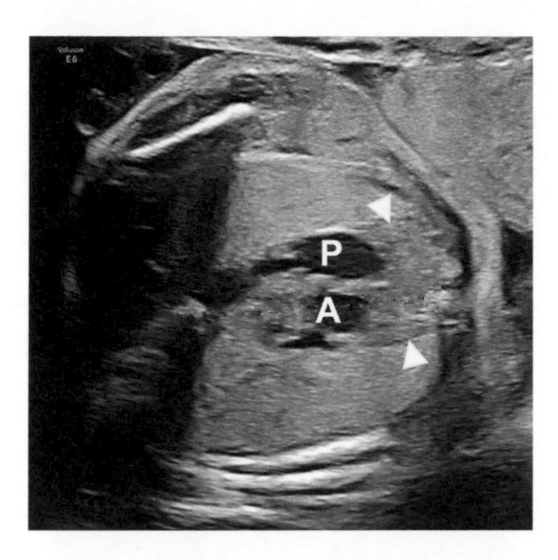

Fig. 3.3.3 Transverse view of the thorax at the level of the three vessel view showing the normal thymus as a hypoechoic structure in the anterior mediastinum (arrowheads). The pulmonary artery (P) and aorta (A) are seen posterior to the thymus.

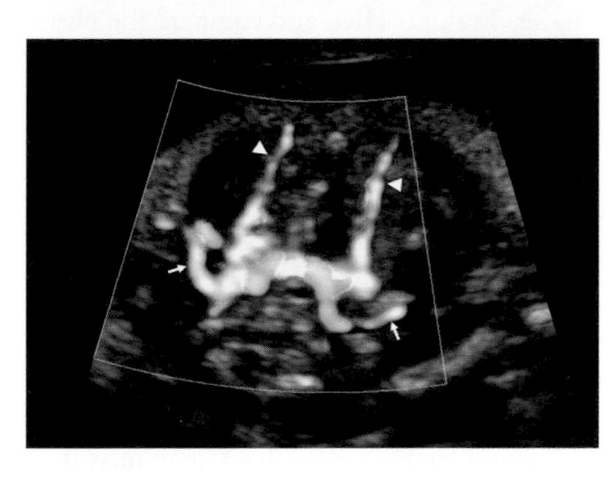

Fig. 3.3.4 The 'thybox' view. The transducer is moved just above the three vessel view and the colour Doppler PRF set at 0.6 KHz. The two internal mammary arteries (arrowheads) are close to the boundaries of the thymus. The origin of the two subclavian arteries is seen on both sides (arrows).

DIAPHRAGMATIC HERNIA

Definition and Characteristics

- A defect or deficiency in the diaphragm allows herniation of the abdominal contents into the chest
- The three basic types of diaphragmatic hernia are:
  - posterolateral Bochdalek hernia (most common, predominantly on the left side)
  - the anterior Morgagni hernia (Fig. 3.3.5)
  - hiatus hernia (very rarely diagnosed antenatally)
- Prevalence of the Bochdalek type diaphragmatic hernia is ~1 in 4,000 births

Ultrasound Assessment

- Where is the defect?
  - Left side defects are more common (~85%) and easier to visualise
  - Right side: it is often difficult to discriminate lung and liver based on their respective echogenicity

- Which viscera have herniated?
  - Stomach: single cyst, left side of chest
  - Small bowel: multiple small 'cysts'
  - Liver: usually less echogenic than lung
  - Gall bladder: single cyst on the right side of the chest
- Is there mediastinal shift?
  - Defined by a shift in cardiac axis
  - Direction is defined by the site of the space-occupying lesion
- Liver up or liver down
  - An additional tool for defining prognosis
- Isolated anomaly?
  - ~40% will have other anomalies
  - Check for craniospinal defects
  - Cardiac defects: be aware that the four chamber view axis will be altered
- What is the residual lung volume?
  - Measure the (contralateral) lung to head ratio (LHR) and compare the observed value to that expected for gestational age (o/e LHR) (Fig. 3.3.6 and Table 3.3.1)
- Polyhydramnios?
  - Affects ~25% of cases >24 weeks

Investigations

- Genetic:
  - Trisomy 18, trisomy 13
  - Tetrasomy 12p (Pallister–Killian syndrome) – amniocentesis is the test of choice. The mosaic isochromosome 12p is mainly present in skin fibroblasts and rarely found in cultured lymphocytes; therefore, CVS and fetal blood analyses may miss it
  - Consider exome testing for genetic syndromes (e.g. Cornelia de Lange, Fryns)
- MRI:
  - Confirm the defect
  - Check for lung 'meniscus' anterior/posterior to herniated viscera and membrane around the herniated tissue (encapsulation). Their presence is consistent with a better prognosis
  - MRI is the best imaging modality to assess liver involvement; aim to measure percentage of liver within the fetal chest
  - Look for evidence of pleural effusion

Counselling

- Survival depends on severity and degree of pulmonary hypoplasia and pulmonary hypertension (Table 3.3.1)
- Discuss the pros and cons of fetal surgery (FETO), if available – see Chapter 17
- Offer termination of pregnancy when o/e LHR <25%
- Optimal postnatal results can only be expected when delivery takes place in a tertiary facility with experience in management of ventilation/ECMO/paediatric surgery
- There will be feeding issues and ongoing gastrointestinal reflux in survivors

Table 3.3.1 The impact on survival of observed versus expected lung to head ratio (o/e LHR) and presence of the liver in the thoracic cavity.

	Survival	
o/e LHR*	**Liver up**	**Liver down**
<25%	~15%	30%
25–45%	~60%	~70%
>45%	>80%	

* Observed/expected lung to head ratio (see Fig. 3.3.6).

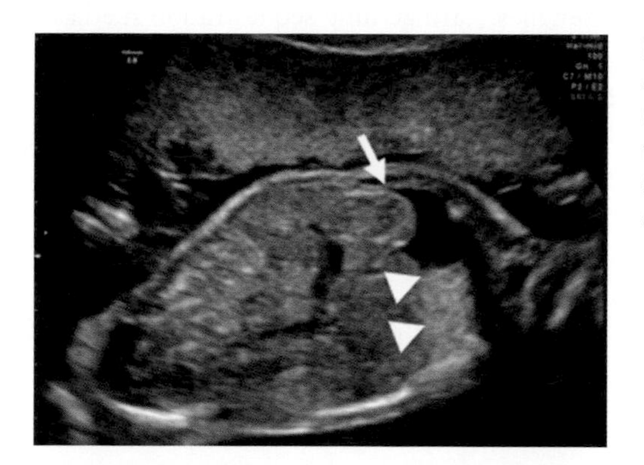

Fig. 3.3.5 Sagittal view of the fetal abdomen showing an anterior diaphragmatic hernia (Morgagni's hernia). The liver is seen herniating through the diaphragm (arrow). Pleural effusion is also seen. The left hemidiaphragm and lung appear intact (arrow heads).

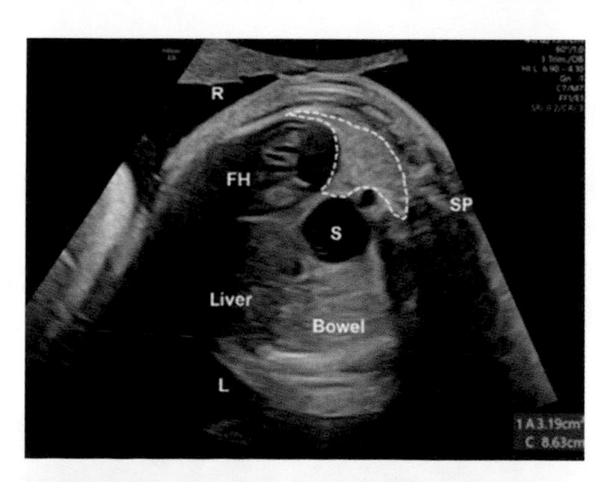

Fig. 3.3.6a Transverse view of the thorax in a case of left-sided diaphragmatic hernia at 28 weeks. The bowel, liver and stomach(s) are seen in the left hemithorax with marked mediastinal shift of the heart to the right (FH). The right lung circumference has been measured using the trace method.

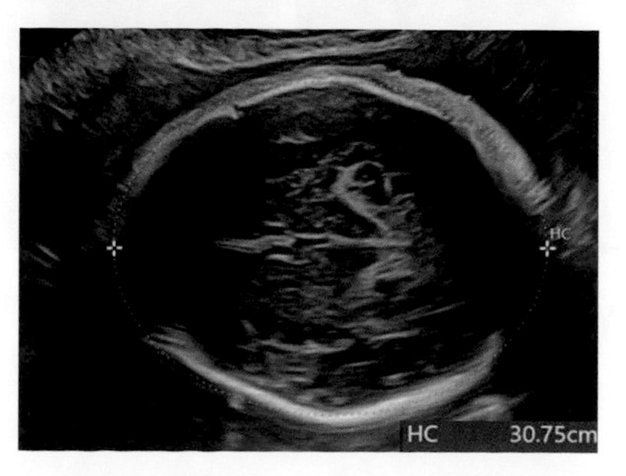

Fig. 3.3.6b Head circumference of the same fetus. The lung to head ratio (LHR) is calculated as the lung area in mm^2 divided by head circumference in mm. In this example LHR is 319 mm^2/307 mm = 1.04. The expected LHR for 28 weeks is 2.76; therefore, the observed to expected LHR (o/e LHR) is 1.04/2.76 = 37.7% (for more calculation see https://perinatology.com/calculators/LHR.htm).

PLEURAL EFFUSIONS

Definitions and Characteristics

- A collection of free fluid within the pleural cavity
- May be unilateral or bilateral
- May cause mediastinal shift
- May develop and become progressively worse, or regress spontaneously at any gestation

Ultrasound Assessment

- Unilateral or bilateral?
- Mild, moderate or severe by subjective assessment? (Fig. 3.3.7)
- Associated with other structural anomalies (cardiac/lung sequestration/mediastinal tumour)?
- Look for evidence of fetal anaemia (check MCA Doppler) and/or evidence of progressive hydrops

Investigations

- Chromosomal microarray
- Exome sequencing, particularly if hydrops and other anomalies are present (Noonan syndrome, hereditary lymphedema or Milroy disease)
- TORCH, parvovirus screen

Counselling

- Small, isolated effusions with no hydrops and no chromosomal abnormality have good prognosis
- Large bilateral effusions that respond to pleural shunting (likely primary chylothorax) have good outcome (see also Chapter 16)
- If large bilateral effusions do not respond to intervention, the prognosis is guarded due to likely complex underlying pathology and significant risk of pulmonary hypoplasia

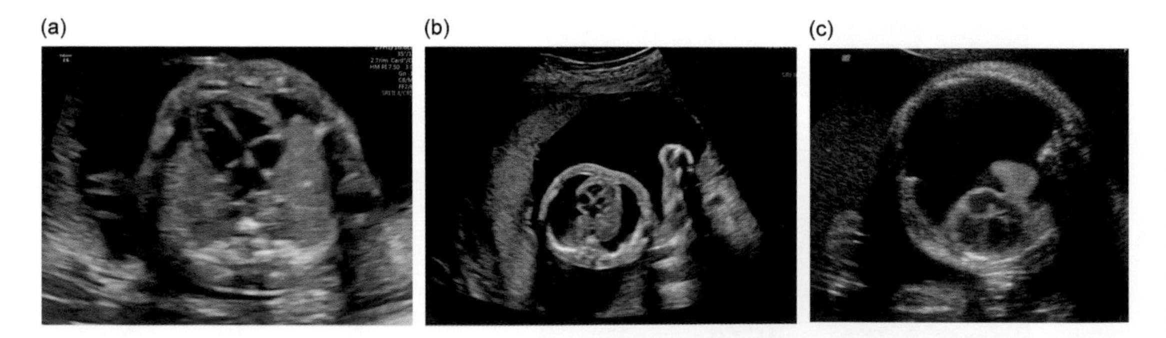

Fig. 3.3.7 Transverse views of the thorax showing (a) mild pleural effusion, (b) moderate bilateral pleural effusion and (c) severe unilateral effusion.

ANOMALIES OF LUNG PARENCHYMA

Definitions and Characteristics

- **Congenital pulmonary airway malformation (CPAM):** nomenclature changed from CCAM (congenital cystic adenomatous malformation) as some types are not cystic and others are not adenomatous (Figs. 3.3.8 and 3.3.9)
- **Bronchogenic cyst:** single cyst, centrally placed (Fig. 3.3.10)
- **Pulmonary sequestration:** hyperechogenic mass in the lung with identifiable feeding vessel. Can be extralobar and below diaphragm (Fig. 3.3.11)
- **Bronchial atresia:** enlarged hyperechogenic lung. Dilated bronchial tree. Normal contralateral lung
- **CHAOS – congenital high airway obstruction syndrome**: laryngeal atresia or tracheal obstruction (Fig. 3.3.12)
- **Unilateral pulmonary agenesis:** scimitar syndrome

Ultrasound Assessment

- Does it affect both lungs?
- Is it lobular?
- Are there cystic lesions?
- Is the lung enlarged and/or echogenic?
  - Multiple small cysts are echogenic
  - Upper airway agenesis leads to expansion of the lung
- Is there a mediastinal shift or compression?
- Is there polyhydramnios or hydrops?
- Is there vascular supply to the lesion?
  - If yes, pulmonary sequestration is likely

Investigations

- Not generally recognised as being associated with aneuploidy
- MRI can help identify parenchymal changes that are not visible on ultrasound

Counselling

- CHAOS – likely to have lethal outcome. Consider genetic pathology (e.g. Fraser syndrome)
- Large space-occupying lesions may cause hydrops and compromise respiration at delivery. Discuss EXIT procedure for delivery
- Macrocystic CPAM
  - Can be shunted (see Chapter 16)
  - Antenatal corticosteroids may relieve mediastinal compression (two doses betamethasone 12 mg IM given 24 hours apart; repeat course every 2–3 weeks, maximum reported four courses)
- Bronchogenic cysts generally have good prognosis. They may improve or resolve spontaneously with advancing gestation, but are likely to be still visible on postnatal MRI
- Controversy remains over postnatal management of smaller lesions in terms of malignancy risk and value of pneumectomy
- Surgery is nowadays less invasive with endoscopic techniques

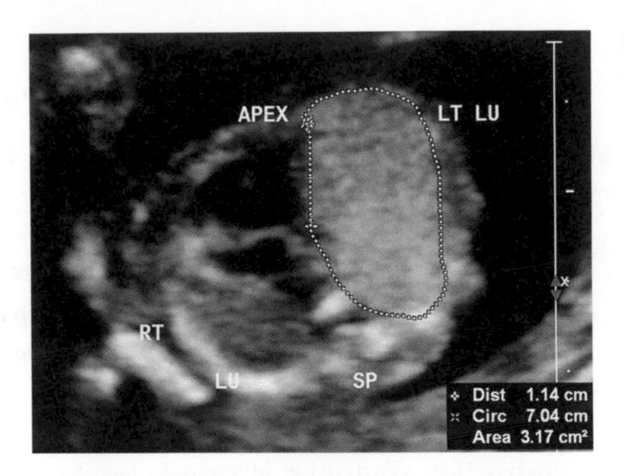

Fig. 3.3.8 Transverse view of the thorax showing enlarged echogenic left lung in a case of microcystic CPAM.

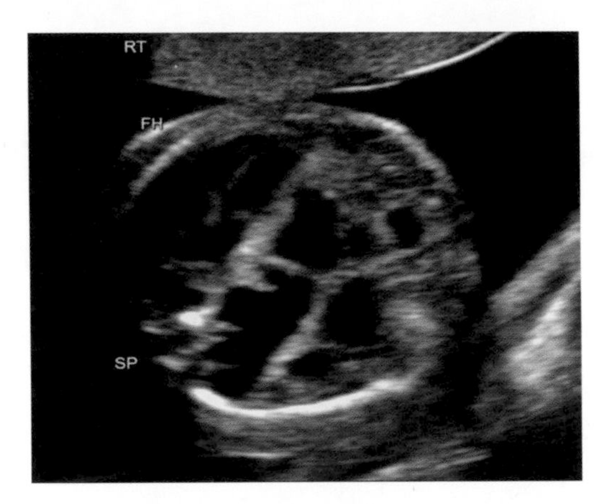

Fig. 3.3.9 A case of macrocystic CPAM on the left side. The heart is pushed to the right.

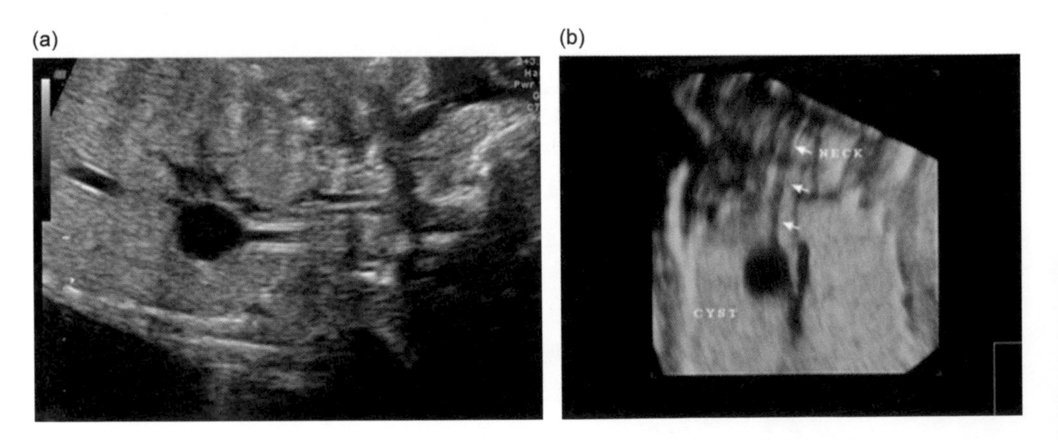

Fig. 3.3.10 Coronal view of the thorax showing a bronchogenic cyst. (a) Typically, they are thin-walled cysts seen in the middle of the thorax. (b) A dilated bronchus is seen just above the cyst (arrowhead) which implies an obstruction.

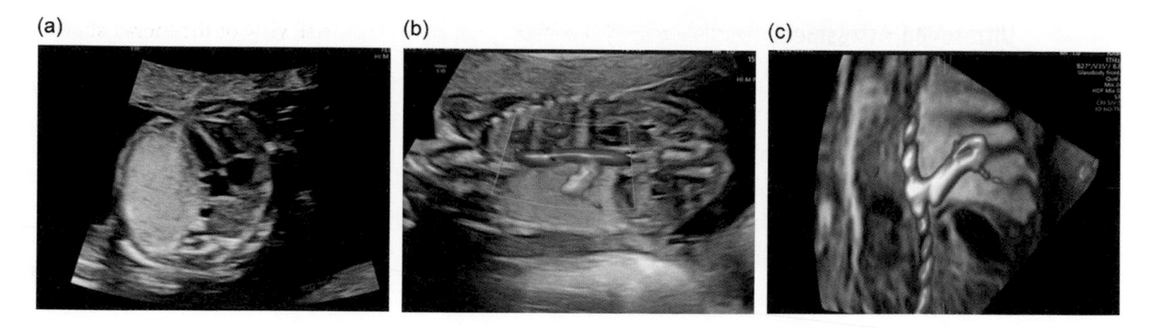

Fig. 3.3.11 (a) Transverse section of the thorax showing an enlarged echogenic lung in the left hemithorax. (b) Colour Doppler shows vascular supply from the descending aorta which confirms the diagnosis of a pulmonary sequestration. (c) 3D picture of the same case showing the vascular supply from the descending aorta. The stomach is seen immediately below the diaphragm.

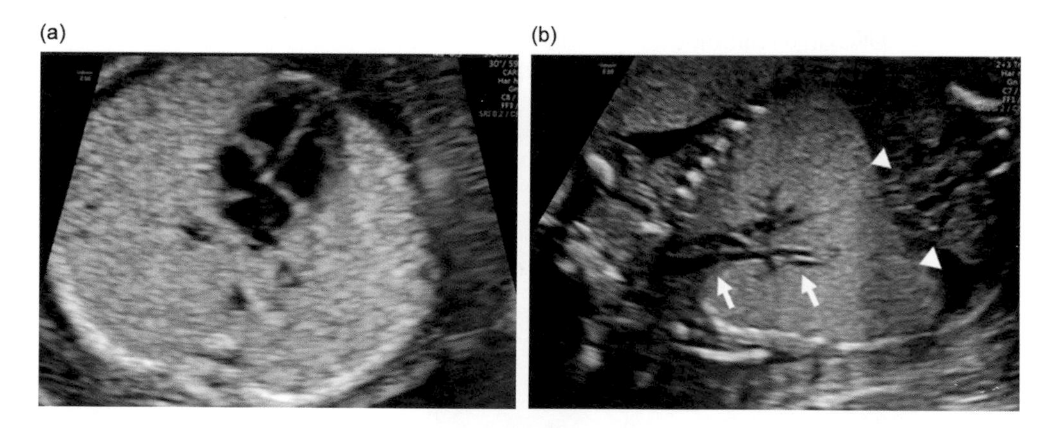

Fig. 3.3.12 (a) Transverse section of the thorax showing bilateral enlarged echogenic lungs in a case of congenital high airway obstruction syndrome (CHAOS). (b) Coronal view showing dilated tracheobronchial tree (arrows) which helps to differentiate CHAOS from large microcystic CPAM. Note the convexity of the diaphragm due to the obstructive pathology (arrowheads)

.

ABSENT THYMUS

Definitions and Characteristics

- Homogeneous quadrangular structure located in the anterior superior mediastinum, anterior to the great arteries (three vessel view) (Fig. 3.3.13)
- Bi-lobed – not readily distinguishable on ultrasound

Ultrasound Assessment

- **Absent/hypoplastic thymus:** assessed in transverse section at the level of the three vessel view
- **Associated cardiac abnormality:** specifically assess for conotruncal anomalies (tetralogy of Fallot, truncus arteriosus, interrupted aortic arch)
- **Associated IUGR:** check fetal biometry

Investigations

- Chromosomal microarray for DiGeorge syndrome
- Consider teratogens (e.g. alcohol)

Counselling

- Normally identified secondary to conotruncal cardiac abnormality – counsel about DiGeorge syndrome

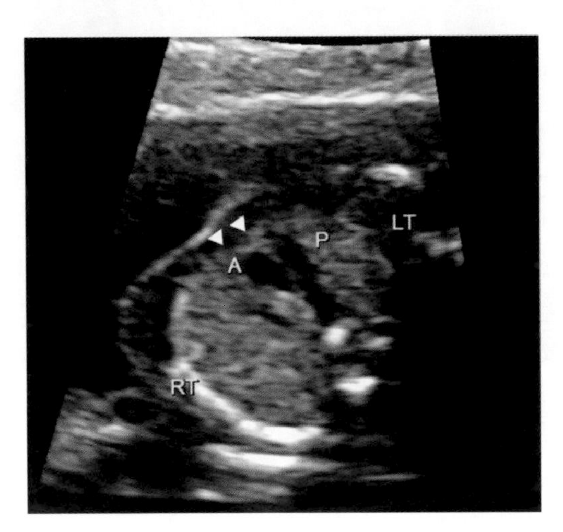

Fig. 3.3.13 Transverse section of the thorax at the level of the three vessel view in a case of Fallot's tetralogy. Note the absence of the thymus. Arrowheads points to the area of the thymus (see Fig. 3.3.3 for comparison). Amniocentesis revealed DiGeorge syndrome microdeletion.

SUGGESTED READING

PRIMARY RESEARCH

Chaoui R, Kalache KD, Heling KS, et al. Absent or hypoplastic thymus on ultrasound: a marker for deletion 22q11.2 in fetal cardiac defects. *Ultrasound Obstet Gynecol* 2002;20(6):546–552.

Deprest JA, Nicolaides KH, Benachi A, et al. Randomized trial of fetal surgery for severe left diaphragmatic hernia. *N Engl J Med* 2021;385(2):107–118.

Derderian SC, Coleman AM, Jeanty C, et al. Favorable outcomes in high-risk congenital pulmonary airway malformations treated with multiple courses of maternal betamethasone. *J Pediatr Surg* 2015;50:515–518.

Nørgaard LN, Nygaard U, Damm JA, et al. OK-432 treatment of early fetal chylothorax: pregnancy outcome and long-term follow-up of 14 cases. *Fetal Diagn Ther* 2019;46(2):81–87.

REVIEWS AND GUIDELINES

Abbasi N, Ryan G. Fetal primary pleural effusions: prenatal diagnosis and management. *Best Pract Res Clin Obstet Gynaecol* 2019;58:66–77.

Basurto D, Russo FM, Van der Veeken L, et al. Prenatal diagnosis and management of congenital diaphragmatic hernia. *Best Pract Res Clin Obstet Gynaecol* 2019;58:93–106.

Chaoui R, Kalache KD, Heling KS, et al. Absent or hypoplastic thymus on ultrasound: a marker for deletion 22q11.2 in fetal cardiac defects. *Ultrasound Obstet Gynecol* 2002;20(6):546–552.

David M, Lamas-Pinheiro R, Henriques-Coelho T. Prenatal and postnatal management of congenital pulmonary airway malformation. *Neonatology* 2016;110(2):101–115.

CHAPTER 3.4

Spine

SUMMARY BOX

ANATOMY ASSESSMENT

Ultrasound Evaluation

- Longitudinal/mid-sagittal views from cervical to sacral parts to:
  - demonstrate intact skin edge (Fig. 3.4.1)
  - evaluate alignment of vertebrae
- Dynamic sweep in transverse section to:
  - check integrity of vertebral bodies throughout the whole length (three ossification centres) (Fig. 3.4.2)
  - confirm intact skin edge
- Coronal views to:
  - exclude scoliosis
  - evaluate sacral tapering

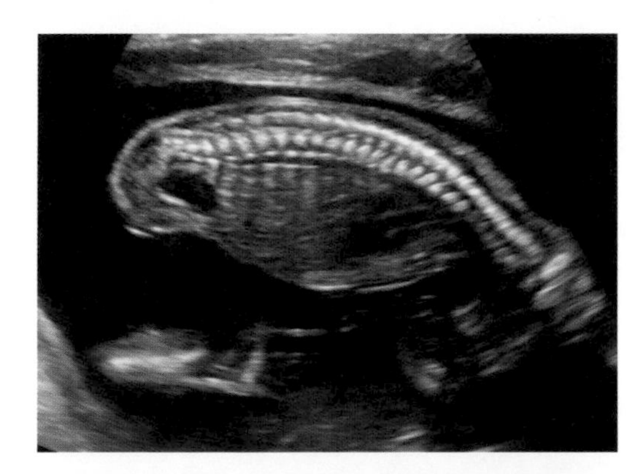

Fig. 3.4.1 Sagittal section of normal spine. Note the sacral tapering and intact skin edge throughout.

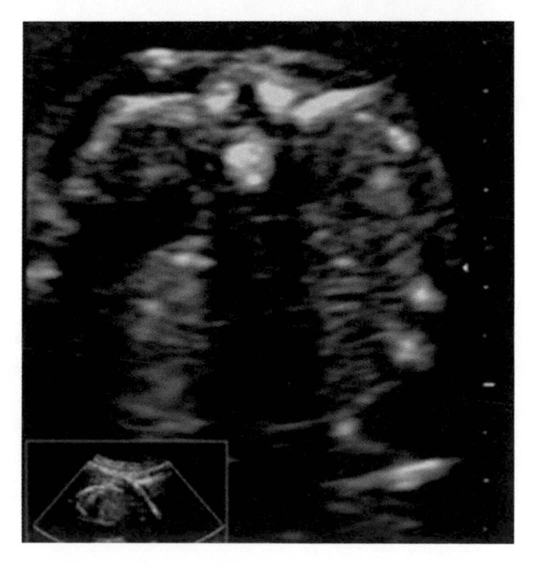

Fig. 3.4.2 Transverse section of a normal thoracic spine. The anterior ossification centre and the two posterior ossification centres are triangular in appearance.

OPEN LESIONS WITH OR WITHOUT BULGING 'CYST'

OPEN SPINA BIFIDA

Definition and Characteristics

- Failure of closure of the neural tube, affecting single or multiple vertebrae at any level
- Prevalence ~1 in 1,000 births
- Most antenatally detected open defects are **meningomyelocele**
- The term **meningocele** should be reserved for fluid-filled lesions that are skin-covered
- When **meningocele** does not appear to be skin-covered and/or is associated with intracranial signs, it is almost certainly a meningomyelocele with as yet invisible neural tissue within the lesion

Ultrasound Assessment

Head

- Scalloping of the frontal bones in transverse section (Fig. 3.4.3)
- Absence or abnormal curvature of the cerebellar hemispheres – Chiari malformation (~95%) (Fig. 3.4.4)
- BPD < 5th centile; ~25% in mid-trimester, more common at later gestations
- Ventriculomegaly ~85%; more prevalent at later gestations

Spine

- U-shaped vertebral bodies are open posteriorly
- Confirming disruption of overlying skin edge is particularly important for counselling **(Fig. 3.4.5)**
- Define level of affected vertebral bodies, using the 12th rib as a marker for thoracolumbar lesions
- Identify talipes/reduced lower limb movement
- May be associated with other structural anomalies; it is particularly important to look for rib abnormalities

Investigations

- Chromosomal microarray, particularly if other anomalies are present
- MRI is particularly useful for distinguishing between open and skin-covered lesions
- Postnatal X-ray is important to look for rib abnormalities (spondylocostal dysostosis)

Counselling and Management

- Prognosis is dependent on level and involvement of neural tube, although the correlation between the neurological deficit and the anatomical level of the defect is not as good as previously thought
- Surgical closure can be done either prenatally (see Chapter 18) or postnatally
- Traditional postnatal closure is associated with:
  - mortality ~5%
  - need for ventriculoperitoneal shunts (~60%), but the rates vary considerably depending on the local surgical practice

- normal or near-normal ambulation ~50%
- normal or near-normal continence ~35%
- IQ >70 ~80%
- cord tethering ~20%

- There is no reduction in morbidity with caesarean delivery
- 1:20 risk of recurrence. Periconceptual high-dose folic acid (5 mg) will reduce this risk
- Spondylocostal dysplasia is commonly (mis)diagnosed as 'isolated' open spina bifida. Only postnatal X-ray will show rib abnormalities. The correct diagnosis is important as recurrence rate is high (~25%)

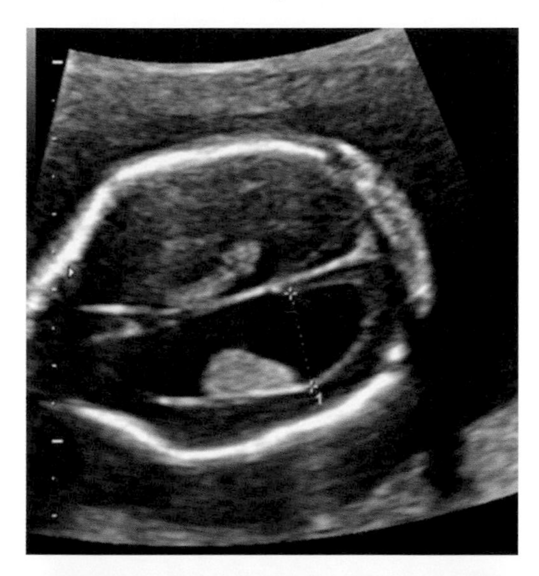

Fig. 3.4.3 Transverse section of the head in the ventricular plane showing the scalloped frontal bones ('lemon sign') in a fetus with open neural tube defect. Note there is also ventriculomegaly.

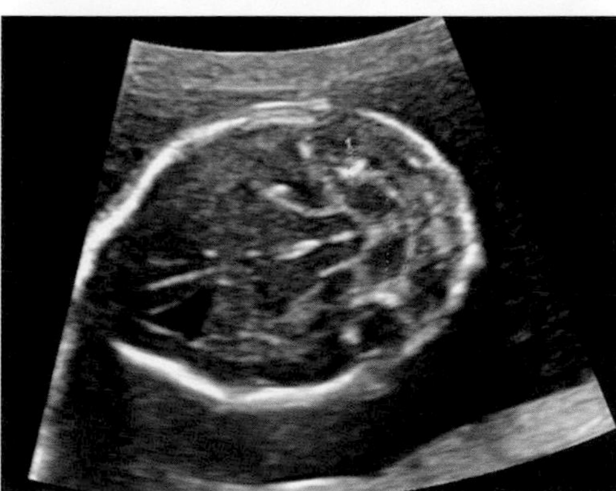

Fig. 3.4.4 Transverse section of the head in the trans-cerebellar plane showing obliterated cisterna magna and abnormal curvature of the cerebellar hemispheres, which gives the cerebellum a 'banana shape'.

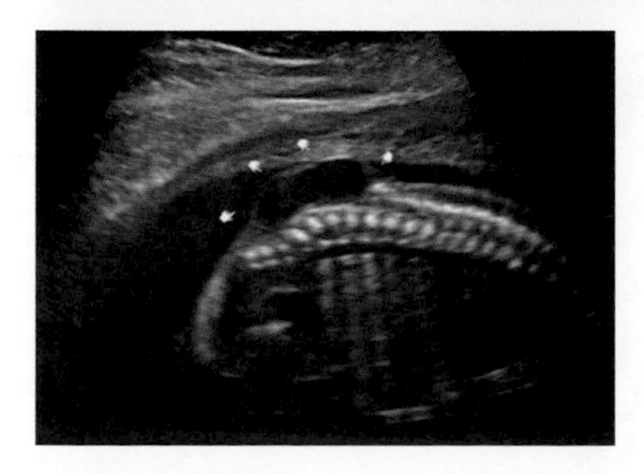

Fig. 3.4.5a Longitudinal scan of the spine showing a large meningomyelocele in the lumbosacral region (finger arrows). A bulge is seen in the lumbosacral region and the skin is disrupted.

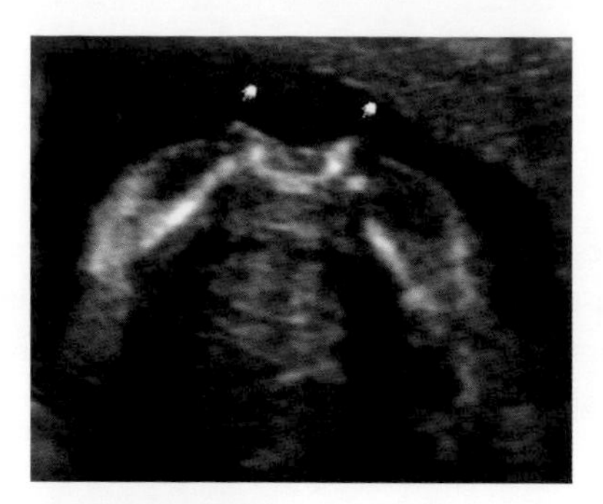

Fig. 3.4.5b Transverse section of the lumbar spine of the same fetus showing a U-shaped vertebrae. There is an obvious absence of the skin covering.

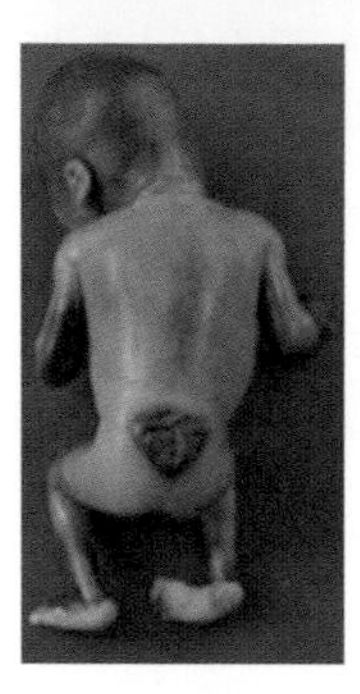

Fig. 3.4.5c Post mortem picture of the same fetus showing a large meningomyelocele in the lumbosacral region. Talipes are also clearly visible.

CRANIORACHISCHISIS

Definition and Characteristics

- Complete failure of closure of the neural tube, including both cranium and spine

Ultrasound Features

- Absent cranial vault
- Abnormality of brain tissue
- Spinal cleft, running the length of the spine (Fig. 3.4.6)

Investigations

- No recognised associations with aneuploidy

Counselling and Management

- Lethal: offer termination of pregnancy
- Folic acid (5 mg periconceptually) for future pregnancies

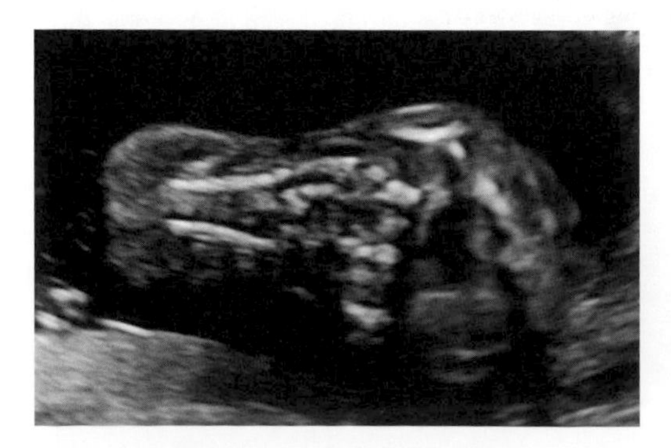

Fig. 3.4.6 Coronal view of the cervical and thoracic spine showing a wide open defect which is typical of craniorachischisis.

SKIN-COVERED LESIONS

SKIN-COVERED MENINGOCELE

Definition and Characteristics

- **Meningocele** is the simplest form of open neural tube defect containing cerebrospinal fluid without any neural tissue
- Fluid-filled, skin-covered meningocele may turn out to be **lipomeningocele** (Fig. 3.4.7); this distinction may not be possible antenatally, even with MRI
- **Limited dorsal myeloschisis (LDM)** is a skin-covered defect with the tethering of the dorsal spinal cord to the overlying skin (fibroneural stalk) (Fig. 3.4.8)

Ultrasound Assessment

- LDM with its liner echogenic stalk can be easily mistaken for meningomyelocele

Counselling and Management

- The prognosis is excellent with a relatively simple surgical repair
- The postnatal management and outcomes of skin-covered meningocele with or without LDM is identical
- Some meningocele can reabsorb by end of pregnancy, representing a different entity called **atretic meningocele**
- Unlike fluid-filled meningocele, atretic meningocele does not require urgent surgical repair and has better prognosis

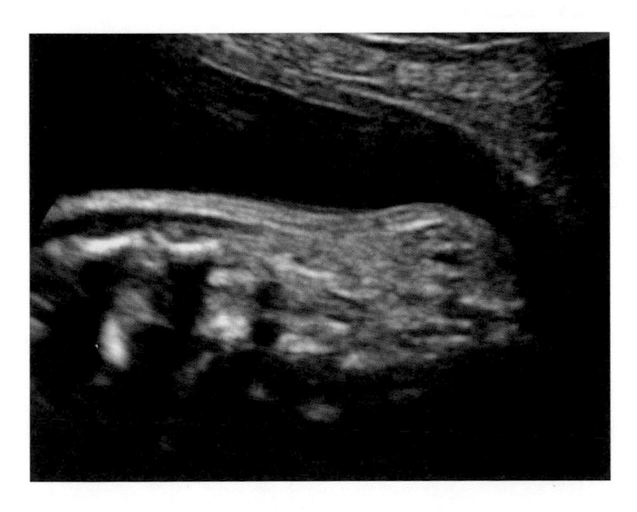

Fig. 3.4.7a Longitudinal section of the sacral spine showing an echogenic bulge with skin covering – lipomeningocele.

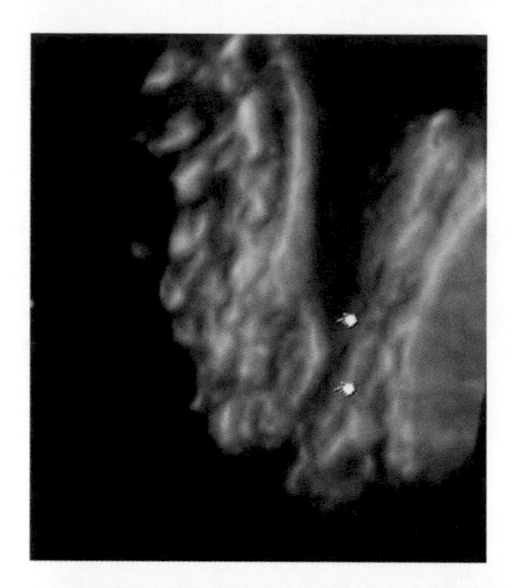

Fig. 3.4.7b 3D picture of the same fetus showing a skin-covered bulge typical of a lipomeningocele.

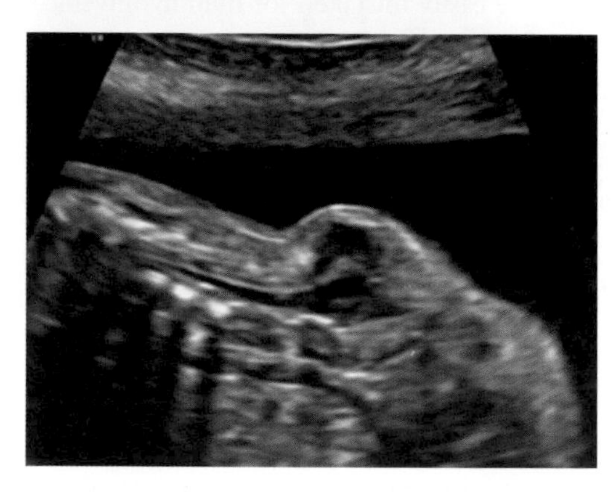

Fig. 3.4.8 Longitudinal section of the sacral spine showing a cystic swelling with skin covering suggestive of LDM. The diagnosis was confirmed postnatally.

CLOSED SPINA BIFIDA

Definition and Characteristics

- Abnormality of the posterior vertebral arch with no open communication
- Prevalence ~5% of neural tube defects

Ultrasound Features

- Absent posterior portion of the vertebral arch
- Intact skin edge
- No protruding neural tissue
- No cranial signs of spinal dysraphism
- Low level of conus medullaris

Investigations

- Invasive testing not indicated as karyotypic anomalies are rare

Counselling and Management

- Low risk of long-term functional effect
- Small risk of false-negative diagnosis of myelomeningocele
- Small risk of requiring surgical repair

HEMIVERTEBRAE

Definition and Characteristics

- Failure of development of one half of a vertebral body
- Prevalence ~1 in 1,000
- Most common in the thoracic region
- May affect multiple vertebral bodies and may 'skip' vertebrae
- Single level are more common in males; multiple level are more common in females
- May be associated with distortion in the shape of the spine (mainly scoliosis)

Ultrasound Assessment

- Absence of one side of the vertebral body (Figs. 3.4.9 and 3.4.10)
- Check for additional skeletal/cardiac/genitourinary anomalies
- The most common association in VACTERL
- Important to exclude spina bifida

Investigations

- Low risk of chromosomal abnormality, but discuss amniocentesis for microarray
- Exome for genetic associations (e.g. Jarcho–Levin)

Counselling and Management

- If isolated, generally good prognosis
- Varying degree of scoliosis may develop, which may become progressively worse (~75% will progress)
- Benefit from early enrolment in orthopaedic/physio follow-up programme for prevention of worsening scoliosis

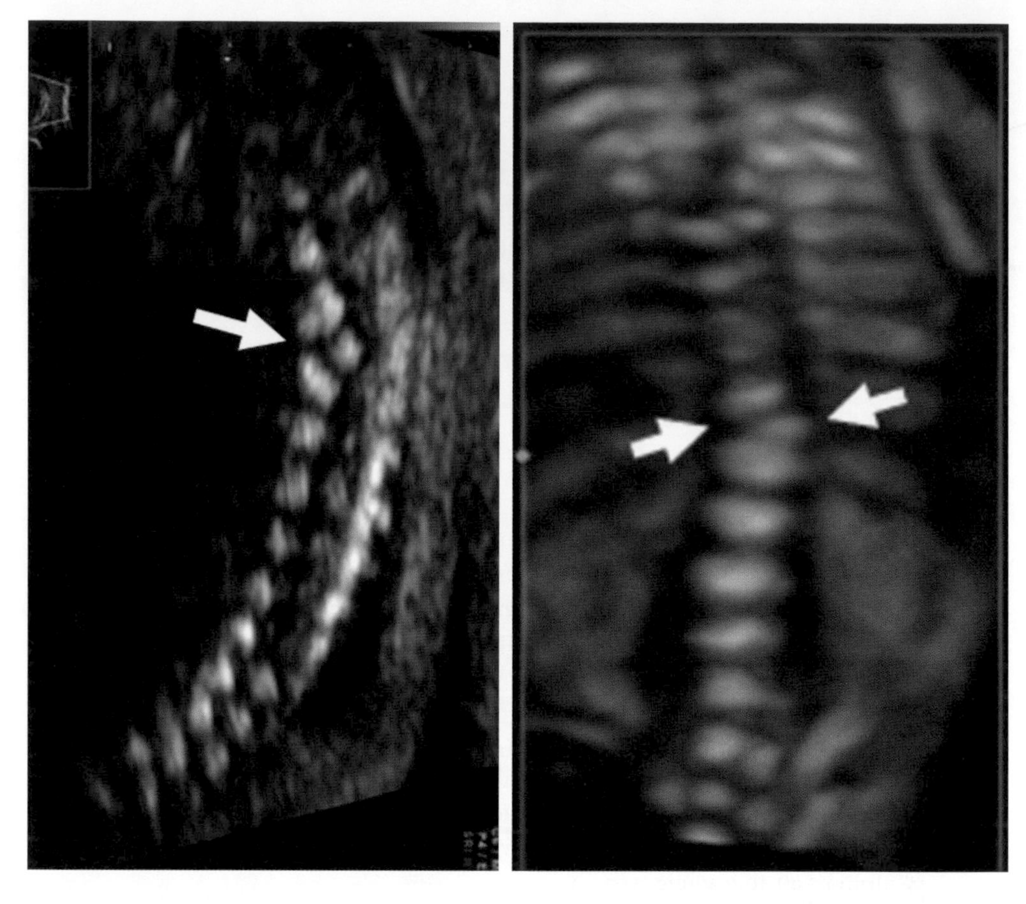

Fig. 3.4.9 2D and 3D images of the spine showing a single vertebra in the thoracic region. Note the mild scoliosis at the level of the hemivertebra (arrows).

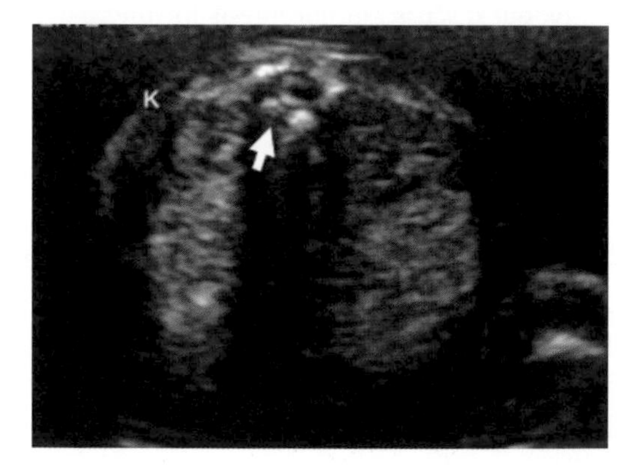

Fig. 3.4.10 Transverse section of the thoracic spine at the level of the hemivertebra. Note the split echoes of the vertebral body (arrow).

SPLIT CORD – DIASTEMATOMYELIA

Definition and Characteristics

- Longitudinal splitting of the cord
- Typically seen in the lumbosacral region
- Rarely cervical

Ultrasound Assessment

- The cord is bisected by a bony (echogenic) focus (Fig. 3.4.11)
- The cord typically reunites distally

Investigations

- No clear chromosomal/genetic association

Counselling and Management

- Generally good outcome
- Can be associated with tethered cord needing surgical intervention

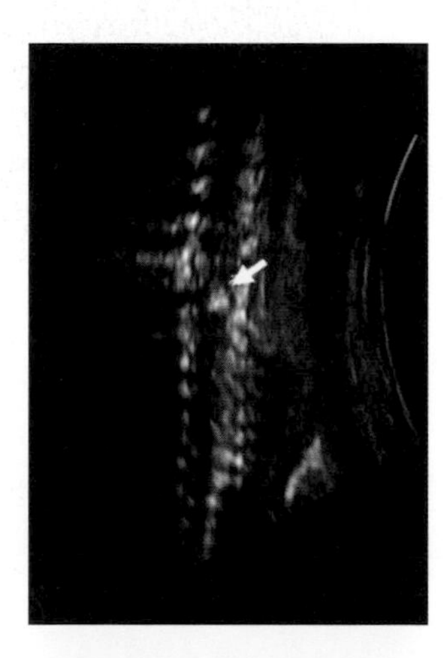

Fig. 3.4.11a Diastematomyelia. Longitudinal section of the spine showing a bony spicule in the thoracic spine (arrow).

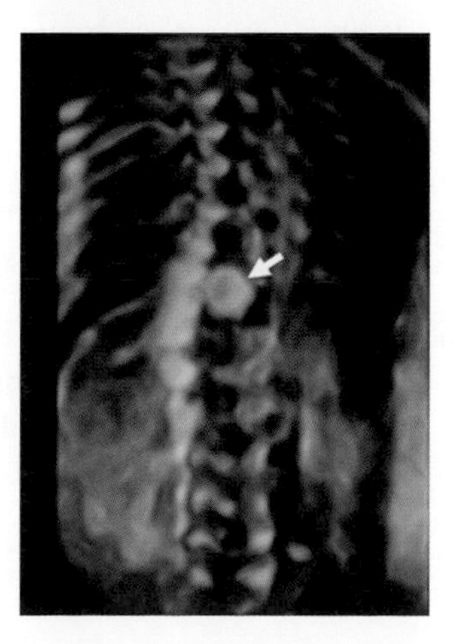

Fig. 3.4.11b Diastematomyelia. 3D rendering of the same fetus showing the bony spicule inside the vertebral canal (arrow).

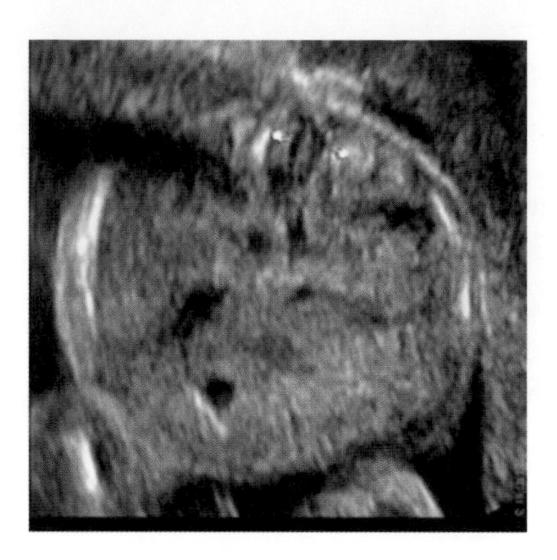

Fig. 3.4.11c Transverse section of the lumbar spine of the same fetus showing the 'split cord' (finger arrows).

SACROCOCCYGEAL TERATOMA

Definition and Characteristics

- A tumour developing at the level of the sacrum and coccyx
- Prevalence ~1 in 10,000 births
- May be only solid, only cystic or both (Fig. 3.4.12)
- May be internal, external or both
- Large, vascular tumours may cause high-output cardiac failure

Ultrasound Assessment

- Often not visible at 11–13^{+6} weeks' scan
- Exclude hydrops
- Exclude anaemia – check MCA PSV
- May cause polyhydramnios
- May cause fetal hydronephrosis

Investigations

- If hydrops develops, look for signs of maternal preeclampsia (mirror syndrome)
- The risk of karyotypic abnormalities is not increased

Counselling and Management

- Small tumours can be delivered vaginally
- Early neonatal surgery reduces risk of malignancy
- Small risk of urogenital complications (incontinence, cosmetic)
- Large tumours (>5 cm before 24 weeks) will have >50% risk of hydrops, anaemia, polyhydramnios and preterm delivery, with >50% risk of mortality – offer termination of pregnancy

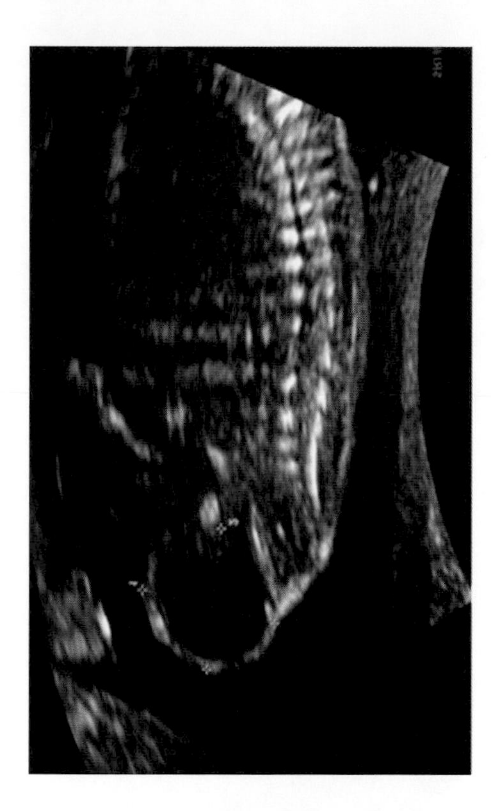

Fig. 3.4.12a Longitudinal section of the fetal spine in a fetus with sacrococcygeal teratoma. The lesion is seen inferior and medial to the sacral spine and appears cystic. These tumours may also have a heterogenous appearance with high vascularity.

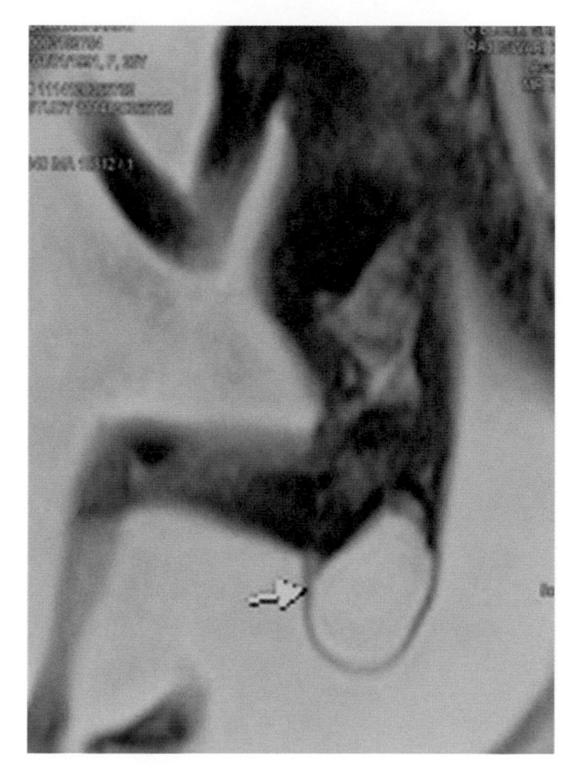

Fig. 3.4.12b A fetogram of the same fetus taken after termination of pregnancy, showing the cystic appearance of the teratoma (arrow).

SUGGESTED READING

PRIMARY RESEARCH

Friszer S, Dhombres F, Morel B, et al. Limited dorsal myeloschisis: a diagnostic pitfall in the prenatal ultrasound of fetal dysraphism. *Fetal Diagn Ther* 2017;41(2):136–144.

CHAPTER 3.5

Abdomen

SUMMARY BOX

ANATOMY ASSESSMENT

- Assessed in three transverse sections:
  - Upper abdomen (stomach, middle third of umbilical vein, ribs laterally) (Fig. 3.5.1):
    - Measure the abdominal circumference
    - Identify the stomach and confirm situs
    - Liver is seen on the right
    - Gallbladder is usually visible
  - Mid-abdomen (umbilical cord anteriorly, kidneys posteriorly) (Fig. 3.5.2)
    - Assess integrity of anterior abdominal wall
    - Identify dilated/hyperechogenic loops of bowel
  - Lower abdomen/pelvic brim
    - Demonstrate presence of bladder
    - Demonstrate bifurcation of umbilical arteries (three vessel cord)
    - Demonstrate intact anal sphincter ('target sign') (Fig. 3.5.3)
- Longitudinal section to confirm the normal cord insertion
- Coronal section to demonstrate left and right hemidiaphragms

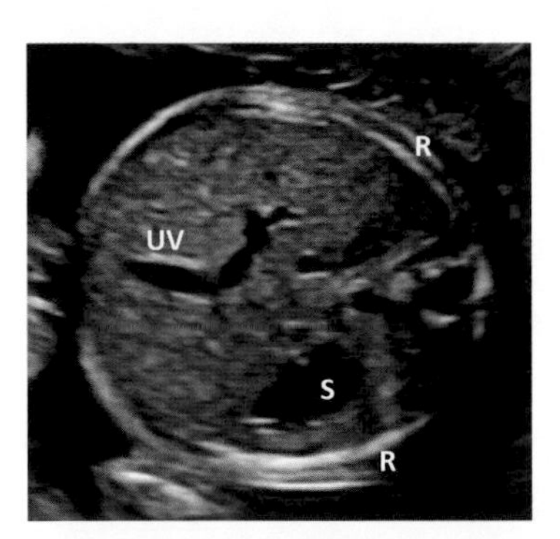

Fig. 3.5.1 Transverse section of upper abdomen in a normal fetus at 20 weeks showing the stomach (S), middle third of umbilical vein (UV) and ribs laterally (R).

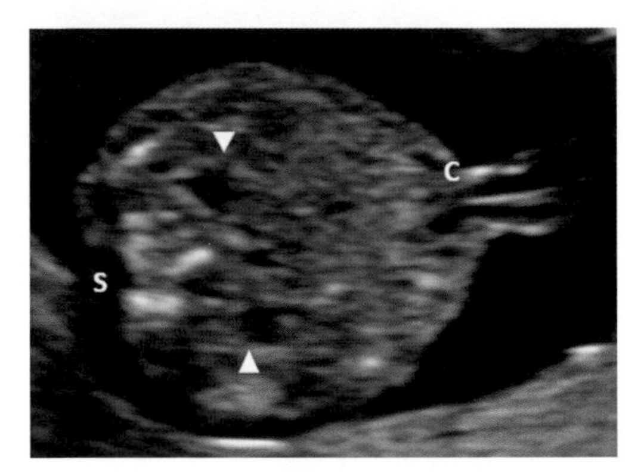

Fig. 3.5.2 Transverse section of mid-abdomen showing the cord insertion in the abdominal wall (C). The transverse section of the kidneys is seen posteriorly by the side of the spine (S) identified by the renal pelvis (arrowheads).

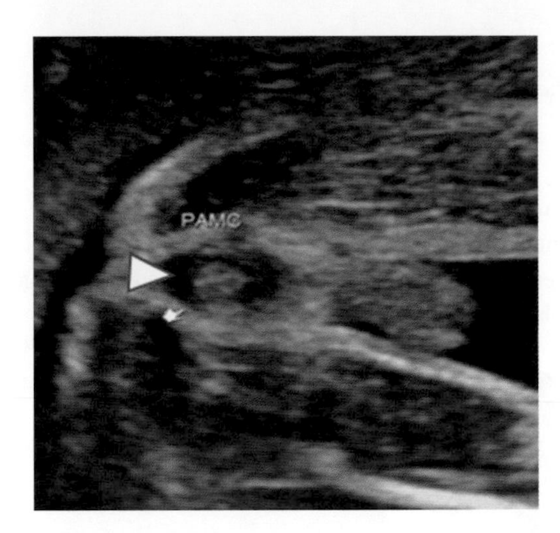

Fig. 3.5.3 Transverse view of the fetal perineum showing the perianal muscular complex (arrowhead), which appears like a 'target'.

ABDOMINAL WALL

EXOMPHALOS

Definition and Characteristics

- Central defect in the anterior abdominal wall at the umbilicus, also described as omphalocele
- Prevalence ~1 in 3,000 births

Ultrasound Assessment

- Herniated abdominal contents should be covered with a membranous sac (Fig. 3.5.4)
- Assess contents: bowel (small and large), stomach, liver
- Diameters of anterior abdominal wall defect and relative sizes of abdomen and herniated sac can be measured, but have little prognostic value (Fig. 3.5.5)
- Look for other structural anomalies, which are reported postnatally in up to 30% of livebirths
- Look for signs of Beckwith–Wiedemann syndrome (macrosomia, macroglossia, large kidneys)
- Look for signs of chromosomal abnormalities (trisomies 18 and 13)

Investigations

- Chromosomal microarray

Counselling

- Prognosis will depend on the presence of chromosomal and structural anomalies
- Type of surgical repair, either primary or secondary with epithelialisation of the sac, will depend on the size of the defect
- Herniated liver reduces the chance of primary closure, but does not appear to influence the long-term neonatal outcome

Small Isolated Exomphalos

- Good prognosis: >90% will make a full recovery

Large Defects

- Risk of pulmonary hypoplasia and need for respiratory support
- Consider termination of pregnancy
- Ideally, delivery should be in a tertiary hospital with facilities for paediatric surgery
- Exomphalos, unless particularly large, is not an indication for caesarean section

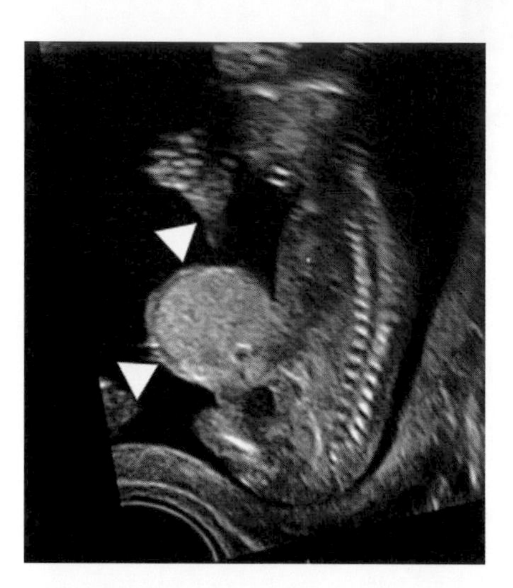

Fig. 3.5.4a Sagittal view of the fetus showing a large exomphalos-containing liver (arrowheads). The membrane covering the defect is clearly visible.

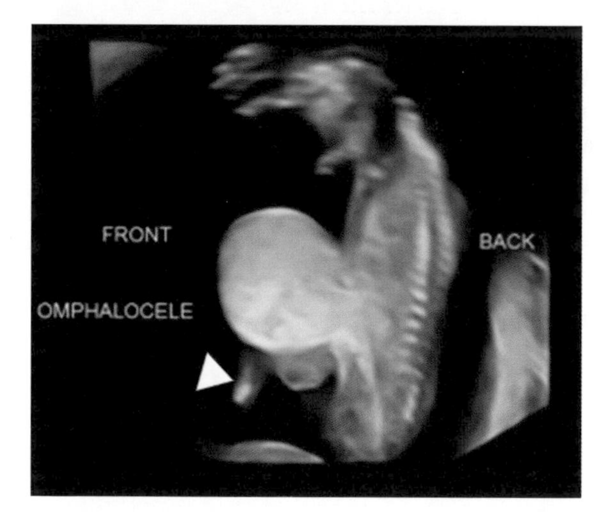

Fig. 3.5.4b 3D picture of the same fetus. The umbilical cord is seen arising from the surface of the exomphalos (arrowhead).

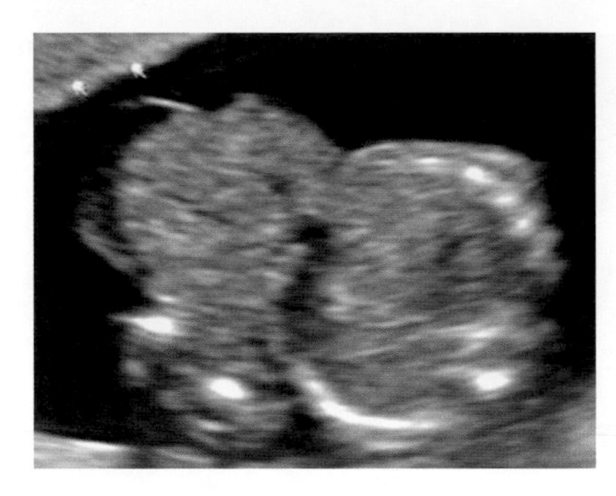

Fig. 3.5.5 Transverse view of the abdomen showing a large exomphalos. The diameter of the omphalocele is almost equal to the abdominal circumference.

GASTROSCHISIS

Definition and Characteristics

- Right paramedial defect in the anterior abdominal wall, allowing herniation of abdominal contents (typically bowel)
- Prevalence ~1 in 4,000 births and rising

Ultrasound Assessment

- Typically the defect is isolated, to the right of the midline
- Herniated abdominal contents should have no membranous covering
- Assess both extra- and intra-abdominal bowel and measure maximum diameters (Fig. 3.5.6)
- Assess amniotic fluid volume
- Monitor fetal growth, but fetal weight estimation may be unreliable as abdominal circumference will be small

Investigations

- Chromosomal microarray; although there is no recognised association with aneuploidy, there is a small increase in risk of pathogenic copy number variants

Counselling

- Intra-abdominal bowel dilatation and polyhydramnios are associated with six-fold increased risk of bowel atresia
- Gastric dilatation associated with a six-fold increased risk of neonatal death
- Elective (vaginal) delivery is indicated at 37^{+0}–37^{+6} weeks because of increased risk of term stillbirths (~5%)
- Delivery is best organised at a tertiary centre with facilities for paediatric surgery
- Primary repair may be delayed until extra-abdominal loops are sufficiently reduced in size
- Surgical repair may require resection of atretic parts of the bowel
- ~3% risk of short gut syndrome which, in most severe cases, can be lethal
- Many infants have difficulties establishing feeding and may need parenteral nutrition

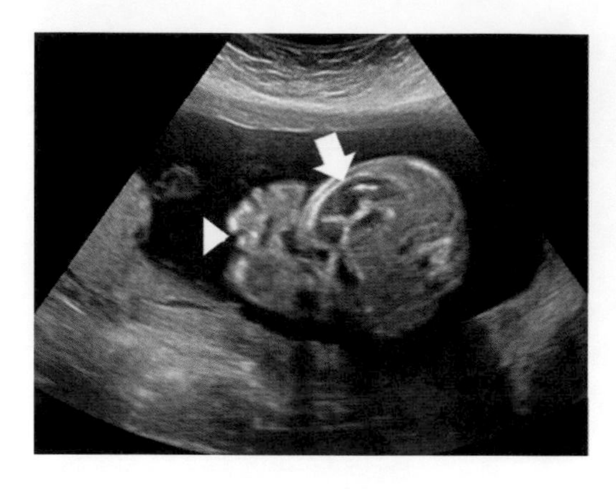

Fig. 3.5.6 Transverse view of the abdomen in a fetus with gastroschisis. Bowel loops are seen floating in the amniotic fluid (arrowhead). Dilated loops of bowel are seen in the abdomen (arrow). Bowel atresia was confirmed postnatally.

INTRA-ABDOMINAL MASSES

Definition and Characteristics

- A solid or cystic mass identified within the abdominal cavity (Table 3.5.1)

Ultrasound Assessment

- Cysts are typically circular rather than tubular (bowel, ureter)
- Single or multiple lesions
- Look for peristalsis (bowel)
- Look for colour Doppler signal within the mass
- Look for 'acoustic shadowing'

Investigations

- Karyotype for duodenal atresia, otherwise not indicated

Counselling

- Differential diagnosis can be refined, but it is difficult to make definitive diagnosis antenatally
- Ensure appropriate neonatal follow-up

Table 3.5.1 Differential diagnosis of intra-abdominal masses.

Initial ultrasound finding	Other ultrasound features	Differential diagnosis	Associations / prenatal testing
Cystic lesions			
'Double bubble'	• In the upper abdomen	• Duodenal atresia • Volvulus • Intussusception	Trisomy 21 – karyotype
Simple cyst	• Sub hepatic	• Choledochal cyst (Fig. 3.5.7)	
	• Lateral / lower abdomen	• Mesenteric / Duplication / Enteric cyst (Fig. 3.5.8) • Ovarian cyst (females)	

Table 3.5.1 (*cont.*)

Initial ultrasound finding	Other ultrasound features	Differential diagnosis	Associations / prenatal testing
Complex cyst	• Retroperitoneal / upper abdomen	• Adrenal haemorrhage (Fig. 3.5.9)	
	• Lateral / lower abdomen	• Ovarian cyst (females)	
Dilated tubular structure	• Contains clear fluid	• Dilated bowel	• Gastroschisis / exomphalos • Cloacal anomalies • Volvulus • Intussusception • Hirschsprung's disease (±trisomy 21)
		• Dilated ureter	• Megacystis microcolon • Bladder outflow obstruction or vesicoureteric reflux
	• Contains echogenic material	• Meconium ileus	• Cystic fibrosis – DNA analysis • Chromosomal anomaly – karyotype
	• Associated with blood flow	• AV malformation • Abnormal ductus venosus	
Solid lesions			
Hyperechogenic bowel	• Dilated loops of bowel	• Bowel obstruction	• Cystic fibrosis – DNA analysis • Trisomy 21 – karyotype
	• Other structural anomalies / markers	• Chromosomal abnormality	• Karyotype
	• CNS anomaly / FGR	• Fetal infection • Chromosomal abnormality	• CMV / toxoplasmosis – maternal TORCH screen • Amniocentesis

Table 3.5.1 (*cont.*)

Initial ultrasound finding	Other ultrasound features	Differential diagnosis	Associations / prenatal testing
	• Abnormal biometry / Doppler (with placental insufficiency)	• Fetal growth restriction	
	• Intraamniotic bleeding	• Ingestion of intra-amniotic blood (Fig. 3.5.11)	
Intra-abdominal calcification	• Within biliary tree	• Biliary atresia	
	• Peritoneal +/− ascites	• Bowel perforation • Meconium peritonitis	• Cystic fibrosis
Intrahepatic calcification	• CNS anomaly / FGR	• Fetal Infection	• CMV / toxoplasmosis – maternal TORCH screen • Amniocentesis

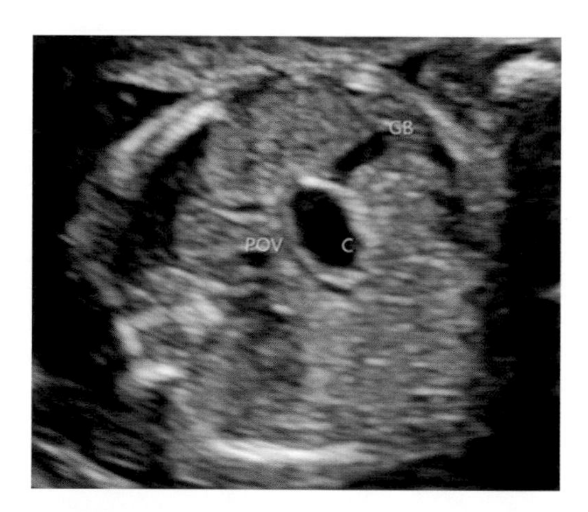

Fig. 3.5.7 Transverse section of the upper abdomen at 21 weeks showing a cyst (C) just adjacent to the portal vein (POV). The gall bladder is seen anteriorly close to the cyst (GB). Postnatally, this was confirmed as a choledochal cyst.

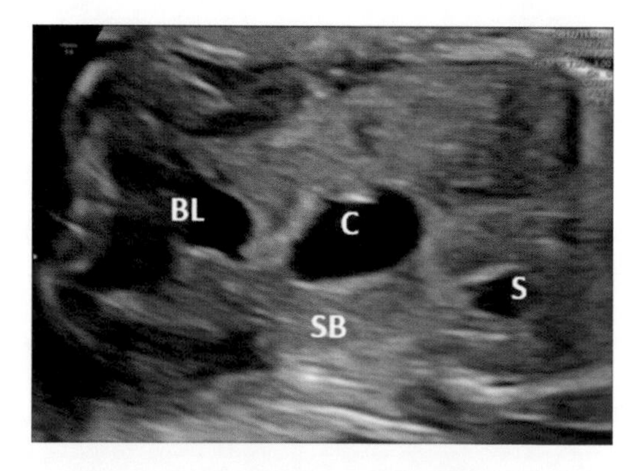

Fig. 3.5.8 Coronal section of the fetal abdomen at 23 weeks showing an elongated cyst (C) adjacent to the small bowel (SB). In relation to the cyst, the stomach is superior (S) and bladder inferior (BL). Postnatally, this was confirmed as a small bowel duplication cyst.

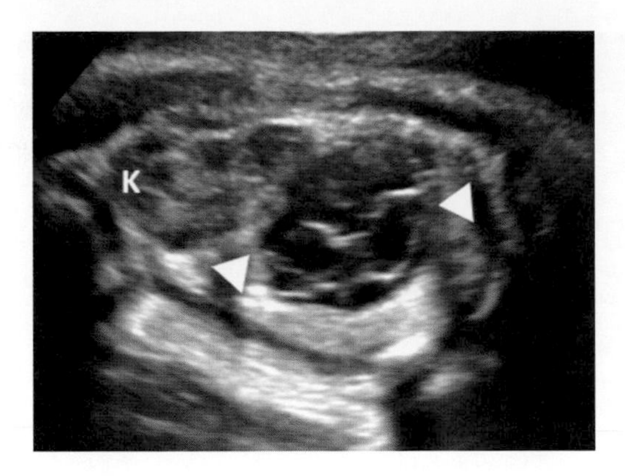

Fig. 3.5.9 Sagittal section of the right side of the abdomen showing a normal right kidney (K). A complex mass with internal echoes and bands is seen superior to the kidney, suggestive of adrenal haemorrhage (arrowheads).

HYPERECHOGENIC BOWEL

Definition and Characteristics

- Loops of bowel that are at least as bright as fetal bony parts
- Potential indicator of a number of different pathologies:
  - bowel obstruction (cystic fibrosis?) (Fig. 3.5.10)
  - chromosomal abnormality
  - severe fetal growth restriction (triploidy?)
  - fetal infection (cytomegalovirus, toxoplasmosis)
  - swallowing of blood-stained amniotic fluid due to intra-amniotic bleeding (Fig. 3.5.11)

Ultrasound Assessment

- It is important to reduce the gain sufficiently to avoid the overdiagnosis (Fig. 3.5.10)
- Look for evidence of fetal growth restriction by using both fetal and uteroplacental Doppler
- Look for intra-amniotic haemorrhage
- Look for signs of aneuploidy (trisomy 21)

Investigations

- Review genetic carrier screening
- Amniocentesis (karyotype, cystic fibrosis panel, cytomegalovirus PCR)

Counselling

- Serial scans to exclude fetal growth restriction
- Negative investigations provide adequate reassurance – no need for postnatal follow-up

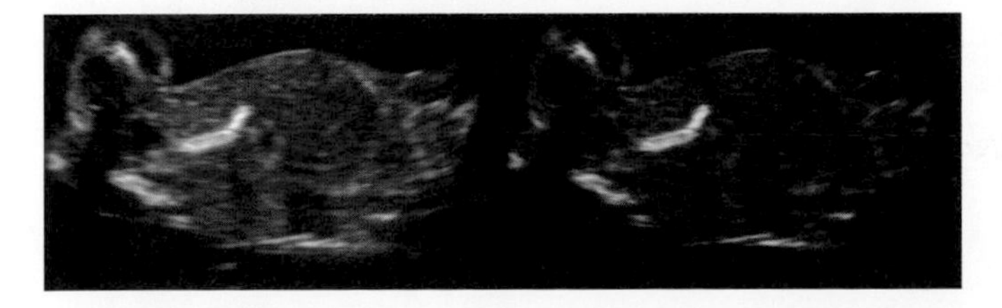

Fig. 3.5.10 Echogenic bowel in a fetus affected by cystic fibrosis. The image on the left shows a linear hyperechogenic loop of bowel with shadowing. The image on the right is with reduced gain. The bowel appears as bright as the pelvic bone below.

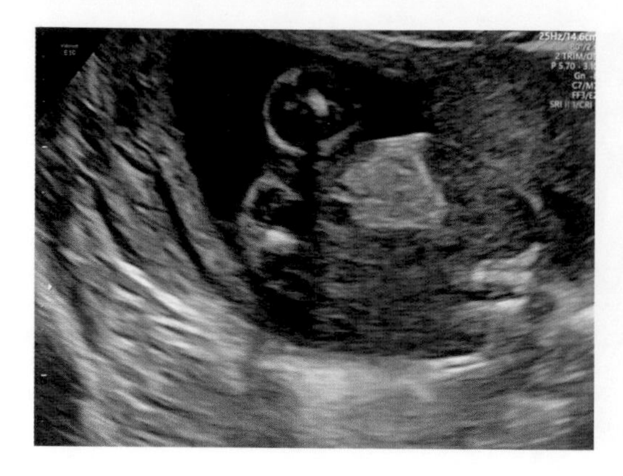

Fig. 3.5.11 Hyperechoic bowel caused by swallowing of blood-stained amniotic fluid. Fetal blood sampling had been done two days previously. Note that there is no shadowing and the echogenicity of the bowel is less bright than the one shown in Fig. 3.5.10. A repeat scan at 34 weeks showed normal-looking bowel.

DILATED LOOPS OF BOWEL

Definition and Characteristics

- Small bowel dilatation is loops >7 mm in the largest cross section diameter
- Large bowel dilatation is loops >18 mm in the largest cross section diameter
- Typically present in the third trimester

Ultrasound Assessment

- Position of dilated loops relate to the level of obstruction – for example, jejunal and upper large bowel obstruction tend to present with dilated loops on the upper abdomen
- Bowel above the obstruction tends to have increased peristalsis and a hyperechogenic wall
- Assess anal sphincter for possible atresia, looking for absent or very small 'target sign' (Fig. 3.5.12)
- Internal echoes within bowel loops suggest recto-urinary fistula
- If anorectal malformation is present, rectum may contain 'meconium pearls' (entherolitiasis) (Fig. 3.5.13)

Investigations

- Chromosomal microarray
- MRI is helpful in distinguishing multiple fluid-filled pelvic structures (rectum, hydrocolpos, hemiuteri)

Counselling

- Caution is needed not to overinterpret imaging findings as exact underlying pathology can be quite complex
- It is best to deliver in a tertiary centre with facilities for paediatric surgery
- Neonatal review should be arranged to confirm prenatal findings and establish the definitive diagnosis as soon as possible

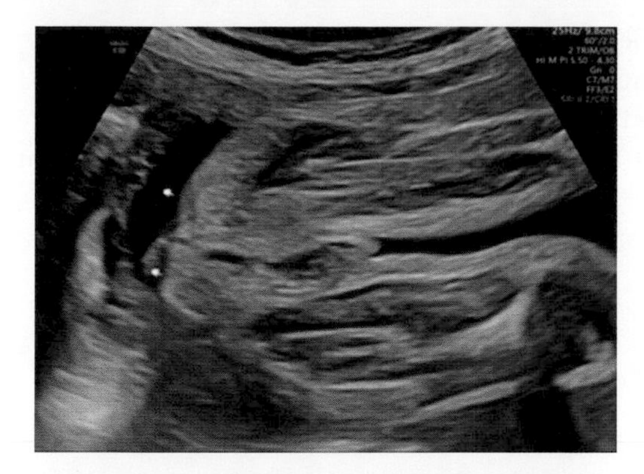

Fig. 3.5.12 Scan of the fetal perineum with absent perianal muscular complex (i.e. no 'target sign'). See Fig. 3.5.3 for comparison. This fetus had anorectal atresia.

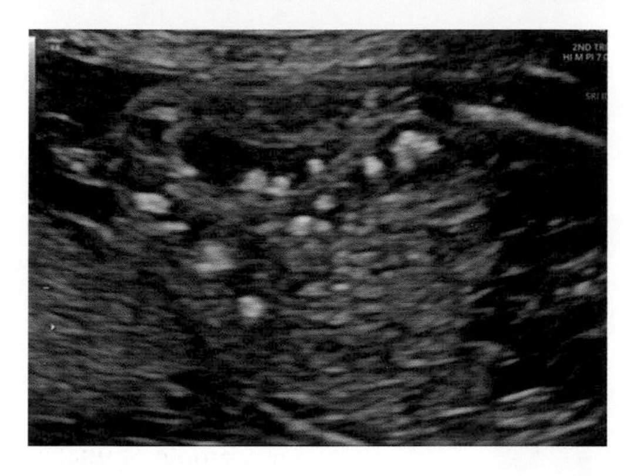

Fig. 3.5.13 Scan of the fetal abdomen showing dilated bowel loops with meconium pellets in a case of anorectal malformation.

LIVER

HEPATOMEGALY

Definition and Characteristics

- The liver size is not routinely measured, but if hepatomegaly is suspected, liver length can be measured and compared with available reference ranges (Fig. 3.5.14)
- Indirect signs of hepatomegaly include the right lobe that is lower than the inferior pole of the right kidney and increased abdominal circumference
- The main causes are:
  - infection (CMV, parvo B19, congenital syphilis)
  - transient abnormal myelopoiesis due to trisomy 21
  - liver storage diseases (Nieman–Pick, congenital haemochromatosis caused by gestational alloimmune liver disease)
  - overgrowth syndromes (Beckwith–Wiedemann)
  - fetal anaemia (hydrops-related congestion or extramedullar haematopoiesis)
  - biliary atresia
  - benign tumours (haemangiomas and hamartomas are the most common, others include simple cysts, focal nodular hyperplasia, haemangioendothelioma)
  - malignant tumours (hepatoblastoma, metastatic neuroblastoma)

Ultrasound Assessment

- MCA Doppler to exclude fetal anaemia
- Look for signs of trisomy 21

- Haemangiomas are usually hypoechoic, often vascular cysts (Fig. 3.5.15)
- Hamartomas tend to be large, multiloculated cysts
- Look for situs inversus associated with biliary atresia
- Large hepatic vessels with colour Doppler signal suggest arteriovenous malformations, or haemangioendothelioma

Investigations

- Maternal infection screen
- Karyotype is indicated if trisomy 21 is suspected
- Maternal alfa-fetoprotein may be raised in haemangioendothelioma

Counselling

- Liver pathology in isolation will rarely, if ever, justify preterm birth
- Neonatal imaging should be arranged
- Long-term outcome will depend on the underlying pathology

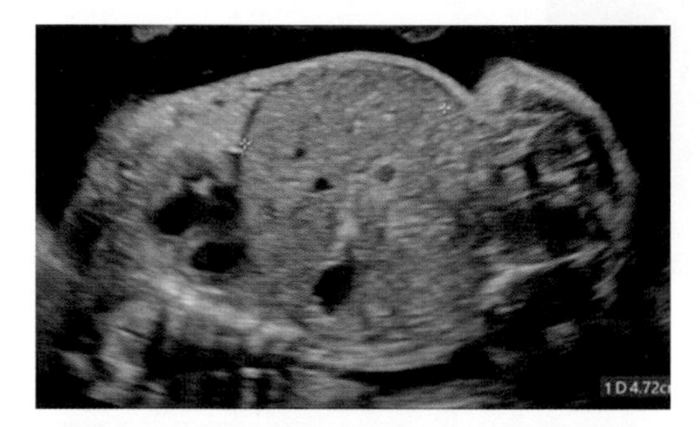

Fig. 3.5.14 Coronal view of the abdomen showing hepatomegaly at 25 weeks. The longitudinal length of the liver is increased (47 mm). Normal liver length at this gestation should be <40 cm.

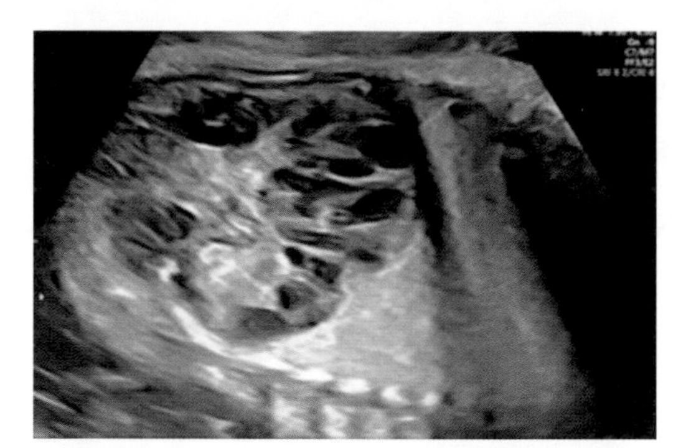

Fig. 3.5.15a Scan of the upper abdomen of a 26-week fetus with a large heterogenous mass in the liver.

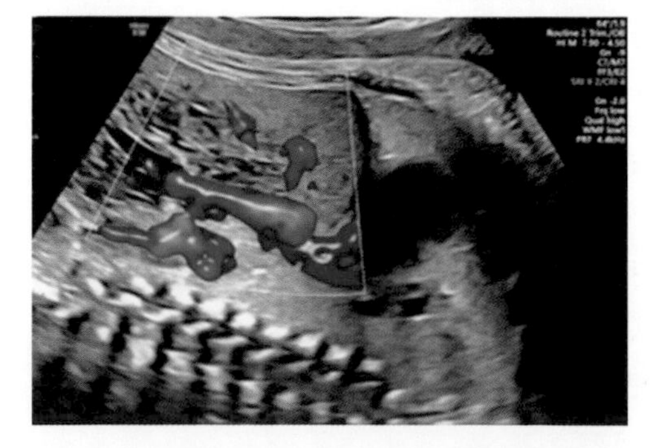

Fig. 3.5.15b On the basis of strong colour Doppler signal within the mass shown in Fig. 3.5.15a, a provisional diagnosis of haemangioma was made. Postnatally, the final diagnosis was haemangioendothelioma.

ABSENT DUCTUS VENOSUS

Definition and Characteristics

- Relatively rare vascular abnormality; ~1 in 2,500 births
- Umbilical vein can be connected to the systemic venous circulation either through the postal sinus via an abnormal venous channel (intrahepatic; Fig. 3.5.16), or by completely bypassing the portal sinus and the liver (extrahepatic; Fig. 3.5.17)
- Associated with aneuploidies (trisomy 21, Turner), Noonan syndrome and various cardiac anomalies

Ultrasound Assessment

- Detailed echocardiography
- Look for signs of aneuploidy
- Look for structural abnormalities
- Look for early signs of hydrops and polyhydramnios
- Serial scans should be arranged to look for signs of cardiac failure

Investigation

- Chromosomal microarray

Counselling and Management

- Postnatal imaging should be arranged to exclude portosystemic shunts or agenesis of the portal system
- If isolated, the outcome is good, irrespective of the type of drainage

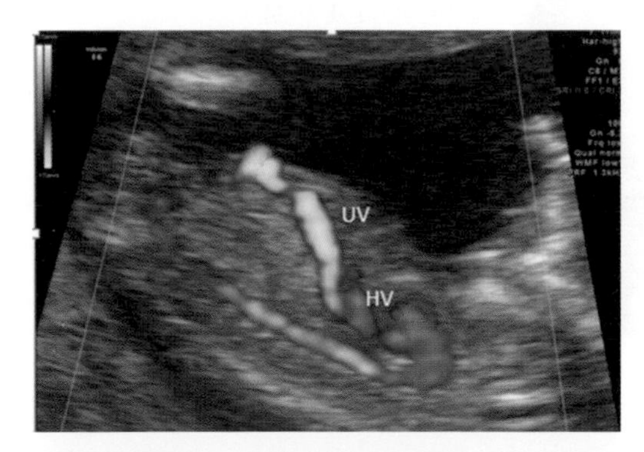

Fig. 3.5.16 Agenesis of ductus venosus. Sagittal view of the fetal abdomen showing the umbilical vein (UV) entering the hepatic vein (HV).

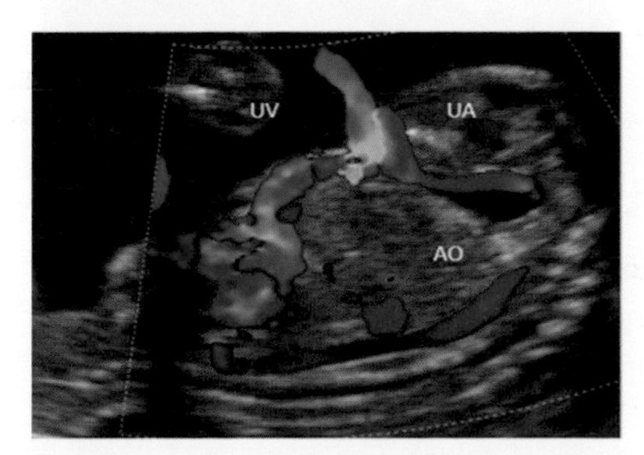

Fig. 3.5.17 Agenesis of ductus venosus. The umbilical vein (UV) is seen directly entering the right atrium. AO, aorta; UA, umbilical artery.

HEPATIC CALCIFICATIONS

Definition and Characteristics

- ~1 in 2,000 pregnancies at 20 weeks
- Generally discrete hyperechogenic foci within parenchyma (Fig. 3.5.18)
- Usually limited to 1–4 foci
- Associated with aneuploidies (trisomy 13 and 21, some atypical) and infection

Ultrasound Assessment

- Two-thirds of cases have other ultrasound anomalies
- Most cases affected by chromosomal abnormality have other anomalies

Investigation

- Chromosomal microarray
- Screen for infection (syphilis, CMV, toxoplasmosis, parvovirus)

Counselling and Management

- If isolated, with no evidence of chromosomal abnormalities or fetal infection, prognosis is good

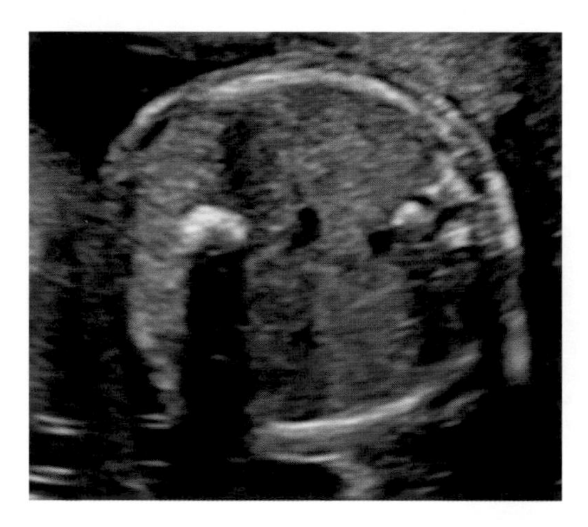

Fig. 3.5.18 Hepatic calcification. Transverse section of the abdomen showing a calcification in the liver as an echogenic focus with acoustic shadowing below. This was an isolated finding and the outcome was good, with no obvious postnatal pathology.

SUGGESTED READING

Heider AL, Strauss RA, Kuller JA. Omphalocele: clinical outcomes in cases with normal karyotypes. *Am J Obstet Gynecol* 2004;190(1):135–141.

Jensen KK, Oh KY, Patel N, et al.. Fetal hepatomegaly: causes and associations. *Radiographics* 2020;40(2):589–604.

Rohrer L, Vial Y, Hanquinet S, Tenisch E, Alamo L. Imaging of anorectal malformations in utero. *Eur J Radiol* 2020;125:108859.

Tongprasert F, Srisupundit K, Luewan S, Tongsong T. Normal length of the fetal liver from 14 to 40 weeks of gestational age. *J Clin Ultrasound* 2011;39(2):74–77.

CHAPTER 3.6

Genitourinary Tract

SUMMARY BOX

ANATOMY ASSESSMENT

Kidneys

- Transverse section of the abdomen demonstrating both kidneys:
  - Most readily imaged with spine anterior (Fig. 3.6.1)
  - Measure size (Table 3.6.1)
  - In most fetuses, anteroposterior diameter of renal pelvis is <7 mm before 28 weeks and <10 mm after 28 weeks (Fig. 3.6.2)
  - Confirm bilateral presence of the kidneys with no fusion in the midline
  - Assess corticomedullary differentiation – clear demarcation between cortex and medulla can be seen at 20 weeks (Fig. 3.6.3)
- Assess echogenicity – renal echogenicity decreases compared to liver and spleen after 20 weeks
- Best practice requires additional sagittal and coronal views to:
  - allow identification of the duplex system
  - allow demonstration of renal arteries (Fig. 3.6.4)

Ureters

Not normally visible on second or third trimester scans

Bladder

- Visible in the pelvis
- Check integrity of the anterior abdominal wall
- If empty, should refill within 30 minutes
- Use colour Doppler to confirm three vessel cord

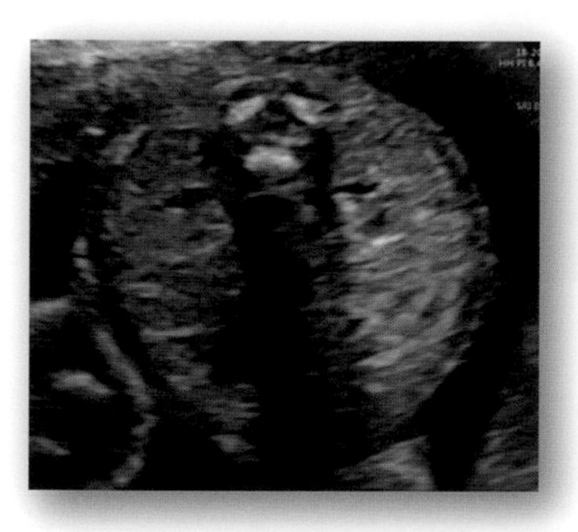

Fig. 3.6.1 Transverse section of the fetal abdomen showing normal fetal kidneys. Note normal renal pelvis on both sides.

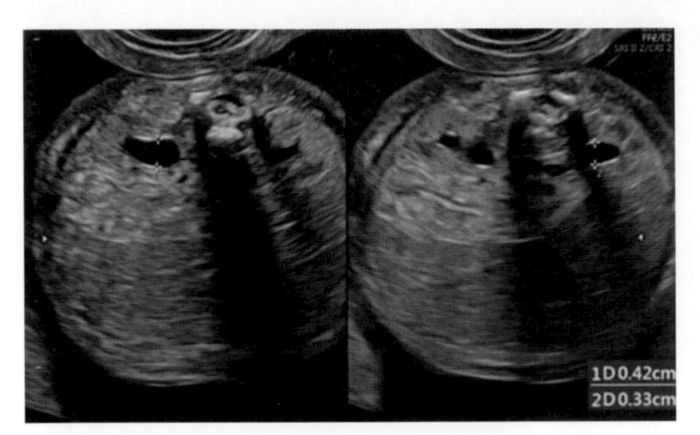

Fig. 3.6.2 Measurement of renal pelvises in anteroposterior diameter.

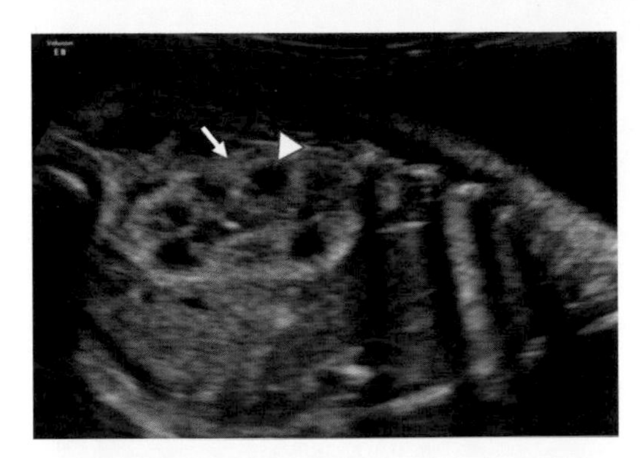

Fig. 3.6.3 Longitudinal section of a normal fetal kidney in the second trimester.
The medullary pyramids are seen as regular, anechoic areas (arrowhead). The relatively brighter cortex surrounds medullary pyramids (arrow). There is an obvious corticomedullary differentiation.

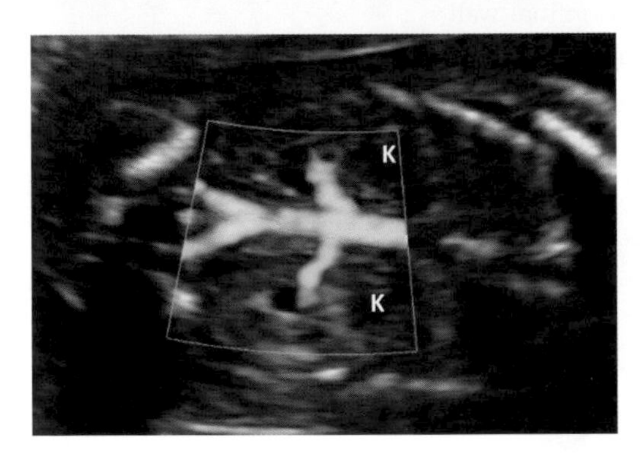

Fig. 3.6.4 Coronal section of the fetal abdomen to demonstrate both kidneys (K). Colour Doppler shows the abdominal aorta and both renal arteries.

Table 3.6.1 Fetal kidneys: normal ranges for length, transverse and anteroposterior (AP) diameter.

	Length (mm)		Transverse (mm)		AP diameter (mm)	
Weeks	Lower	Upper	Lower	Upper	Lower	Upper
18	14	20	7	14	7	13
20	17	23	9	16	9	15
22	19	26	11	18	10	16
24	22	28	13	20	12	18
26	24	31	15	22	13	20
28	27	34	16	24	14	21
30	29	36	18	25	19	23

Modified from van Vuuren SH et al. Size and volume charts of fetal kidney, renal pelvis and adrenal gland. *Ultrasound Obstet Gynecol* 2012;40:659–664.

KIDNEY(S) NOT VISIBLE

UNILATERAL AGENESIS

Definition and Characteristics

- Normal renal development starts around the fifth week of gestation when the ureteric bud starts to interact with the metanephric mesenchyme
- Agenesis is caused by a failure of this interaction, possibly due to an early vascular insult or a failure of renal mesenchyme to form nephrons
- Birth prevalence of unilateral agenesis is 1 in 2,000 births, more common in males
- Unilateral agenesis can be caused by many gene mutations (*RET*, *BMP4*)
- Most cases are sporadic, but can be inherited in an autosomal dominant manner with incomplete penetrance

Ultrasound Assessment

- Check in all three planes
- Use the transvaginal approach if breech
- Use colour Doppler to demonstrate renal arteries (Fig. 3.6.5a)
- Check for pelvic (ectopic) kidney
- The fetal adrenal gland often expands into the renal fossa and can be easily mistaken for a kidney
- Check the other kidney
- Assess amniotic fluid volume
- Exclude associated anomalies (trisomies 18 and 21, Fraser syndrome, Smith–Lemli–Opitz, VACTERL)

Investigations

- Genetic testing by microarray and exome, if available
- The input of clinical geneticists is very important to ensure that appropriate tests are done based on phenotype/genotype correlation

Management and Counselling

- Unilateral isolated renal agenesis has no impact on obstetric care
- Postnatal renal scan should be arranged, usually 7–14 days after birth
- Associated renal abnormalities are relatively common, mainly vesicoureteral reflux (~30%)
- If a neonate has a ureteric dilatation on the contralateral side, antibiotics are usually prescribed (e.g. trimethoprim 2 mg/kg/day) and follow-up arranged
- Long-term prognosis depends mainly on the functional state of the contralateral kidney and the presence of extra-renal anomalies (~30%)
- Hypertension and proteinuria are relatively common in later life (~20%)

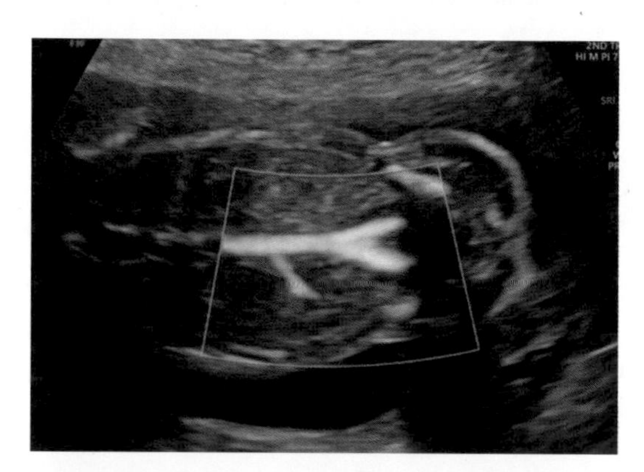

Fig. 3.6.5a Coronal section of the abdomen showing a single kidney and a single renal artery. Unilateral renal agenesis is a likely diagnosis; however, an ectopic kidney should be excluded.

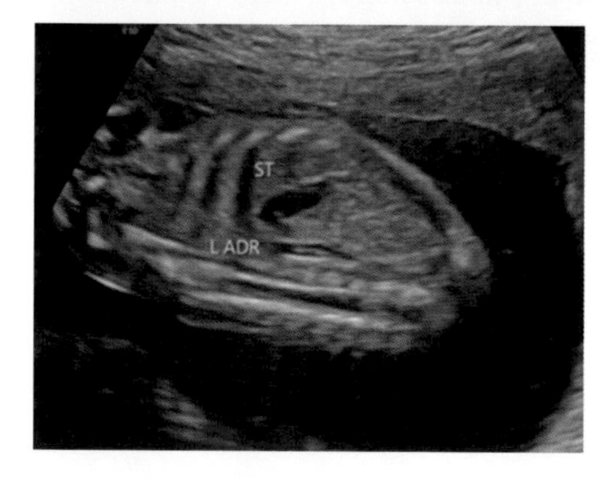

Fig. 3.6.5b Picture from the same case showing empty renal fossa and a "lying down" adrenal gland. The adrenal gland does not change its position in the case of ectopic kidneys. LADR, left adrenal gland; ST, stomach.

BILATERAL AGENESIS

Definition and Characteristics

- Reported fetal prevalence of bilateral agenesis ~1 in 10,000
- Detectable genetic mutations in bilateral agenesis are relatively rare. If present, they are inherited autosomal recessively

Ultrasound Assessment

- Anhydramnios makes detailed assessment very difficult
- Amnioinfusion is often necessary to make the definitive diagnosis, particularly in obese patients
- Fetal adrenal glands are relatively large, with a shape distinctly similar to the fetal kidneys (Fig. 3.6.6)
- Use the transvaginal approach if breech
- Use colour Doppler to demonstrate renal arteries
- Look for associated cardiac and VATER abnormalities (~25%)

Investigations

- Amnioinfusion will not only allow better visualisation and confirmation of suspected diagnosis, but will also exclude PPROM (see Chapter 16)
- MRI may be needed to confirm absence and exclude an ectopic kidney

Counselling

- Anhydramnios causes lethal pulmonary hypoplasia, joint contractures and Potter's facies (a flat nose, recessed chin, prominent epicanthal folds and abnormal, low-set ears)
- Consider termination of pregnancy
- Rare reports of survival with repeated amnioinfusions, but the repeated procedures can cause chorioamnionitis and significant maternal morbidity

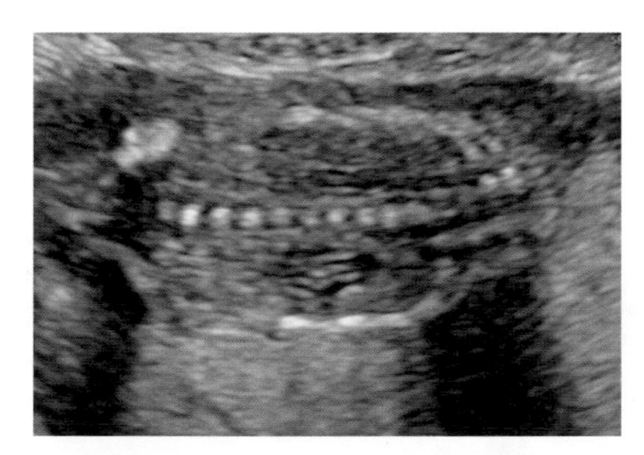

Fig. 3.6.6a Coronal view of fetal abdomen showing bilateral renal agenesis. The empty renal fossae with 'lying down' adrenal glands.

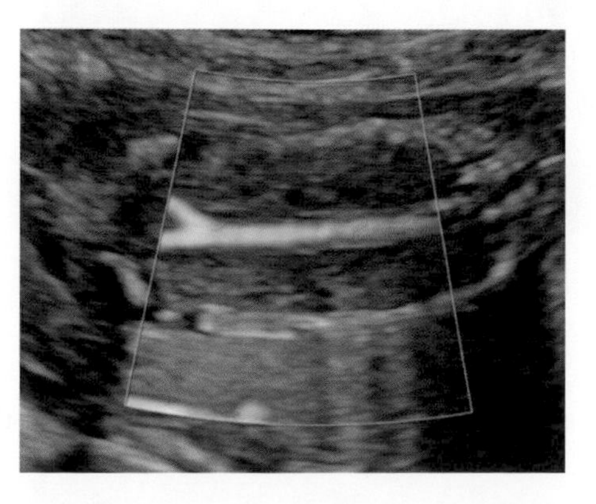

Fig. 3.6.6b Colour Doppler of the same case showing bilateral absence of renal arteries.

DISTORTED RENAL ANATOMY

DUPLEX KIDNEY

Definition and Characteristics

- Duplication of ureteric bud, normally with fusion, resulting in a large duplex kidney with upper and lower poles
- May be unilateral or bilateral

Ultrasound Assessment

- Sagittal or coronal sections reveal duplication of renal parenchyma (Fig. 3.6.7)
- Transverse cross section usually appears normal, although hydronephrosis may be present
- Check if unilateral or bilateral
- Ureters may merge or run separately
- Exclude other structural anomalies including ureterocele (Fig. 3.6.7b)

Investigations

- Genetic testing by microarray and exome, if available
- The input of clinical geneticists is very important to ensure that appropriate tests are done based on phenotype–genotype correlation

Counselling

- Long-term prognosis depends on the presence of associated pathologies, including significant hydronephrosis, ureterovesical reflux, ureterocoele and ureteropelvic junction obstruction
- Full extent of renal abnormalities may not be determined until infancy
- Good prognosis, if isolated

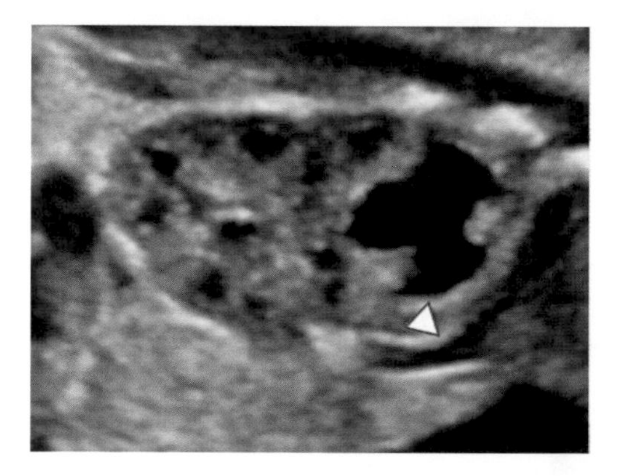

Fig. 3.6.7a Longitudinal section of the fetal kidney showing a double moiety. The lower moiety shows dilatation of the pelvis (arrowhead).

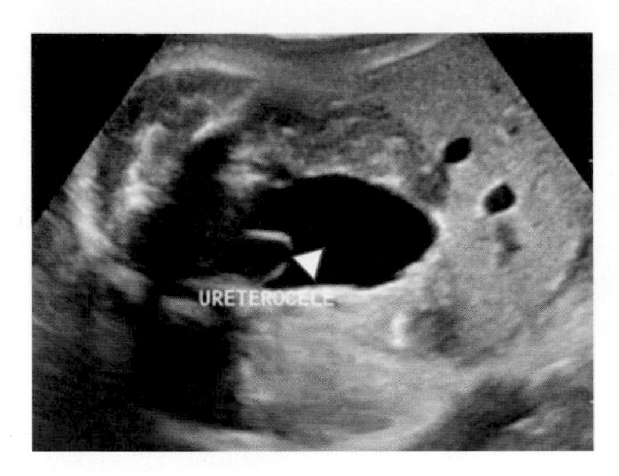

Fig. 3.6.7b Distended bladder in the same patient with double moiety. Ureterocoele is seen as a "bladder within a bladder" (arrowhead).

HORSESHOE KIDNEY

Definition and Characteristics

- Fused lower poles of fetal kidneys
- Prevalence ~1 in 500 births, more common in males
- Mostly sporadic, but also associated with syndromic pathology, or chromosomal abnormalities (Turner syndrome, trisomies)

Ultrasound Assessment

- Best visualised on the transverse and coronal views (Fig. 3.6.8)
- The fused lower pole sits in front of the aorta
- Look for the most common associated anomalies (caudal regression syndrome with sacral agenesis and anal atresia, CNS, cardiac)
- Look for signs of common trisomies (13, 18, 21) and Turner syndrome
- Look for hydronephrosis

Investigations

- If ultrasound exam suggests an isolated horseshoe kidney, no other tests are needed

Counselling

- No impact on obstetric care
- Postnatal follow-up is needed because of association with infections, hydronephrosis due to ureteropelvic junction obstruction and nephrolithiasis

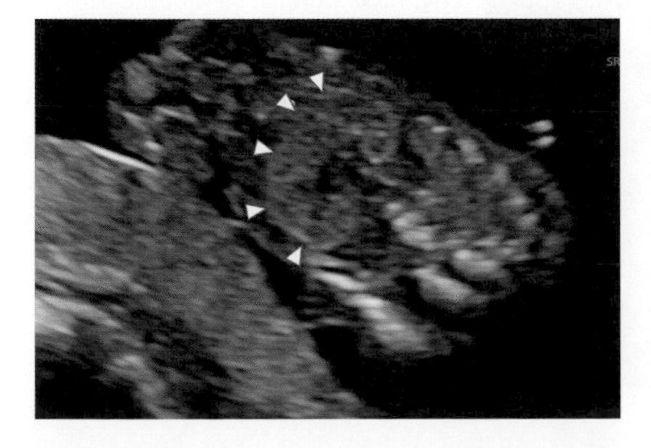

Fig. 3.6.8a Coronal section of the fetal abdomen showing horseshoe kidney (arrowheads). A band of tissue is seen bridging across the midline.

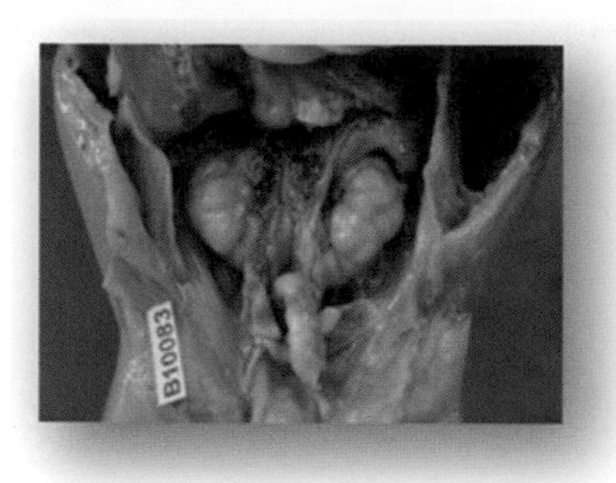

Fig. 3.6.8b Autopsy picture of the same case showing horseshoe kidney.

PELVIC KIDNEY

Definition and Characteristics

- The most common location of an ectopic kidney
- It is caused by a failure of the fetal kidney to migrate upwards from the fetal pelvis during embryological development
- Relatively common (1 in 700–1,000 livebirths)

Ultrasound Assessment

- The kidney lies below the aortic bifurcation (Fig. 3.6.9)
- The kidney's size and shape are usually normal
- The renal fossa is empty and the renal artery cannot be seen in its usual place; therefore, a false diagnosis of unilateral agenesis is easily made
- If pelvic kidney is isolated, amniotic volume should be normal

Investigations

- If ultrasound exam suggests an isolated pelvic kidney, no other tests are needed

Counselling

- No impact on obstetric care
- Normal renal function is highly likely

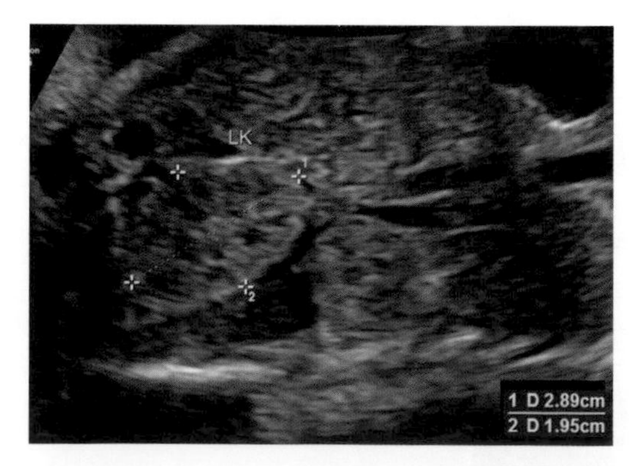

Fig. 3.6.9a Coronal view of the pelvis with a pelvic kidney.

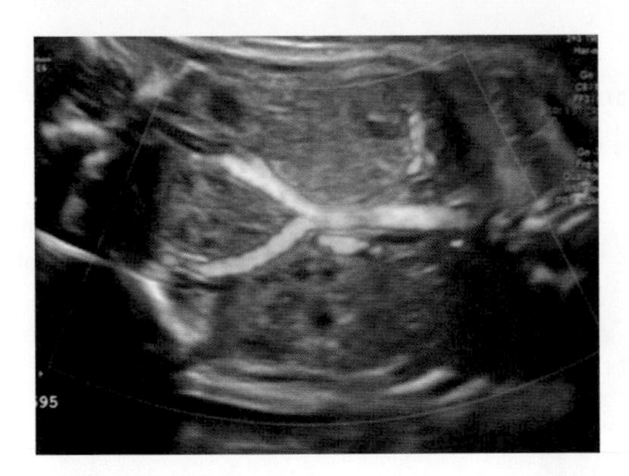

Fig. 3.6.9b Colour Doppler of the same patient showing a widened aortic bifurcation angle which could be an indicator for the presence of a pelvic kidney.

RENAL CYSTS

MULTICYSTIC DYSPLASTIC KIDNEY DISEASE

Definition and Characteristics

- Multicystic dysplastic kidney disease (MCDK) is a result of an abnormal interaction between the ureteric bud and metanephros, possibly due to an ischaemic insult
- Multiple non-communicating, thin-walled cysts arise from immature glomeruli and primitive tubules
- Prevalence ~1 in 4,000 livebirths

Ultrasound Assessment

- Assess the size and regularity of cysts
- In MCDK, kidney(s) have increased length and thin-walled, non-communicating cysts of varying size (Figs 3.6.10 and 3.6.11)
- Assess amniotic fluid volume serially
- In isolated unilateral MCDK, amniotic fluid volume is normal
- In bilateral MCDK, amniotic fluid volume will be reduced or absent
- Look for ureterocele as it is relatively common in MCDK
- Look for other anatomical anomalies
- Look for markers of common trisomies

Investigations

- Invasive testing for isolated unilateral MCDK is not indicated as the risk of chromosomal abnormalities is not increased
- If MCDK is bilateral, the risk of chromosomal abnormalities is ~15%

Counselling

Unilateral MCDK

- The affected kidney usually has no or minimal function
- Risk of renal or other associated anomalies is ~20%
- In the absence of associated pathology, most affected kidneys will regress (~70%) with good long-term prognosis
- If symptomatic, can be removed laparoscopically in early childhood
- The risk of malignancy is low

Bilateral MCDK

- In bilateral disease, oligo/anhydramnios is always present and prognosis is poor
- Termination of pregnancy should be offered, if legally permissible

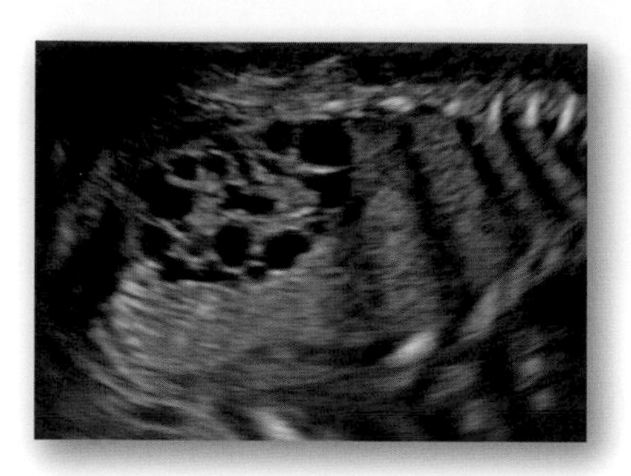

Fig. 3.6.10 Longitudinal section of the multicystic dysplastic kidney with multiple cysts of varying sizes.

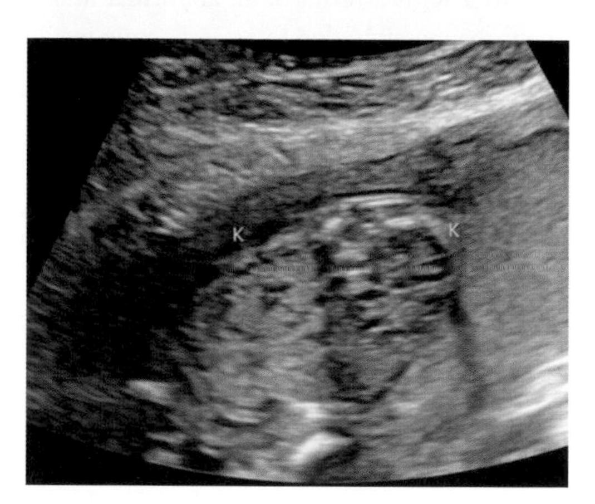

Fig. 3.6.11 Transverse section of the abdomen showing bilateral multicystic dysplastic kidneys. The bladder was not visualised and anhydramnios was present.

OBSTRUCTIVE UROPATHY

- 'Cystic kidneys' may be seen in obstructive uropathy but will be associated with dilation of the collecting system and / or bladder

COMPLEX CYSTS

- Complex renal cysts can be caused by:
  - renal lymphangioma
  - cystic changes within tumours (hamartoma)

ABNORMAL SIZE AND ECHOGENICITY

- Abnormal kidneys will usually have all three measurements outside the normal range (Table 3.6.1)
- Renal echogenicity gradually decreases with gestation and should not be brighter than the liver after 17 weeks' gestation

- Abnormal corticomedullar differentiation is more difficult to define. Normally, renal cortex should be clearly distinguishable from the inner, more hypoechogenic medulla (Fig. 3.6.3)

LARGE BRIGHT KIDNEYS

Differential Diagnosis

Autosomal Recessive Polycystic Kidney Disease (ARPKD)

- *PKD1* gene mutation on chromosome 6
- Classically presents with bilateral, huge hyperechoic kidneys without corticomedullary differentiation and oligo/anhydramnios (Fig. 3.6.12)
- Less frequently, kidneys may be only moderately large with echogenic medulla, hypoechoic cortex ('reversed corticomedullary differentiation') and normal amniotic fluid

Autosomal Dominant Polycystic Kidney Disease (ADPKD)

- *PKD1,2,3* gene mutation; ~10% de novo
- Kidneys are moderately large, with exaggerated corticomedullary differentiation (hyperechoic cortex and hypoechoic medulla)

Other Causes

- Trisomies 13 and 18 (renal cortical microcysts)
- *TCF2* gene mutation (also known as *HNF1b*)
- Overgrowth syndromes (Beckwith–Wiedemann, Perlman)
- Ciliopathies (Bardet–Biedl, Meckel–Gruber)
- Zellweger syndrome
- Renal vein thrombosis – rarely diagnosed prenatally, only in the third trimester
- Congenital nephrotic syndrome (Finnish type) – microcysts caused by dilated proximal tubules

Ultrasound Assessment

- Measure the size of both kidneys
- High-frequency probe may reveal dilated (spindle-like) tubules which are characteristic for ARPKD
- Assess corticomedullary differentiation. ADPKD may look similar to ARPKD, but corticomedullary differentiation is usually visible in ADPKD
- Look for polydactyly (often present in ciliopathies)
- Look for other associated anomalies, especially extremities, posterior fossa, thorax and spine
- Look for FGR or macrosomia

Investigation

- Detailed family history and renal scan of both parents, if indicated
- Genetic testing, including exome testing, if available

Counselling

- Generally, large echogenic kidneys with anhydramnios diagnosed before 24 weeks have poor prognosis and termination of pregnancy should be offered, if legally permissible
- For most cases the prognosis will depend on the underlying pathology
- ARPKD diagnosed in utero has poor prognosis, although less severe cases with normal amniotic fluid have better prognosis
- The prognosis for ADPKD is variable. When there is no family history (de novo cases) ~40% of babies will die within the first year of life

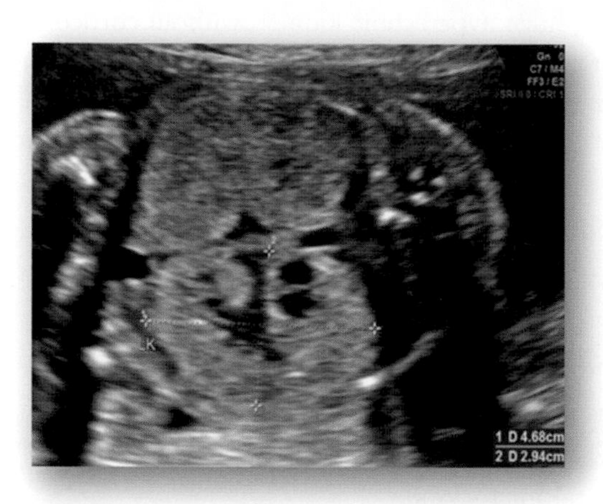

Fig. 3.6.12a Coronal section of a fetus at 21 weeks showing bilateral enlarged echogenic kidney in a case of autosomal recessive polycystic kidneys (ARPKD). Renal pelvis is seen on the right side.

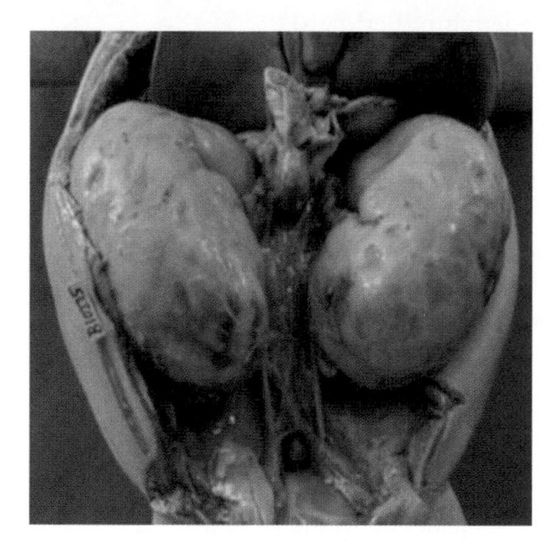

Fig. 3.6.12b Autopsy picture of the same fetus showing bilateral enlarged kidneys.

BRIGHT KIDNEYS, NORMAL SIZE

- Bright kidneys are sometimes seen in normal fetuses; the aetiology is yet to be determined
- Similarly, transient medullary echogenicity is a recognised entity in neonates and is considered a normal variant
- Obstructive uropathy can present with increased echogenicity caused by reduction in glomerular numbers and interstitial fibrosis
- Cytomegalovirus may cause renal echogenicity due to tubular dilatation

SMALL KIDNEYS

Definition and Characteristics

- The diagnosis should be made when all three measurements are repeatedly below the normal range (see Table 3.6.1)
- Isolated hypoplasia is rare and may be caused by mainly sporadic gene mutations (*HNF1Bm*, *PAX2*, *PBX1*)
- Small kidneys can sometimes be seen in severe fetal growth restriction

Ultrasound Assessment

- Isolated hypoplasia should be suspected prenatally when no other pathology has been found on repeated assessments
- Corticomedullary architecture is typically normal

Investigations

- If isolated, karyotyping is not usually offered

Counselling

- Long-term follow-up is needed due to higher risk of hypertension and proteinuria. End-stage renal disease in childhood is rare

EXCESS FLUID IN THE RENAL TRACT

RENAL PELVIS DILATATION AND HYDRONEPHROSIS

Definition and Characteristics

- There is no international consensus on terminology and definitions
- For management and counselling purposes, we prefer to make a distinction between mild renal pelvic dilatation (RPD) and hydronephrosis:
  - **Mild RPD:** renal pelvis measures 4–6 mm with no calyceal involvement and normal corticomedullary differentiation. In most cases these will resolve spontaneously and, therefore, we do not consider this a reportable ultrasound finding
  - **Hydronephrosis:** AP diameter is $\geq$7 mm. Calyceal dilatation may or may not be visible
  - **Severe hydronephrosis:** $>$10 mm before 28^{+0} weeks and $>$15 mm after 28^{+0} weeks

Ultrasound Assessment

- Repeated measurements of the AP diameter (Fig. 3.6.13a)
- Assessment of renal parenchyma (cortex and medulla) (Fig. 3.6.13b)
- Unilateral or bilateral?
- Exclude associated genitourinary and other structural abnormalities (Fig. 3.6.13c)
- Check for aneuploidy markers

Investigations

- Genetic testing by microarray and exome, if available
- The input of clinical geneticists is very important to ensure that appropriate tests are done based on phenotype–genotype correlation

Management and Counselling

- If fetal hydronephrosis is detected, postnatal follow-up should be arranged
- Postnatal ultrasound assessment should be delayed for at least 48 hours, because the neonate may be dehydrated soon after birth and full phenotype may not be apparent soon after birth
- ~45% of babies will have significant postnatal pathology, mainly ureteropelvic junction obstruction, vesicoureteric reflux and low urinary tract obstruction (LUTO)
- The risk of significant postnatal pathology increases to ~90% if renal pelvis AP diameter was >15 mm in the third trimester

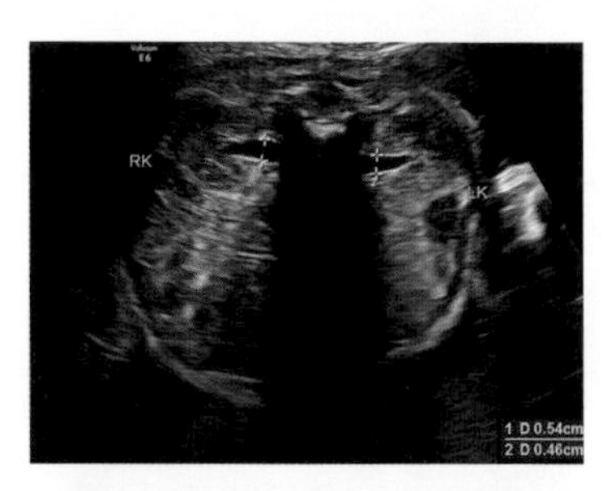

Fig. 3.6.13a 21-week fetus with normal renal pelvis on both sides.

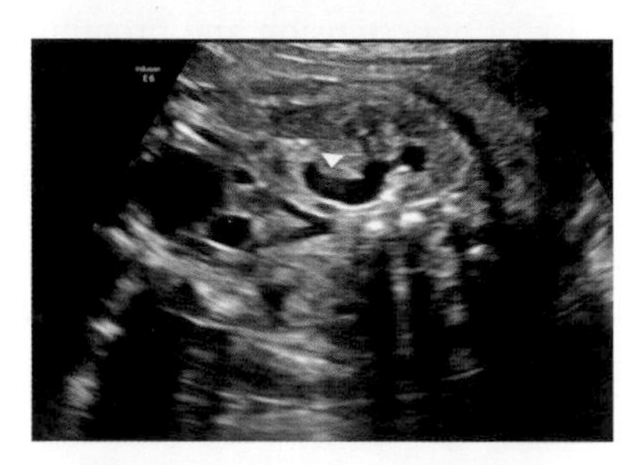

Fig. 3.6.13b Coronal section of the abdomen of the same fetus showing the right kidney and bladder. The ureter appears dilated (arrowhead). Ureteric peristalsis was seen in real time. There were no signs of bladder outlet obstruction or ureterocele. Vesicoureteric reflux was confirmed after birth.

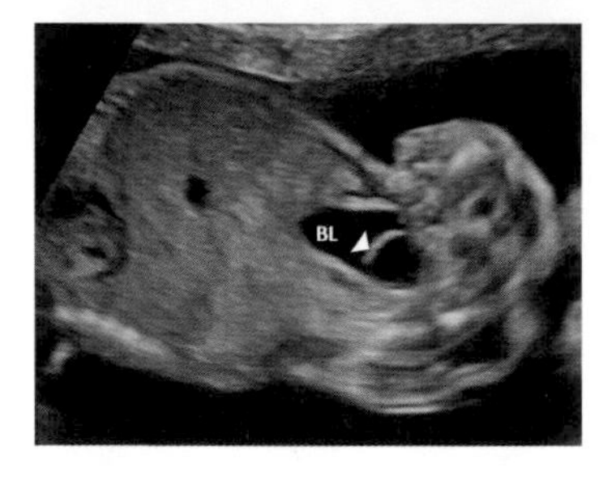

Fig. 3.6.13c Ureterocele is seen as an echogenic ring within the bladder (arrow). BL = bladder.

DILATED URETER(S) WITH NORMAL BLADDER

Definition and Characteristics

- The ureters are not normally seen on prenatal scans – if they can be seen then they are dilated
- The term primary (congenital) megaureter should be used when the underlying pathology is thought to be intrinsic to the ureter and not a consequence of other (more distal) pathology like posterior urethral valve obstruction

- Primary megaureters can be caused by an obstruction (usually at the level of the ureterovesical junction), vesicoureteric reflux (VUR), or combination of both
- Ureteropelvic junction (UPJ) obstruction usually presents with dilated renal pelvis, but without visible urethral dilatation
- Although fetal VUR presents mostly only with dilated renal pelvis, severe cases will have distended ureters and bladder. Family history is important. If parents have VUR, ~35% of offspring will also have it
- It is important to note that fetal megaureter can be both unobstructed and non-refluxing. In fact, this form is the most common in neonates

Ultrasound Assessment

- Unilateral or bilateral?
- Measure the largest transverse diameter for later comparison
- Look for signs of bladder outflow obstruction or ureterocoele (Fig. 3.6.13c)
- If obstructive renal dysplasia is present, the cortex will be hyperechoic, cysts may be present, but corticomedullary differentiation is often absent
- Look for possible duplex kidney and/or ectopic ureter
- Check that dilatation is tubular and not circular (e.g. ovarian cyst)

Investigations

If isolated, there is no indication for invasive testing

Counselling

- Most primary megaureters will resolve spontaneously in the postnatal period (~70%)
- Long-term prognosis, however, is difficult to ascertain based on antenatal features
- The prognosis depends on the underlying pathology and long-term impact on bladder and kidney(s)

ABNORMAL BLADDER

DISTENDED BLADDER

Definition and Characteristics

- The most commonly used definition is subjective but pragmatic: 'large bladder failing to empty during an ultrasound examination lasting ≥40 minutes'
- The enlarged fetal bladder (megacystis) in the second half of pregnancy can be confirmed using the following formula: Megacystis = sagittal diameter (mm) > gestation at diagnosis in weeks + 12
- Possible causes include:
  - LUTO due to posterior urethral valve in boys or urethral stenosis/atresia (Fig. 3.6.14)
  - prune belly syndrome (absent or weak abdominal muscles, bilateral cryptorchism and dilated renal system, often with reflux; aetiology unknown)
  - anorectal malformations including VACTERL, caudal regression and cloacal extrophy
  - overgrowth syndromes (Beckwith–Wiedemann, Sotos)

- megacytis–microcolon–intestinal hypoperistalsis syndrome (MMIHS); this is a functional, usually fatal, obstruction of the gastrointestinal system
- vesicoureteric reflux
- duplex collecting system
- major chromosomal abnormalities (more likely when megacystis is found in the first trimester)
- neurogenic bladder

Ultrasound Assessment

- Confirm that large bladder persists for >40 minutes
- Measure amniotic fluid volume
- Look for bladder wall hypertrophy (Fig. 3.6.15)
- Look for ureteric dilatation and/or ureterocele
- Look for 'keyhole sign', but bear in mind that the sign is not pathognomonic for LUTO; it has also been reported in vesicoureteric reflux (VUR), primary megaureter and prune belly syndrome
- Look for evidence of obstructive renal dysplasia. If present, cortex will be hyperechoic, cysts may be present, but corticomedullary differentiation is usually absent
- Detailed fetal echocardiography (22q11 deletion syndrome)
- Exclude congenital diaphragmatic hernia
- Look for evidence of VACTERL
- Look for signs of MMHIS (thin bladder wall, dilated stomach and bowel loops; amniotic fluid is likely to be normal)

Investigations

- Genetic testing by microarray and exome, if available
- The input of clinical geneticists is very important to ensure that appropriate tests are done based on phenotype–genotype correlation
- The authors do not use (serial) vesicocentesis in the diagnostic work-up of megacystis. The management is based on the phenotypic characteristics rather than biochemistry
- MRI may be useful to exclude anorectal anomalies

Counselling

- If resolution occurs before 23 weeks, the condition is unlikely to be clinically significant
- Any resolution after 23 weeks is still associated with a significant risk of postnatal urological pathology (~70%)
- Ultrasound phenotype is not a very good predictor of long-term outcome; therefore, every effort should be made to ascertain the underlying pathology
- The pros and cons of vesicoamniotic shunting are discussed in Chapter 16

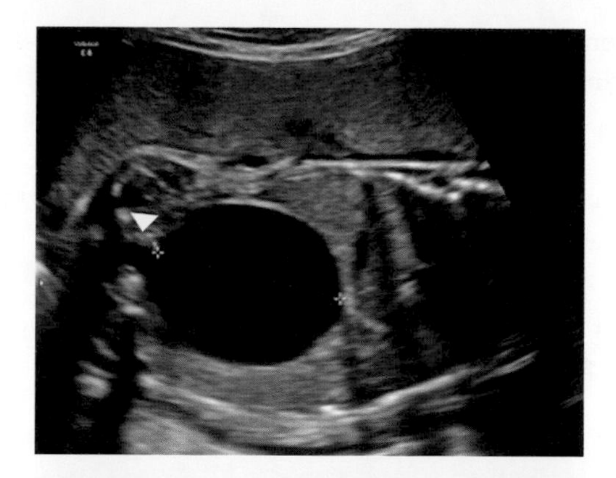

Fig. 3.6.14a Distended bladder with dilated posterior urethra in a fetus with lower urinary tract obstruction (LUTO).

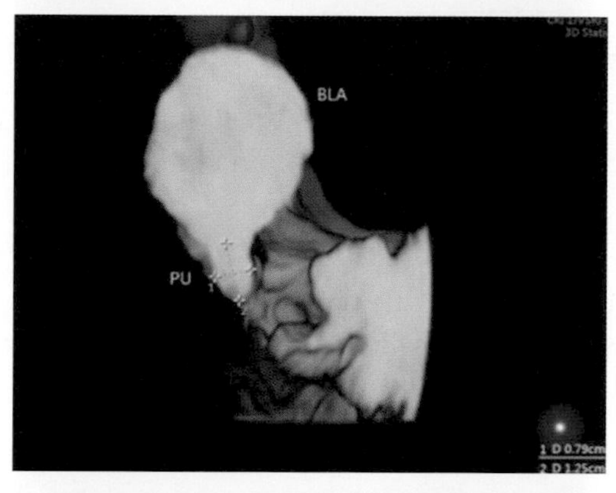

Fig. 3.6.14b 3D rendering in inversion mode of the same fetus, showing distended bladder and a dilated posterior urethra.

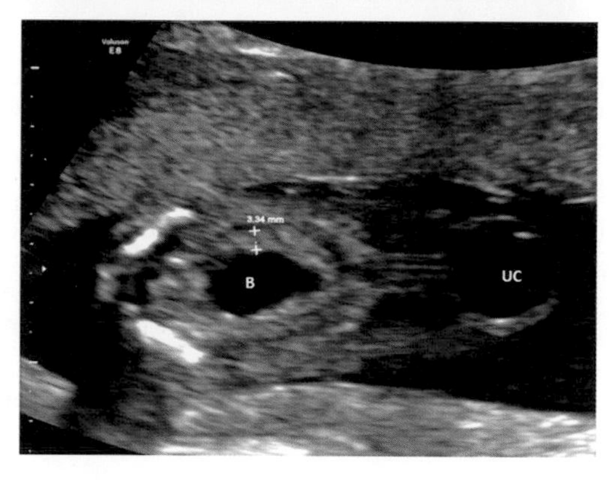

Fig. 3.6.15 Thick-walled bladder (B) of 3.3 mm in a case of bladder outlet obstruction. The fetus has bilateral hydronephrosis. An umbilical cord cyst (UC) was also visible.

SMALL OR NOT VISIBLE BLADDER

Bladder Exstrophy

Definition and Characteristics

- Anterior bladder wall is missing and posterior wall is exposed
- Rare: ~1 in 30,000–50,000 births

Ultrasound Assessment

- Usually presents with an absent bladder and a solid mass in the lower abdomen (Fig. 3.6.16)
- Umbilical arteries run alongside the 'bulge'

- Misdiagnosis of gastroschisis or omphalocele is common
- Amniotic fluid volume is usually normal
- Widely separated pubic bones
- Kidneys are usually normal
- External genitalia are usually difficult to visualise

Invasive Testing

- Not associated with chromosomal abnormalities, but karyotyping may be offered in the work-up of presumed ambiguous genitalia

Management and Counselling

- Long-term prognosis after neonatal surgical repair is good
- It is critical to exclude OEIS, in which case in utero transfer to a specialist surgical centre is preferable

OEIS Complex (Cloacal Exstrophy)

Definition and Characteristics

- OEIS complex is the preferred term for this specific cluster of anomalies: omphalocele, bladder (cloacal) exstrophy, imperforate anus, malformations of the spine (absent sacral vertebrae, spina bifida) (Fig. 3.6.17)
- Very rare: ~1 in 300,000 births

Ultrasound Assessment

- Bladder is not visible as it is split into two halves
- Look for an omphalocele that is attached to the top of the 'bulge' and may contain not just bowel and liver, but also stomach and other parts of the genitourinary tract
- Detailed examination of the whole spine (most defects are skin-covered)
- Look for other associated anomalies, including abnormally formed genitalia, and talipes
- A single umbilical artery is common

Investigations

- Not associated with chromosomal abnormalities, but karyotyping may be offered in the work-up of presumed ambiguous genitalia

Management and Counselling

- Counselling is best done by local experts in surgical repair and long-term follow-up
- Multiple operations are needed, but in the best centres long-term outcome is good for many children
- If optimal postnatal care is not readily available, termination of pregnancy should be discussed

Other Causes

- Renal agenesis
- Fetal growth restriction
- Twin–twin transfusion syndrome

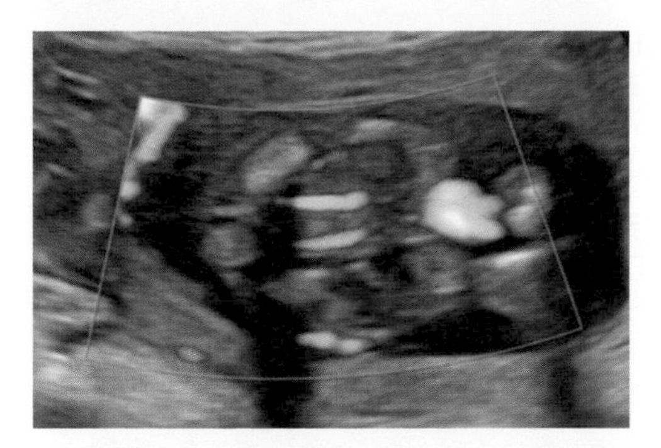

Fig. 3.6.16a Bladder exstrophy. The two umbilical arteries are clearly seen but the bladder is not visible.

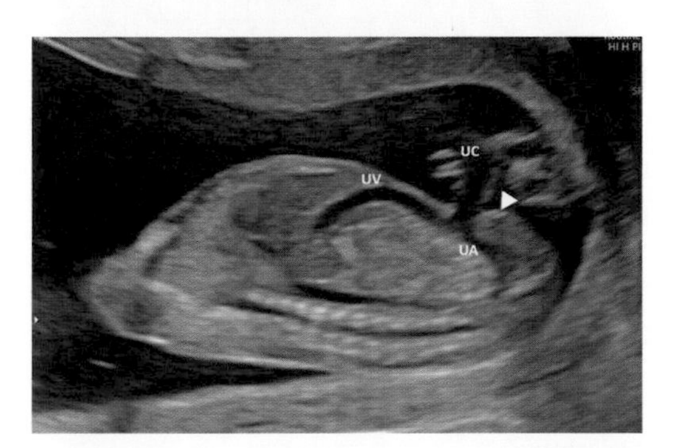

Fig. 3.6.16b Sagittal view of the same case. Bladder exstrophy is seen as a small echogenic bulge (arrowhead) just inferior to the umbilical cord insertion. Note the absence of bladder in the pelvis and normal liquor. UA, umbilical artery; UV, umbilical vein.

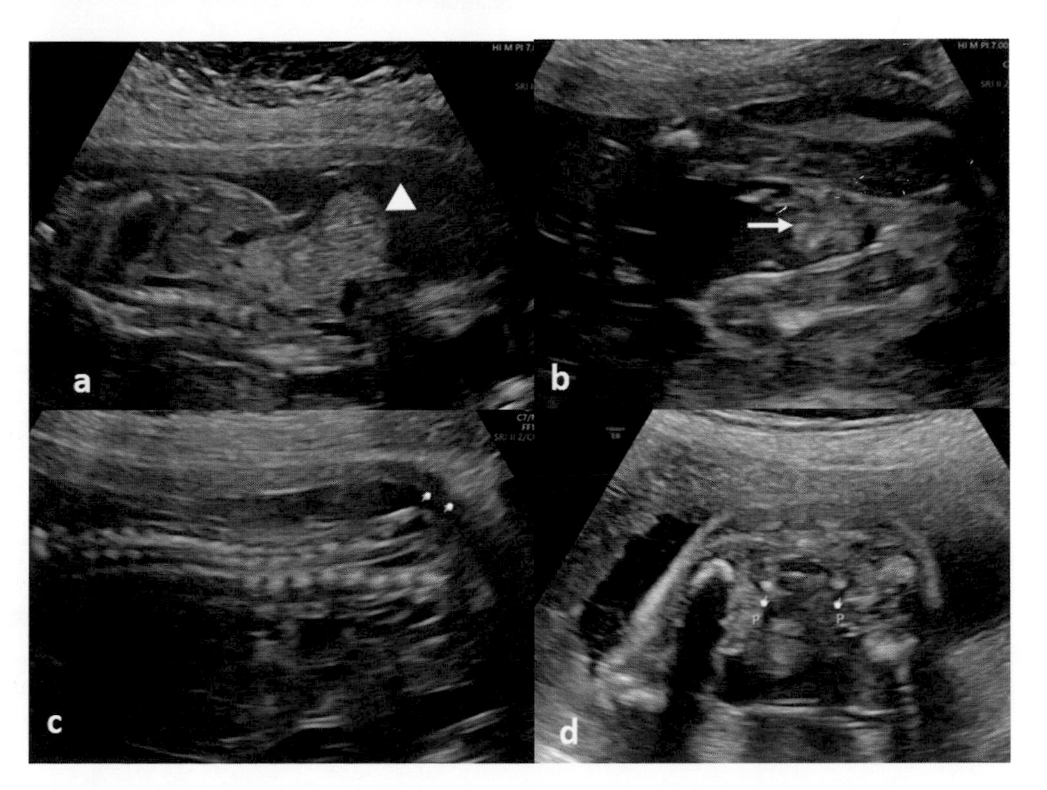

Fig. 3.6.17 OEIS complex. (a) Omphalocele (arrowhead). (b) Bladder exstrophy (arrow). (c) Spina bifida. (d) Coronal view of the pelvis showing widened pubic rami as two echogenic dots (small finger arrows).

'DOUBLE RING' WITHIN BLADDER (URETEROCELE)

Definition and Characteristics

- Abnormal dilatation of the distal portion of the ureter is called ureterocele
- Most ureterocele are extravesical ('ectopic') and associated with a duplicated collecting system, most commonly in the upper moiety
- Also associated with MCDK (~20%) and vesicoureteric reflux
- Bilateral in ~10%

Ultrasound Assessment

- Echogenic ring within the bladder is virtually diagnostic (Fig. 3.6.18)
- Look for evidence of a duplex kidney (upper moiety) or other renal anomalies (e.g. MCDK)
- Serial scanning is indicated because large ureterocele may obstruct the contralateral collecting system, causing hydronephrosis

Investigations

- Genetic testing by microarray and exome, if available
- The input of clinical geneticists is very important to ensure that appropriate tests are done based on phenotype–genotype correlation

Counselling

- Good prognosis, if isolated
- Prophylactic antibiotics are prescribed in the neonatal period followed by regular follow-up
- Surgery may be needed for severe, symptomatic cases
- Recurrence risk is low

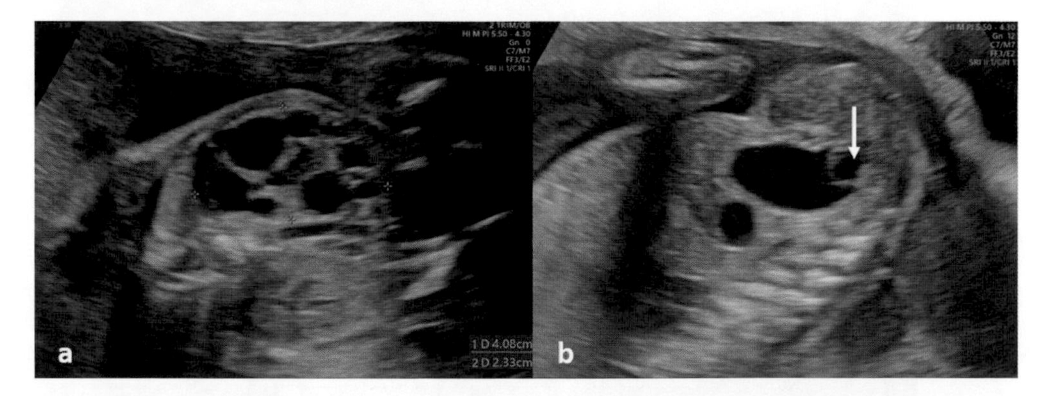

Fig. 3.6.18 (a) Unilateral MCDK at 21 weeks. (b) There was also an ureterocele seen as an echogenic ring (arrow) within the bladder.

GENITALIA APPEAR AMBIGUOUS

Definition and Characteristics

- Embryological sexual differentiation occurs from 6 weeks' gestation
- Differentiation into male phenotype is driven by the *SRY* gene
- Ambiguous genitalia may be identified through:
  - discrepancy between genetic (NIPT or karyotype) and ultrasound-based gender identification
  - identification of a small penis or large clitoris
  - identification of large labial/scrotal folds (Fig. 3.6.19)

Ultrasound Assessment

- Exclude other structural anomalies
- Expanded skeletal survey (Chapter 3.7)
- Look for phenotypic characteristics of Smith–Lemli–Opitz and Fraser syndrome (Chapter 19)

Investigations

- Amniocentesis for chromosomal microarray

46XY But Not Clearly Male Phenotype

- Whole-exome sequencing may be useful to identify genetic mutation
- Gene mutation testing:
  - *SRY*
  - *AR* for androgen insensitivity syndrome
  - *SRD5A2* for 5-alpha reductase deficiency
  - *AMH*/*AMHR2* for persistent Mullerian duct syndrome
  - *LHCGR* for Leydig cell failure
- Other tests:
  - amniotic fluid 7-8-dehydrocholesterol (7/8-DHC) levels for Smith–Lemli–Opitz syndrome

46XX But Not Clearly Female Phenotype

- Whole-exome sequencing may be useful to identify genetic mutation
- Gene mutation testing:
  - *CYP21A2* for congenital adrenal hyperplasia (>90% of cases are due to impaired activity caused by this mutation). NIPT is also available
  - *SRY*, *SOX3*, *SOX9*, *NROB1*, *NR5A1* for ovotesticular syndrome
  - *CYP19A1* for placental aromatase deficiency
- Other tests:
  - Maternal serum testosterone for androgen-secreting metastatic ovarian Krukenberg tumour

Management and Counselling

- Avoid assigning gender/gender-based pronouns
- Input from clinical geneticists and endocrinologists will be invaluable to identify the best time for investigations (antenatal versus postnatal)
- Involve neonatologist/paediatric endocrinologist for postnatal review and management

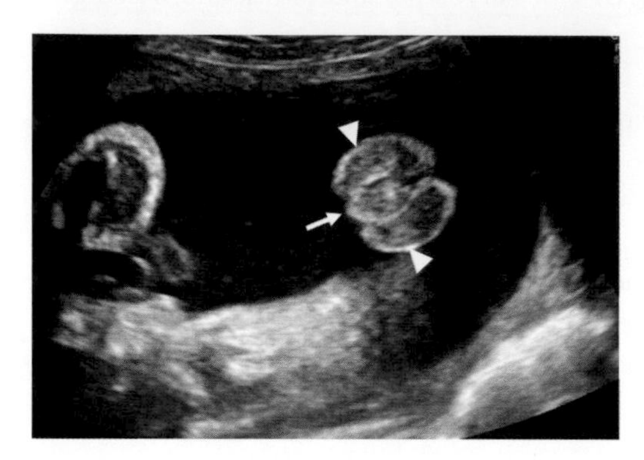

Fig. 3.6.19 Ambiguous genitalia in a fetus with congenital adrenal hyperplasia. The two labial folds are seen (arrowheads) and an enlarged clitoris (arrow). This patient had a previously affected baby.

SUGGESTED READING

PRIMARY RESEARCH

Al Naimi A, Baumüller JE, Spahn S, Bahlmann F. Prenatal diagnosis of multicystic dysplastic kidney disease in the second trimester screening. *Prenat Diagn* 2013;33(8):726–731.

Fontanella F, Duin L, Adama van Scheltema PN, et al. Fetal megacystis: prediction of spontaneous resolution and outcome. *Ultrasound Obstet Gynecol* 2017;50(4):458–463.

Turkyilmaz G, Cetin B, Sivrikoz T, et al. Antenatally detected ureterocele: associated anomalies and postnatal prognosis. *Taiwan J Obstet Gynecol* 2019;58:531–535.

REVIEWS AND GUIDELINES

Cheung KW, Morris RK, Kilby MD. Congenital urinary tract obstruction. *Best Pract Res Clin Obstet Gynaecol* 2019;58:78–92.

Dias T, Sairam S, Kumarasiri S. Ultrasound diagnosis of fetal renal abnormalities. *Best Pract Res Clin Obstet Gynaecol* 2014;28(3):403–415.

Gimpel C, Avni FE, Bergmann C, et al. Perinatal diagnosis, management, and follow-up of cystic renal diseases: a clinical practice recommendation with systematic literature reviews. *JAMA Pediatr* 2018;172(1):74–86.

Huber C, Shazly SA, Blumenfeld YJ, Jelin E, Ruano R. Update on the prenatal diagnosis and outcomes of fetal bilateral renal agenesis. *Obstet Gynecol Surv* 2019;74(5):298–302.

Liu DB, Armstrong WR 3rd, Maizels M. Hydronephrosis: prenatal and postnatal evaluation and management. *Clin Perinatol* 2014;41(3):661–678.

Nguyen HT, Herndon CD, Cooper C, et al. The Society for Fetal Urology consensus statement on the evaluation and management of antenatal hydronephrosis. *J Pediatr Urol* 2010;6(3):212–231.

Rosenblum S, Pal A, Reidy K. Renal development in the fetus and premature infant. *Semin Fetal Neonatal Med* 2017;22(2):58–66.

Stambough K, Magistrado L, Perez-Milicua G. Evaluation of ambiguous genitalia. *Curr Opin Obstet Gynecol* 2019;31:303–308.

Taghavi K, Sharpe C, Stringer MD. Fetal megacystis: a systematic review. *J Pediatr Urol* 2017;13(1): 7–15.

Talati AN, Webster CM, Vora NL. Prenatal genetic considerations of congenital anomalies of the kidney and urinary tract (CAKUT). *Prenat Diagn* 2019;39(9):679–692.

Westland R, Schreuder MF, Ket JCF, van Wijk JAE. Unilateral renal agenesis: a systematic review on associated anomalies and renal injury, *Nephrol Dialy Transplant* 2013;28(7):1844–1855.

CHAPTER 3.7

Skeletal Anomalies

SUMMARY BOX

ANTENATAL DIAGNOSTIC WORK-UP

- Skeletal dysplasias are most commonly suspected during routine mid-trimester scan that should include visualisation of all long bones and normal-looking hands and feet
- More than 450 different skeletal dysplasias have been described
- While ultrasound remains the main method for prenatal diagnosis of skeletal dysplasia, given the difficulties with fetal dysmorphology due to overlapping phenotypes (Table 3.7.1), early recourse to molecular diagnosis is recommended
- While whole-exome sequencing is important for discovery of new disease-causing genes, targeted exome sequencing (TES) is currently the preferred method for prenatal diagnosis of skeletal dysplasias
- Currently >350 causative genes have been identified; therefore, detailed and accurate fetal phenotyping is critically important to maximise the clinical utility of genetic testing
- Increasingly, genetic testing of skeletal dysplasias can be done by cffDNA analysis (NIPT), including testing for *FGFR* and *COL* mutations

Table 3.7.1 Differential diagnosis of skeletal abnormalities based on phenotypic characteristics that can be identified antenatally with ultrasound.

Phenotype	Differential diagnosis before 24 weeks	Differential diagnosis after 24 weeks
Skull		
• Hypomineralisation (Fig. 3.7.1a)	Osteogenesis imperfecta (OI) type 2, Achondrogenesis, Cleidocranial dysplasia, Hypophosphatasia,	
• Deformation under pressure (Fig. 3.7.1b)	OI type 2/3, Hypophosphatasia	
• Cloverleaf shape (Fig. 3.7.2)	Thanatophoric dysplasia type 2	Crouzon and other craniosynostosis syndromes
• Microcephaly	Rhizomelic chondrodysplasia punctata	Cockayne, Microcephalic osteodysplastic primordial dwarfism, Seckel syndrome
• Macrocephaly relative	Achondrogenesis, Thanatophoric dysplasia, Campomelic dysplasia	Achondroplasia, hypochondroplasia

Table 3.7.1 (*cont.*)

Phenotype	Differential diagnosis before 24 weeks	Differential diagnosis after 24 weeks
Face		
• Hypotelorism (Fig. 3.7.3)		
• Hypertelorism (Fig. 3.7.4)	Atelosteogenesis (usually subtle)	
• Cataract (solid, echogenic disc) (Fig. 3.7.5)	Rhizomelic Chondrodysplasia punctata	
• Nasal bone		
• Cleft lip/palate	Roberts	
• Frontal bossing (unusually pronounced forehead) (Fig. 3.7.6)	Achondrogenesis, Atelosteogenesis, Acromesomelic dysplasia	Achondroplasia
• Sloping forehead (Fig. 3.7.7)		Seckel syndrome
• Midface hypoplasia (Fig. 3.7.8)	Chondrodysplasia punctata, Stickler syndrome	
• Micrognathia	Achondrogenesis, Atelosteogenesis, Campomelic dysplasia, Diastrophic dysplasia	Stickler, Spondyloepiphyseal dysplasia congenita, Seckel syndrome
Shoulder girdle		
• Clavicle short or absent (Fig. 3.7.9)	Cleidocranial dysostosis	
• Scapulae small or absent (Figs. 3.7.10 and 3.7.11)	Campomelic dysplasia	
Thorax		
• Very short and narrow (Fig. 3.7.12)	Achondrogenesis, Thanatophoric dysplasia, OI, Atelosteogenesis, Hypophosphatasia, Short rib polydactyly syndrome, Jeune, Ellis–Van Creveld	
• Champagne cork appearance (Fig. 3.7.13)	Thanatophoric dysplasia	

Table 3.7.1 (*cont.*)

Phenotype	Differential diagnosis before 24 weeks	Differential diagnosis after 24 weeks
• Long and narrow	Campomelic dysplasia, Jarcho–Levin	Ellis–van Creveld
• Short ('head on neck')	Jarcho–Levin	Spondyloepiphyseal dysplasia congenita, Klippel–Feil, Goldenhar
Ribs		
• Short straight (Fig. 3.7.14)	Thantophoric dysplasia, Short rib polydactyly syndrome, Jeune, Ellis–van Creveld, Achondrogenesis type 2	
• Rib fractures/beading (Fig. 3.7.15)	OI, Achondrogenesis type 1	
• Ribs – fusion	Jarcho–Levin, Gorlin	
Spine		
• Kyphoscoliosis – excessive outward and sideways curvature of thoracic spine (Fig. 3.7.16a,b)	Spondylocostal dysplasia, Jarcho–Levin	Achondroplasia
• Lordosis – lumbar part arches too far inward		Achondroplasia, hypochondroplasia
• Hypomineralisation	OI type 2; Hypophosphatasia, Achondrogenesis type 1	
• Diastematomyelia – split cord (Figs. 3.7.17 and 3.7.18)		
• Vertebral bodies – fusion (Fig. 3.7.19)	Jarcho–Levin, Klipper–Feil (cervical), VATER	
• Hemivertebrae (Fig. 3.7.20)	Goldenhar, VATER	
• Sacral agenesis/caudal regression (Fig. 3.7.21)		

Table 3.7.1 (*cont.*)

Phenotype	Differential diagnosis before 24 weeks	Differential diagnosis after 24 weeks
Long bones		
• Present/absent		
• Length		
• Shortening – entire limb (micromelia) (Fig. 3.7.22a,b)	Achondrogenesis, OI type 2, Atelosteogenesis, Diastrophic dysplasia, Hypophosphatasia, Short rib polydactyly, Thanatophoric dysplasia, Roberts	Achondroplasia, spondyloepiphyseal dysplasia congenita
• Shortening – humerus or femur (rhizomelia)	Achondroplasia, Atelosteogenesis, Rhizomelic chondrodysplasia punctata	Jeune
• Shortening – radius, ulna, tibia or fibula (mesomelia)	Ellis–van Creveld	Ellis–van Creveld, SHOX deficiency
• Shortening of bones in hands and feet (acromelia)		Achondroplasia, Ellis–van Creveld
• Bowing/angulation (Fig. 3.7.23)	Thanatophoric dysplasia type 1 (telephone receiver), OI type 2/3, Campomelic dysplasia (femur/tibia)	
• Fractures (Fig. 3.7.24)	OI, Hypophosphatasia	
• Hypomineralisation (Fig. 3.7.24)	Hypophosphatasia, OI type 2	
• Epiphyseal stippling – multiple ossification centres that severely deform the long bone and give it a stippled (multiple specks) appearance and a thickened shaft Fig. 3.7.25)	Chondrodysplasia punctata	
• Bone spurs	Hypophosphatasia, Campomelic dysplasia, Jeune, Short rib polydactyly	

Table 3.7.1 (*cont.*)

Phenotype	Differential diagnosis before 24 weeks	Differential diagnosis after 24 weeks
Hands and feet		
• Syndactyly (fused fingers) (Fig. 3.7.26)	Apert	
• Postaxial polydactyly – the extra digit is on the ulnar (little finger) side of the hand – most common (Fig. 3.7.27)	Ellis–van Creveld, Short rib polydactyly, Jeune, Acrocallosal syndrome	
• Preaxial polydactyly – radial (thumb) or tibial side (Fig. 3.7.28)	Short rib polydactyly, VATER/VACTERL, Acrocallosal syndrome (feet)	
• Central polydactyly – middle three fingers (very rare)		Bardet–Biedl
• Oligodactyly (Fig. 3.7.29)	Roberts, Ectrodactyly ectodermal dysplasia	
• Trident hand – short with stubby fingers, with a separation between the middle and ring fingers (Fig. 3.7.30)	Acromesomelic dysplasia	Achondroplasia
• Radial/ulnar club hand deformity (Fig. 3.7.31)	Diastrophic dysplasia, Thrombocytopenia – absent radius (TAR), Holt–Oram, Okihiro, Fanconi, Roberts	
• Hitchhiker thumb and toes (Fig. 3.7.32)	Atelosteogenesis type 2, Diastrophic dysplasia	
• Sandal gap (Fig. 3.7.33)	Diastrophic dysplasia	
• Talipes (club foot)	Atelosteogenesis, Dystrophic dysplasia, Campomelic dysplasia	
• Joint contractures	Rhizomelic chondrodysplasia punctata, Roberts, Arthrogryposis	

Table 3.7.1 (*cont.*)

Phenotype	Differential diagnosis before 24 weeks	Differential diagnosis after 24 weeks
Skin		
• Nuchal thickness, oedema	Achondrogenesis, Thanatophoric dysplasia, Noonan, Short rib polydactyly	
• Hydrops	Thanatophoric dysplasia, Achondrogenesis, Short rib polydactyly syndrome, Noonan	
Liquor		
• Polyhydramnios	Achondrogenesis, Thanatophoric dysplasia	Achondroplasia
Gender		
• Discordance between genetic and phenotypic sex	Campomelic dysplasia (male to female), Carpenter, Antley–Bixler	

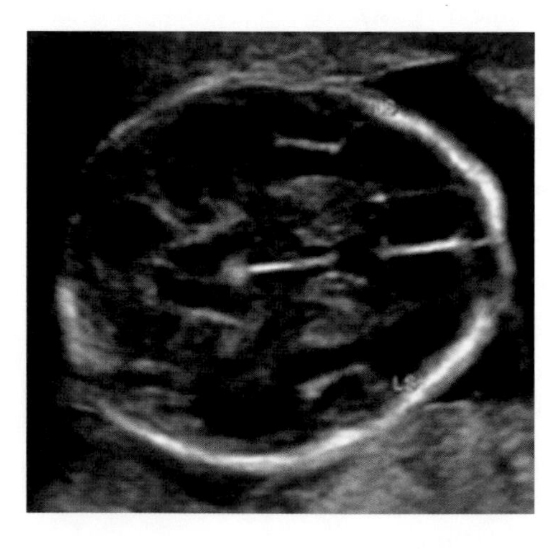

Fig. 3.7.1a Hypomineralisation in a fetus with osteogenesis imperfecta. Note the thinning of the skull and clearly visible near-field intracranial anatomy due to lack of reverberation artefacts from the skull.

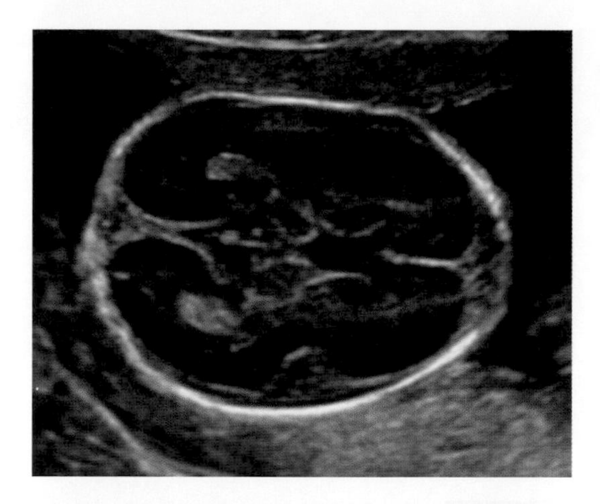

Fig. 3.7.1b Image of the skull of the same fetus showing deformation (flattening) of the parietal bone when pressure is applied with the ultrasound probe.

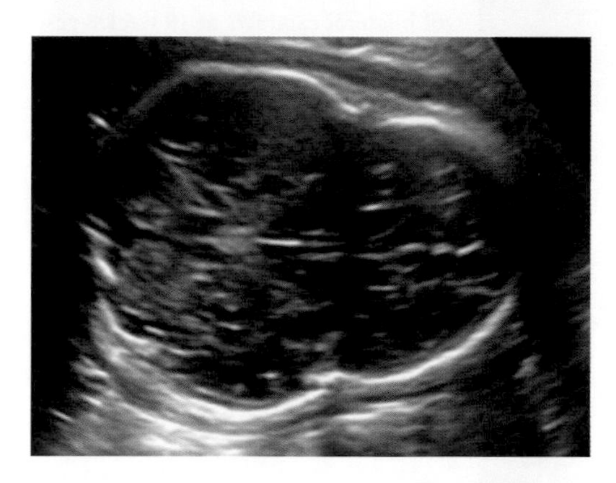

Fig. 3.7.2 Typical cloverleaf skull in a fetus with thanatophoric dysplasia caused by fusion of the coronal sutures.

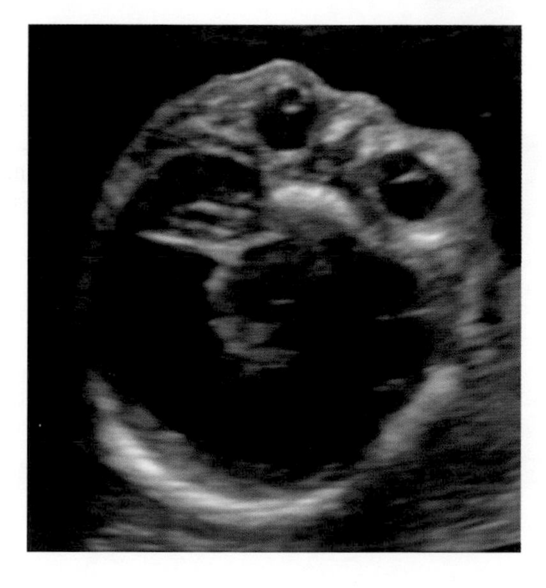

Fig. 3.7.3 Hypotelorism in a fetus with alobar holoprosencephaly. Both orbits are seen close to each other with reduced interorbital space. Normally, the diameter of the interorbital space is the same as the orbital diameter.

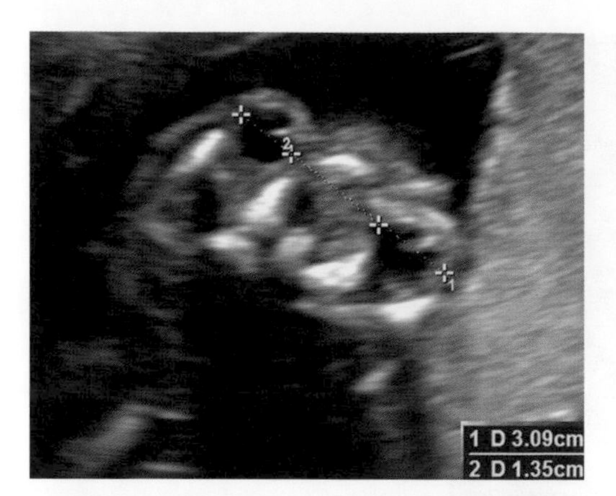

Fig. 3.7.4 Hypertelorism showing widened interorbital space in a fetus with Apert syndrome.

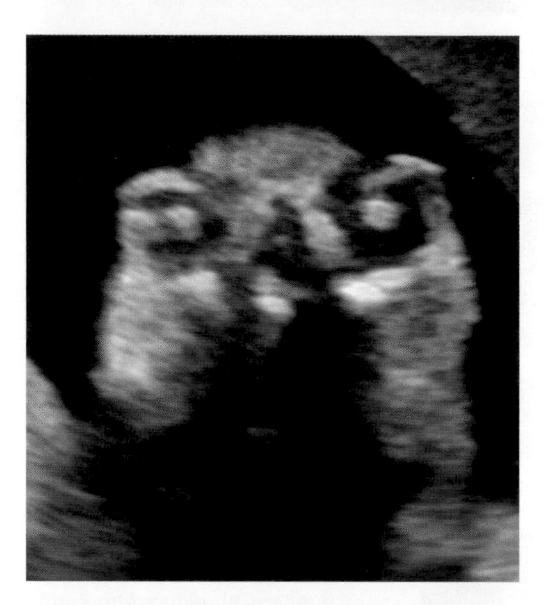

Fig. 3.7.5 Bilateral, hyperechoic lenses suggestive of bilateral cataracts at 18 weeks' gestation. This fetus also had severe microcephaly and was diagnosed with Neu–Laxova syndrome postnatally.

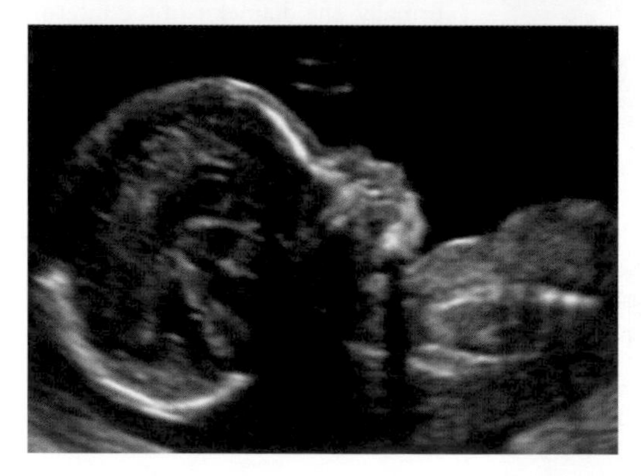

Fig. 3.7.6 Mid-sagittal view of the face showing prominent forehead (frontal bossing) in a fetus with achondroplasia.

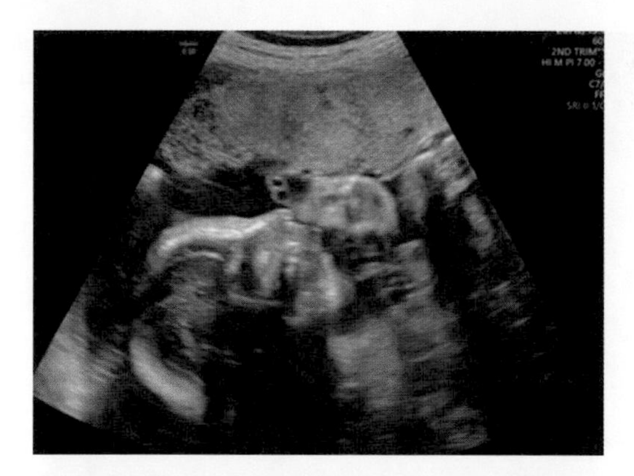

Fig. 3.7.7 Fetus with Seckel syndrome showing sloping forehead, microcephaly and micrognathia.

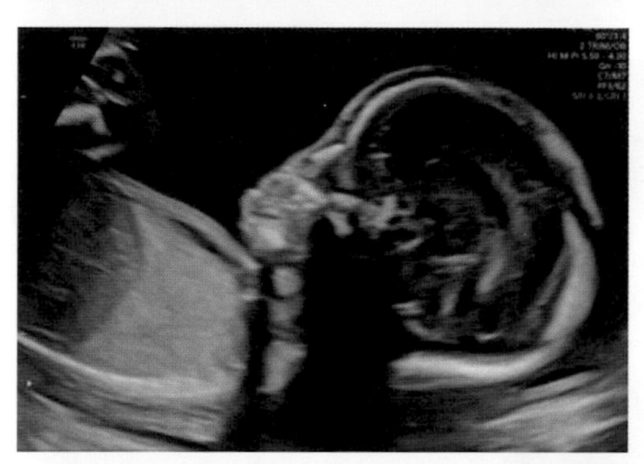

Fig. 3.7.8 Midfacial hypoplasia in a fetus with chondrodysplasia punctata. Epiphyseal stippling was seen in the long bones.

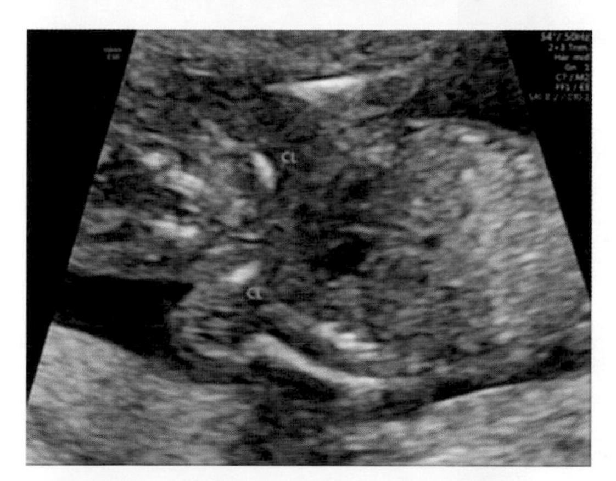

Fig. 3.7.9a Hypoplastic clavicles (CL) in a fetus with cleidocranial dysostosis at 26 weeks. The fetus had poorly mineralised skull bones, widened metopic sutures and abnormal teeth.

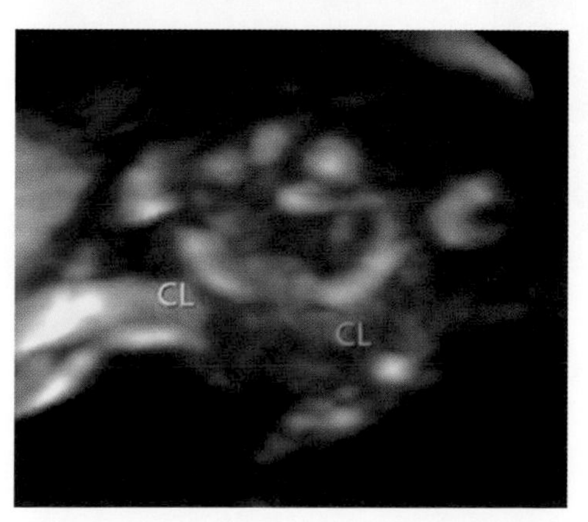

Fig. 3.7.9b 3D image of hypoplastic clavicles (CL) in the same fetus.

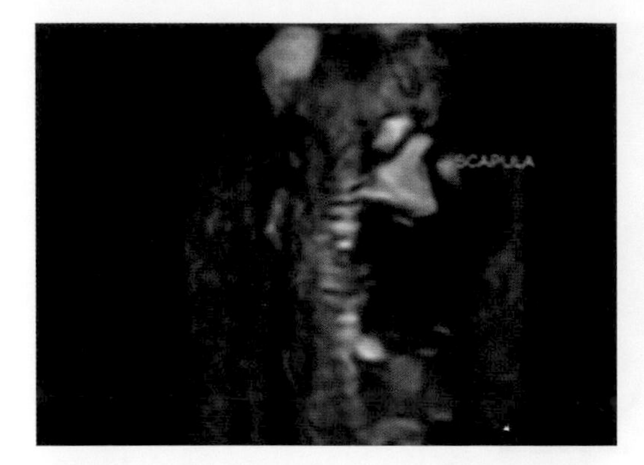

Fig. 3.7.10 3D image of a normal scapula at 20 weeks. The mean scapular length at this gestation is 16 mm (normal range 12–20 mm).

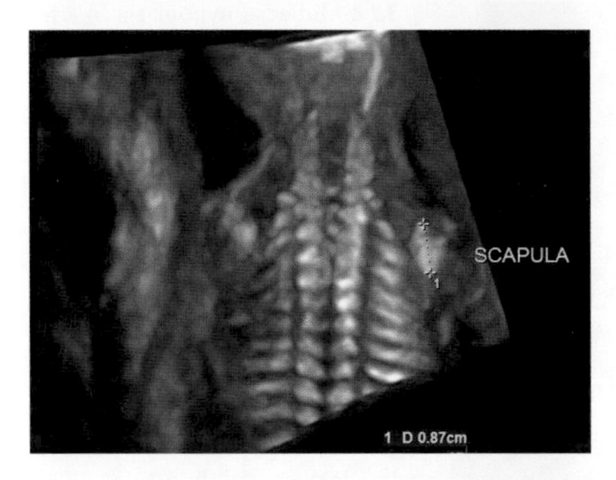

Fig. 3.7.11 3D image of a hypoplastic scapula. This fetus had ulnar mammary syndrome.

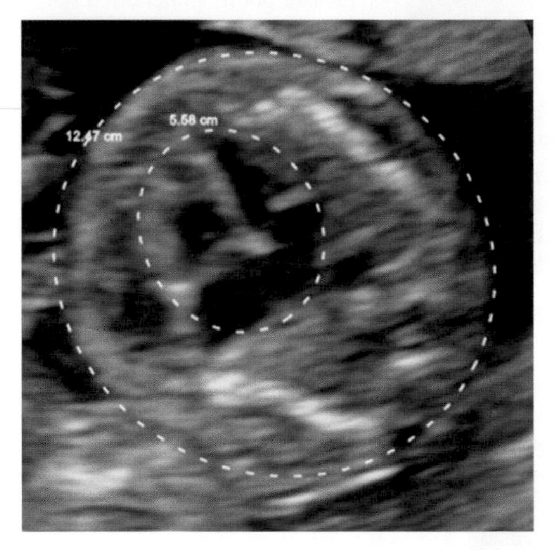

Fig. 3.7.12 Very short and narrow thorax with normal CT ratio of 0.45 at 23 weeks in a fetus with osteogenesis imperfecta.

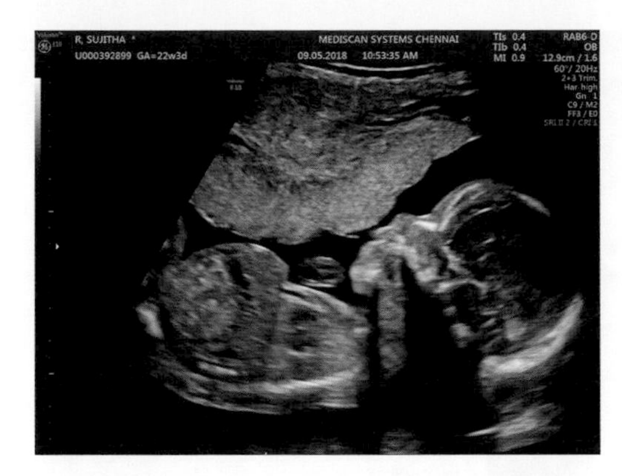

Fig. 3.7.13 Champagne cork appearance of fetal thorax with protuberant abdomen at 22 weeks. Fetus affected by thanatophoric dysplasia.

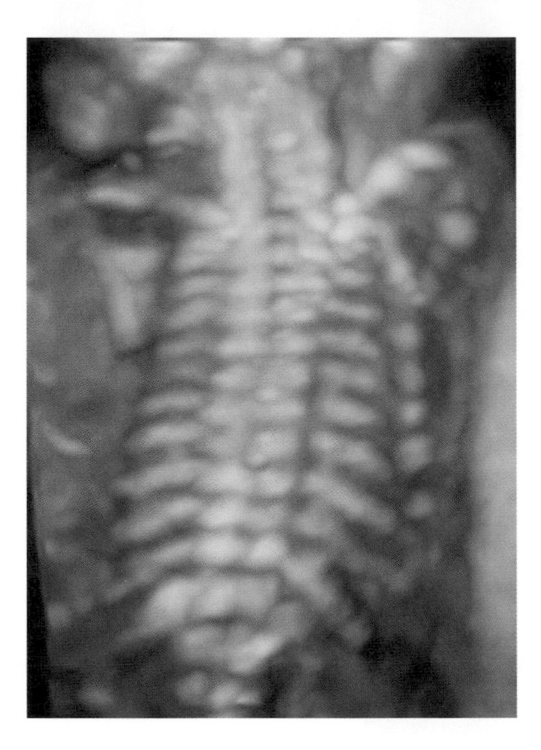

Fig. 3.7.14 Short, straight ribs with narrow thorax with normal mineralisation at 20 weeks in a fetus with Ellis–van Creveld syndrome.

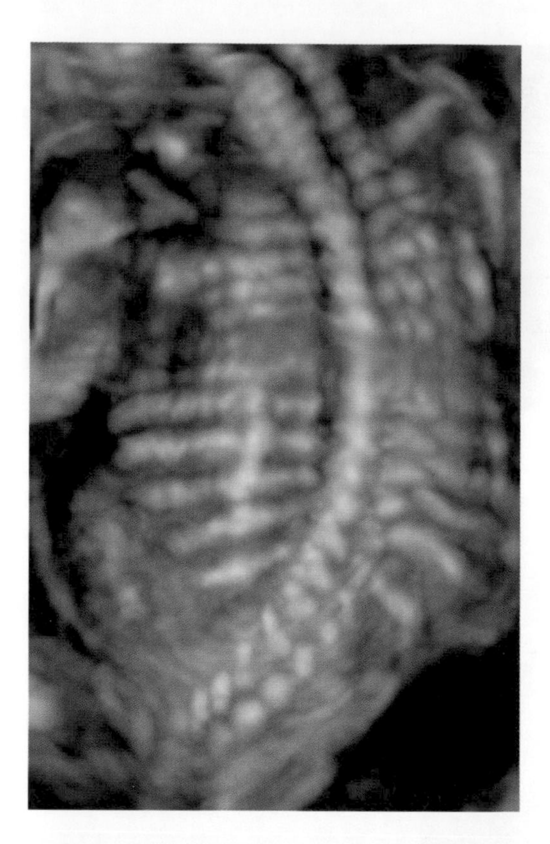

Fig. 3.7.15 Thin and beaded ribs in a 22-week fetus with osteogenesis imperfecta.

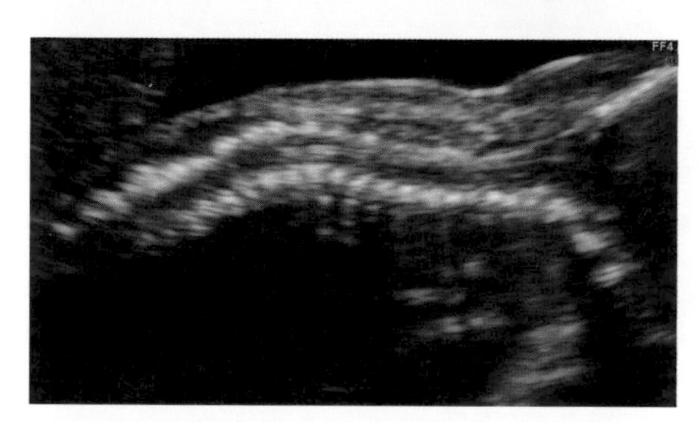

Fig. 3.7.16a Kyphosis of the lumbar spine with hemivertebrae.

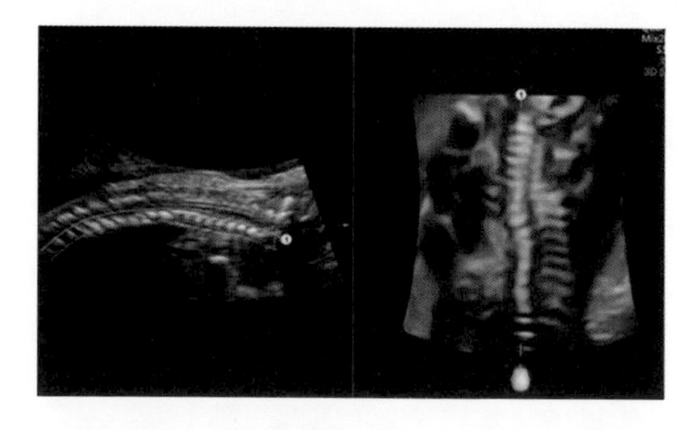

Fig. 3.7.16b Scoliosis was also present, but this was much better visualised using the 3D omni-view technique.

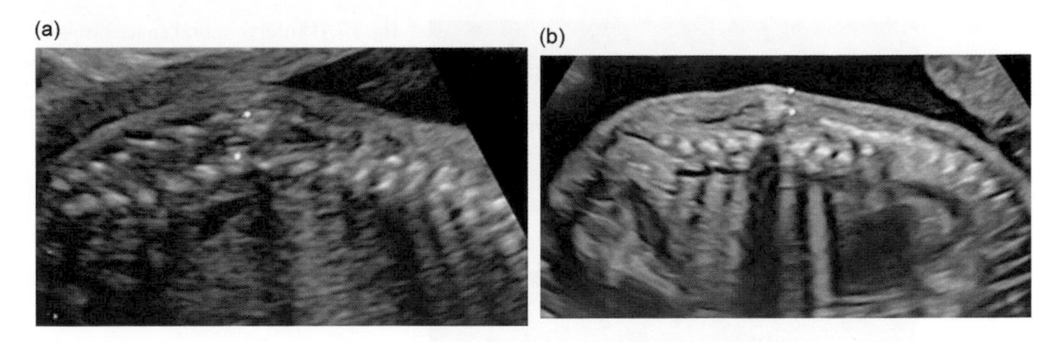

Fig. 3.7.17 Diastematomyelia seen in a fetus at 23 weeks' gestation. (a) Bony spur is clearly visible in the lumbar spine (L2–L3 level) with widening of the vertebral arches. (b) Splitting of the spinal cord at the same level is clearly visible.

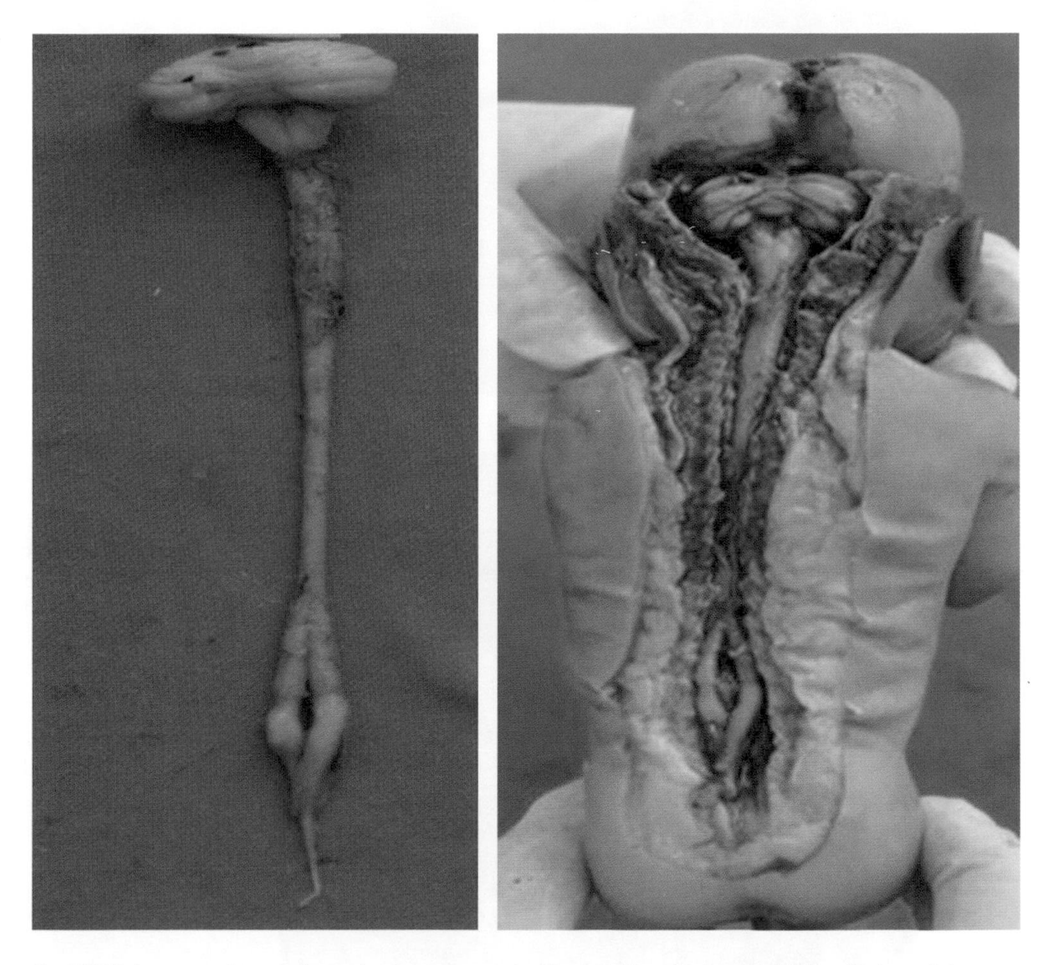

Fig. 3.7.18 Autopsy pictures from the fetus shown in Fig. 3.7.17 with clearly visible splitting of the spinal cord.

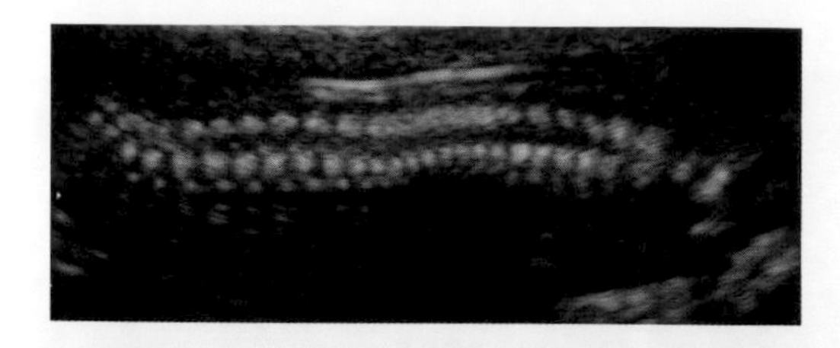

Fig. 3.7.19 Intervertebral space not seen distinctly in the thoracic region due to the fusion of the vertebral bodies. This was an isolated finding with no other pathology postnatally.

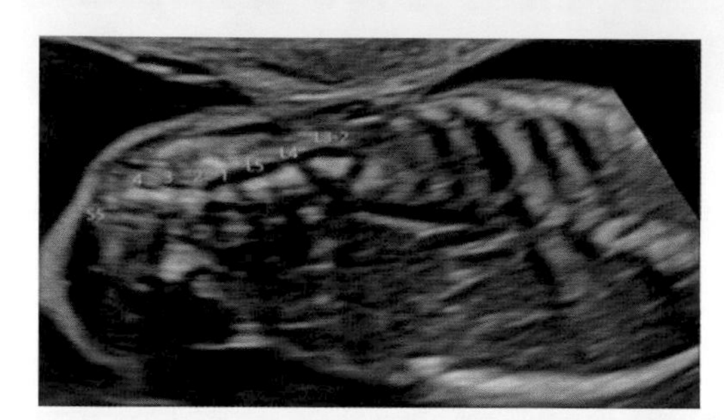

Fig. 3.7.20 Single-level hemivertebra seen at the L2–L3 level at 20 weeks' gestation.

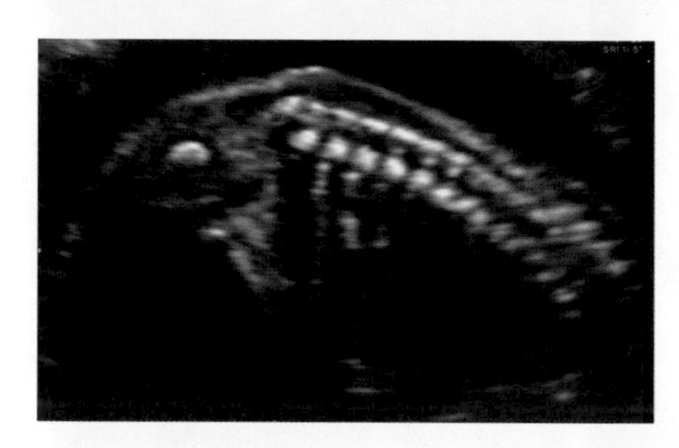

Fig. 3.7.21 Only two lumbar vertebrae seen at 23 weeks in a case of lumbosacral agenesis in a patient with uncontrolled pregestational diabetes. Her HBA1c was 10.5% at 11 weeks.

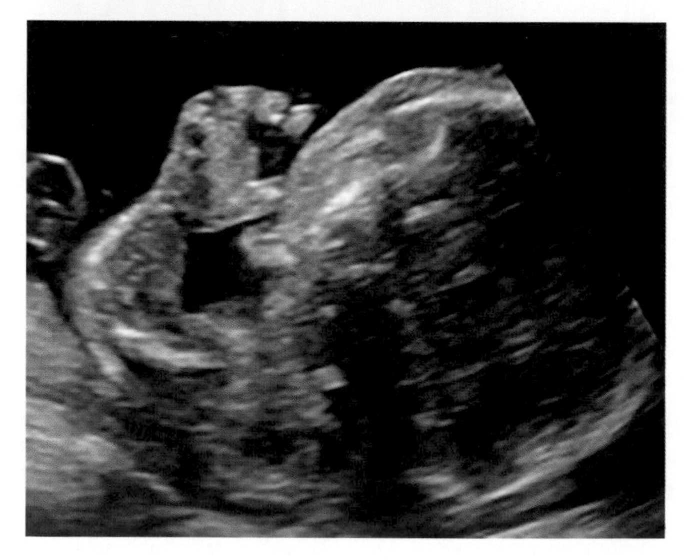

Fig. 3.7.22a Micromelia at 23 weeks' gestation. All long bones appeared short and bent. Decreased mineralisation was seen in some long bones. Femur/foot length ratio was 0.5 (normal range is 0.8–1.1). Fetus was diagnosed with osteogenesis imperfecta type II.

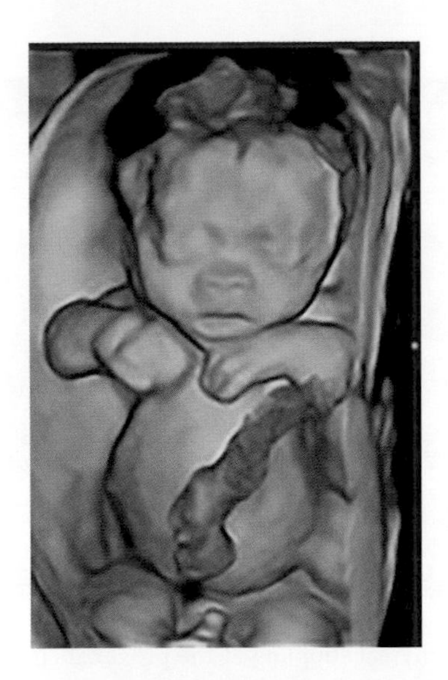

Fig. 3.7.22b 3D picture of the same fetus with micromelia.

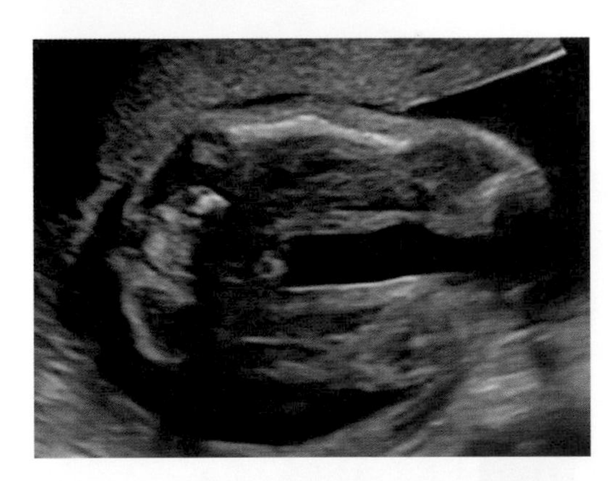

Fig. 3.7.23 Bowed and short femur at 20 weeks' gestation. This fetus had rhizomelic shortening of the long bones and micrognathia. Echogenicity of the bones appeared normal. The definitive diagnosis was not established – the patient was lost to follow-up.

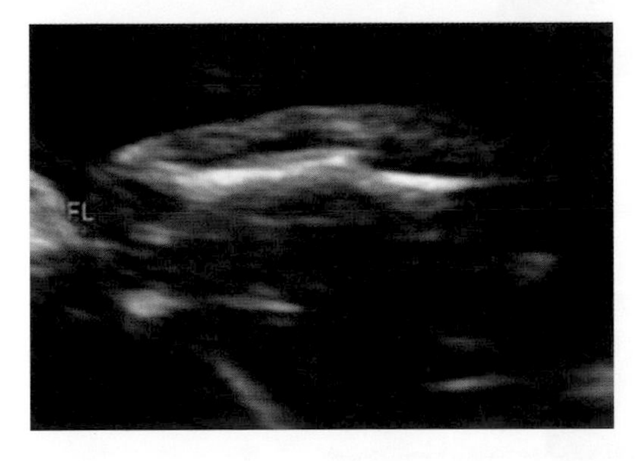

Fig. 3.7.24 Fractured femur in a case of hypophosphatasia. Note the poor mineralisation as evidenced by poor shadowing from the femur.

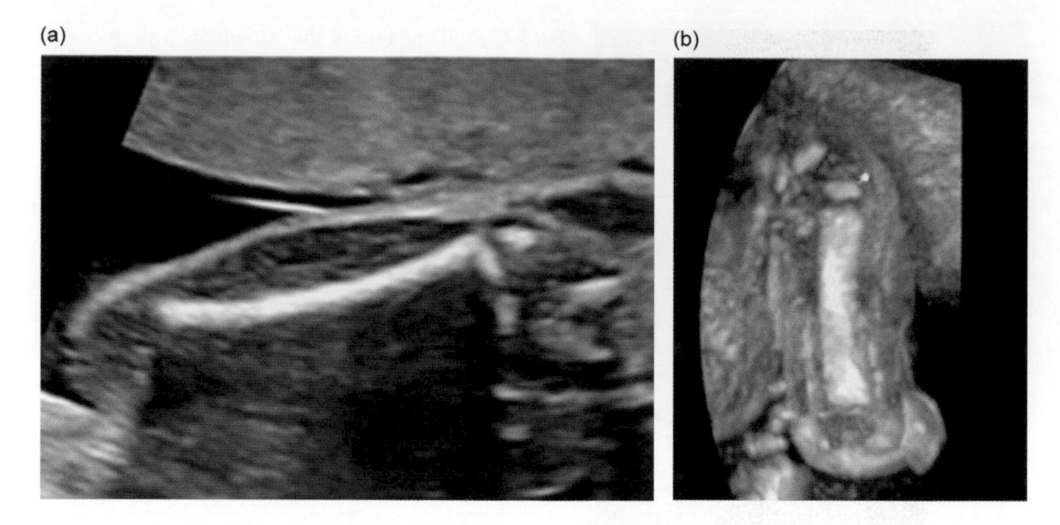

Fig. 3.7.25 (a) 2D and (b) 3D scan of femur showing epiphyseal stippling at the proximal end. This is typically seen in chondrodysplasia punctata.

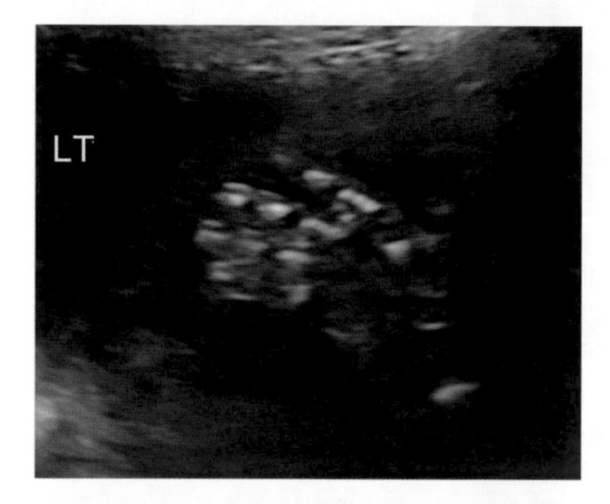

Fig. 3.7.26 Isolated syndactyly between the fourth and fifth fingers of the right hand at 20 weeks' gestation.

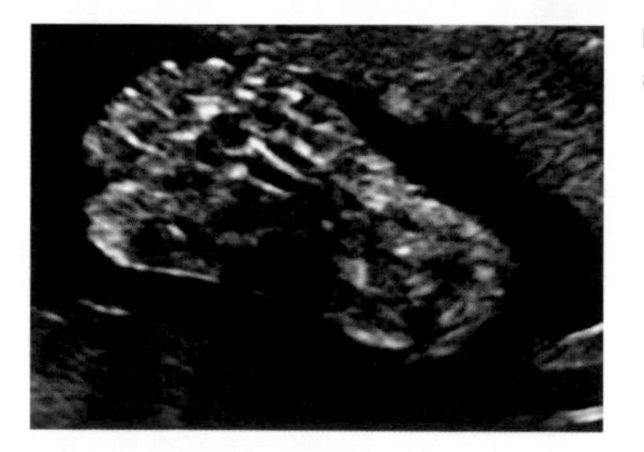

Fig. 3.7.27a Fetal foot with postaxial (fibular side) polydactyly.

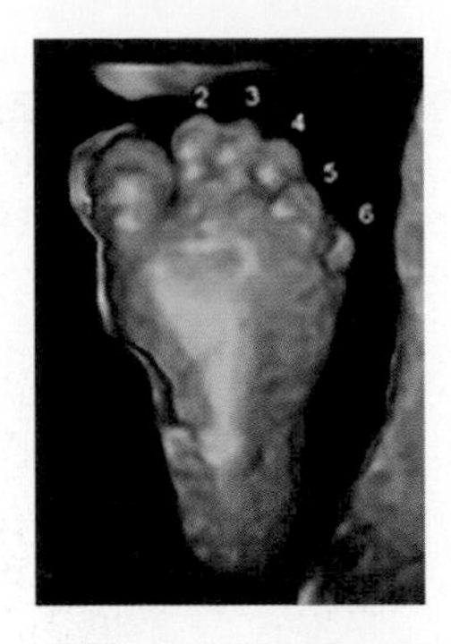

Fig. 3.7.27b 3D view of the same foot.

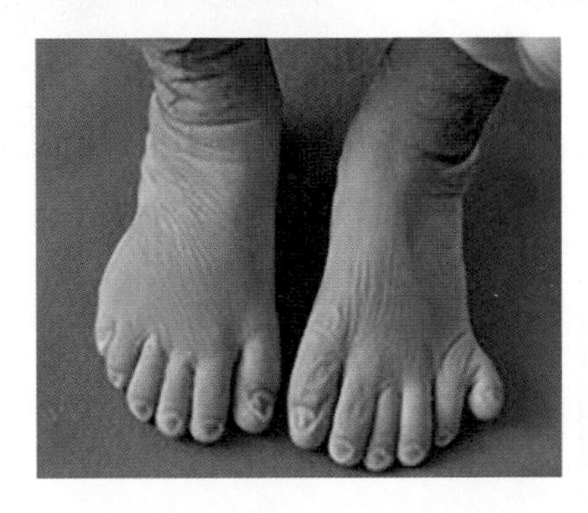

Fig. 3.7.27c Postaxial polydactyly was present in both feet.

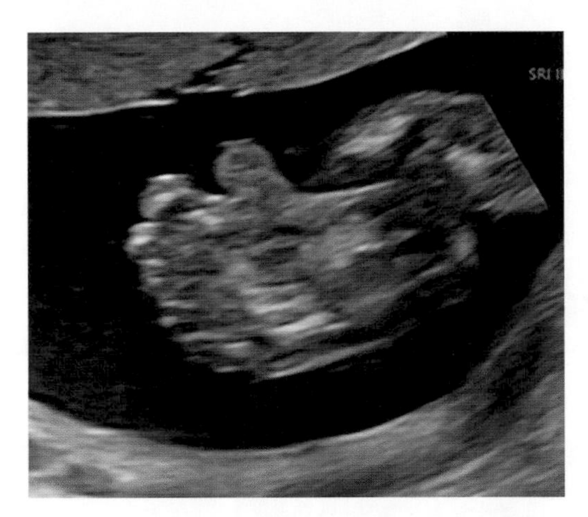

Fig. 3.7.28 Isolated preaxial (radial side) polydactyly seen in a fetus with family history of polydactyly.

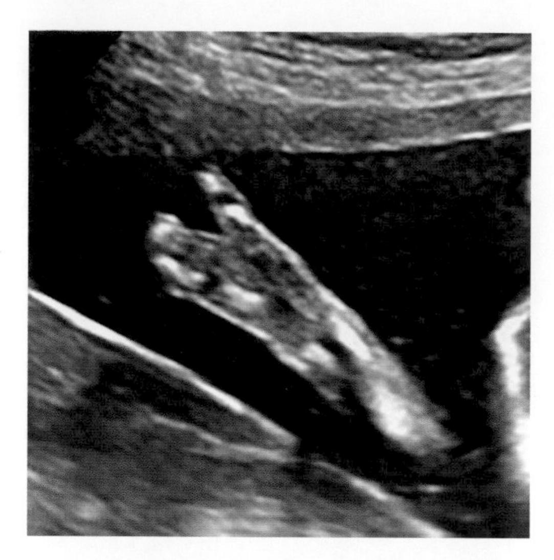

Fig. 3.7.29 Fetal hand with oligodactyly – fused fourth and fifth fingers with absent thumb and second finger. Fetus had mesomelia of the right upper limb and oligodactyly of the left hand. This was an isolated longitudinal limb defect.

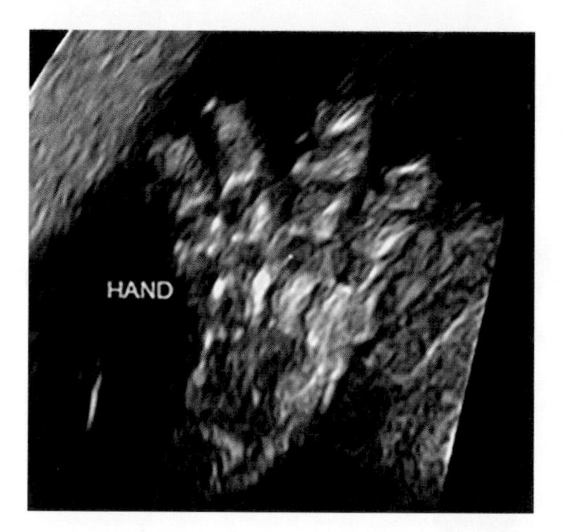

Fig. 3.7.30 Trident hand in a fetus with achondroplasia. Note short fingers (brachydactyly) with increased gap between the third and fourth fingers.

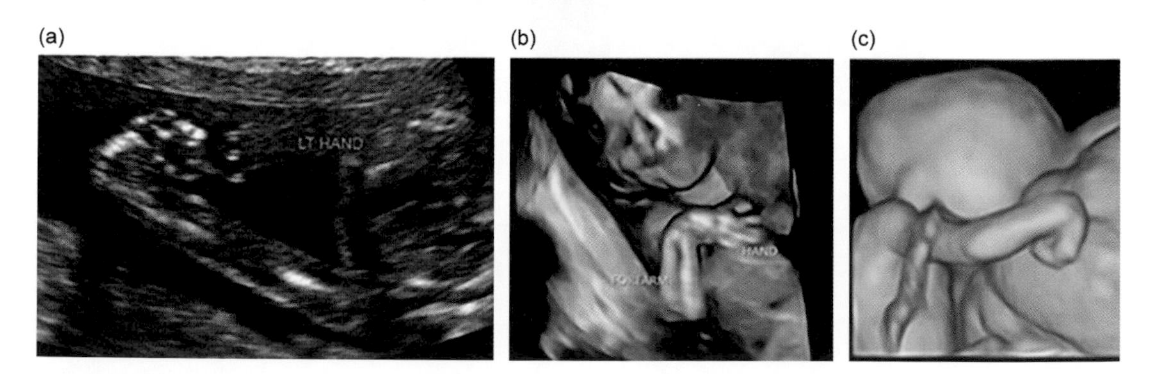

Fig. 3.7.31 (a) 2D and (b,c) 3D images of the right club hand in a fetus with Holt–Oram syndrome.

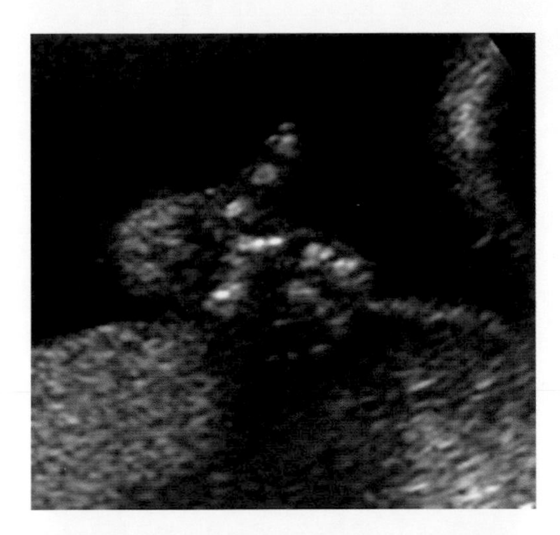

Fig. 3.7.32 Right hand with a hitchhiker thumb in a 21-week fetus with ventriculomegaly, fibular hypoplasia and posteriorly rotated feet. The definitive diagnosis was not established postnatally.

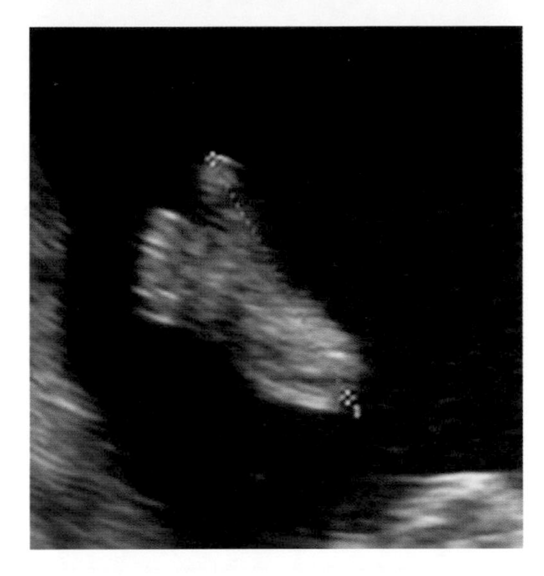

Fig. 3.7.33 Sandal gap – increased gap between great toe and the other toes. There was no syndromic association in this case.

SKELETAL DYSPLASIAS MOST COMMONLY DIAGNOSED ANTENATALLY

See Table 3.7.2.

Table 3.7.2 Skeletal dysplasias most commonly diagnosed antenatally.

Condition	Epidemiology	Genetics*	Long bones	Chest	Head	Spine	Hands/Feet	Other
Achondrogenesis (Figs. 3.7.34 and 3.7.35)	• 1 in 40,000 • Uniformly lethal	**Type 1**: AR • 1a – *TRIP11* mutation • 1b – *SLC26A2* mutation **Type 2:** AD • *COL2A1*	• Very short	• Narrow • Rib fractures (type 1a)	• Macrocephaly • Hypomineralisation of skull (type 1a, not 1b) • No ossification (type 2) • Cleft palate • Midface hypoplasia	Hypomineralisation of the spine	• Short fingers • Hitchhiker thumbs (type 1b) • Talipes	• Facial abnormalities (type 1a) • Fetal hydrops and polyhydramnios (type 2)
Achondroplasia (heterozygous) (Fig. 3.7.36)	• 1 in 25,000 • Most common non-lethal dysplasia	• *FGFR3* group • AD • Homozygous form is uniformly lethal	• Short after 22 weeks	• Usually smaller than average due to anteroposterior narrowing of the ribs	• Macrocephaly • Frontal bossing	• Lumbar lordosis • Champagne glass pelvis	• Short fingers • 'Trident hand'	
Asphyxiating thoracic dystrophy (Jeune syndrome) (Fig. 3.7.37)	~1 in 100,000	• AR • Ciliopathy • Genetically heterogeneous (several mutations)	• Short after 22 weeks with mild bowing and metaphyseal spurs • Trident acetabular roof	• Narrow and elongated, can be bell-shaped	Normal		• Polydactyly (~10%)	
Campomelic dysplasia	• Very rare • Almost always lethal	• AD • *SOX9*	• Tibia and fibula worst affected – short and bowed with osseous spikes • Femur also short and bowed • Arms normal	• Narrow, bell-shaped • 11 rib pairs • Hypoplastic scapulae	• Macrocephaly • Cleft palate • Micrognathia • Flat face short nose	Scoliosis	Marked talipes	• Ambiguous genitalia/sex reversal in males • Hydronephrosis • Cardiac anomalies (septal defects)

Chondrodysplasia punctata								
X-linked dominant	• Mildest form seen only in females • Heterozygous form in males is lethal	Xp11; EBP	• Asymmetrical (mild) shortening • Epiphyseal stippling					
X-linked recessive	• Heterozygous female carriers are normal	Xp22; ARSE	• Moderate shortening • Stippling in femora			• Paravertebral stippling may look like a disorganised spine		
Rhizomelic	1 in 100,000	Three distinct genetic types	• Humerus is affected the most with very prominent epiphyseal stippling • Fixed flexion deformities may be present		• Progressive microcephaly • Cataracts • Midface hypoplasia			
Diastrophic dysplasia	Very rare	• AR • *DTDST* gene mutations	• Very short and bowed in severe cases, but in milder cases can be minimal.	Usually normal	• Cleft palate • Micrognathia • Abnormal ears	• Cervical spina bifida occulta • Scoliosis	• Hitchhiker thumb • Wrist deviation • Talipes	
Ellis–van Creveld (Fig. 3.7.38)	Very rare	• AR • *EVC* and *EVC2* mutations	• Mesomelic shortening (forearms and lower legs) • Trident acetabulum	• Narrow with horizontal ribs	• Normal skull • Posterior fossa cyst		• Polydactyly (hands almost 100%, feet ~10%)	• Cardiac, mainly ASD (60%)

Table 3.7.2 (*cont.*)

Condition	Epidemiology	Genetics*	Long bones	Chest	Head	Spine	Hands/Feet	Other
Hypophosphatasia (Figs. 3.7.39 and 3.7.40)	• Heterogenous group caused by alkaline deficiency		• Short, may be bowed • Osseous spurs	• Thin ribs, may be fractured	Hypomineralised similar to OI type 2	• Demineralised		
Osteogenesis imperfecta (Fig. 3.7.41)	• Overall ~1 in 15,000 • Type 2 ~1 in 50,000	• AD and AR • 85% collagen types *COL1A1*, *COL1A2* • 15% non-collagen	• Type II: short, fractured • Type III: bowed, almost normal length, fractured	• Type II: narrow, fractured ribs • Type III: barrel-shaped	• Type 2: hypomineralisation of skull, micrognathia	• Not demineralised • Type III: scoliosis	• Type II: wrist deviation, talipes	
Short rib polydactylies		Ciliopathies						
Type 1: Saldino–Noonan	Rare, lethal	• AR • *DYNC2H1* mutation	• Severe shortening • Femur is short and wide with pointed end (narrow metaphyses)	• Small	• Normal		Polydactyly	• Generalised skin oedema • Urogenital anomalies
Type II: Majewski	Rare, lethal	• AR • *PTGSS1* mutation	Very short oval tibia	Small, short horizontal ribs	• May have cloverleaf appearance/flat nasal bridge • Midline facial clefts		Polydactyly	• Omphalocele • Bladder obstruction • Skin oedema
Type III: Verma–Naumoff	Rare, lethal	• AR • *NEK1* mutation	• Less severe shortening • Wide metaphyses with spurs	Narrow	Midline cleft lip		Polydactyly (postaxial)	• Cardiac anomalies

Type IV: Beemer–Langer (Fig. 3.7.42)	Rare, lethal	• AR • *IFT80* mutation	• Micromellic shortening • Ulna and radius may be bowed • Tibia longer than fibula	• Narrow, horizontal ribs • Small scapulae	• May have cloverleaf skull • Micrognathia • Medial cleft lip/palate		Talipes	• Omphalocele • Skin oedema • Ambiguous genitalia
Spondyloepiphyseal dysplasia	Rare	• *COL2A1*	• Moderately short throughout	• Chest appears small because of short spine		• Short spine • Platyspondyly		
Spondylocostal dysplasia (Jarcho–Levin syndrome) (Fig. 3.7.43)	~ 1 in 40,000	• Mostly AR (*DLL3*, *MESP2*, *LFNG*, *HES7*) • *TBX6* is known to cause AD form	Arms and legs are usually of normal length	• Fused ribs, or missing in chaotic manner		• Scoliosis, kyphosis, vertebral defects		
Thanatophoric dysplasia (Fig. 3.7.44)	• 1 in 20,000 • Most common lethal dysplasia	• AD • *FGFR3* group	• Curved, telephone receiver femora (type 1) • Short, straight long bones (type 2)	Narrow, short ribs	• Large but not cloverleaf (type 1) • Cloverleaf skull (type 2) • Frontal bossing	Platyspondyly	Short fingers	Polyhydramnios

* AD, autosomal dominant; AR, autosomal recessive.

ACHONDROGENESIS

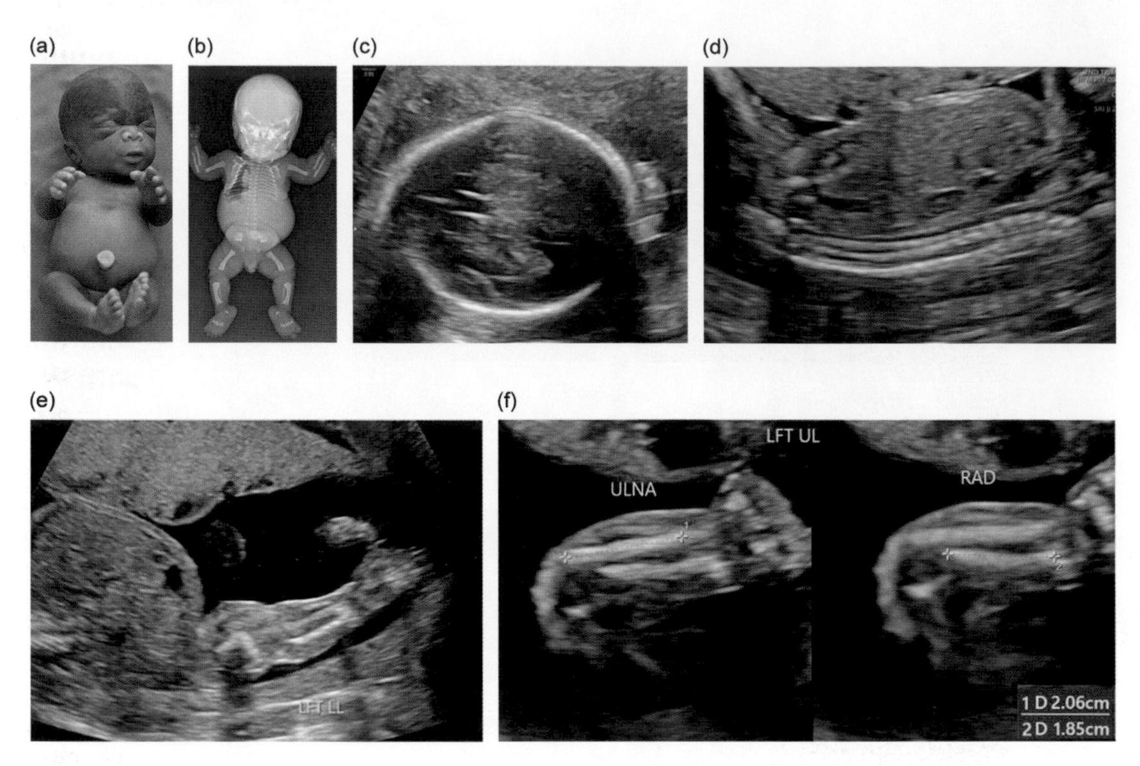

Fig. 3.7.34 Phenotype of a fetus at 22 weeks affected with **achondrogenesis type 1**. (a) Note the short trunk and limbs, short neck, protuberant abdomen, inward rotation of the feet and disproportionally large head. (b) Fetogram shows severe micromelia and narrow chest. The vertebral bodies are poorly ossified. The skull and long bones are ossified in this fetus but variable degrees of ossification may be present in this condition. (c–f) Ultrasound pictures of the same fetus show ossification of the skull, spine and long bones. The long bones are extremely short. The poor ossification of the vertebral body is better seen in the fetogram. Some fetuses may have cleft palate, umbilical or inguinal hernia and a thickened nuchal fold.

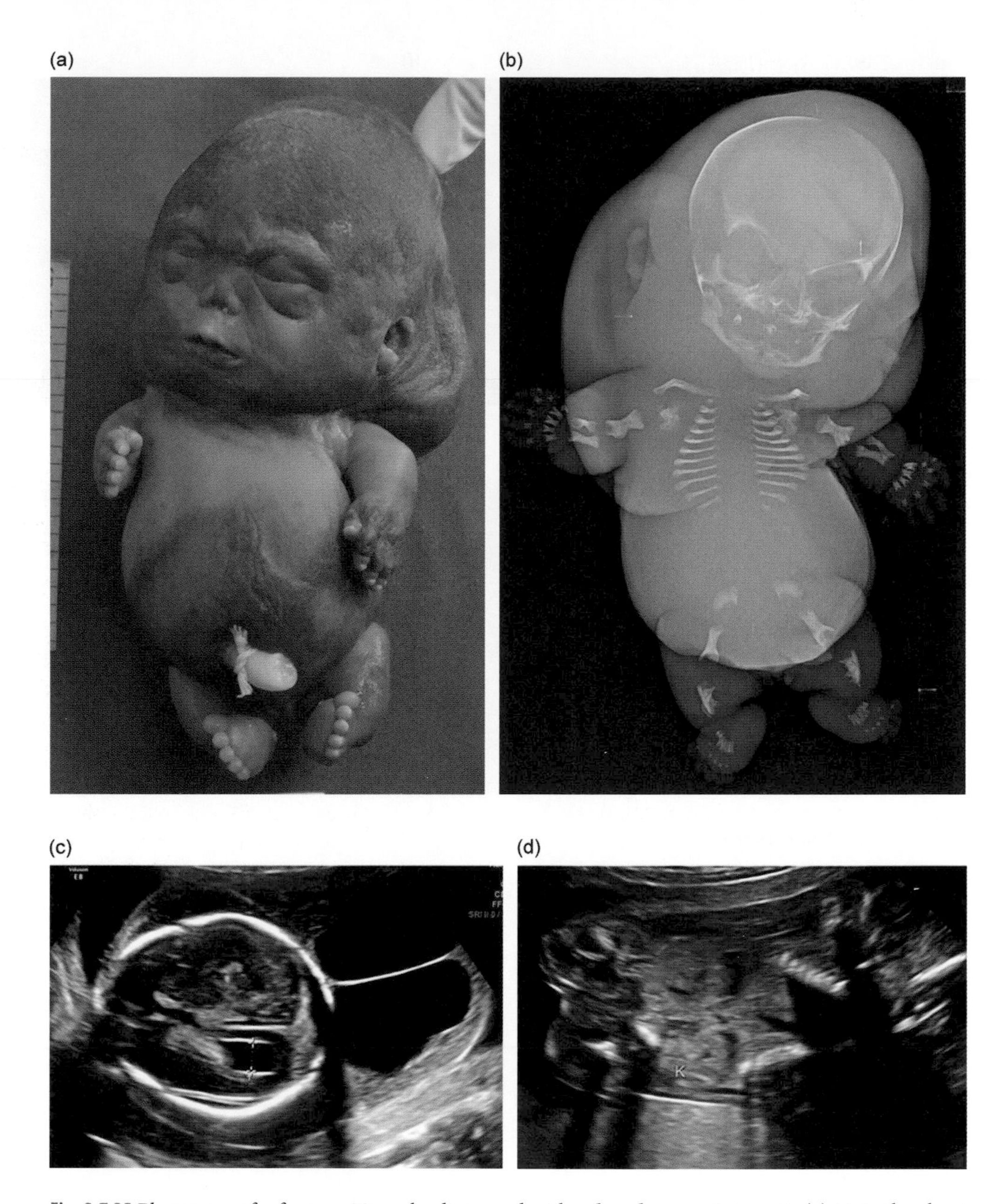

Fig. 3.7.35 Phenotype of a fetus at 20 weeks diagnosed with **achondrogenesis type 2**. (a) Note the short trunk, severe limbs shortening, short neck, large cystic hygroma, protuberant abdomen, inward rotation of feet and disproportionally large head. (b) Fetogram confirmed severe micromelia, narrow chest with poor ossification of the skull, vertebrae and long bones. Ultrasound pictures of the same fetus show (c) large cystic hygroma, (d) short trunk with narrow thorax, (e) short spine with poor ossification and (f,g) severely short, deformed and poorly mineralised long bones.

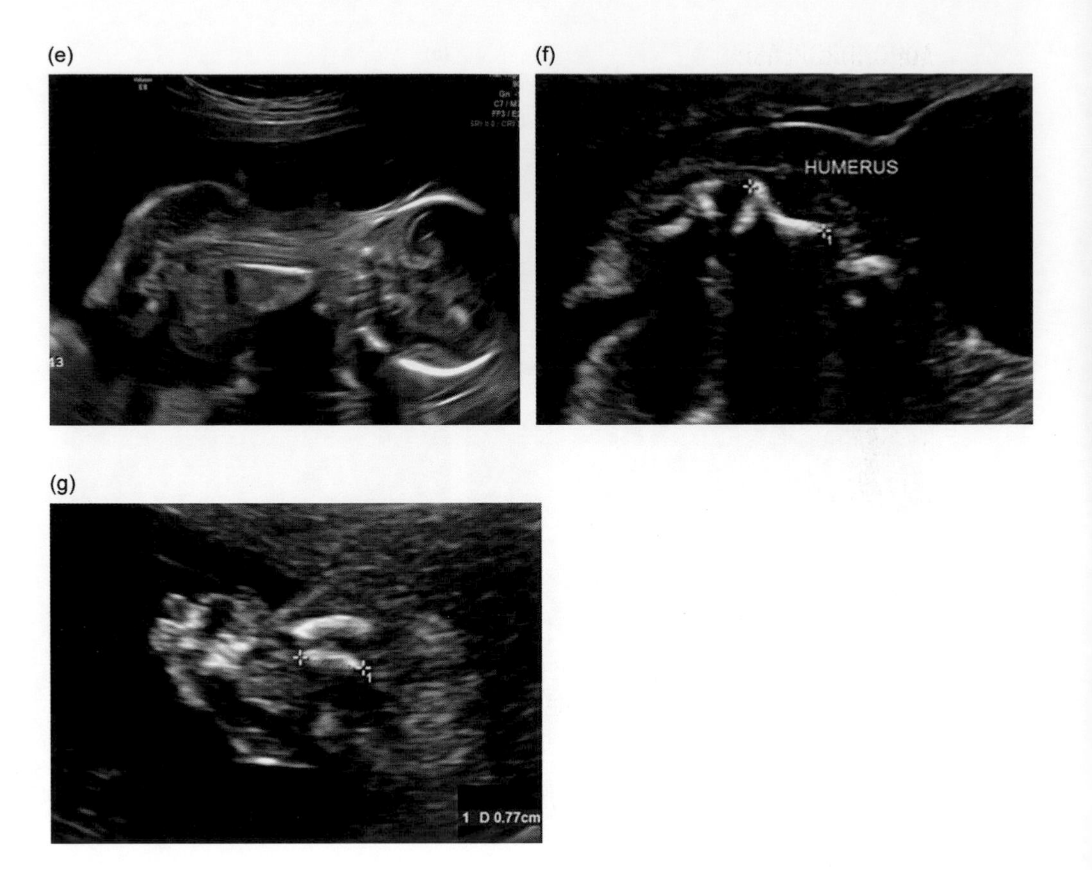

Fig. 3.7.35 (*cont.*)

ACHONDROPLASIA

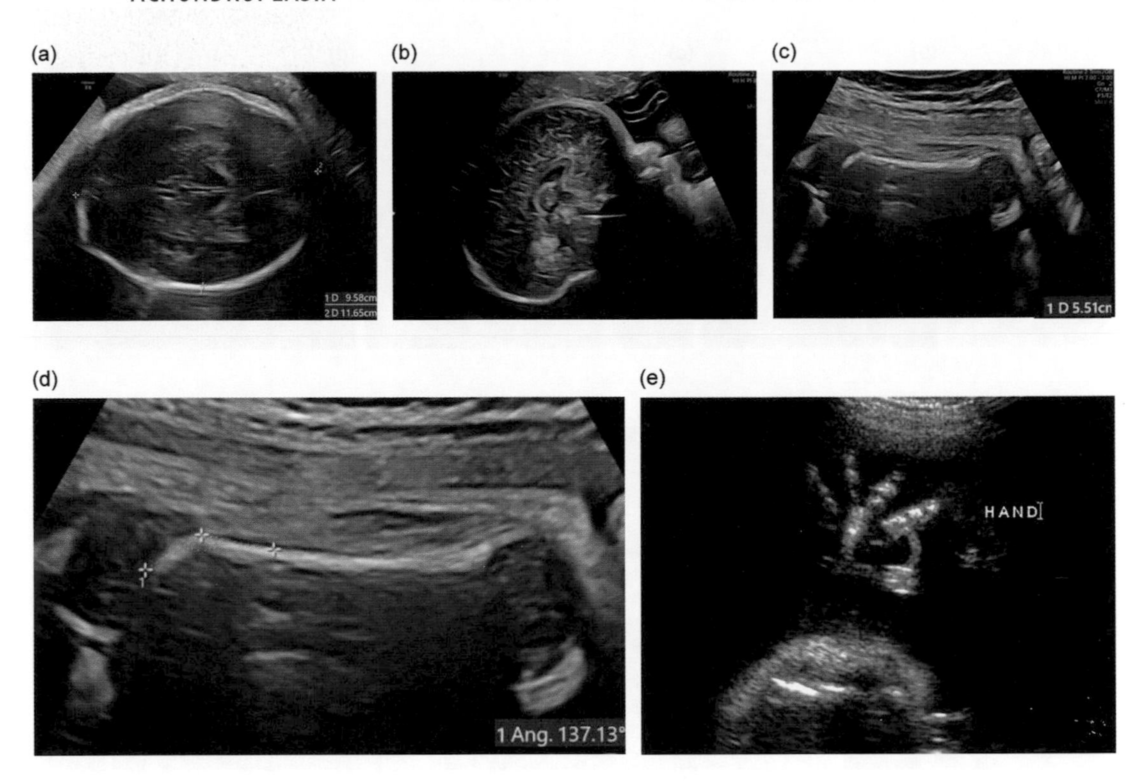

Fig. 3.7.36 (a) Macrocephaly with normal intracranial anatomy in a 34-week fetus affected with **achondroplasia**. (b) Profile view of the face showing frontal bossing and depressed nasal bridge. (c) Short femur has normal mineralisation and shape, but (d) proximal diaphyseal/metaphyseal angle is wide (>130°). In normal and SGA fetuses this angle increases with gestational age but is always less than 130°. (e) Trident hand for another fetus with achondroplasia which is evident when the fetus opens its hands.

ASPHYXIATING THORACIC DYSTROPHY (JEUNE SYNDROME)

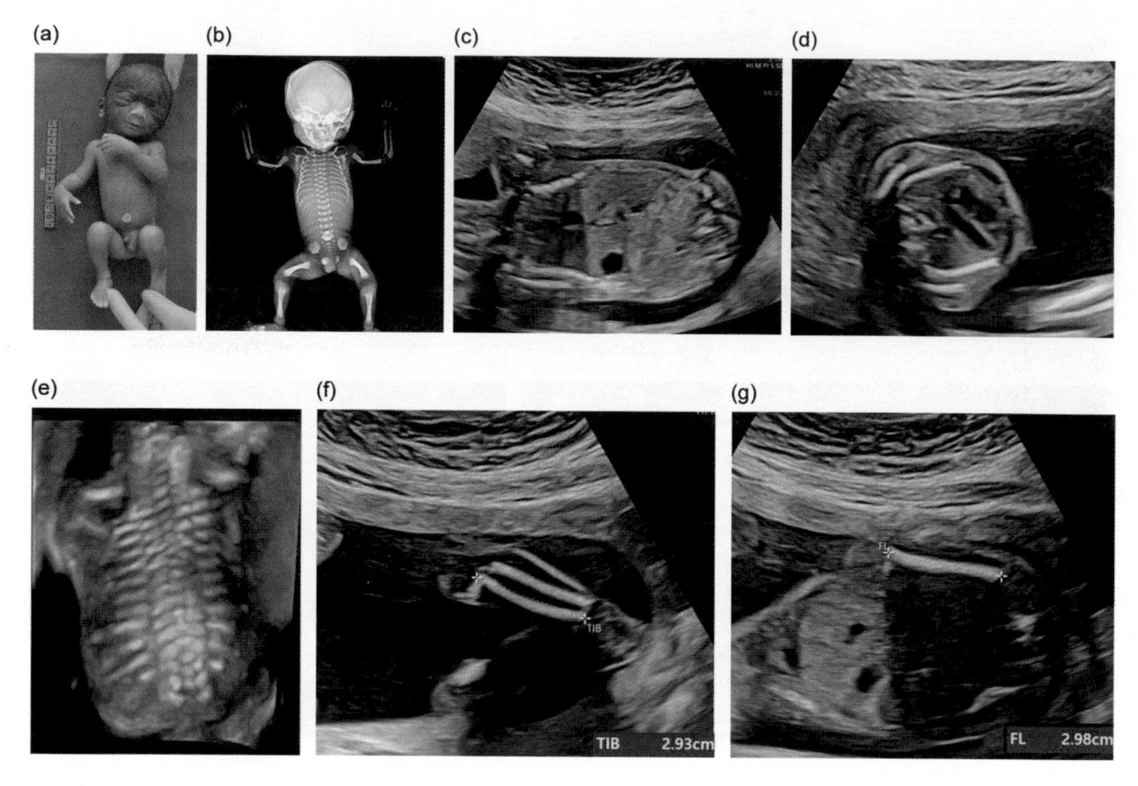

Fig. 3.7.37 (a) Phenotype of a fetus at 19 weeks with **asphyxiating thoracic dystrophy** (also known as Jeune syndrome) showing mild narrowing of the thorax and short limbs with no polydactyly. (b) Fetogram shows well-ossified skeleton with short ribs and long bones. (c) Coronal view of the fetus showing narrow thorax. (d) Transverse view of the thorax showing hypoplastic lungs with the heart appearing relatively large. (e) 3D image of the chest showing short ribs. (f,g) Short long bones. Polydactyly may be seen in some cases. If present, short rib polydactyly has to be considered in the differential diagnosis.

ELLIS–VAN CREVELD SYNDROME

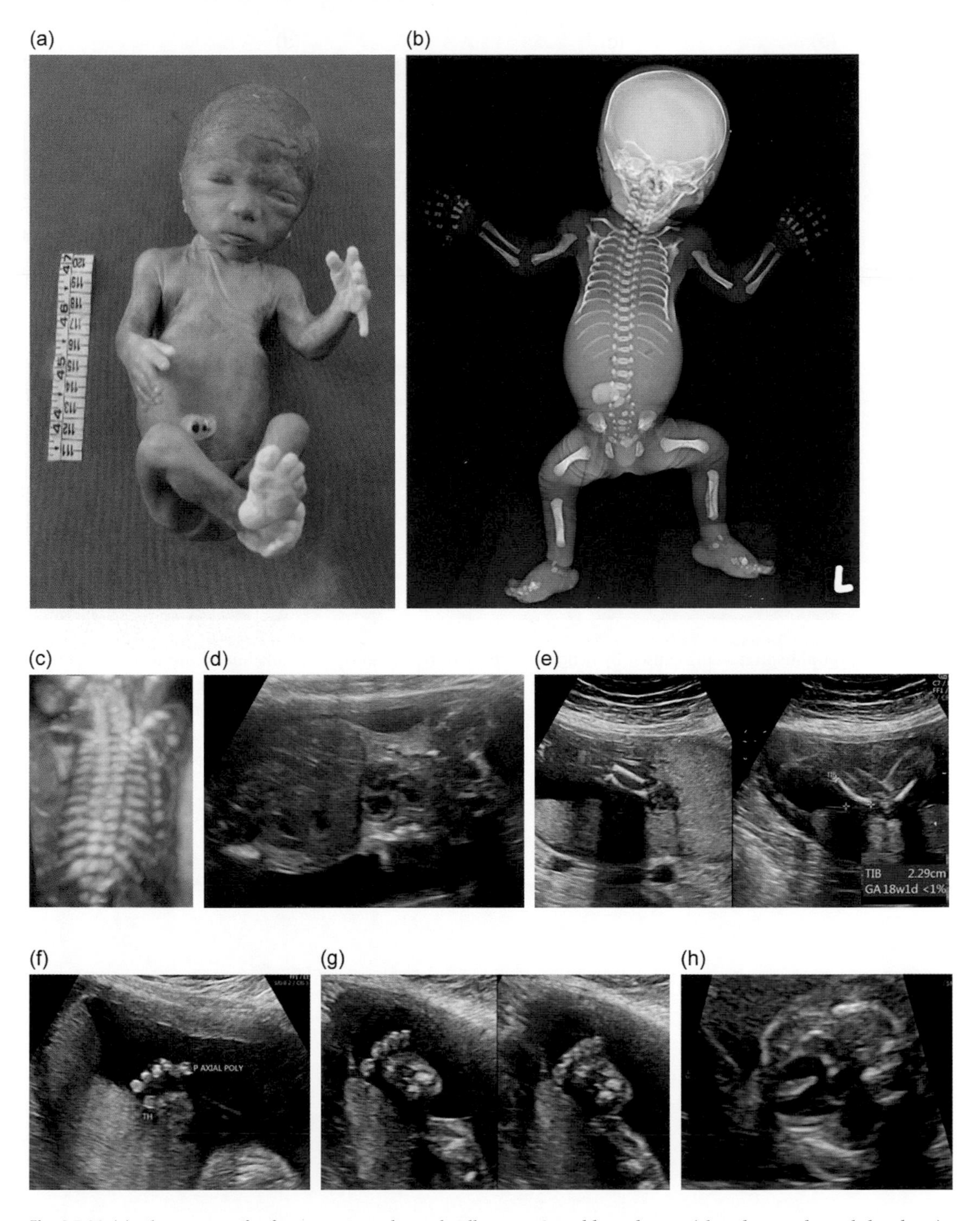

Fig. 3.7.38 (a) Phenotype of a fetus at 23 weeks with Ellis–van Creveld syndrome (chondroectodermal dysplasia) showing narrow thorax and postaxial polydactyly of hands. (b) Fetogram of the same fetus shows well-ossified skeleton, short long bones with cone-shaped epiphyses, flared iliac bones and mild bowing of the humeri. (c) 3D view showing narrow thorax and short straight ribs. (d) Coronal view showing narrow thorax. (e) Long bones are short but mineralisation is normal. (f) Polydactyly of the hands is consistent with the diagnosis. (g) There is no polydactyly of the feet in this fetus; feet polydactyly may be seen in ~10% of cases. (h) Apical four chamber view of the heart showing AVSD. Cardiac defects are seen in ~50% of fetuses, mainly AVSD, VSD or a single atrium.

HYPOPHOSPHATASIA

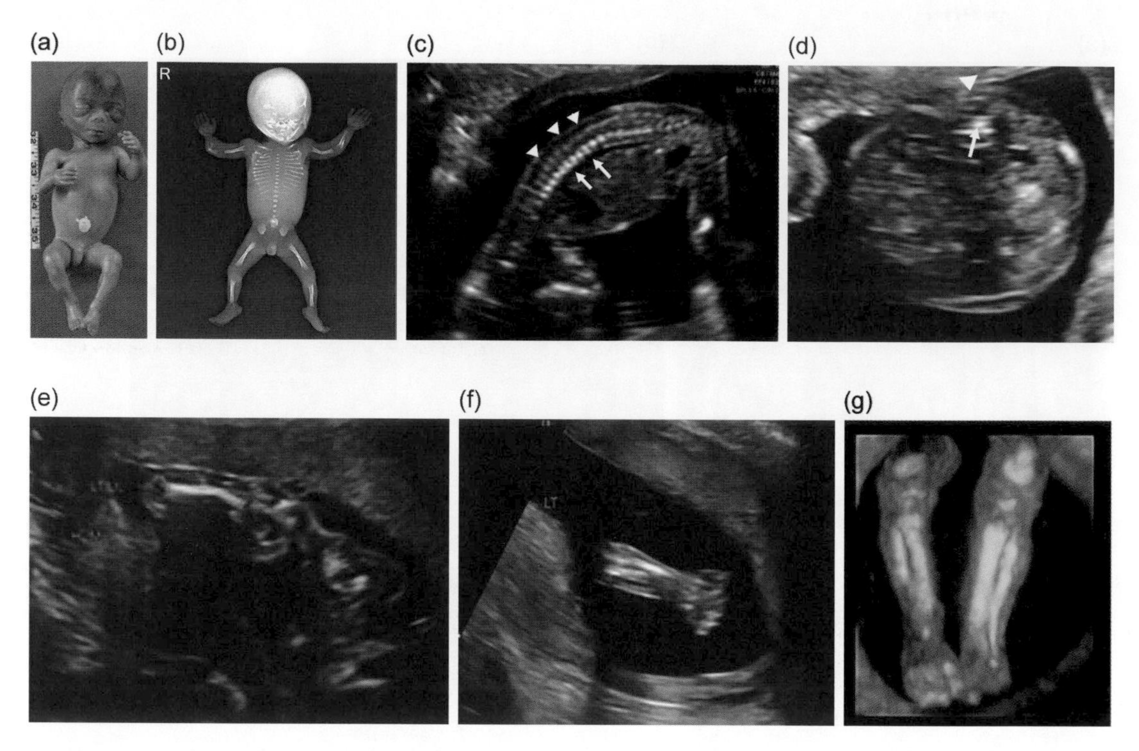

Fig. 3.7.39 Hypophosphatasia is caused by deficient activity of tissue nonspecific alkaline phosphatase enzyme (TNSALP) of varying degree. (a) In this fetus there is a mild bowing of the upper limbs. (b) Fetogram confirmed rhizomesomelic shortening with bowing of the left humerus. The radius and ulna are extremely short. Ribs are also short and flat. The vertebral bodies are ossified but the vertebral arches are completely unossified. (c,d) Sagittal and transverse sections of the spine showing ossified vertebral body (arrows) and poor ossification of the lamina (arrowheads). (e) Humerus is bowed and (f) forearm bones are short. (g) 3D skeleton mode highlights abnormal tibia and fibula.

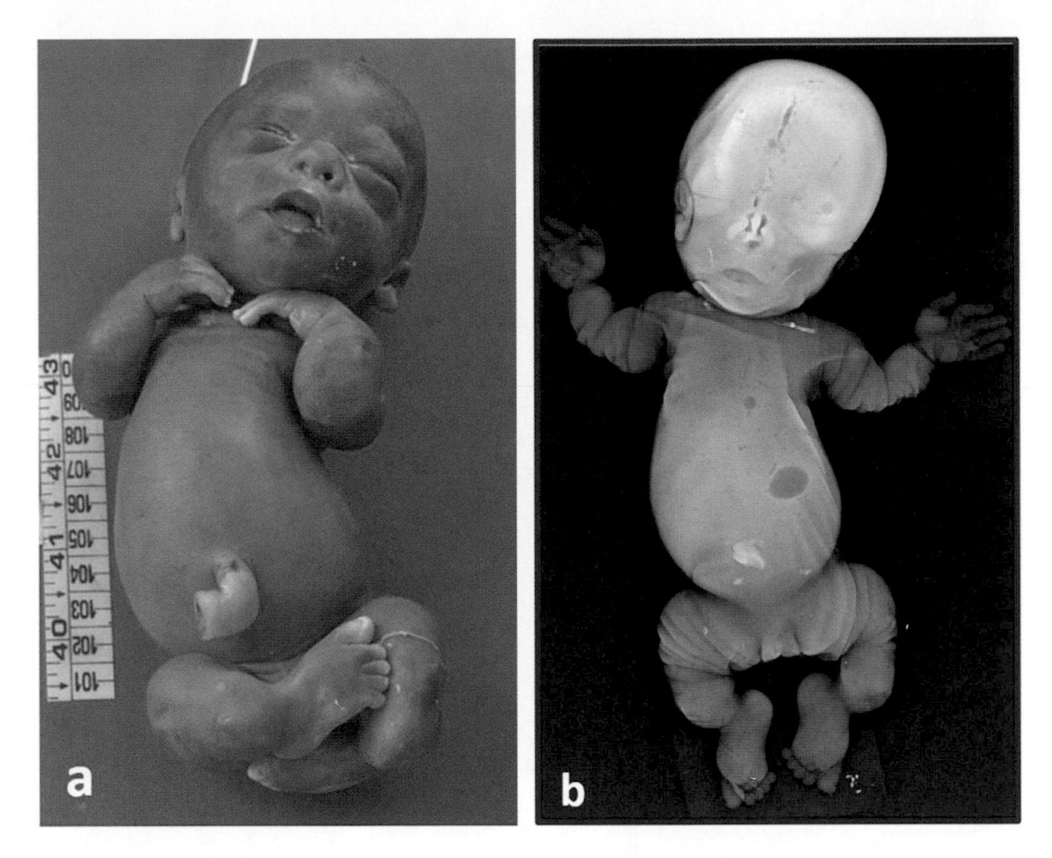

Fig. 3.7.40 Hypophosphatasia – severe lethal type. This fetus was examined in a perinatal pathology department, but prenatal ultrasound pictures were not available. (a) Phenotype shows very short limbs, deformed feet and very narrow thorax. (b) Fetogram shows non-ossified skull, spine and long bones.

OSTEOGENESIS IMPERFECTA

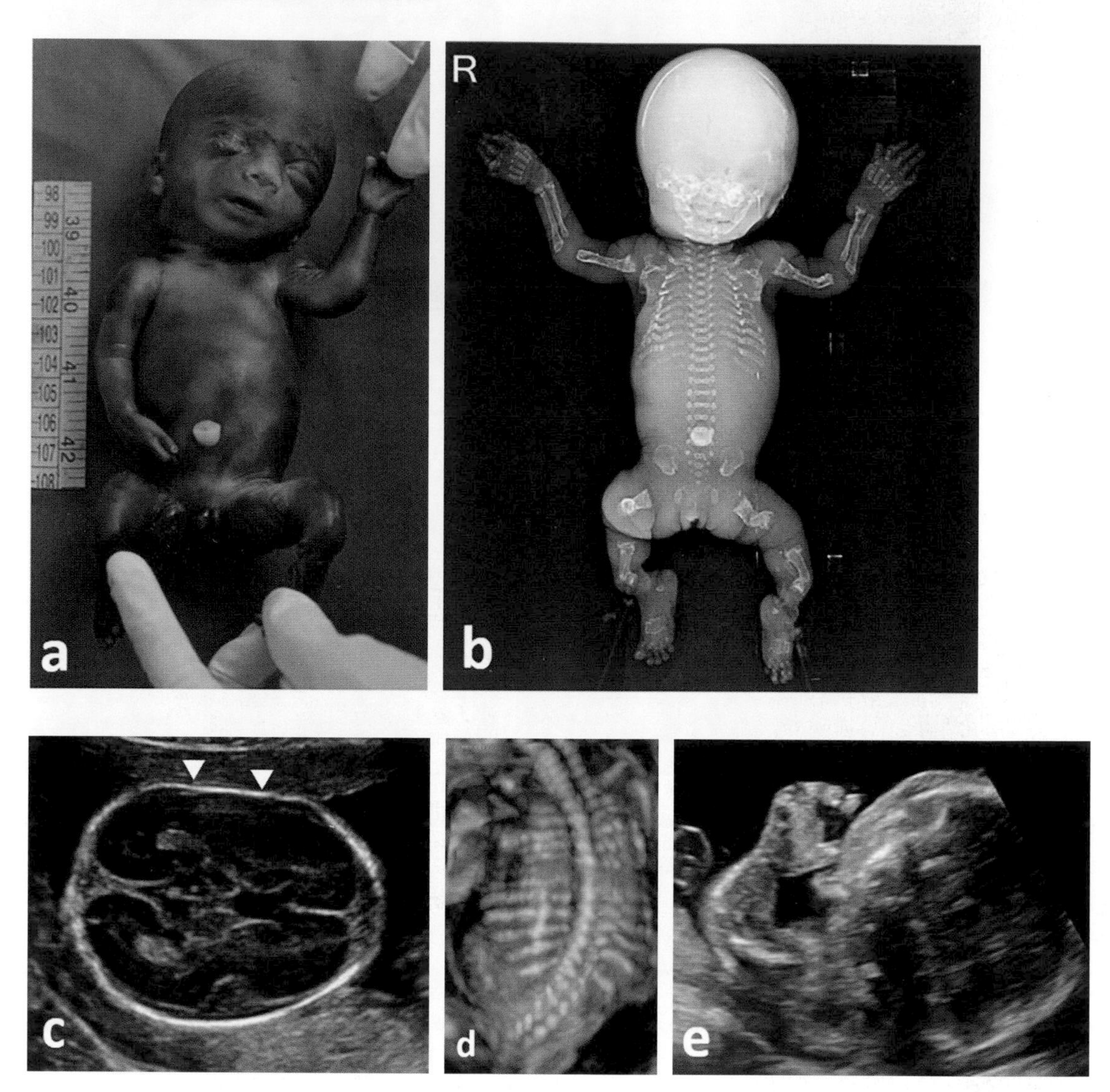

Fig. 3.7.41 (a) Phenotype of a fetus affected with **osteogenesis imperfecta type 2**. Limbs are short and bowed. Thorax is not very narrow but the lungs were hypoplastic. (b) Fetogram shows generalised osteopenia of all the bones, including the skull. The spine is ossified but poorly mineralised. The ribs appear thin and irregular due to fractures. The long bones are short and show fractures in the femur and tibia. (c) Ultrasound of the skull shows poor mineralisation. Note the flattening of the parietal bone when probe pressure is applied (arrowheads). (d) 3D of the chest shows thin beaded ribs. (e–g) Ultrasound pictures show micromelia with thin deformed long bones and fractures. (h) 3D image of the same fetus with micromelic limbs.

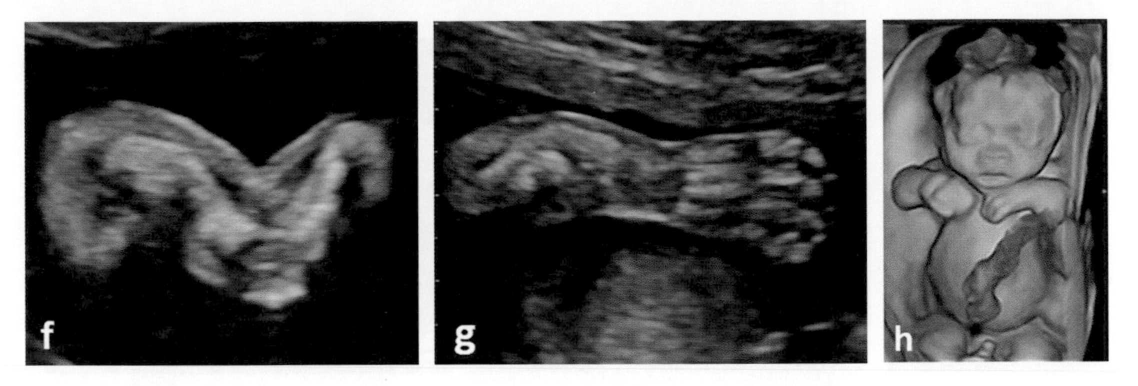

Fig. 3.7.41 *(cont.)*

SHORT RIB POLYDACTYLY SYNDROME

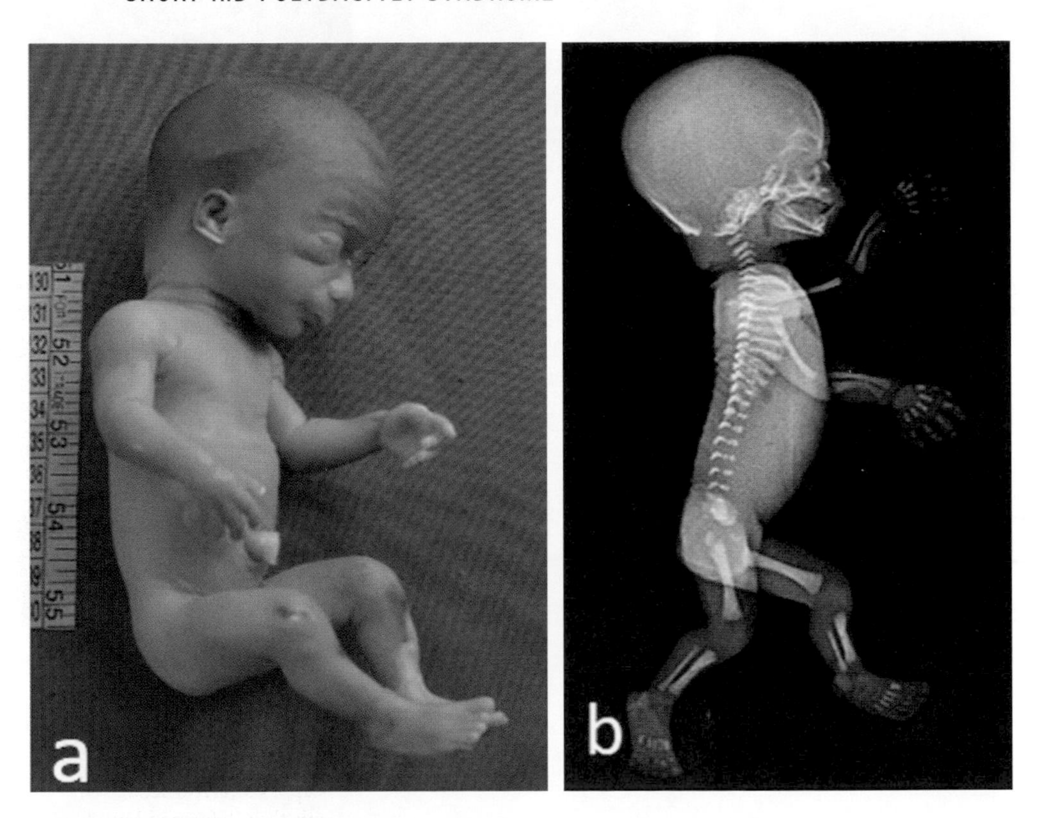

Fig. 3.7.42 (a) A 22-week fetus with **short rib polydactyly syndrome** showing narrowing of the thorax and polydactyly of hands and feet. (b) Fetogram shows a well-ossified skeleton. The ribs and long bones are short but well ossified. (c) 3D view of the same fetus showing narrow thorax and short ribs. (d) Transverse view of the thorax showing hypoplastic lungs and very short ribs. (e) Long bones are short with tibia longer than fibula and (f) mild bowing of radius and ulna. Polydactyly of (g) hand and (h) foot. Even though four types have been described, there is a significant overlap in phenotypes. In this case the tibia is longer than the fibula, which suggests type 4 (Beemer–Langer). However, in type 4 midline facial clefts may be seen but polydactyly is usually not present.

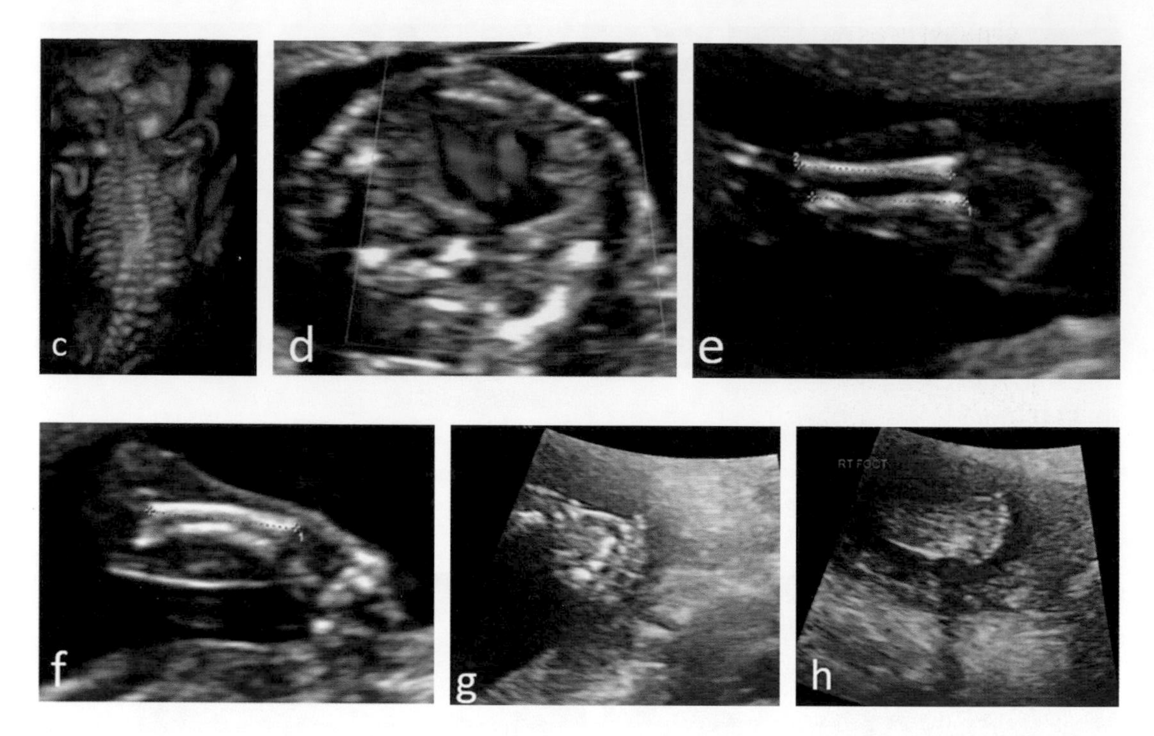

Fig. 3.7.42 (*cont.*)

SPONDYLOCOSTAL DYSPLASIA (JARCHO–LEVIN SYNDROME)

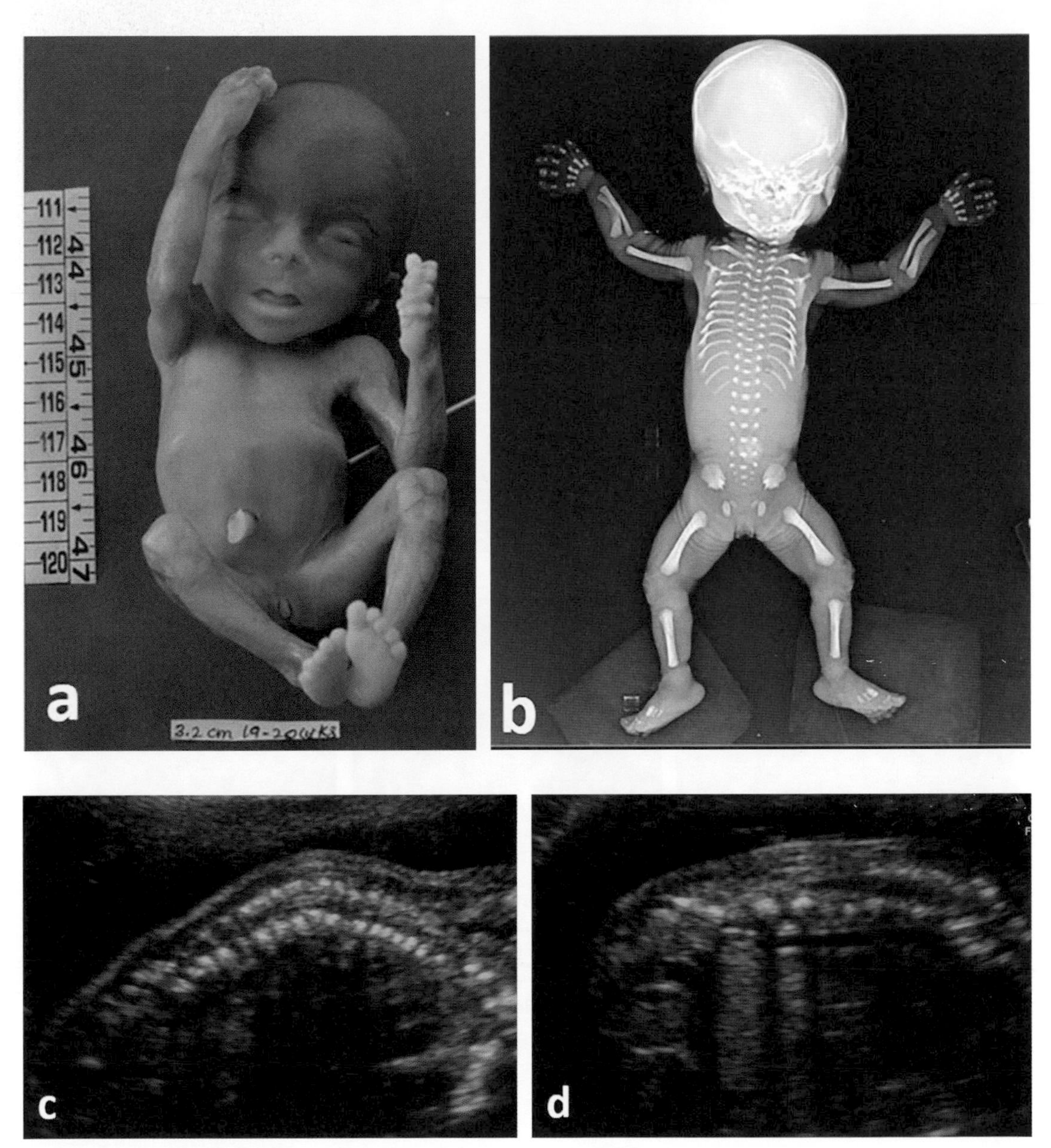

Fig. 3.7.43 (a) A 22-week fetus affected with spondylocostal dysplasia (Jarcho–Levin syndrome). (b) Fetogram shows multiple vertebral defects giving a "pebble like" appearance. The ribs are misshaped, with fusion at the costovertebral junction. The chest shows a 'crab-like deformity'. The long bones have normal appearance. (c,d) Sagittal views of the spine show multiple vertebral defects and kyphosis.

THANATOPHORIC DYSPLASIA

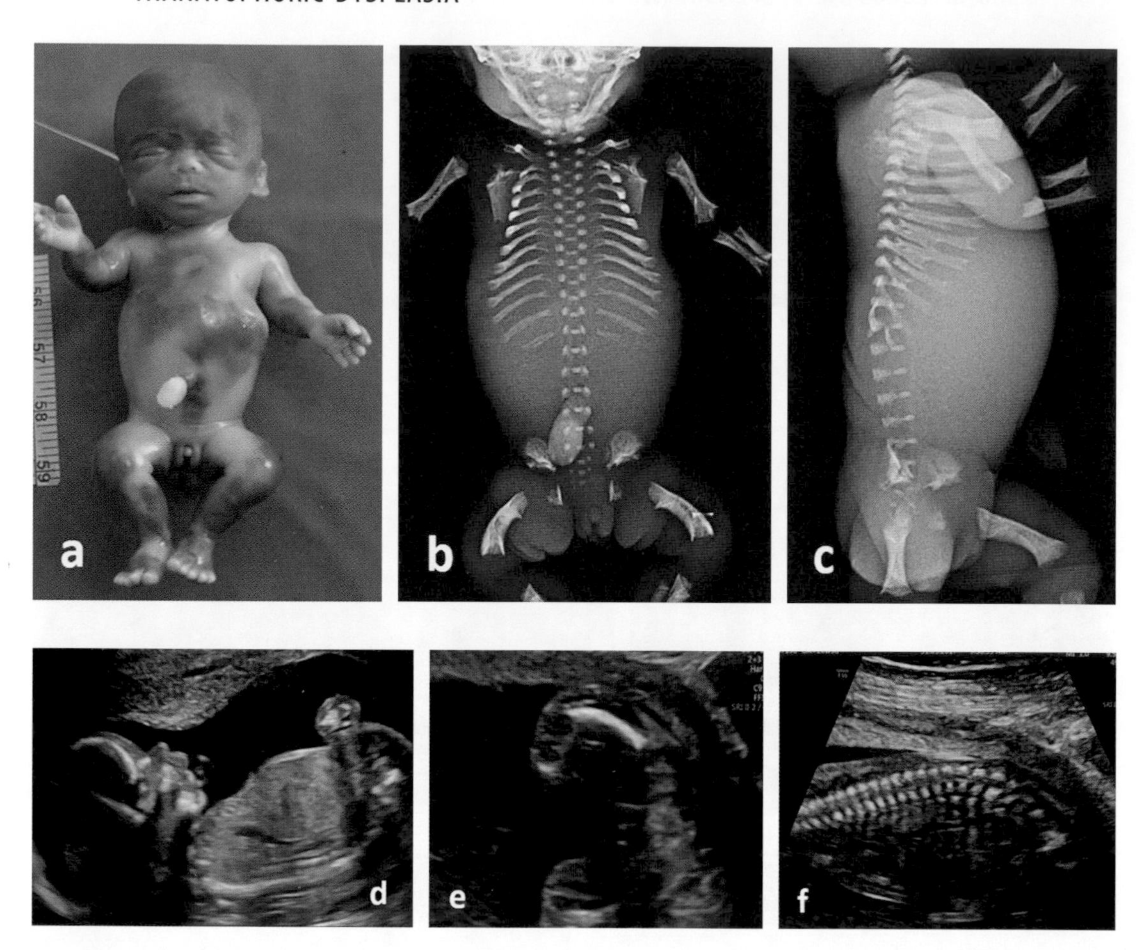

Fig. 3.7.44 (a) Phenotype of a fetus affected with **thanatophoric dysplasia**. Thorax is narrow and limbs are short. The hands appear short and stubby (brachydactyly). (b,c) Anteroposterior and lateral fetograms show short long bones with bowing of the femur. The metaphyseal ends of the long bones are flared. The iliac bones are abnormal and the vertebral bodies are flat (platyspondyly). Ribs appear short with metaphyseal flaring. (d) Sagittal section of the fetus shows very narrow thorax and protuberant abdomen. (e) Although long bones are extremely short and bowed, mineralisation is good. (f) Sagittal section of spine showing platyspondyly of all vertebral bodies with wide intervertebral spaces.

ABNORMAL FEET

Talipes (Club Foot)

- Equinovarus – deviation inward and downward:
  - the most common foot deformity
  - isolated (idiopathic) in most cases
  - syndromic (Table 3.7.1)
  - neurological disorders (e.g. spina bifida, spinal muscular atrophy)

- Calcaneovalgus – extreme dorsiflexion (foot maybe touching the shin):
  - most commonly positional due to oligohydramnios
  - can be repositioned relatively easily after birth
  - usually resolves spontaneously after a few months

Rocker Bottom Foot

- Convex foot (congenital vertical talus)
- Rigid due to structural deformity
- Main causes:
  - trisomy 13/18
  - spina bifida
  - arthrogryposis

Is Karyotyping Indicated?

- Even in the best centres, apparently isolated talipes will have other structural abnormalities in ~7% and chromosomal in ~4% of cases
- There are no clinically important differences in these risks between unilateral and bilateral talipes
- Our recommendation is, therefore, to offer invasive testing, even when talipes are unilateral and apparently isolated

ISOLATED SHORT FEMUR

Differential Diagnosis

- Short stature
- Fetal growth restriction
- Trisomy 21 (even with negative first trimester screening)
- Other chromosomal abnormalities (unbalanced, trisomy 13/18, Turner, mosaicisms)

Look for the Features:

- Proximal femoral focal deficiency:
  - commonly bilateral, can be unilateral
  - external hip rotation may cause altered movements
- Femur–fibula–ulna complex:
  - striking asymmetry of long bones, more commonly upper limb and unilateral (right)
- Femoral hypoplasia–unusual facies syndrome:
  - also cleft palate, micrognathia, abnormal vertebrae

ABSENT RADIUS

Differential Diagnosis

- Baller–Gerold syndrome
  - also craniosynostosis, hypertelorism, cardiac defects
- Cat eye syndrome
  - also coloboma and abnormal facial features, anal atresia/stenosis, heart defects, renal anomalies, ambiguous genitalia

- Fanconi anaemia
  - also growth restriction, horseshoe kidney and vertebral anomalies
- Holt–Oram syndrome:
  - also heart anomalies
- Nager syndrome
  - also micrognathia and microtia
- Thrombocytopenia absent radius (TAR) syndrome
  - also absent or hypoplastic ulna, heart and renal anomalies
- VACTERL association
  - costovertebral anomalies, anal atresia, heart defects, trachea–oesophageal anomalies, renal and limb abnormalities (radial)

LIMB REDUCTION DEFECTS

Diagnosis and Characteristics

- Terminal transverse defects; more common in the upper limbs
- ~1 in 2,000 births
- Most cases are non-genetic, caused by a vascular injury or amniotic band sequence
- Bowing and shortening suggest underlying skeletal dysplasia

Look for Phenotypic Characteristics

- Proximal femoral focal hypoplasia (Fig. 3.7.45)
- femoral hypoplasia–unusual facies syndrome

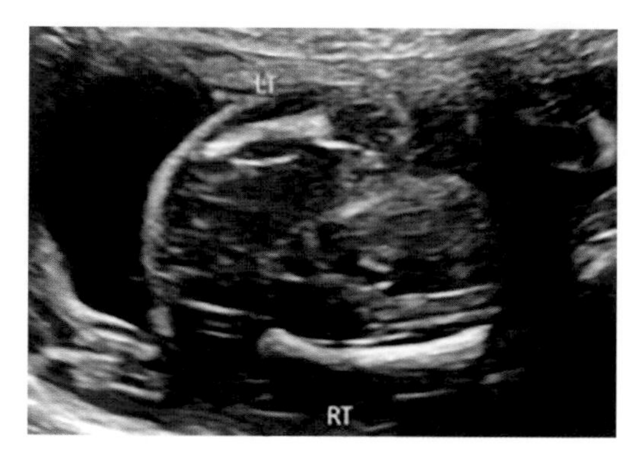

Fig. 3.7.45 Fetus with proximal focal femoral hypoplasia. The left femur is very short. The right femur is appropriate for gestation.

SUGGESTED READING

PRIMARY RESEARCH

Mathiesen JM, Aksglaede L, Skibsted L, et al. Outcome of fetuses with short femur length detected at second-trimester anomaly scan: a national survey. *Ultrasound Obstet Gynecol* 2014;44(2):160–165.

REVIEWS AND GUIDELINES

Chitty LS, Everett F, Usakov F. Songoraphic diagnosis of skeletal anomalies. In: *Fetal Medicine* (Kumar B, Alfirevic Z, eds), Cambridge University Press, Cambridge, 2016; 161–181.

Di Mascio D, Buca D, Khalil A, et al. Outcome of isolated fetal talipes: a systematic review and meta-analysis. *Acta Obstet Gynecol Scand* 2019;98(11):1367–1377.

CHAPTER 4

Small for Gestational Age (SGA) and Fetal Growth Restriction

SUMMARY BOX

DEFINITIONS AND CHARACTERISTICS

- The main concern about the small for gestational age (SGA) fetus comes from its association with stillbirths – in some published cohorts up to 50% of stillbirths were judged to be SGA
- SGA is most commonly defined as an estimated fetal weight (EFW) or abdominal circumference (AC) <10th centile
- SGA is detected by plotting fetal biometry on locally generated charts, customised charts (e.g. https://perinatal.org.uk/FetalGrowth/home), or standardised population-based charts (e.g. (https://intergrowth21.tghn.org/fetal-growth)
- The 10th centile for EFW near term can vary quite considerably between various charts (>100 g)
- There is no good-quality evidence that any of the currently available charts, customised or population-based, are superior to others in reducing perinatal mortality and morbidity
- Fetal growth restriction (FGR) is a pathological subgroup of SGA, most commonly defined as an EFW <10th centile with abnormal fetal Dopplers or EFW <3rd centile irrespective of Doppler findings
- FGR fetuses are most likely to be associated with iatrogenic early preterm birth and perinatal mortality and morbidity
- Reduced growth velocity is defined as a fall of more than 50 centiles in EFW or AC between consecutive scans
- Accurate dating by first trimester ultrasound is essential for appropriate management of SGA/FGR

MATERNAL RISK FACTORS

- Preeclampsia
- Previous history of SGA/FGR
- Previous stillbirth
- Previous hypertensive disease of pregnancy
- Low PAPP-A (<5th centile, <0.415 MoM)
- Abnormal uterine artery Doppler at 18–24 weeks
- Smoking
- Age >40 years

FETAL CAUSES

- Prevalence of various fetal causes depends on the timing of presentation
- Placental insufficiency is the most common cause (>80%), but when SGA is detected at 18–24 weeks only 20% will be due to a placental cause
- Most common chromosomal abnormalities are triploidies before 26 weeks and trisomy 18 after 26 weeks
- In ~5% of fetuses with early severe growth restriction and common aneuploidies excluded, microarray can reveal significant pathology
- Genetic syndromes (Table 4.1)
- Infection (CMV)

Table 4.1 Ultrasound features of the most common genetic conditions associated with severe FGR.

Triploidy – diandric	Large cystic placenta (molar?), relative microcephaly, structural abnormalities (CNS, cardiac, renal, syndactyly), oligohydramnios
Triploidy – digynic	Small, non-cystic placenta, relative macrocephaly, oligohydramnios
Trisomy 18, 21, 13, 16, 7	Multiple structural abnormalities
Cornelia de Lange syndrome	Microcephaly, long convex philtrum, upturned nose with anteverted nostrils, micrognathia, mandibular spur, excessive hair growth, long eyelashes, limb abnormalities (mainly hands, often asymmetrical), atrial and ventricular septal defects, anomalous systemic venous drainage, ectopic kidneys, diaphragmatic hernia (25%)
Smith–Lemli–Opitz syndrome	Increased nuchal translucency, microcephaly, CNS, cardiac and renal abnormalities, ambiguous genitalia, fused second and third toes, postaxial polydactyly, clubfoot
Russell–Silver syndrome	Small triangular face with relative macrocephaly, short long bones and narrow thorax may mimic skeletal dysplasias, ambiguous genitalia, curved fifth finger (clinodactyly)

INITIAL ULTRASOUND ASSESSMENT

- Every effort should be made to establish correct gestational age by reviewing previous scans, menstrual history and any assisted conception procedures
- Detailed survey of anatomy including fetal echocardiography to exclude structural anomalies
- If femur length is <5th centile, full skeletal survey should be done (see Chapter 3)
- Fetal Doppler (umbilical artery, middle cerebral artery, ductus venosus)
- Look for signs of fetal infection (e.g. echogenic bowel, calcifications)
- Look for placental causes, including velamentous cord insertion, extensive calcifications and abnormal uterine artery Doppler (mean pulsatility index >95th centile, or >1.45, bilateral diastolic notching)

INVESTIGATIONS

- Infection screen (CMV, toxoplasma, syphilis and malaria in high-risk populations)
- Microarray for severe SGA <3rd centile, unless there is clear evidence of placental insufficiency
- If suspected, Smith–Lemli–Opitz syndrome can be confirmed by elevated amniotic fluid 7-8-dehydrocholesterol (7/8-DHC) level, which is normally undetectable

MANAGEMENT

<24^{+0} WEEKS, STRUCTURALLY NORMAL, NO EVIDENCE OF FETAL INFECTION

- Genetic testing (microarray) is indicated if EFW <3rd centile, unless uterine and fetal Doppler strongly suggest placental cause
- Repeat growth scan and fetal Doppler when viability is reached (23–24 weeks)
- If uterine artery Doppler is abnormal, 150 mg aspirin at night is indicated
- There is no good evidence to support any other intervention to promote fetal growth (bed rest, low molecular weight heparin, sildenafil, L-arginine)
- If uterine artery Doppler is abnormal, look for early signs of preeclampsia by more frequent antenatal visits
- **Most fetuses in this group will have normal growth trajectory and normal outcome**

24^{+0} TO 32^{+0} WEEKS, STRUCTURALLY NORMAL, NO EVIDENCE OF FETAL INFECTION

- Genetic testing (microarray) is indicated if EFW <3rd centile, unless there are obvious signs of placental insufficiency
- Growth scans and fetal Doppler should be repeated every 2 weeks
- If fetal Doppler is abnormal, intensive fetal monitoring is indicated (Table 4.2)
- There is no good evidence to support use of middle cerebral artery Doppler for clinical decision-making before 32 weeks
- Antenatal steroids should be prescribed only when elective delivery is planned within 72 hours
- **Gestational age at birth remains the best predictor of long-term outcome (Fig. 4.1 and Table 4.3)**
- **With intensive fetal monitoring more than 90% of babies will be born alive and have no neurological impairment at the age of 2 years**

>32^{+0} WEEKS, STRUCTURALLY NORMAL, NO EVIDENCE OF INFECTION

Fetal Monitoring

- Fetal biometry:
  - head circumference
  - abdominal circumference
  - femur length
  - estimated fetal weight
  - maximum vertical amniotic pool depth (cm)
- Extensive placental calcifications (Y/N)
- Umbilical artery:
  - pulsatility index
  - absent/reversed end diastolic flow
- Middle cerebral artery:
  - pulsatility index/cerebroplacental ratio
- Ductus venosus:
  - pulsatility index
  - ‘a’ wave present/absent/reversed
- Computerized CTG (cCTG) (when fetal Doppler is abnormal)

Frequency of Assessments

- EFW 3rd to 10th centile + Doppler normal = every 2 weeks
- EFW <3rd + Doppler normal = once per week (Doppler weekly, fetal biometry every 2 weeks)
- Fetal Doppler abnormal = every 48–72 hours

Indications for Delivery

- Fetuses that are found to have reversed or absent EDV in the umbilical artery after 32^{+0} weeks should be delivered irrespective of other findings
- There is no good evidence to support elective delivery before 37^{+0} weeks just because middle cerebral Doppler is abnormal (PI <5th centile, low cerebro-placental ratio)
- Fetuses with persistently raised umbilical artery PI should be delivered by 37^{+0} weeks
- Fetuses with no increase in EFW over 3 weeks should be delivered
- Fetuses with EFW <3rd centile should be delivered no later than 37^{+6} weeks
- Fetuses with EFW 3rd to 10th centile should be delivered no later than 38^{+6} weeks

Labour and Delivery

- Fetuses with reversed or absent umbilical artery EDV should be delivered by caesarean section
- Fetuses with abnormal fetal Doppler but present umbilical artery EDV can be induced with continuous CTG monitoring through induction process
- SGA is not a contraindication for antenatal corticosteroids
- A second course of corticosteroids can be given if delivery is planned before 34^{+0} weeks and the first course was given more than 14 days previously
- The neonatal team should be involved in the decision regarding timing of delivery
- Placental histology is important to exclude recurrent pathology (e.g. villitis of unknown aetiology, chronic histiocytic intervillositis, maternal vascular under-perfusion, massive perivillous fibrin deposition) (see Chapter 9)

Table 4.2 Liverpool management protocol for SGA with abnormal fetal Doppler before 32 weeks

	Ductus venosus PI normal	Ductus venosus PI >95th centile	Ductus venosus absent/ reversed 'a' wave
Umbilical artery PI >95th centile	Follow-up 7 days	Follow-up 3 days	Repeat within 24 h; if persists, deliver
Umbilical artery absent EDV	Follow-up 3 days	Follow-up 3 days	Repeat within 24 h; if persists, deliver
Umbilical artery reversed EDV	Follow-up 3 days	Follow-up daily	Repeat within 24 h; if persists, deliver

- 60 min computerised CTG at each visit – deliver if persistent decelerations are present or short-term variability is <2.6 ms before 29^{+0} weeks, or <3.0 ms $\geq 29^{+0}$ weeks (Dawes–Redman criteria)
- If computerised CTG is not available, indication for delivery has to be subjective using locally agreed criteria for abnormal (pathological) CTG
- If antenatal steroids were given within 72 hours, above cCTG criteria don't apply. Only recurrent unprovoked recurrent decelerations should be considered clinically significant

Table 4.3 Neurodevelopmental outcomes affected by fetal growth. Note that the neurodevelopmental impact of FGR is exacerbated by the severity of FGR and confounded by the association with preterm birth

Neurodisability	Impact of FGR
Cerebral palsy	↑
Spasticity	↑
Dyskinesia	↑
Postnatal head size	↓
IQ	↓
Gross and fine motor skills	↓
Muscle tone	↓
Cognition	↓

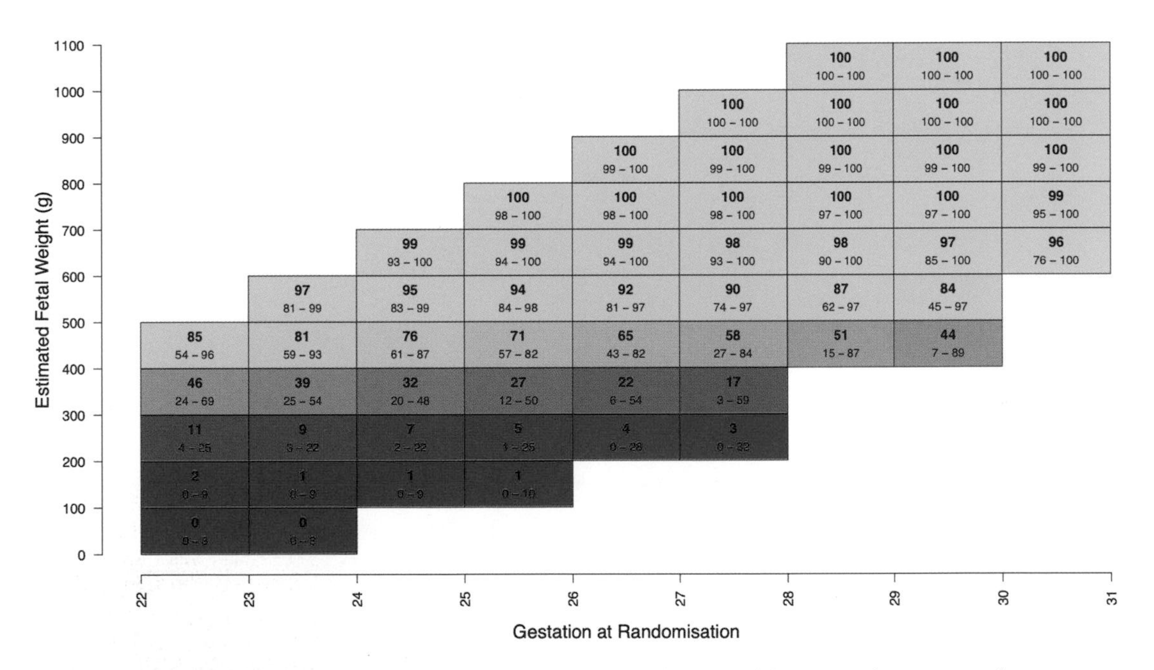

Fig. 4.1 Overall survival by estimated fetal weight and gestation at the time of diagnosis of severe growth restriction before 32 weeks. Reproduced with permission from Sharp A, et al. A prediction model for short-term neonatal outcomes in severe early-onset fetal growth restriction. *Eur J Obstet Gynaecol* 2019;241:109–118.

SUGGESTED READING

Lees CC, Stampalija T, Baschat AA, et al. ISUOG Practice Guidelines: diagnosis and management of small-for-gestational-age fetus and fetal growth restriction. *Ultrasound Obstet Gynecol* 2020;56:298–312.

Meler E, Sisterna S, Borrell A. Genetic syndromes associated with isolated fetal growth restriction. *Prenat Diagn* 2020;40(4):432–446.

CHAPTER 5

Large for Gestational Age (LGA) Fetus

SUMMARY BOX

DEFINITIONS AND DETECTION

- Large for gestational age (LGA) fetus is most commonly defined as estimated fetal weight (EFW) >90th centile using either customised charts (e.g. https://perinatal.org.uk/FetalGrowth/home) or population-based charts e.g. (https://intergrowth21.tghn.org/fetal-growth)
- There is no good-quality evidence showing that any chart is better than the other in terms of diagnostic accuracy or reduction in adverse perinatal outcomes
- Fetal macrosomia is defined as EFW of 4,000 g, irrespective of gestational age
- Diagnostic accuracy of antenatal ultrasound to detect LGA/macrosomia in the general obstetric population is not good enough to justify routine screening; therefore, ultrasound as a diagnostic test for LGA should be limited to women with risk factors

MATERNAL RISK FACTORS

- Diabetes
- LGA/macrosomia in previous pregnancy
- Obesity
- Excessive weight gain in pregnancy
- High symphysis fundal height

FETAL RISK FACTORS

- Overgrowth syndromes (Beckwith–Wiedemann, Costello, Perlman, Simpson–Golabi–Behmel, Sotos, Weaver)

INVESTIGATIONS

- Maternal diabetes should be excluded with a glucose tolerance test and/or HBA1c
- If available, offer genetic testing when phenotypic features suggest a possibility of an overgrowth syndrome (Table 5.1)

Table 5.1 Ultrasound findings associated with overgrowth syndromes.

Beckwith–Wiedemann	Polyhydramnios, large kidneys, macroglossia, omphalocele placentomegaly
Simpson–Golabi–Behmel	Polyhydramnios, cystic hygroma, craniofacial abnormalities, renal anomalies, congenital diaphragmatic hernia, polydactyly, single umbilical artery
Sotos	Polyhydramnios, macrocephaly, ventriculomegaly, large cisterna magna, hypoplastic corpus callosum, renal abnormalities, increased nuchal translucency in the first trimester
Perlman	Polyhydramnios, ascites, large kidneys

COUNSELLING AND MANAGEMENT

- When fetus is macrosomic, at or after 36 weeks, elective delivery should be offered at 38^{+0} to 38^{+6} weeks, irrespective of possible underlying cause. This is because of the potential risk of shoulder dystocia and perineal damage
- When EFW is >4,500 g (4,000 g for diabetics) an elective caesarean section is preferable to induction of labour, accepting that the false-positive rate for LGA near term can be as high as 15%
- Women who opt for vaginal birth should be managed in an obstetric unit with experienced staff and facilities to manage shoulder dystocia

SUGGESTED READING

Robinson R, Walker KF, White VA, et al. The test accuracy of antenatal ultrasound definitions of fetal macrosomia to predict birth injury: a systematic review. *Eur J Obstet Gynecol Reprod Biol* 2020;246:79–85.

Vora N, Bianchi DW. Genetic considerations in the prenatal diagnosis of overgrowth syndromes. *Prenat Diagn* 2009;29(10):923–929.

CHAPTER 6

Rhesus Disease

SUMMARY BOX

DEFINITIONS AND PRESENTATION

- Each human red cell has 39 blood group systems with more than 300 antigens, but only a few of them can cause fetal disease
- The incidence of fetal anaemia caused by anti-D IgG antibodies to RhD antigen has decreased dramatically due to postnatal and, more recently, antenatal anti-D prophylaxis
- Relatively common causes of immune fetal anaemia nowadays include other Rh antibodies (c, C, e, E) or atypical antibodies against Kell, Duffy, Kidd or MNS antigens
- Antibody quantification requires specific equipment and measurements against a national standard. It is currently available only for anti-D and anti-c antibodies, and reported as IU/ml
- Concentration of other antibodies is assessed by titration. Doubling dilutions (1 in 2, 4, 8, 16, 32, etc.) of a patient's plasma are tested using reagent red cells that express relevant antigens. The reported titre is of the highest dilution that gives a positive reaction
- Only an increase of more than one dilution (i.e. 1 in 8 rising to 32, or 1 in 64 rising to 1 in 256) should be considered clinically significant
- Clinically important thresholds are listed in Table 6.1
- Thresholds for intensive monitoring are lower in the presence of multiple antibodies (e.g. combination of 6 IU/ml of anti-D and 10 IU/ml of anti-C)
- The '10 weeks rule' is useful as a guide to decide the timing of the next follow-up scan. If in a previously affected pregnancy the first intrauterine transfusion was performed at 30 weeks, in the next pregnancy intensive weekly monitoring should start around 20 weeks

Table 6.1 Antibodies to red cell antigens that may cause fetal anaemia with threshold levels for fetal monitoring. The threshold for intensive monitoring is lower in the presence of multiple antibodies.

Antibodies likely to cause fetal anaemia	Antibody levels/titre requiring serial MCA PSV monitoring	Antibody levels requiring intensive monitoring (weekly or twice each week)
Anti-D	4 IU/ml or 1:16	• More than 15 IU/ml • Significant rise in antibodies** • <10 weeks from the gestation when previous baby was affected
Anti-c	>7.5 IU/ml or 1:16	• More than 20 IU/ml • Significant rise in antibodies** • <10 weeks from the gestation when previous baby was affected
Kell blood group system (Anti-K, -k, -Kp^{a}, -Js^{a}, -Js^{b})	1:1*	• Significant rise in antibodies** • <10 weeks from the gestation when previous baby was affected
Anti-C, -E, -e, Duffy blood group system (anti-Fy^{a}, -Fyb), Kidd blood group system (anti-Jk^{a}, -Jk^{b}), anti-M	1:32	• Significant rise in antibodies** • <10 weeks from the gestation when previous baby was affected

* Anti-K, -k, -KP^{a} do not correlate well with the severity of the disease. Low titres have been reported in severely affected fetuses.

** One-step rise in titres from 1:32 to 1:64, 1:256 to 1:512 or 1:1,024 to 1:2,048 is not considered significant as it is within margins of a laboratory error.

INVESTIGATIONS

- Check paternal Rh status
- If the father is heterozygous for Rh antigens (D, c, C, E) or Kell (K) antigen, fetal genotype can be determined from cffDNA in maternal blood after 11 weeks
- Most recent reports show that false-negative results for fetal Rh status (D, c, C, E) are very rare (<1 in 1,000)
- False-negative results for fetal Kell (K1) status may be as high as 1 in 200. It is, therefore, advisable to repeat fetal Kell genotyping around 24 weeks
- If fetal genotyping is not available, amniocentesis should be offered to avoid intensive monitoring and a possibility of a false-positive high MCA PSV that may trigger an unnecessary intervention
- If fetal Rh genotyping is negative for the offending antigen, our policy is to check antibody levels around 32 weeks to exclude significant rise in antibodies, but we do not perform serial MCA PSV monitoring

ANTENATAL MANAGEMENT

FETUS IS ANTIGEN POSITIVE OR FATHER IS HOMOZYGOUS, BUT THERE IS NO HISTORY OF IMMUNE ANAEMIA

- Start MCA PSV monitoring and antibody monitoring every 2 weeks from 24 weeks, then weekly from 28 weeks (Fig. 6.1; Table 6.2)
- If there is a significant rise in maternal antibodies or MCA PSV is rising close to 1.5 MoM, scans should be done *weekly* before 28 weeks and *twice per week* after 28 weeks
- Many fetal medicine teams do not check antibody levels/titre once the threshold for regular MCA PSV monitoring has been reached
- Antenatal CTGs are of no value in monitoring of Rhesus disease
- Delivery should be arranged at 37^{+0} weeks

FETUS ANTIGEN IS POSITIVE OR FATHER IS HOMOZYGOUS WITH HISTORY OF IMMUNE ANAEMIA

- *Weekly* MCA PSV monitoring should start 10 weeks before gestation at which previous child needed therapy (phototherapy or transfusion) – the '10 week rule'
- If intrauterine transfusion was needed before 28 weeks in previous pregnancy, first assessment should be arranged as early as 16^{+0} weeks as severe anaemia with ascites may be already present
- If MCA PSV remains below 1.5 MoM, delivery can be delayed until 37^{+0} weeks

MCA PSV >1.5 MOM OR FETAL ASCITES

- Delivery is indicated after 34^{+0} weeks
- Intrauterine intravascular transfusion* is indicated before 34^{+0} weeks
- If MCA PSV is >36 cm/s or ascites is present before 18 weeks and intravascular approach is not feasible, an intraperitoneal transfusion (10–15 ml) is indicated – it can be repeated weekly until the intravascular approach is possible
- Once the first intrauterine transfusion is given, we do not monitor antibody levels anymore as the levels are of little clinical value
- The follow-up transfusions should be timed using a combination of MCA PSV values and calculated drop in haemoglobin between the first and second transfusion

HOW TO TIME A FOLLOW-UP INTRAUTERINE TRANSFUSION

Second Transfusion

- Assuming that the post-transfusion haemoglobin after the first transfusion was ~14–15 g/dl, the second transfusion is done 3–4 weeks later
- Twice-weekly MCA PSV monitoring should start 2 weeks after the first transfusion
- If MCA PSV is >1.5 MoM within 3 weeks of the first transfusion, MCA PSV should be repeated a few hours later to confirm that the MCA PSV is persistently high (i.e. to avoid a false-positive result)
- If MCA PSV remains normal 4 weeks after the first transfusion, our preference is to perform the second transfusion 'electively' at that point to avoid a false-negative Doppler result

Subsequent Transfusions

- A combination of daily haemoglobin drop and MCA PSV is used to determine the timing of subsequent transfusions, aiming to prolong the gap between the procedures as much as possible
- Daily haemoglobin drop is calculated by dividing the difference between post- and pre-transfusion Hb with the number of days between two transfusions
- The assumption is that daily haemoglobin drop is the highest between the first and second transfusion and slows thereafter

* The technical aspects of intrauterine transfusion are described in Chapter 16

- For example, if fetal haemoglobin dropped from 14.5 g/dl immediately after the first transfusion to 8.2 g/dl in 21 days, the daily Hb drop was 14.5 – 8.2/21 = 0.3 g/dl. If post-transfusion haemoglobin after successful second transfusion was 15 g/dl, a gap of at least 4 weeks should be safe. It is extremely unlikely that haemoglobin will drop by more than 8.4 g/dl (28 days × 0.3) – that is, fetal haemoglobin after 4 weeks should be higher than 6.6 g/dl
- The last intrauterine transfusion is timed around 34 weeks with elective delivery planned 10–14 days later
- Babies who have had an intrauterine transfusion require admission to a neonatal unit to manage ongoing haemolysis

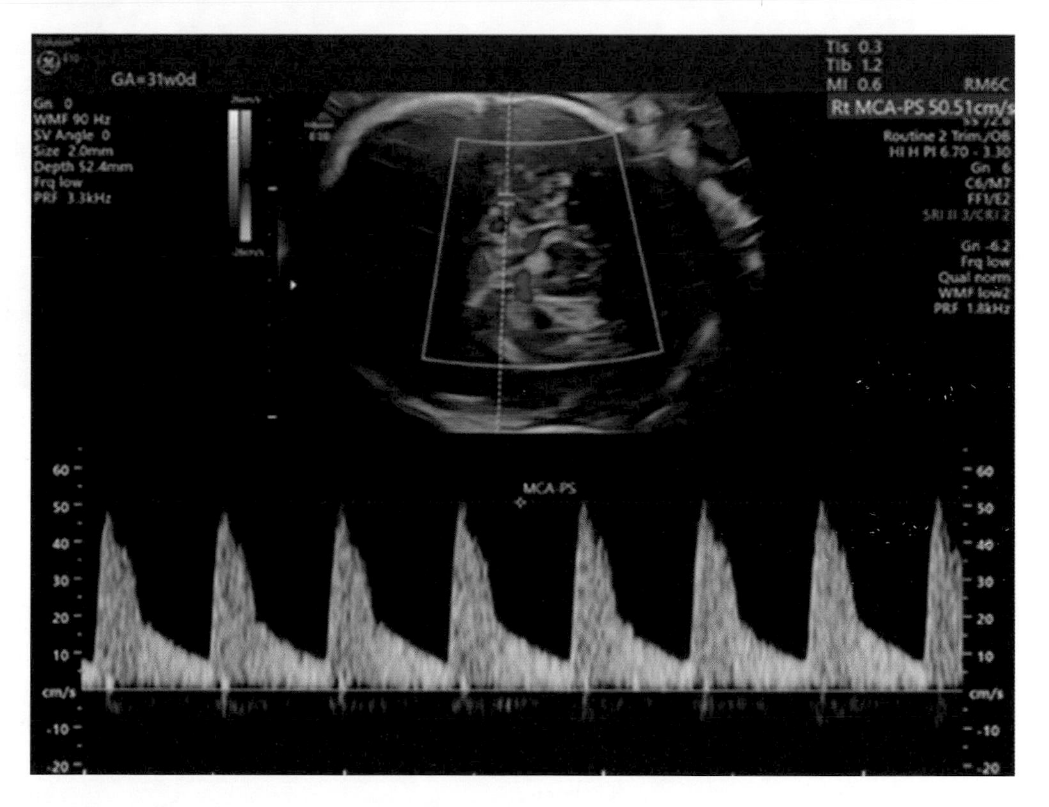

Fig. 6.1a Middle cerebral artery peak systolic measurement (MCA PSV). Note that the angle between the ultrasound beam and the vessel is effectively zero. The peak velocity is measured by aligning the PSV measurement line with the highest peaks.

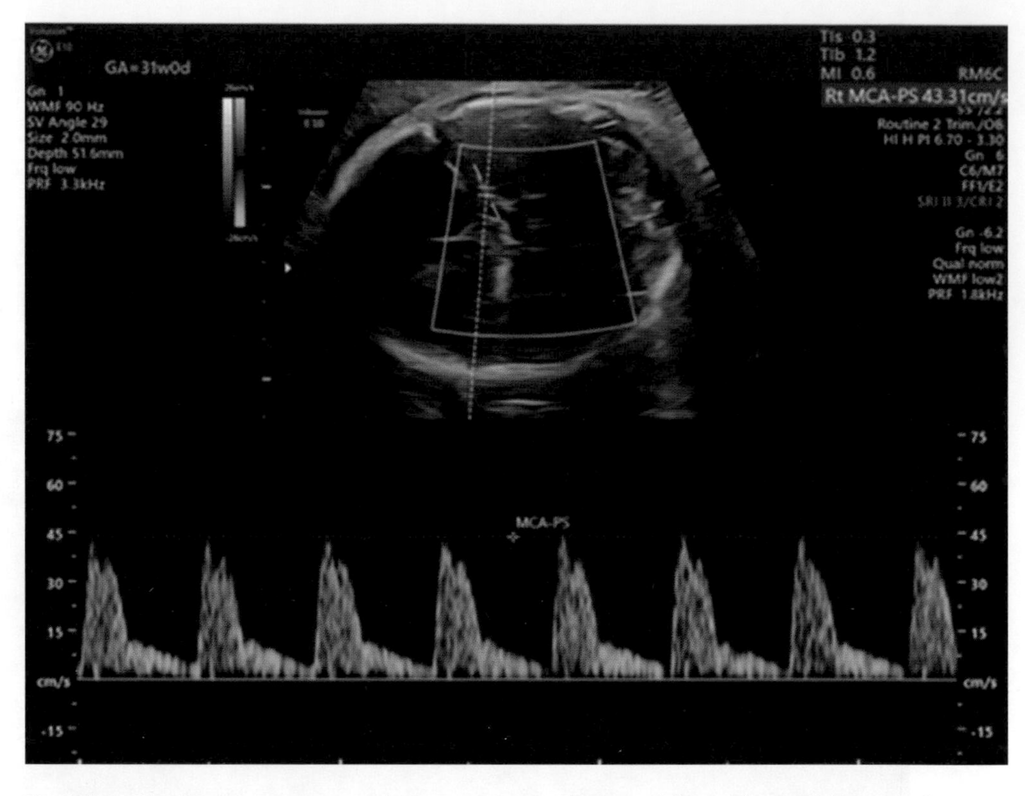

Fig. 6.1b MCA PSV measurement in the same patient only seconds later. The angle between the ultrasound beam and the vessel is suboptimal. Despite the 'angle correction', the PSV is significantly lower. Such 'angle corrections' are best avoided – every effort should be made to align the ultrasound beam with the vessel with the zero angle.

Table 6.2 Reference range of fetal MCA-PSV median and 1.5 multiples of the median (MoM) values during pregnancy.

	MCA PSV (cm/s)	
Gestational age (weeks)	**Median**	**1.5 MoM**
14	19	29
15	20	30
16	21	32
17	22	33
18	23	35
19	24	36.5
20	25	38
21	27	40

Table 6.2 (*cont.*)

Gestational age (weeks)	MCA PSV (cm/s)	
	Median	1.5 MoM
22	28	42
23	29	44
24	31	46
25	32	48
26	34	50
27	35	53
28	37	55
29	39	58
30	40.5	61
31	42	64
32	44	67
33	46.5	70
34	49	73
35	51	77
36	53.5	80
37	56	84
38	59	88

Modified from Mari G, et al. Noninvasive diagnosis by Doppler ultrasonography of fetal anemia due to maternal red-cell alloimmunization. *N Engl J Med* 2000;342:9–14, with permission. Copyright © 2000 Massachusetts Medical Society.

NEONATAL MANAGEMENT

- Rhesus disease presents postnatally with anaemia and jaundice
- Cord blood is sent for direct Coombs test (detects antibodies attached to the surface of red blood cells), haemoglobin and bilirubin levels
- In most settings, high-risk babies will be admitted to the neonatal unit; 4-hourly bilirubin measurements will be plotted on gestation-specific bilirubin charts
- Folic acid supplementation is commonly prescribed due to its role in proliferation of erythroblasts
- The management strategy aims to prevent the complication of acute bilirubin encephalopathy and kernicterus, and includes phototherapy, immunoglobulin (IVIg) and blood transfusion

Phototherapy

- Photo-isomerisation of unconjugated bilirubin in the skin to water-soluble isomers
- Intensified phototherapy is performed in the neonatal unit and is not interrupted for feeding
- Prophylactic phototherapy is not beneficial

Immunoglobulin (IVIg)

- Blood product is from healthy human donors
- Reduces the breakdown of antibody-coated red cells by blockage of Fc receptors
- May be used as an adjunct to phototherapy if serum bilirubin rises >8.5 μmol/L/h or when transfusions are not possible or deemed too high risk. However, good-quality evidence that IVIg reduces the need for transfusions is lacking

Blood Transfusions

- Indicated when cord haemoglobin is low or serum bilirubin levels are too high
- Associated morbidity is due to catheter complications, thrombocytopenia and infections
- Around 20% of babies that have required an intrauterine transfusion will need postnatal transfusion(s)
- Late anaemia is a known complication; therefore, monitoring for several weeks after birth is required
- Intrauterine transfusions increase the risk of late anaemia due to a transient suppression of neonatal erythropoiesis
- Top-up transfusions may be necessary in around 50% of babies

SUGGESTED READING

Mari G. Middle cerebral artery peak systolic velocity for the diagnosis of fetal anemia: the untold story. *Ultrasound Obstet Gynecol* 2005;25(4):323–330.

Ree IMC, Smits-Wintjens VEHJ, van der Bom JG, et al. Neonatal management and outcome in alloimmune hemolytic disease. *Expert Rev Hematol* 2017;10(7):607–616.

CHAPTER 7

Fetal Alloimmune Thrombocytopenia

SUMMARY BOX

DEFINITION AND PRESENTATION

- Clinically important (severe) fetal thrombocytopenia is defined as platelet count below 50×10^9/L
- Fetal alloimmune thrombocytopenia (FAIT) is often under-reported with incidence around 1:1,000 pregnancies; however, severe forms causing intracranial bleeding are very rare
- FAIT is caused by maternal IgG antibodies against human platelet antigens (HPA); the two most common HPAs are HPA-1a and HPA-5b
- Only 10% of HPA-1a negative women who carry an HPA-1a positive fetus will produce a detectable amount of anti-HPA antibodies
- Antenatal antibody screening programmes are not cost-effective
- Prophylaxis against FAIT, similar to the anti-D prophylaxis, is still in the development phase

PRE-PREGNANCY COUNSELLING

- Fetal medicine specialists will be alerted to the possibility of FAIT because of:
  - previously affected child (in utero or soon after birth)
  - presence of anti-platelet antibodies in maternal blood
  - a first-degree relative affected by the disease
- It is important to establish the severity of the disease in an affected child as objectively as possible (timing, lowest platelet count, clinical symptoms, imaging)

Investigations

- Maternal HPA antigen/antibody status should be reviewed and repeated if necessary
- HPA testing should be offered in all cases of confirmed fetal intracranial haemorrhage or severe neonatal thrombocytopenia, regardless of presumed aetiology
- First-degree female relatives of reproductive age should also be offered HPA testing
- Paternal HPA status for the offending antigen should be established; if the father is heterozygous, discuss available options for fetal genotyping in subsequent pregnancy
- Options for fetal genotyping include:
  - cffDNA from maternal serum (already available in several European countries)
  - amniocentesis
- CVS is best avoided to minimise the risk of further alloimmune reaction
- Antibody titres are not predictive and, therefore, repeated testing before or during pregnancy has no clinical value

MANAGEMENT

- Discuss the risks, treatment options, antenatal imaging and mode of delivery in subsequent pregnancies, taking into account severity of the disease
- Only around 10% of fetuses with severe thrombocytopenia will develop intracranial haemorrhage
- Side effects of intravenous immune globulin (IVIg) are common (headache). Allergic-type reactions requiring medical intervention can be expected in up to 5% of patients

PREVIOUSLY AFFECTED CHILD WITHOUT INTRACRANIAL HAEMORRHAGE

- Offer fetal genotyping if the father is heterozygous

Treatment

- Start IVIg infusions at 20 weeks (1 g/kg) over 4 hours once a week until birth
- For mild cases (e.g. asymptomatic neonatal thrombocytopenia) treatment can be delayed until 24 weeks

Monitoring

- Four-weekly ultrasound scans
- Antenatal MRI is not needed if scans are normal
- Antenatal cordocentesis to determine whether vaginal delivery is contraindicated is best avoided – the risks associated with fetal blood sampling outweigh the benefits

Labour and Delivery

- If there are no obstetric contraindications, offer induction of labour between 37^{+0} and 38^{+0} weeks
- Avoid use of fetal scalp electrode and intrapartum fetal blood sampling
- Instrumental deliveries are best avoided, particularly use of ventouse
- If operative delivery is urgently needed when the fetal head is low in the pelvis, a careful decision is needed on the gentlest method
- Liaise with the neonatal team to ensure matched platelets are available for immediate transfusion if cord blood platelets are low
- Neonatal platelets should be monitored for 5 days; if normal, no further tests/ interventions are needed
- Breastfeeding is not contraindicated

PREVIOUSLY AFFECTED CHILD WITH INTRACRANIAL HAEMORRHAGE

- Offer fetal genotyping if the father is heterozygous

Treatment

- Start IVIg transfusion at 16 weeks (1 g/kg over 4 hours once a week) until birth
- If intracranial haemorrhage occurred before 28 weeks, we recommend IVIg (2 g/kg/week) from 12 weeks

Monitoring

- Risks of fetal blood sampling and platelet transfusions outweigh any potential benefits
- Four-weekly ultrasound scans
- MRI is not indicated if scans are normal

Labour and Delivery

- Elective caesarean section should be arranged around 37^{+0} weeks with antenatal corticosteroid cover

- Neonatal platelets should be monitored for 5 days; if normal, no further tests/ interventions are needed
- Breastfeeding is not contraindicated

FETUS WITH NEWLY DIAGNOSED INTRACRANIAL HAEMORRHAGE

- Fetal MRI is useful to determine the severity and impact of haemorrhage
- Start IVIg treatment (2 g/kg/week)
- Termination of pregnancy may be appropriate
- Around 25% in this group will either die in utero or during the neonatal period, or will have severe neurological sequalae

SUGGESTED READING

Kamphuis MM, Oepkes D. Fetal thrombocytopenia. In: *High-Risk Pregnancy* (James D, Steer P, Weiner C, et al., eds), Cambridge University Press, Cambridge, 2020.

CHAPTER 8

Hydrops in Second and Third Trimester

SUMMARY BOX

DEFINITION AND CHARACTERISTICS

- There is no consensus on the definition of hydrops – the most common requires accumulation of fluid in at least two fetal compartments. While ascites, pleural effusion and pericardial effusion are easily identified on ultrasound, the diagnosis of skin oedema is very subjective
- Some studies have included placentomegaly and even polyhydramnios in the definition, which adds to the confusion and heterogeneity of epidemiological data
- For clinical purposes, it is much more informative to identify the compartments separately (e.g. pleural effusion, pericardial effusion, ascites, skin oedema, or any combination of these)
- Distribution and progression of the fluid accumulation can help in identifying the underlying cause. Severe anaemia usually presents with ascites, while pleural effusions without ascites suggest chylothorax, Noonan or Down syndrome
- Immune hydrops is caused by red cell antibodies
- Non-immune causes include chromosomal abnormalities (trisomies, Turner syndrome), infection (parvo B19, CMV), cardiac causes (structural, arrhythmias), fetal tumours and inborn errors of metabolism
- Exome sequencing can identify pathogenic genetic variants in up to 30% of cases of previously unexplained non-immune hydrops
- Quoted prevalence is around 1 in 2,000, but varies both regionally and seasonally (e.g. seasonal variation caused by peaks of parvo B19 infections)

INITIAL ULTRASOUND ASSESSMENT

- Detailed anatomical survey, including fetal echocardiography and placental assessment
- Middle cerebral artery Doppler peak systolic velocity (MCA PSV)

INVESTIGATIONS

MATERNAL INVESTIGATIONS

- Infection screen to exclude congenital viral infections (parvo B19, CMV)
- Red cell antibodies
- Exclude haemoglobinopathies (alpha thalassemia)
- Exclude stomatocytosis

FETAL INVESTIGATIONS

- Full blood count and direct Coombs test if MCA PSV is raised above 1.5 MoM
- Microarray testing
- Exome sequencing, if available, when other tests are negative
- Ascitic fluid analysis should be offered if invasive testing is accepted by a patient and the cause is still uncertain
- Ascitic fluid analyses should include cytology and biochemistry

Cytology

- High lymphoid cell count >80% suggests chylous effusions
- Vacuolated lymphocytes suggest glycogen storage disorders

Biochemistry

- High gamma-glutamyl transferase (GGT) is found in bowel perforation
- Low total protein levels are found in urinary ascites

MANAGEMENT AND COUNSELLING

RAISED MCA DOPPLER

Differential Diagnosis

- Rhesus disease
- Infections (parvo B19, CMV)
- Trisomies
- Alpha thalassemia
- Hereditary stomatocytosis
- Cardiac hypertrophy (poorly controlled diabetes, Pompe disease) – fetal Hb will be normal
- Congenital dyserythropoetic anaemia (rare)
- Leukaemia (rare)

Counselling

- If fetal anaemia is the presumed cause, intrauterine transfusion should be carried out as soon as possible
- Survival of children after intrauterine transfusions for Rhesus incompatibility or parvo B19 is >90%, but lower cognitive functioning and behavioural difficulties are more common than in the general population
- Hydropic fetuses due to Hb Bart's treated with intrauterine transfusion have high perinatal mortality (≥30%), but may survive with acceptable neurocognitive outcome

NORMAL MCA DOPPLER

Differential Diagnosis

- **Cardiac** abnormalities, cardiomyopathies and/or arrhythmias
- **Bowel** perforation/meconium peritonitis due to volvulus, intestinal atresia, colon atresia. Look for polyhydramnios. Exclude cystic fibrosis
- **Urinary** ascites (lower urinary tract obstruction, persistent urogenital sinus, bladder rupture)
- **Lymphatic** malformations
- **Inborn error of metabolism** (Gaucher, Niemann–Pick)
- Ovarian cyst rupture
- Umbilical vein varix thrombosis
- Congenital nephrotic syndrome
- Placental chorioangioma

Counselling

- Long-term outcome will depend on the specific underlying disease and its severity; therefore, counselling should involve multidisciplinary teams

- Urinary ascites and ascites caused by bowel perforation generally have favourable outcome
- Exome sequencing can identify an underlying pathology in up to 30% of otherwise unexplained cases with varying long-term prognosis (RASopathies, inborn errors of metabolism, musculoskeletal disorders)
- Counselling for pathogenic genetic variants, if found, is complex and should involve clinical geneticists

SUGGESTED READING

PRIMARY RESEARCH

Nagel HT, de Haan TR, Vandenbussche FP, Oepkes D, Walther FJ. Long-term outcome after fetal transfusion for hydrops associated with parvovirus B19 infection. *Obstet Gynecol* 2007;109(1):42–47.

Sparks TN, Lianoglou BR, Adami RR, et al. Exome sequencing for prenatal diagnosis in nonimmune hydrops fetalis. *N Engl J Med.* 2020;383(18):1746–1756.

van Klink JM, Lindenburg IT, Inklaar MJ, et al. Health-related quality of life and behavioral functioning after intrauterine transfusion for alloimmune anemia. *J Pediatr* 2015;167(5):1130-5.e2.

CHAPTER 9

Abnormal Placenta

SUMMARY BOX

PLACENTAL SIZE

- A large placenta (placentomegaly) is usually defined as placental thickness >4 cm, while a small placenta measures <2 cm perpendicular to the uterine wall in the midportion of the placenta (Fig. 9.1)

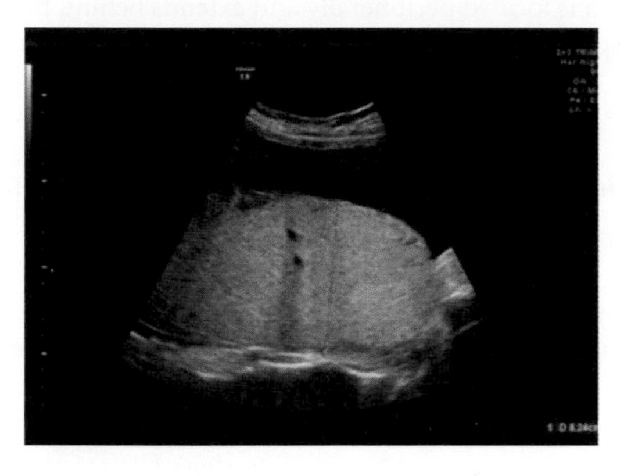

Fig. 9.1 Placental thickness is measured at the level of the umbilical cord insertion with the calliper perpendicular to the uterine wall. In cases of marginal or velamentous insertion, the measurement is done at the level of maximum thickness with the probe perpendicular to the uterine wall.

LARGE PLACENTA

Mother

- Diabetes
- Anaemia

Fetus

- Hydrops
  - intrauterine infections
  - fetal anaemia
- Fetal abnormalities
  - Beckwith–Wiedemann
  - triploidy – diandric
  - congenital nephrotic syndrome

SMALL PLACENTA

- Preeclampsia
- Growth restriction
- Trisomy
- Triploidy – digynic
- Infection
- Smoking
- Drug abuse

ABNORMAL TEXTURE

PLACENTAL HAEMATOMA

Definition and Characteristics

- Retroplacental haematoma elevates the placenta from the underlying myometrium
- Marginal subchorionic haematoma is located peripherally and extends behind the chorion
- Intraplacental haematoma is caused by bleeding inside the placenta (Fig. 9.2)

Ultrasound Assessment

- Haematoma may be (1) hyperechoic (acute), (2) isoechoic, (3) echolucent (chronic), or a combination of all three
- Acute and subacute haematomas may look very similar to placental tissue
- Colour Doppler should be used to confirm absence of internal vascularity
- Myometrial contractions may have very similar appearance to retroplacental haematoma

Counselling and Management

- Size and ultrasound appearance of placental haematoma should not be used to determine pregnancy outcome, particularly if the patient is asymptomatic
- If placental abruption is suspected clinically, presence of haematoma on scan is enough to confirm the diagnosis, but absence of a visible haematoma does not exclude the diagnosis
- The timing of the follow-up scan will depend on the gestation and severity of clinical symptoms, ranging from a few days in a symptomatic third trimester patient to 4 weeks in an asymptomatic women in the first trimester

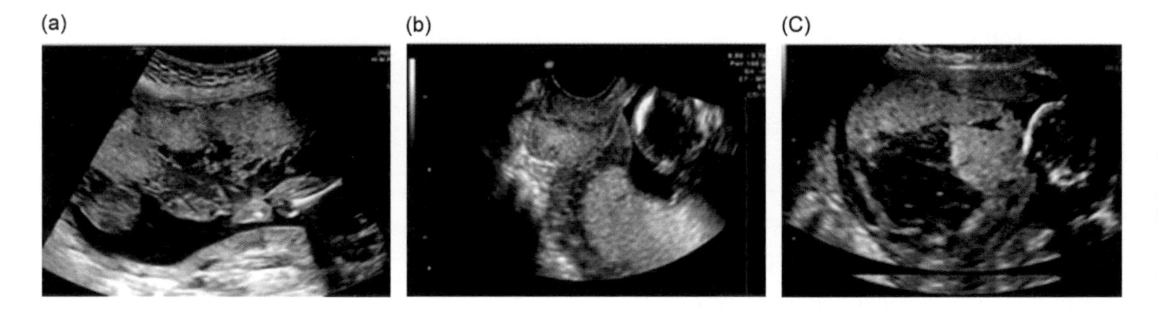

Fig. 9.2 Placental haematoma. (a) Subchorionic, (b) marginal and (c) intraplacental.

PLACENTAL LAKES

Definition and Characteristics

- Cystic changes within areas of subchorionic fibrin deposition

Ultrasound Assessment

- Hypoechoic cystic spaces filled with maternal blood
- Colour Doppler imaging may show low-velocity venous flow (Fig. 9.3)
- Look for signs of placenta accreta spectrum (PAS)

Counselling and Management

- Multiple lakes detected in early pregnancy have been associated with fetal growth restriction (FGR), so serial growth scans should be arranged
- If placenta accreta is excluded, placental lakes that appear in the second half of the pregnancy are a normal finding

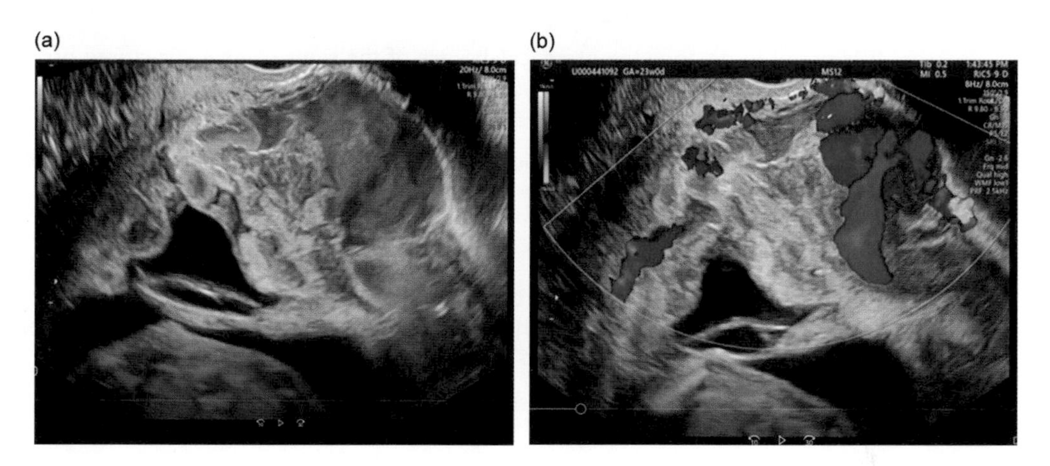

Fig. 9.3 Placental lakes with low-velocity venous flow seen on (a) B-mode and (b) colour Doppler images.

PLACENTA ACCRETA SPECTRUM

Definition and Characteristics

- The PAS includes attachment of the placenta to the myometrium (accreta), invasion of the trophoblast into the myometrium (increta) and invasion into surrounding structures (percreta)
- True incidence, although rising, is difficult to estimate because the diagnosis of PAS remains subjective
- Overestimates are common as they often include retained placentas and uterine dehiscence
- Clinically significant PAS is unlikely in the absence of important risk factors (praevia or previous uterine surgery including caesarean section, curettage, endometrial ablation and manual removal of the placenta)

Ultrasound Assessment

- As most cases will include placenta praevia, a combination of transvaginal and transabdominal scan in combination with colour Doppler should be used to look for signs of PAS
- The most important ultrasounds signs are:
  - loss or irregularity of hypoechoic plane underlying placental bed (loss of clear zone)
  - thinning of myometrium overlying placenta to <1 mm
  - abnormal placental lacunae
  - bladder wall interruption

  - placental bulge
  - focal exophytic placental tissue breaking through serosa most often seen inside filled maternal bladder
- Colour Doppler signs are:
  - uterovesical and subplacental hypervascularity (Fig. 9.4)
  - vessels extending from placenta into bladder or other organs (bridging vessels)
  - placental lacunae feeder vessels
- It is useful to describe the presence/absence of the signs using a structured proforma (https://obgyn-onlinelibrary-wiley-com.liverpool.idm.oclc.org/doi/epdf/10.1002/uog.15810)
- For asymptomatic patients, it is best to delay the full assessment until 28 weeks

Investigations

- MRI may be particularly useful in cases of posterior placenta praevia, or to assess potential bladder and parametrial invasion, but it should be interpreted only by experts in placental imaging (Fig. 9.5)
- Sensitivity and specificity of ultrasound and MRI are comparable and the two methods should be considered synergistic
- Placental biomarkers, including maternal hCG levels, are not helpful for diagnostic purposes, although aneuploid screening markers may be significantly elevated in pregnancies affected by PAS

Counselling and Management

- Timing and place of birth, type of abdominal and uterine incision, any co-interventions including use of ureteral stents, and decision on whether it is best to leave placenta in situ or attempt to remove placenta by gentle cord traction should be individualised, agreed and documented in advance, with input from a multidisciplinary team
- The multidisciplinary team should include an experienced pelvic surgeon, anaesthetist and other specialists, depending on additional risk factors and local circumstances
- Despite significant morbidity, leaving placenta in situ should be considered a treatment of choice if peripartum hysterectomy is unacceptable to the patient, or deemed unsafe (e.g. in an out-of-hours emergency)
- When placenta is left in situ (complete or partial), up to 75% will resorb spontaneously, but this takes on average 3 months and may take more than 12 months
- There is no good-quality evidence to support use of methotrexate to hasten resorption

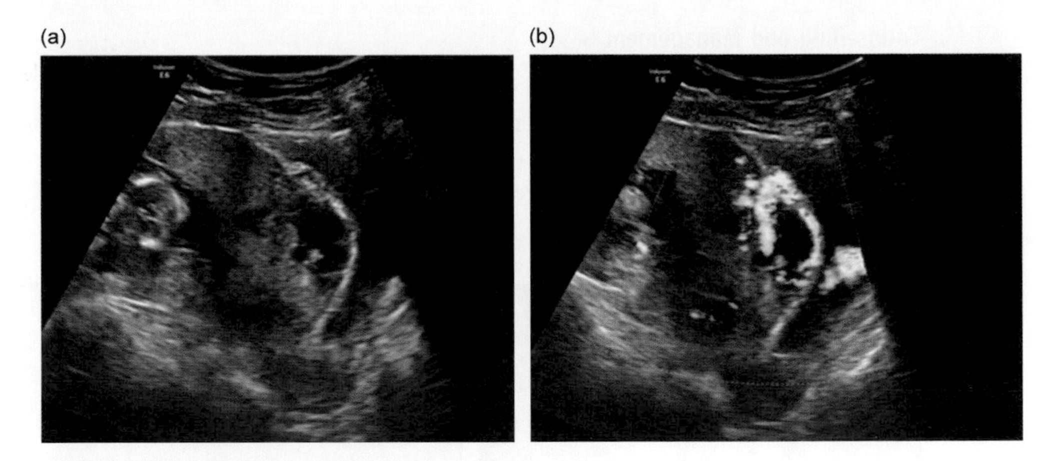

Fig. 9.4 2D image of a placenta accreta spectrum (a) with superimposed colour Doppler (b).

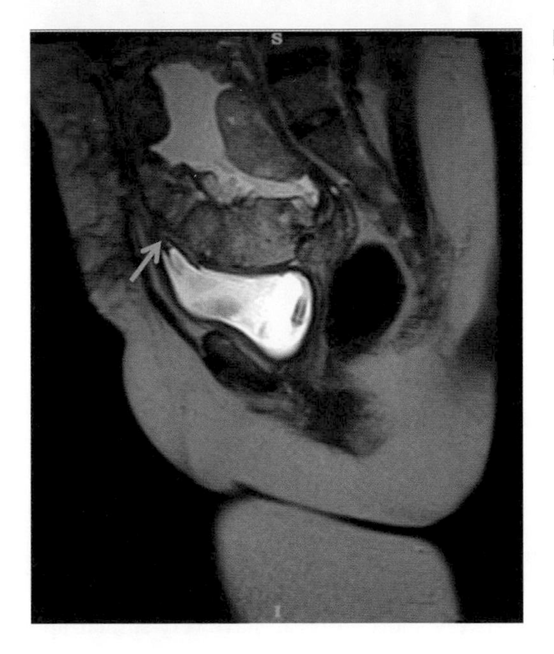

Fig. 9.5 MRI of the placenta that has invaded the bladder (arrow).

CHORIOANGIOMA

Definition and Characteristics

- The most common non-trophoblastic vascular tumour of the placenta
- Incidence is around 1%, but most are small and not clinically important

Ultrasound Assessment

- Look for a hypoechogenic, well-circumscribed placental mass on the fetal surface of the placenta
- Feeding vessels entering the placental mass should be visible with colour Doppler (Fig. 9.6)
- High-output cardiac failure (cardiomegaly, high middle cerebral artery velocity, hydrops) is present in around 20% of large tumours

Counselling and Management

- Outcome correlates with the mass size and presence of fetal hydrops
- If signs of cardiac failure are present, occlusion of a feeder vessel(s) with laser or embolisation should be offered, if expertise is available
- If intervention is not indicated, pregnancy loss is around 10%

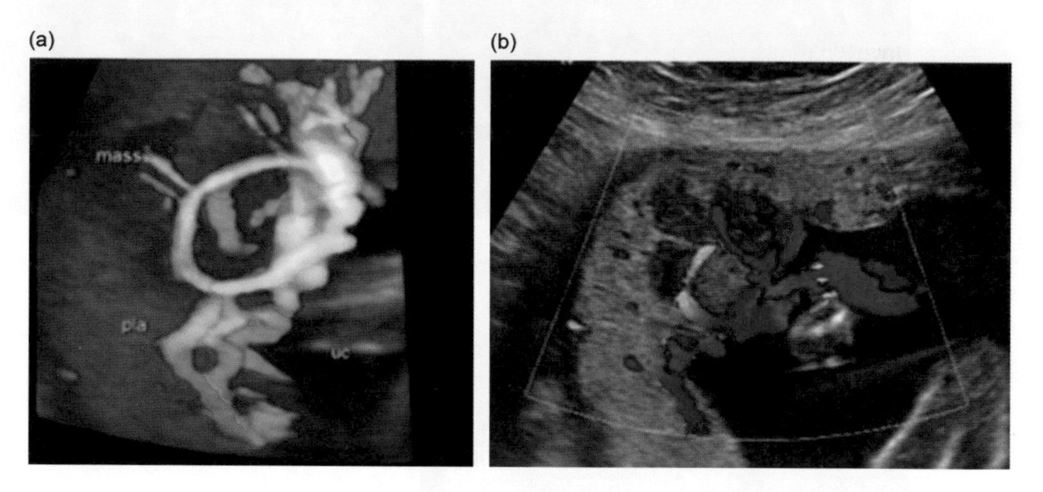

Fig. 9.6 Chorioangioma with (a) hypervascularity on 2D and (b) colour Doppler images.

PLACENTAL TERATOMA

Definition and Characteristics

- Rare tumours arising from the abnormal migration of embryonic germ cells

Ultrasound Assessment

- Calcifications, fat and fluid within a teratoma will have variable echogenicity
- Usually positioned between the amnion and chorion on the fetal surface of the placenta
- Fetus in fetu (fetus amorphous) with very short cord can have very similar appearance

Counselling and Management

- Benign
- No need for any obstetric intervention

PLACENTAL MESENCHYMAL DYSPLASIA

Definition and Characteristics

- Benign cause of placentomegaly
- It can be easily misdiagnosed on ultrasound as a molar pregnancy with coexisting live fetus
- Rare (<0.1%), but likely to be under-reported

Ultrasound Assessment

- Common signs include placentomegaly in ~50% of cases, hypoechoic cysts in ~80% and dilated chorionic vessels in ~15% (Fig. 9.7)
- Colour Doppler signal within the cystic lesions has been described as 'stained glass' mosaic of varying colours due to blood flow of differing speed and directions

Investigations

- As a rule, fetal karyotype is normal, although coincidental aneuploidies have been reported
- Serum AFP is raised
- hCG is normal or only slightly raised

Counselling and Management

- Definitive diagnosis can only be made by histology
- 25% of placental mesenchymal dysplasias are associated with Beckwith–Wiedemann syndrome
- Fetal growth restriction and preeclampsia are common in the third trimester (50%)

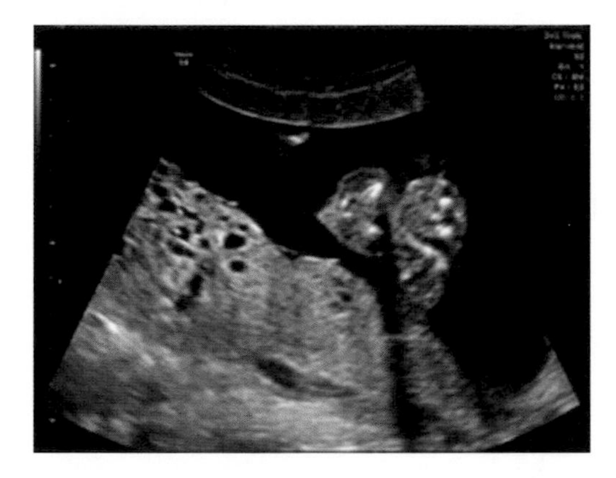

Fig. 9.7 Mesenchymal dysplasia with hypoechoic cysts.

MOLAR-LOOKING PLACENTA WITH A LIVE FETUS

Definition and Characteristics

- Molar pregnancy very rarely presents with a live fetus: <1 in 20,000 births
- *Singleton pregnancy with a partial mole* presents with a structurally abnormal triploid (diandric) fetus, although diploid fetuses have also been reported
- *Twin pregnancy with a complete hydatidiform mole* usually presents with an anatomically normal fetus and coexisting molar placenta

Ultrasound Assessment

- Detailed anatomy scan using transvaginal probe in the first trimester
- Look for triploidy features (severe growth restriction, oligohydramnios, relative microcephaly)

- Look for Beckwith–Wiedemann features (exomphalos, macroglossia, macrosomia, organomegaly, midfacial hypoplasia, renal abnormalities, Wilms tumour, hepatoblastoma)
- Chorioangiomas and placental mesenchymal dysplasia have detectable colour Doppler flow within anechogenic areas, while complete hydatidiform mole shows very little or no blood flow

Investigations

- Check maternal serum hCG and AFP
- Offer amniocentesis after 15 weeks

Karyotype Is Abnormal

Counselling and Management

- Offer termination of pregnancy
- If triploidy is confirmed, placental histology must be performed to confirm/exclude molar changes
- Obtain parental blood to confirm parental origin
- If molar changes are confirmed histologically, gestational trophoblastic neoplasia (GTN) must be excluded by serial hCG in the postnatal period
- Frequency and duration of postnatal hCG testing should be agreed in accordance with local/national guidelines

Anatomy, Karyotype and hCG Are All Normal

Differential Diagnosis

- Chorioangioma
- Placental mesenchymal dysplasia
- Subchorionic haematoma
- Teratoma
- Atypical placental lakes
- Placenta accreta spectrum

Ultrasound Assessment

- Follow-up scan to look for Beckwith–Wiedemann syndrome (macroglossia, cardiac anomaly, organomegaly/macrosomia)

Investigations

- Repeat hCG after 4 weeks
- Maternal AFP levels are often raised in placental mesenchymal dysplasia

Counselling and Management

- If follow-up scans, hCG and AFP are normal, a clinically important pathology is unlikely

Normal Fetal Anatomy and Karyotype but hCG Is High (>3 MoM)

Differential Diagnosis

- This is likely to be a twin pregnancy with one normal conceptus and complete mole (Fig. 9.8)
- Partial mole (focal or diffuse) with a diploid fetus has also been reported

Counselling and Management

- Termination of pregnancy will not reduce the risk of malignancy
- Antenatal complications are common, including vaginal bleeding (70%), early-onset preeclampsia (20%) and hyperthyroidism (20%)
- Livebirth rate is ~60%
- If molar changes are histologically confirmed, 20% of women will need chemotherapy due to persistently high hCG – liaise with a specialist centre

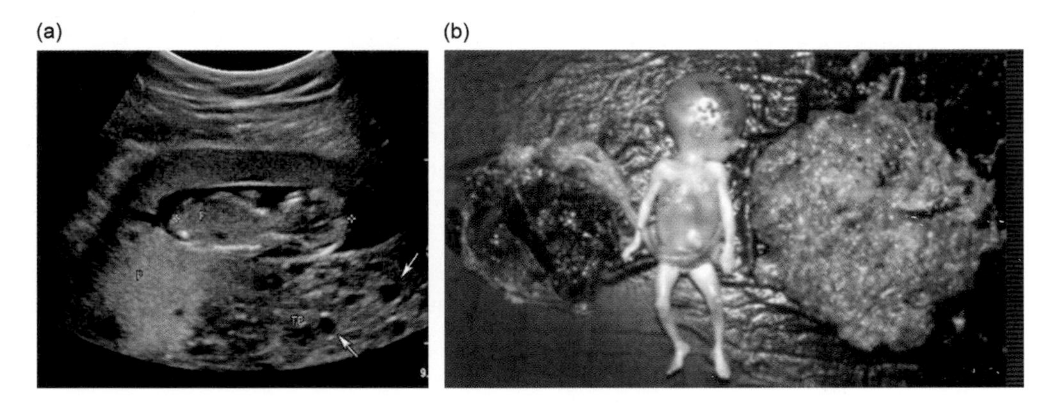

Fig. 9.8 (a) Twin pregnancy (TP) with a molar placenta. (b) Coexisting fetus had a normal karyotype.

CALCIFICATIONS

Definition and Characteristics

- Calcifications may be visible on a third trimester scan in >75% of pregnancies
- Less than 5% of low-risk pregnancies will have extensive calcifications

Ultrasound Assessment

- Our practice is to report only extensive calcification defined as irregular echogenic foci casting acoustic shadows with echogenic connections dividing placenta into ‘cotyledons’ (Fig. 9.9)

Counselling and Management

- If there are no signs of FGR, placental calcifications are not associated with adverse pregnancy outcome and should be considered a normal finding
- If calcifications are extensive, labour induction at 38^{+0} to 38^{+6} weeks is preferable to serial assessments of fetal wellbeing

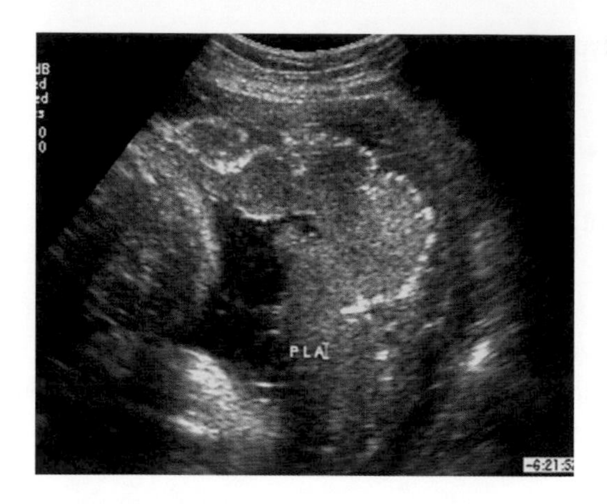

Fig. 9.9 Extensive placental calcifications.

ABNORMAL SHAPE

CIRCUMVALLATE (SURROUNDED) PLACENTA

Definition and Characteristics

- The chorionic plate is smaller than the basal plate; therefore, fetal membranes do not insert at the edge of the placenta but towards the umbilical cord
- Incidence ~1%, but rarely reported antenatally

Ultrasound Appearance

- Peripheral rim of chorionic tissue appearing as an echodense raised placenta margin (Figs. 9.10 and 9.11)
- Fetal membranes folding towards the fetus (shouldering)
- Rarely diagnosed before 20 weeks

Counselling and Management

- Look for early signs of placental abruption
- At risk for fetal growth restriction, antepartum haemorrhage and preterm premature rupture of membranes (PPROM)
- Elective delivery should be planned at 37^{+0} to 37^{+6} weeks

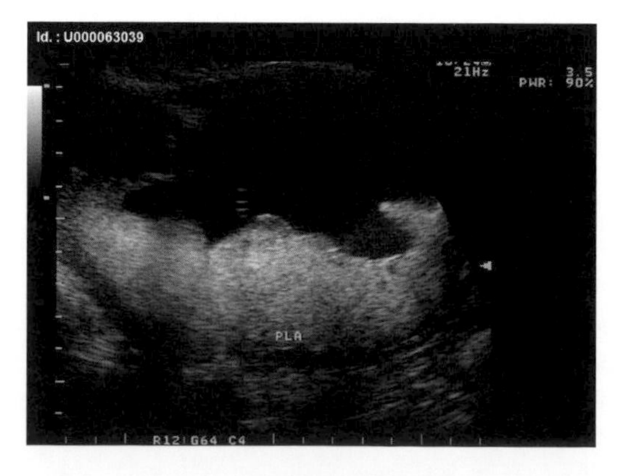

Fig. 9.10 Classic ultrasound appearance of a circumvallate placenta.

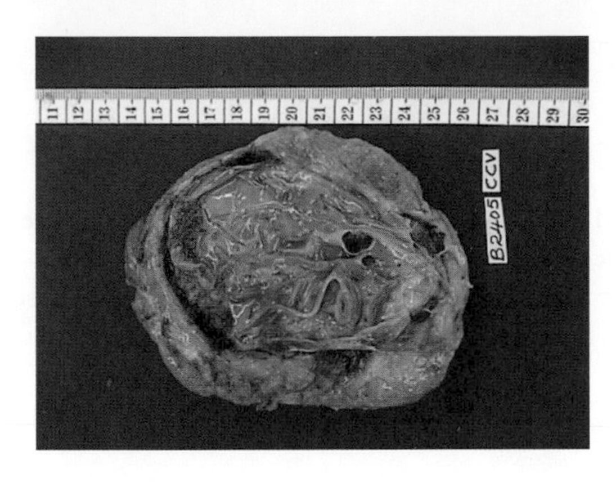

Fig. 9.11 Pathological specimen of circumvallate placenta.

SUCCENTURIATE (ACCESSORY) LOBE

Definition and Characteristics

A variant of bilobed placenta (Figs. 9.12 and 9.13)

Ultrasound Appearance

- It is important to use colour Doppler to exclude vasa praevia

Counselling and Management

- If vasa praevia has been excluded, additional antenatal monitoring is not indicated
- Higher risk of retained placenta

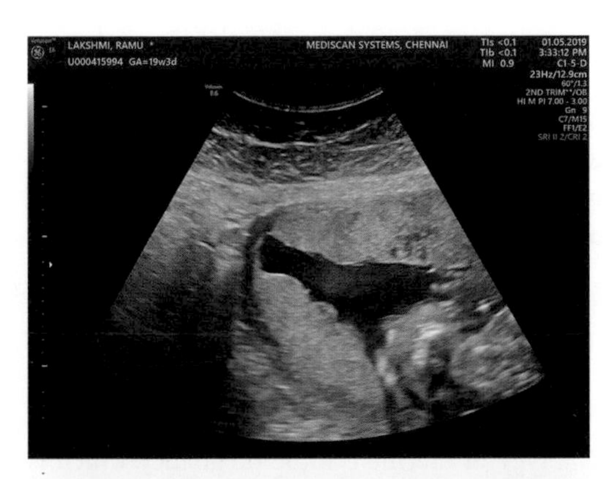

Fig. 9.12 Succenturiate lobe giving an impression of two separate placentas.

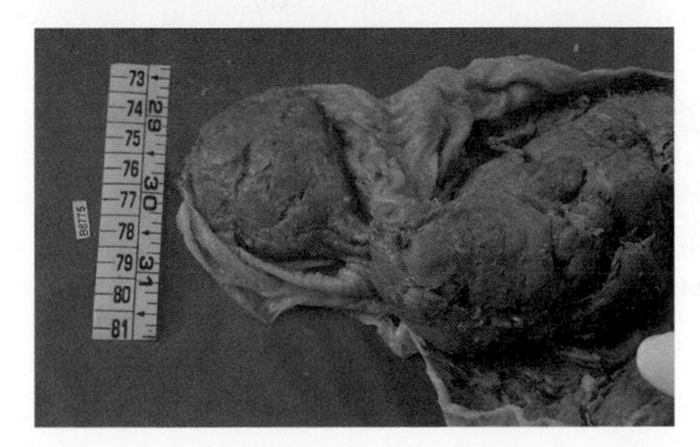

Fig. 9.13 Pathological specimen of the same placenta

ABNORMAL LOCATION

LOW-LYING PLACENTA

Definition and Characteristics

- The placenta should be described as low-lying when the shortest distance between the placental edge and internal cervical os is <20 mm
- The term *placenta praevia* has important clinical implications and should be used only when transvaginal scan confirms that, after 28 weeks of gestation, the placenta is still low-lying

Ultrasound Assessment

- The diagnosis of low-lying placenta should always be with transvaginal ultrasound as this is the only method to reliably measure the shortest distance between the leading edge of the placenta and the internal cervical os
- Every effort should be made to avoid false-negative diagnoses with a posterior placenta
- The placental cord insertion should be identified and colour Doppler used to exclude vasa praevia, or PAS

Counselling and Management

- Antenatal care of women with placenta praevia should be individualised
- Some women with placenta praevia and easy access to hospital may choose to stay at home in the third trimester
- Asymptomatic women with low-lying placenta >10 mm from the internal os can be offered a trial of vaginal birth
- For asymptomatic women, caesarean section should be planned at 38^{+0} to 38^{+6} weeks, or earlier if antepartum haemorrhage keeps recurring in the third trimester
- Women should be counselled about the possible need for blood transfusion and hysterectomy if bleeding cannot be stopped

SUSPECTED CAESAREAN SCAR PREGNANCY

Definition and Characteristics

- Caesarean scar pregnancy (CSP) is a type of uterine ectopic pregnancy which is partially or completely implanted into uterine defect following previous lower segment caesarean section (CS) (Fig. 9.14)
- Prevalence varies according to the proportion of CS births in a population:
  - risk after one previous CS is 1 in 400
  - risk after multiple CS is 1 in 50
  - risk after previous CSP is 1 in 20
- Live first trimester scar pregnancies are considered precursors of abnormally adherent placenta

Diagnostic Criteria

- Combination of transvaginal and transabdominal ultrasound is the diagnostic method of choice
- There is a defect, or a partial loss, of the anterior myometrial layer
- Hypoechoic areas within placenta, usually filled with slow-moving blood (lacunae), are often present (Fig. 9.15)
- Blood supply to the gestational sac/placenta is increased on colour Doppler examination
- *Sliding organs sign* is negative – when pressure is applied to the uterus with ultrasound probe, gestational sac appears fixed. In a cervical phase of a miscarriage, gestational sac will move when pressure is applied with ultrasound probe to the uterus at the level of the internal os (Fig. 9.16)
- Maternal serum hCG levels have no diagnostic value

Clinically Unstable

$<12^{+0}$ Weeks

- *Transcervical suction curettage* alone or with additional haemostatic measures (cervical suture, Foley balloon)

$>12^{+0}$ Weeks

- *Transcervical evacuation* (if expertise available) or *transabdominal hysterotomy* (open or laparoscopic) $\pm$ uterine artery embolisation

Clinically Stable (Asymptomatic or Mild Symptoms) – NO LIVE FETUS

Transcervical Suction Curettage

- It can be done alone or with additional haemostatic measures (cervical suture, Foley balloon)
- We do not recommend expectant management – resolution may take many weeks and surgery for prolonged or acute severe bleeding may still be needed (~30%)

Clinically Stable (Asymptomatic or Mild Symptoms) – LIVE FETUS

$<14^{+0}$ Weeks

- Discuss the options of expectant management versus termination
- Pregnancies located at or above the internal os with no evidence of cervical shortening/ dilatation are more likely to reach viability
- Surgical or medical treatment with methotrexate could be offered, depending on local expertise and available resources
- Surgical evacuation complications ~35%
- Medical management success rate ~50%; complications ~60%

14–24 Weeks

- Termination of pregnancy should not be offered as the risk of major haemorrhage is very high
- Overall risk of hysterectomy is 50–80%, with ~25% occurring before 24^{+0} weeks

>24 Weeks

- Local PAS protocol should be followed

Future Pregnancies

- When the uterus is preserved, fertility is unaffected and healthy intrauterine pregnancy rates are similar to women of comparable age with no history of scar implantation
- The risk of scar rupture is not increased compared to other women with history of previous CS

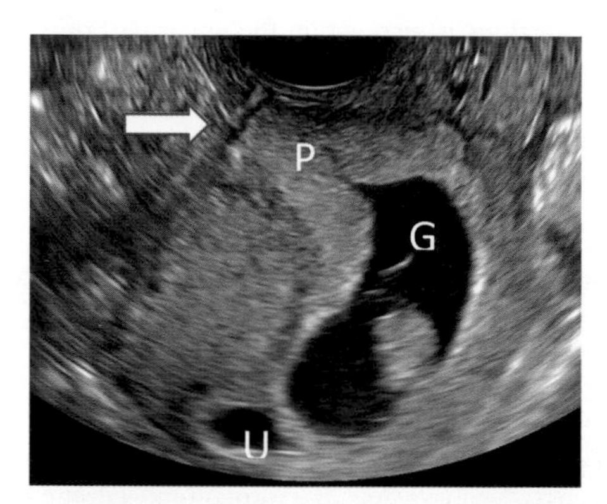

Fig. 9.14a A longitudinal section of the uterus showing an 8-week pregnancy implanted into an anterior myometrial defect caused by poor healing of CS scar. G, gestational sac; P, placenta; U, uterine cavity; thick arrow is the myometrial defect.

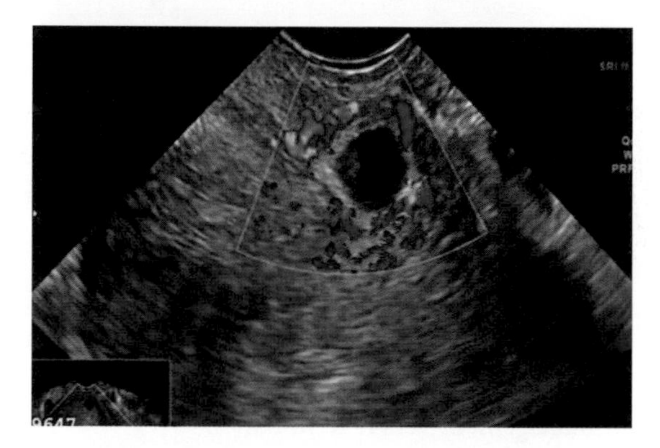

Fig. 9.14b Colour Doppler demonstrates increased blood supply at the placental implantation site.

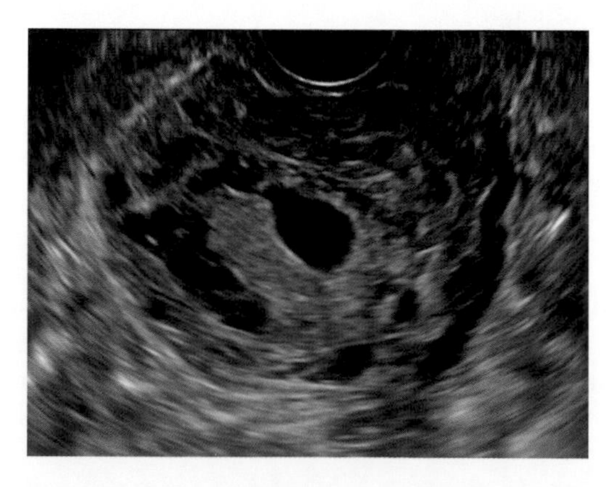

Fig. 9.15 Extensive placental lacunae in caesarean scar ectopic pregnancy.

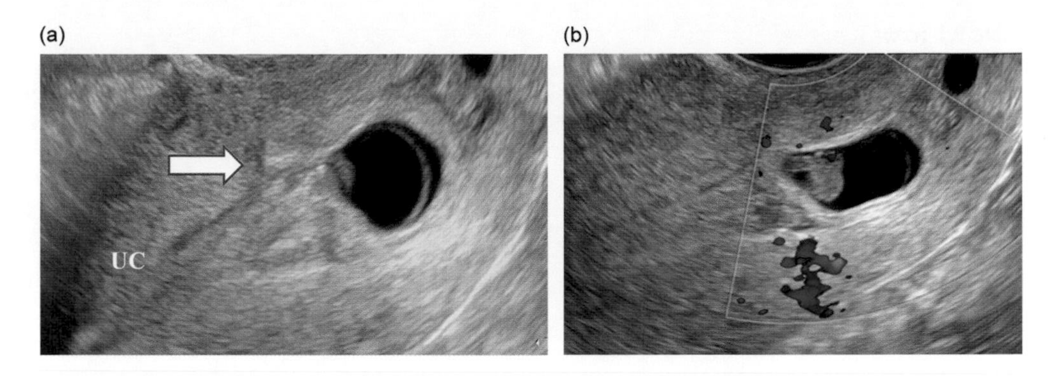

Fig. 9.16 Cervical phase of miscarriage. (a) Gestational sac is seen within the upper part of the cervical canal (thick arrow is the CS scar, UC is the uterine cavity). (b) Ultrasound colour Doppler shows no evidence of increased peritrophoblastic flow, which indicates that the gestational sac was displaced from the implantation site and is only passing through the cervix.

ABNORMAL PLACENTAL HISTOLOGY

See Table 9.1.

Table 9.1 Abnormal placental histology.

	Villitis of unknown aetiology (VUE)	Chromic histiocytic intervillositis (CHI)	Massive perivillous fibrin deposition
Counselling	• Chronic villitis is relatively common in third trimester – seen in up to 1 in 3 term placentas (Fig. 9.17) • Likely to be an immune component • Estimated recurrence is 10–15%	• Best described as an extreme variant of VUE (Fig. 9.18) • Recurrence is very high ≥70%	• Reaction to trophoblastic damage/ necrosis (Fig. 9.19) • Prevalence <1% • May be also immunological aetiology • Estimated recurrence around 50%
Postnatal tests after adverse pregnancy outcome	• Look for evidence of infection in the index pregnancy • Review TORCH results and repeat if needed to look for seroconversion • Exclude antiphospholipid syndrome, particularly if recurrent • Other thrombophilias are unlikely, but best to be excluded	• As with VUE, exclude infections (chlamydia psittaci, CMV, *listeria*, tularemia coccidioidomycosis, rickettsiosis, blastomycosis, schistosomiasis and Zika) • Exclude autoimmune disorders and thrombophilias	• Exclude thrombophilias and autoimmune disorders • Coxsackie virus has been implicated

Table 9.1 (*cont.*)

	Villitis of unknown aetiology (VUE)	Chromic histiocytic intervillositis (CHI)	Massive perivillous fibrin deposition
Treatment options for future pregnancy	• Low-dose aspirin from 12 weeks • If recurrent, add low-dose prednisolone • IVIg has been tried but should only be used in a research setting	• Low-dose aspirin and low-dose prednisolone • Consider adding hydroxychloroquine 200 mg bd, particularly if recurrent	• Low-dose aspirin and low molecular weight heparin • IVIg was tried but should only be used in a research setting

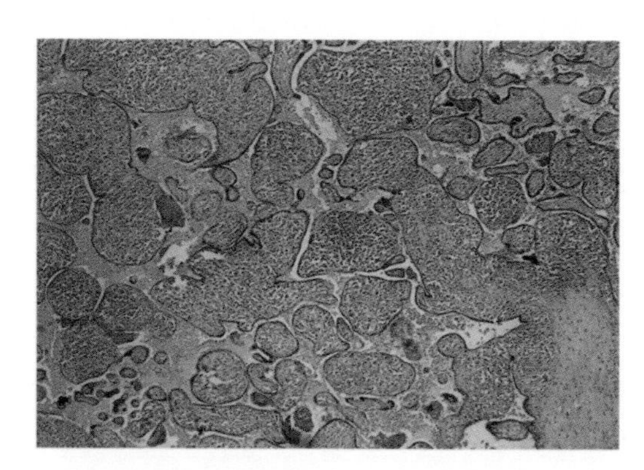

Fig. 9.17 Chronic villitis. Diffuse enlargement of villi with diffuse stromal hypercellularity due to infiltration with mononuclear cells.

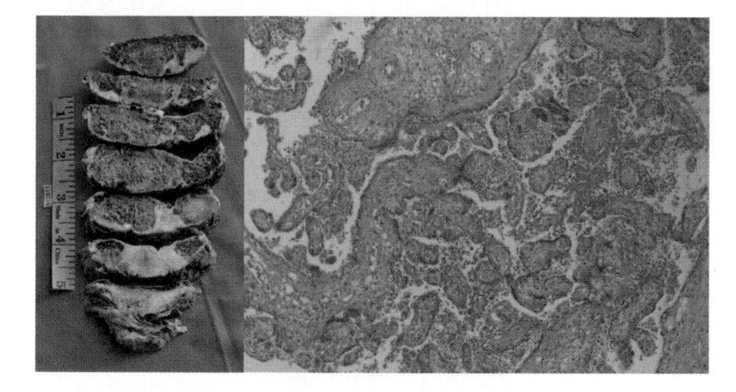

Fig. 9.18 Chronic histiocytic intervillositis. Multiple areas of old infarction and maternal floor fibrin deposition can be seen on the pathological specimen (left). Histology shows villi with hypercellular stroma and intervillous space with diffuse histiocytic infiltration. Stromal calcifications are also present (right).

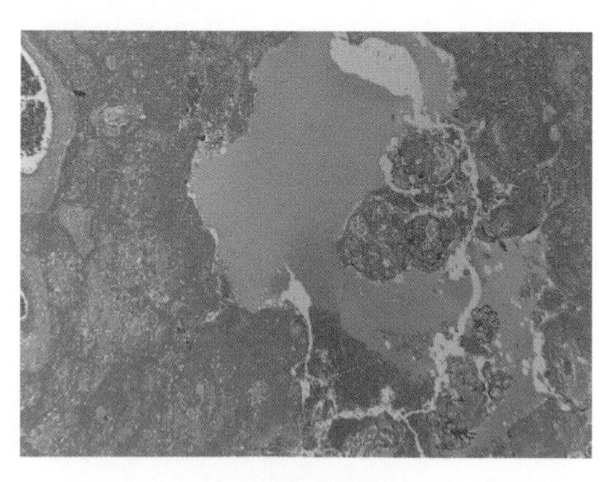

Fig. 9.19 Massive fibrin deposition surrounding sclerosed villi with small islands of viable villi between the fibrin.

SUGGESTED READING

PRIMARY RESEARCH

Ben Nagi J, Helmy S, Ofili-Yebovi D, et al. Reproductive outcomes of women with a previous history of Caesarean scar ectopic pregnancies. *Hum Reprod* 2007;22(7):2012–2015.

Harb HM, Knight M, Bottomley C, et al. Caesarean scar pregnancy in the UK: a national cohort study. *BJOG* 2018;125:1663–1670.

REVIEWS AND GUIDELINES

Buca D, Iacovella C, Khalil A, et al. Perinatal outcome of pregnancies complicated by placental chorioangioma: systematic review and meta-analysis. *Ultrasound Obstet Gynecol* 2020;55(4):441–449.

Chen A, Roberts DJ. Placental pathologic lesions with a significant recurrence risk – what not to miss! *APMIS* 2018;126:589–601.

Colpaert RM, Ramseyer AM, Luu T, et al. Diagnosis and management of placental mesenchymal disease: a review of the literature. *Obstet Gynecol Surv* 2019;74(10):611–622.

Fadl SA, Linnau KF, Dighe MK. Placental abruption and hemorrhage: review of imaging appearance. *Emerg Radiol* 2019;26(1):87–97.

Jauniaux E, Alfirevic Z, Bhide AG, et al. Placenta praevia and placenta accreta: diagnosis and management: Green-top Guideline No. 27a. *BJOG* 2019;126(1):e1–e48.

Liu L, Ross WT, Chu AL, Deimling TA. An updated guide to the diagnosis and management of caesarean scar pregnancies. *Curr Opinn Obstet Gynecol* 2020;32:255–262.

Mirza FG, Ghulmiyyah LM, Tamim H, et al. To ignore or not to ignore placental calcifications on prenatal ultrasound: a systematic review and meta-analysis. *J Matern Fetal Neonatal Med* 2018;31(6):797–804.

Morlando M, Buca D, Timor-Tritsch I, et al. Reproductive outcome after cesarean scar pregnancy: a systematic review and meta-analysis. *Acta Obstet Gynecol Scand* 2020;99(10):1278–1289.

Sentilhes L, Kayem G, Silver RM. Conservative management of placenta accreta spectrum. *Clin Obstet Gynecol* 2018;61(4):783–794

Zilberman Sharon N, Maymon R, Melcer Y, Jauniaux E. Obstetric outcomes of twin pregnancies presenting with a complete hydatidiform mole and coexistent normal fetus: a systematic review and meta-analysis. *BJOG* 2020;127(12):1450–1457.

CHAPTER 10

Umbilical Cord Abnormalities

SUMMARY BOX

SINGLE UMBILICAL ARTERY

Definition and Characteristics

- Left artery is more commonly absent
- More common in multiple pregnancies
- Incidence is ~0.5%
- Single umbilical artery (SUA) is associated with increased risk of gastrointestinal atresias/stenosis, renal agenesis, heart defects, trisomies and fetal growth restriction

Ultrasound Assessment

- SUA is best identified on a transverse bladder view (Fig. 10.1a) and confirmed on a transverse section of a free loop (Fig. 10.1b)
- Detailed anatomical survey is indicated in the second and third trimesters

Counselling and Management

- If a third trimester scan (30–32 weeks) has confirmed that SUA is isolated, follow-up scans should be arranged to exclude fetal growth restriction (FGR)
- If there is no evidence of FGR, elective delivery is not indicated

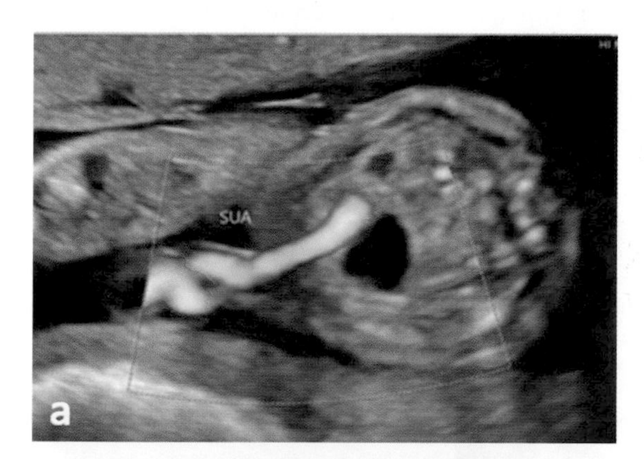

FIG 10.1a Single umbilical artery (SUA, in blue) at the level of the fetal bladder. This view is ideal to identify SUA in the first trimester.

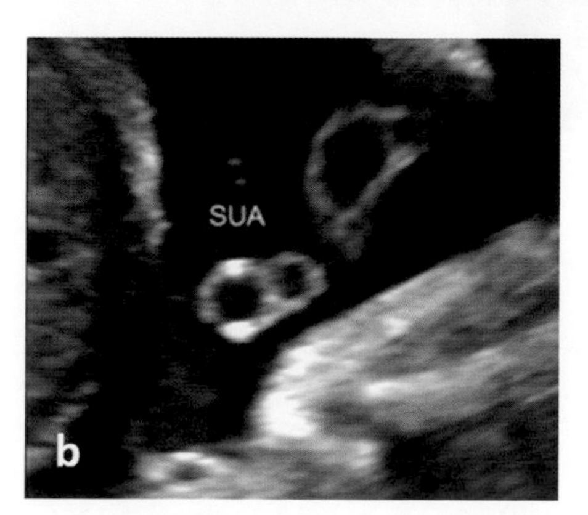

Fig. 10.1b A transverse section of the umbilical cord in a second trimester fetus showing a two-vessel cord.

UMBILICAL CORD CYST

Definition and Characteristics

- True cysts are derived from the allantois or the omphalomesenteric duct. They tend to be located close to the fetal cord insertion
- Pseudocysts, caused by oedema and liquefaction of Wharton's jelly, have no epithelial lining. They can be found anywhere on the cord
- ~20% of cord cysts seen in the first trimester will still be present in the second trimester
- Incidence is 0.5–3%

Ultrasound Assessment

- Size and presence/absence of colour Doppler signal should be noted (Fig. 10.2)
- It is not possible to confidently differentiate true cysts from pseudocysts during the antenatal period

Counselling and Management

- In the absence of structural abnormalities, fetal karyotyping is not indicated
- Isolated small umbilical cord cysts (<3 cm) have no clinical significance, regardless of their size or location
- Large cysts have been associated with sporadic intrauterine deaths
- When large cysts are present (>3 cm), the authors advise 2-weekly monitoring in the third trimester, including colour Doppler to look for evidence of compromised blood flow followed by induction of labour at 36^{+0} to 36^{+6} weeks

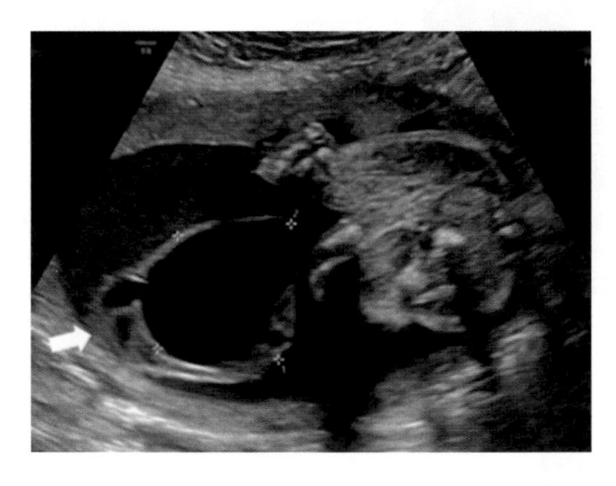

Fig. 10.2 A large cord cyst is seen near the fetal end of the umbilical cord. Note the umbilical vessels to one side of the cyst (arrow).

CORD KNOTS

Definition and Characteristics

- True knots are rare (<1% of pregnancies) and most of them are loose

Ultrasound Assessment

- True knots are rarely diagnosed antenatally
- If suspected, use colour Doppler to look for the 'hanging noose' sign – transverse section of the umbilical cord surrounded by a loop of umbilical cord

- 3/4D scans may help to confirm the true knot
- If a true knot is confirmed, normal umbilical artery flow should be confirmed by pulsed wave Doppler

Counselling and Management

- Although there is no consensus on how to manage true knots antenatally, we advise weekly assessments of umbilical artery blood flow after 34 weeks and induction of labour at 38^{+0} to 38^{+6} weeks

NUCHAL CORD

Definition and Characteristics

- This term is used when the umbilical cord is wrapped around the fetal neck

Ultrasound Assessment

- Colour Doppler should be used to confirm the umbilical cord is completely encircling the neck at two consecutive scans, at least 2 weeks apart (Fig. 10.3)

Counselling and Management

- No antenatal intervention is indicated if there are no other concerns regarding fetal wellbeing (e.g. abnormal fetal movements, heart rate decelerations), but continuous intrapartum CTG monitoring, even in the latent phase, is advisable

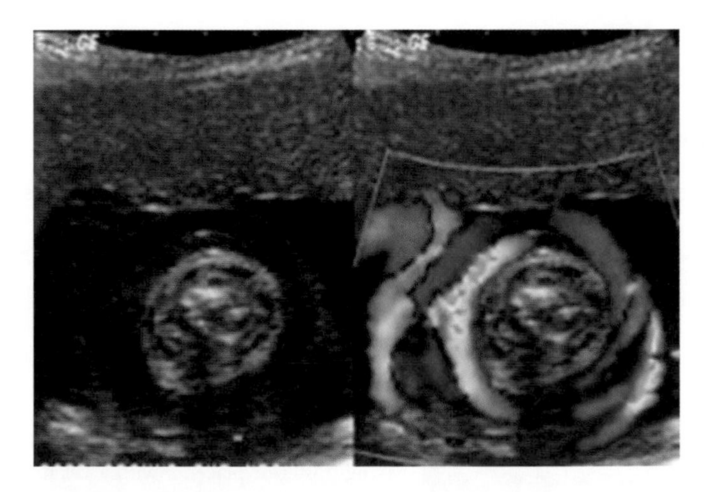

Fig. 10.3 Transverse section of the fetal neck in B-mode (left) and colour Doppler (right) showing two loops of cord around the neck.

CORD TUMOURS

Definition and Characteristics

- Isolated cord tumours are very rare; most likely haemangioma or teratoma

Ultrasound Assessment

- *Haemangioma* may be echogenic or multicystic with demonstrable colour Doppler blood flow. They are commonly seen near the placental cord insertion

- *Teratoma* may be solid or cystic. Colour Doppler signal within a teratoma is very unlikely (Fig. 10.4)

Counselling and Management

- The authors advise 2-weekly monitoring in the third trimester with colour Doppler, looking for evidence of compromised blood flow
- Induction of labour should be offered at 36^{+0} to 36^{+6} weeks

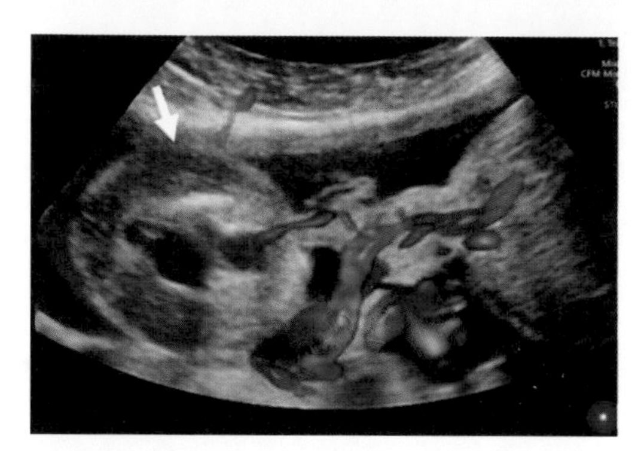

Fig. 10.4 Transverse section at the level of the fetal end of the cord showing a large teratoma (arrow) attached to the umbilical cord.

VASA PRAEVIA

Definition and Characteristics

- Aberrant fetal vessel(s) running through the membranes, either across or close (<2 cm) to the internal cervical os
- Fetal vessel(s) are typically connected to velamentous cord, or a succenturiate lobe
- Reported prevalence is ~1 in 5,000 births

Ultrasound Assessment

- All low-lying placentae should be carefully examined with transvaginal scans, using both colour and pulse wave Doppler (Fig. 10.5)

Counselling and Management

- Once vasa praevia in confirmed, elective caesarean section should be offered at 36^{+0} to 36^{+6} weeks

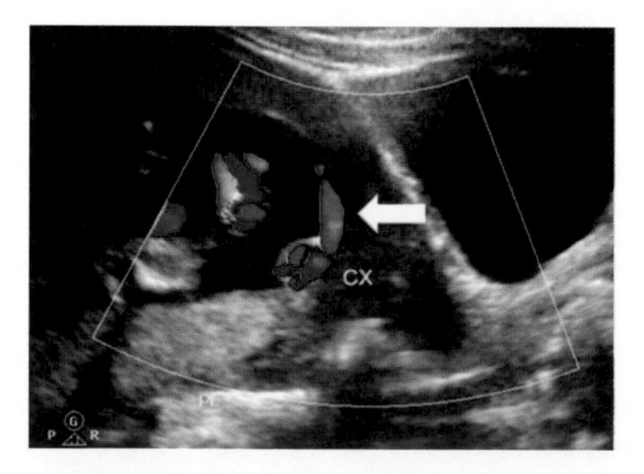

Fig. 10.5 Transabdominal image showing a low-lying posterior placenta with a velamentous insertion of the cord. The cord vessels are crossing the internal os (arrow). CX, cervix.

VELAMENTOUS CORD INSERTION

Definition and Characteristics

- Umbilical cord and placenta are connected with diverging vessels that are not surrounded by Warton's jelly
- The vessels are situated between the amnion and the chorion

Ultrasound Assessment

- Findings of cord insertion at the placental periphery with splaying of the vessels on colour Doppler are diagnostic (Fig. 10.6)

Counselling and Management

- Serial third trimester growth scans (e.g. 32 and 36 weeks) should be offered because of somewhat higher risk of FGR
- Induction of labour should be offered at 38^{+0} to 38^{+6} weeks

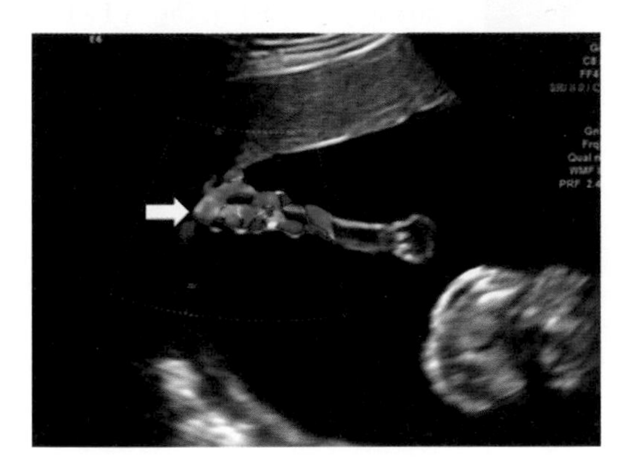

Fig. 10.6 Transabdominal image of an anterior placenta with a velamentous insertion of the cord at the upper end (arrow).

MARGINAL CORD INSERTION

Definition

- A cord insertion is within 2 cm of the placental edge, but still supported by some placenta tissue

Ultrasound Assessment

- Formal assessment of cord insertion is not usually carried out during routine ultrasound exam
- In most cases it is described in the presence of abnormal-looking or small placenta, or FGR
- It is important to differentiate from velamentous insertion and/or vasa praevia

Counselling and Management

- Serial third trimester growth scans (e.g. 32 and 36 weeks) should be offered because of somewhat higher risk of FGR

HYPER/HYPOCOILING OF THE UMBILICAL CORD

Definition

- Umbilical cord coiling pattern can be identified either antenatally or postnatally by correlating the number of coils with umbilical cord length
- Umbilical coil index (UCI) is calculated as the reciprocal of the distance between the two coils
- Hypercoiling is defined as UCI >0.6 (>90th centile) (Fig. 10.7)
- Hypocoiling is defined as UCI <0.2 (<10th centile)

Counselling

- There is no good-quality evidence to support the suggestion that cord coiling index >90th centile or <10th centile is associated with adverse clinical outcome in an otherwise uncomplicated pregnancy

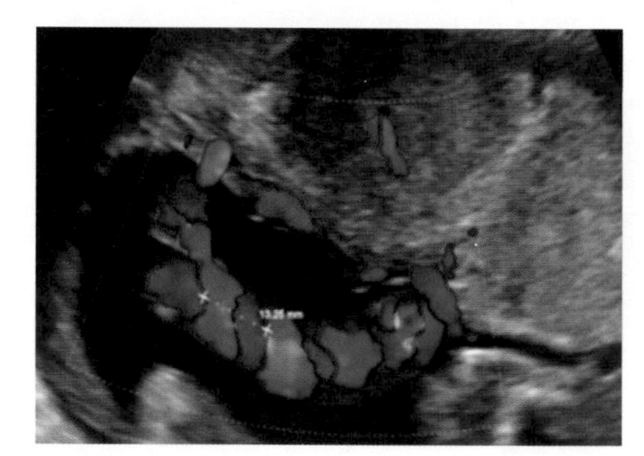

Fig. 10.7 A long section of the umbilical cord showing hypercoiling. The UCI is 0.75 (1/1.325), which is above the 0.6 threshold.

PRIMARY RESEARCH

SUGGESTED READING

Ebbing C, Kessler J, Moster D, Rasmussen S. Single umbilical artery and risk of congenital malformation: population-based study in Norway. *Ultrasound Obstet Gynecol* 2020;55(4):510–515.

REVIEWS AND GUIDELINES

Jessop FA, Lees CC, Pathak S, Hook CE, Sebire NJ. Umbilical cord coiling: clinical outcomes in an unselected population and systematic review. *Virchows Arch* 2014;464(1):105–112.

Kim HJ, Kim JH, Chay DB, Park JH, Kim MA. Association of isolated single umbilical artery with perinatal outcomes: systemic review and meta-analysis. *Obstet Gynecol Sci* 2017;60(3):266–273.

Melcer Y, Maymon R, Jauniaux E. Vasa previa: prenatal diagnosis and management. *Curr Opin Obstet Gynecol* 2018;30(6):385–391.

Moshiri M, Zaidi SF, Robinson TJ, et al. Comprehensive imaging review of abnormalities of the umbilical cord. *RadioGraphics* 2014;314:179–196.

CHAPTER 11

Amniotic Fluid Abnormalities

SUMMARY BOX

POLYHYDRAMNIOS

Definition and Characteristics

- We use the term *polyhydramnios* when the maximum single pool depth is >10 cm, although referrals to fetal medicine specialists are often made when the maximum pool depth is ≥8 cm, or the amniotic fluid index is ≥25 cm
- There is no clinical advantage in measuring the amniotic fluid index compared to the maximum pool depth

Causes

- **Fetal ~15%:**
  - Infections:
    - parvo B19
    - cytomegalovirus
    - toxoplasmosis
  - CNS abnormalities
  - Neck masses:
    - goitre
    - teratoma
  - Thoracic obstruction:
    - congenital pulmonary airways malformations (CPAM)
    - congenital high airways obstruction syndrome (CHAOS)
    - congenital diaphragmatic hernia
  - Gastrointestinal obstructions:
    - atresias
    - volvulus
    - abdominal wall defects
  - Cardiovascular compromise:
    - sustained fetal tachycardia
    - twin-to-twin transfusion syndrome
  - Skeletal abnormalities
  - Hydrops
  - Genetic conditions:
    - fetal akinesia–dyskinesia syndrome (incl. Pena–Shokeir syndrome)
    - myotonic dystrophy
    - Prader–Willi syndrome
    - Bartter syndrome (impairment of renal salt absorption)
    - fetal diabetes insipidus caused by lithium
    - Beckwith–Wiedemann syndrome
- **Idiopathic** ~60%
- **Maternal** ~25% (mainly diabetes)
- **Placental chorioangioma**

Ultrasound Assessment

- Detailed anatomical survey
- Measure the maximum pool depth (Fig. 11.1)

- Estimated fetal weight (small for gestational age (SGA), large for gestational age (LGA))
- Combination of SGA and polyhydramnios is particularly worrying; look for signs of trisomy 18
- Middle cerebral artery Doppler to exclude fetal anaemia
- Confirm normal fetal movements

Investigations

- Glucose tolerance test
- Maternal infection screen
- We offer microarray testing if polyhydramnios is associated with structural abnormalities, or a structurally normal SGA fetus (<5th centile)
- Microarray testing is not indicated for idiopathic polyhydramnios

Counselling and Management

- For asymptomatic women with 'idiopathic' polyhydramnios we recommend routine antenatal care and do not advise early induction as there is no evidence that induction before term will improve perinatal outcome
- Symptomatic women can be considered for therapeutic amnio-drainage
- We do not recommend use of pharmacological treatments (indomethacin, sulindac, intra-amniotic arginine vasopressin)

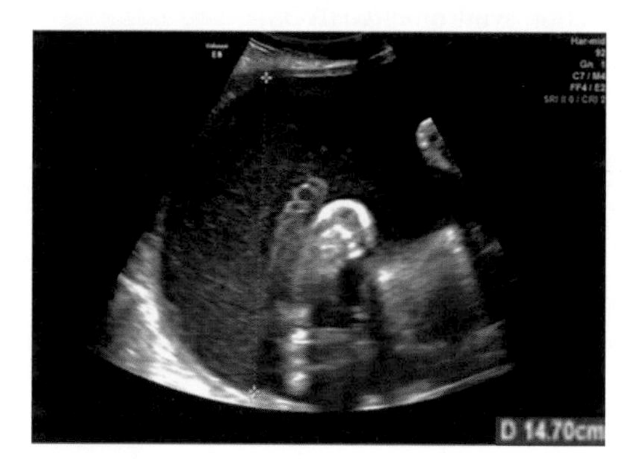

Fig. 11.1 Idiopathic polyhydramnios with maximum pool depth of 14.7 cm.

OLIGOHYDRAMNIOS

Definition and Characteristics

- Amniotic fluid volume should be quantified with ultrasound by measuring maximum (vertical) pool depth
- Oligohydramnios is defined as maximum pool depth <2 cm
- There is no clinical advantage from using amniotic fluid index (four quadrant technique)

Ultrasound Assessment

- In order to accurately measure maximum pool depth, colour Doppler should be used to avoid umbilical cord loops

- Full fetal anatomical survey should be carried out, with particular emphasis on the genitourinary tract to exclude renal anomalies
- Assessment of fetal growth, including uteroplacental and fetal Doppler, should be carried out

Investigations

- Every effort should be made to exclude prelabour rupture membranes by taking careful history, performing a targeted clinical examination including, if necessary, point of care testing for preterm prelabour rupture of membranes (PPROM) (e.g. Actim PROM™ – insulin-like growth factor binding protein-1 and Amnisure™ placental alpha microglobulin-1)
- In the absence of structural abnormality or fetal growth restriction, fetal karyotyping is not indicated

Counselling and Management

- For an apparently isolated oligohydramnios, a follow-up scan should be arranged every 2–3 weeks to provide further reassurance
- If there is no evidence of fetal growth restriction or reduced fetal movements, antenatal cardiotocography is not indicated
- We do not recommend additional fluid intake to increase amniotic fluid volume
- If isolated oligohydramnios is still present at term, we advise induction of labour at 38^{+0} to 38^{+6} weeks with continuous intrapartum CTG monitoring

ANHYDRAMNIOS

Definition and Characteristics

- This term should only be used when there is no measurable pool of amniotic fluid
- Persistent anhydramnios cannot be 'physiological' and every effort should be made to ascertain the underlying pathology

Ultrasound Assessment

- Look for signs of bilateral renal agenesis, cystic kidney disease, or lower urinary tract obstruction (Fig. 11.2)
- If the urinary tract looks normal, PPROM is the most likely diagnosis

Investigations

- If history and scans are inconclusive, point of care testing for PPROM (e.g. Actim PROM – insulin-like growth factor binding protein-1 and Amnisure placental alpha microglobulin-1) should be used
- If fetal anatomy is difficult to assess and there are no obvious signs of PPROM, diagnostic amnioinfusion with 500 ml of saline should be considered (see Chapter 16)
- Following an amnioinfusion, if anhydramnios is caused by PPROM, infused fluid will start leaking vaginally almost immediately

Counselling and Management

Non-obstructive Renal Causes

- Persistent anhydramnios caused by a non-obstructive renal disease is likely to have a lethal outcome
- We do not offer *serial (therapeutic) amnioinfusions* for non-obstructive renal disease as there is no good-quality evidence of improved outcome

Obstructive Renal Causes (LUTO)

- Anhydramnios is not a contraindication for bladder shunting in LUTO (see Chapter 16)

PPROM

- Counselling and management plans are gestation-dependent

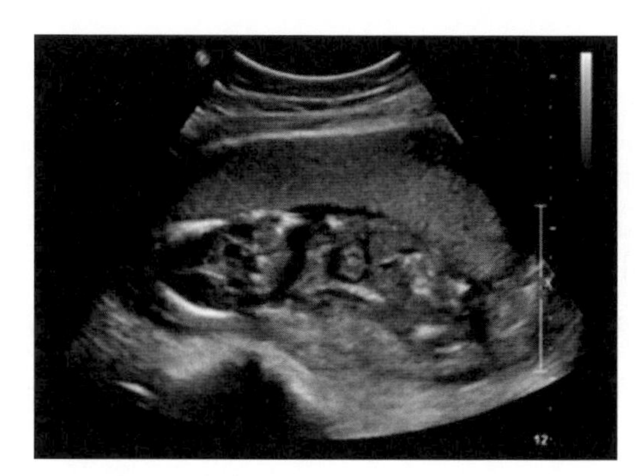

Fig. 11.2 Anhydramnios due to bilateral renal agenesis

PRETERM PRELABOUR RUPTURE OF MEMBRANES (PPROM)

Definition and Characteristics

- PPROM is best defined as either:
  - PPROM to onset of labour interval of >12 hours, or
  - PPROM to delivery interval of >24 hours
- PPROM occurs before 22 weeks in ~10%, between 22 and 26 weeks in ~30% and after 26 weeks in ~60%
- Pregnancy outcomes and management are gestation-dependent and should be reassessed every 1–2 weeks, particularly before 26 weeks

PPROM $<22^{+0}$ WEEK (PREVIABLE)

Counselling and Management

- >50% risk of pregnancy loss within 7 days
- As the chances of intact survival after expectant management are low (~10–15%), the option of termination of pregnancy should be discussed
- If termination of pregnancy is not an option, outpatient management is the norm, unless there are signs of chorioamnionitis, bleeding or labour
- Prophylactic antibiotics are not indicated for asymptomatic women

- There is no good evidence to support the use of amniotic fluid volume to guide clinical decision-making
- Amnioinfusion is not justified as there is no good evidence of improved perinatal outcome
- Follow-up should be arranged around 22 weeks to estimate fetal weight and assess viability
- Once viability is established, women need to be managed in a setting that provides access to tertiary-level neonatal intensive care

PPROM 22^{+0} TO 25^{+6} WEEKS (BORDERLINE VIABILITY)

Ultrasound Assessment

- Estimate fetal weight
- Exclude fetal growth restriction
- Look for placental haematomas
- Maximum pool depth can be recorded, although it has no value in guiding clinical management
- Cord presentation should be excluded

Investigations

- Full blood count and CRP weekly or more frequent if clinically indicated
- Urine testing to exclude asymptomatic bacteriuria
- Amniotic fluid glucose (>1.5 mmol/L) and lactate dehydrogenase (>419 IU/L) can be useful to exclude suspected chorioamnionitis and prevent an unnecessary iatrogenic very early preterm delivery

Counselling and Management

- Stillbirths are uncommon (~5%)
- ~50% of babies will be alive at discharge from hospital
- There is no good evidence to support the use of amniotic fluid volume to guide clinical decision-making
- Amnioinfusion is not justified as there is no good evidence of improved perinatal outcome
- The most important prognostic factor for long-term outcome is gestation at birth, rather than gestation when PPROM occurred or presence of antenatal complications
- The management plan should be agreed with the neonatal team and clearly documented
- Corticosteroids should be prescribed once the baby is judged to be viable and delivery is likely to occur within 48–72 hours
- Good-quality evidence does not support use of regular repeated courses of antenatal corticosteroids
- Erythromycin is prescribed for 10 days (250 mg 6-hourly), but there is no good evidence to support further courses or 'cycling' of antibiotics
- Co-amoxiclav should not be prescribed due to increased risk of neonatal necrotising enterocolitis
- There is no good evidence to support antibiotic treatment of vaginal colonisation in the absence of clinical symptoms; the benefit of testing is to allow antibiotic cover in labour and early neonatal interventions

- $MgSO_4$ for fetal neuroprotection is indicated if early preterm delivery is judged to be imminent (within 12 hours)
- If antenatal steroids and $MgSO_4$ are indicated, continuous electronic fetal monitoring in labour and emergency caesarean section for fetal distress should be offered and maternal choice clearly documented
- Outpatient management should be agreed only in exceptional circumstances, with easy access to tertiary-level neonatal intensive care in case of obstetric emergency (precipitate labour, cord prolapse, abruption)

PPROM $\geq 26^{+0}$ WEEKS (VIABLE)

Counselling and Management

- The management plan should be agreed with the neonatal team and clearly documented
- Outpatient monitoring is a reasonable option for women with easy access to tertiary-level neonatal intensive care and should be individually discussed and agreed
- In otherwise asymptomatic women, weekly normal full blood count and CRP are reassuring
- Amniotic fluid glucose (>1.5 mmol/L) and lactate dehydrogenase (>419 IU/L) can be useful to exclude suspected chorioamnionitis and prevent an unnecessary iatrogenic very early preterm delivery
- Antenatal corticosteroids should be prescribed in accordance with the local guidelines
- Prophylactic antibiotics (erythromycin 250 mg 6-hourly for 10 days) improve neonatal outcome
- Co-amoxiclav should not be prescribed due to increased risk of neonatal necrotising enterocolitis
- If birth is judged to be imminent, $MgSO_4$ should be given for neuroprotection and continued until delivery. If uterine contractions stop, $MgSO_4$ infusion should be stopped and restarted if necessary. Upper gestational age for $MgSO_4$ is 32^{+0} weeks in most units, but can be extended to 33^{+6} weeks if locally agreed
- Good-quality evidence does not support use of tocolysis
- Most babies will be liveborn; gestation at birth is by far the most important predictor of long-term outcome
- Our advice for asymptomatic women without GBS colonisation is to delay elective delivery until 37^{+0} weeks, although, depending on the individual circumstances and woman's preferences, elective delivery at any time after 34^{+0} is reasonable
- For GBS-positive women the risk of early onset neonatal infection is too high with expectant management; therefore, induction at 34^{+0} to 34^{+6} weeks should be offered

SUGGESTED READING

PRIMARY RESEARCH

Lorthe E, Torchin H, Delorme P, et al. Preterm premature rupture of membranes at 22–25 weeks' gestation: perinatal and 2-year outcomes within a national population-based study (EPIPAGE-2). *Am J Obstet Gynecol* 2018;219(3):298.e1–298.e14.

REVIEWS AND GUIDELINES

Etyang AK, Omuse G, Mukaindo AM, Temmerman M. Maternal inflammatory markers for chorioamnionitis in preterm prelabour rupture of membranes: a systematic review and meta-analysis of diagnostic test accuracy studies. *Syst Rev* 2020;9(1):141.

Sim WH, Araujo Júnior E, Da Silva Costa F, Sheehan PM. Maternal and neonatal outcomes following expectant management of preterm prelabour rupture of membranes before viability. *J Perinat Med* 2017;45(1):29–44.

Thomson AJ, on behalf of the Royal College of Obstetricians and Gynaecologists. Care of women presenting with suspected preterm prelabour rupture of membranes from 24^{+0} weeks of gestation. *BJOG* 2019;126e:152–116.

CHAPTER 12

Multiple Pregnancy

SUMMARY BOX

TWINS

ZYGOSITY, CHORIONICITY, AMNIONICITY

ZYGOSITY

- 70% of twin pregnancies are *dizygotic* (DZ) resulting from fertilisation between two ova and two spermatozoa. Dizygotic twins are genetically different
- 30% of twin pregnancies are *monozygotic* (MZ) resulting from splitting of a single fertilised ovum. In most circumstances monozygotic twins are genetically 'identical'
- Zygosity can be inferred through ultrasound, but not proven
- SNP-based cffDNA (NIPT) testing can be used to define zygosity

CHORIONICITY

- *Chorionicity* describes placentation within a twin pregnancy
- Twin pregnancy may be dichorionic (two placental beds) or monochorionic (single placental bed)
- All dizygotic twins are dichorionic. They also contain two amniotic sacs and are described as dichorionic–diamniotic (DCDA)
- For monozygotic twins, chorionicity is dependent on the timing of the single fertilised ovum split (Fig. 12.1)
  - Early splitting (1–3 days post-conception) results in dichorionic placenta (~30% of monozygotic twins). These twins are also diamniotic (DCDA) and are, therefore, indistinguishable by ultrasound from dizygotic twin pregnancies
  - Splitting that occurs 4–7 days post-conception results in monochorionic placenta. These twins are still diamniotic (MCDA)
  - Splitting after day 8 of conception also results in monochorionic placentation. These twins are also monoamniotic (MCMA)
  - Splitting after day 14 of conception results in conjoined twins that are MCMA
  - 75–80% of twins will be dichorionic. Dichorionic twins may be either dizygotic (85%) or monozygotic (15%)
  - 20–25% of twins will be monochorionic. They can be assumed to be monozygotic in almost all situations
  - ~0.1% of twins will be both monochorionic and monoamniotic
  - Ultrasound can accurately identify chorionicity before 11 weeks' gestation, but this is rarely done as ultrasound screening in very early pregnancy is not routine
  - Ultrasound is 97% accurate at defining chorionicity between 11^{+0} and 13^{+6} weeks' gestation

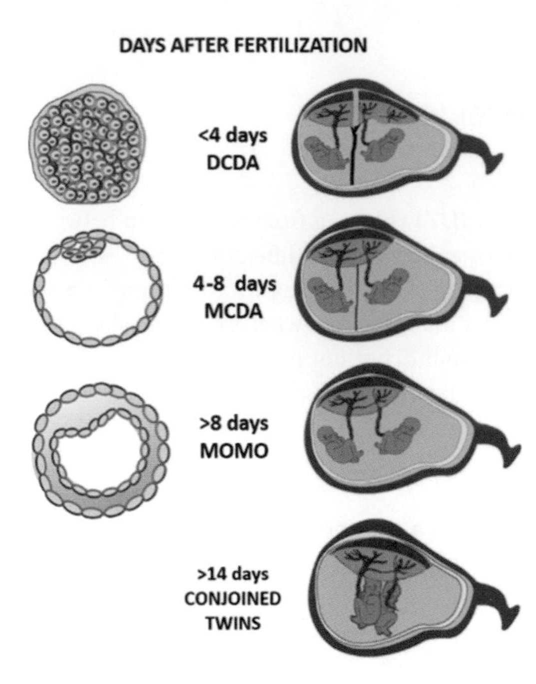

Fig. 12.1 Monozygous splitting after fertilisation.

DEFINING CHORIONICITY AND AMNIONICITY

- Most obstetric pathologies in multiple pregnancies relate to chorionicity rather than zygosity
- Accurate early diagnosis of chorionicity and amnionicity is important for risk assessment and determines the pathway for ongoing surveillance
- In clinical practice, chorionicity is best determined by ultrasound assessment of the placenta and inter-twin membrane at the routine 11^{+0} to 13^{+6} week scan
- DCDA twins have two placental masses. These may be completely separate or may abut one another. If they abut one another then the margin of one placenta rides up the other
- The inter-twin membrane forms a 'twin peak' or 'lambda' sign (Fig. 12.2)
- MCDA twins have a single placental mass with a thin inter-twin membrane that forms a T-shaped intersection with the placenta (Fig. 12.3)
- MCMA twins have a single placental mass and no inter-twin membrane. The lack of an inter-twin membrane means both fetuses will be dependent on gravity. This is best demonstrated by rolling the patient and establishing that both twins fall to the lowest part of the uterus
- Colour Doppler can be used to identify both umbilical cords as cord entanglement is a hallmark finding for monoamniotic pregnancy
- If chorionicity cannot be readily confirmed, the sonographer should perform a transvaginal scan, or ask another experienced colleague to review the findings

What if Chorionicity Was Not Defined by 13^{+6} Weeks' Gestation?

- Fetal gender should be assessed – if these are not the same the twins are typically dichorionic
- Placental site should be assessed – two completely separate placentas will be typically dichorionic, although a possibility of MCDA with bipartite placenta must be borne in mind

- Although the inter-twin membrane is thicker in DCDA twins, ultrasound assessment of membrane thickness is not an effective method for determining chorionicity in the second trimester
- If doubt remains about chorionicity in the second trimester, genetic evaluation with an SNP-based cffDNA (NIPT) may be informative. Alternatively, the pregnancy should be managed as monochorionic due to the consequences of failure to recognise developing twin–twin transfusion syndrome

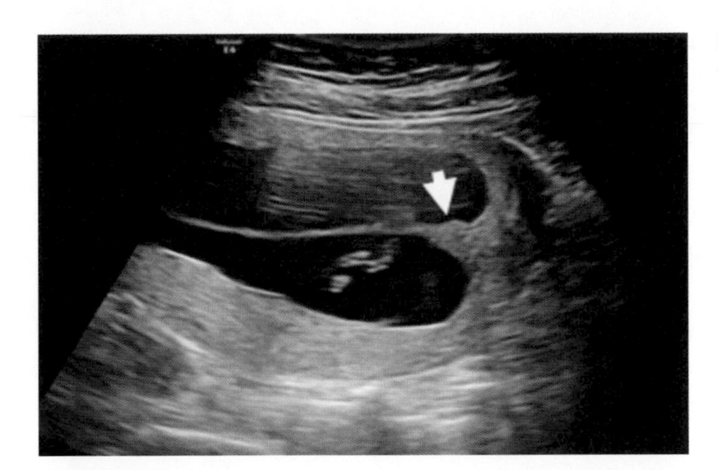

Fig. 12.2 DCDA twins showing the lambda sign (arrow).

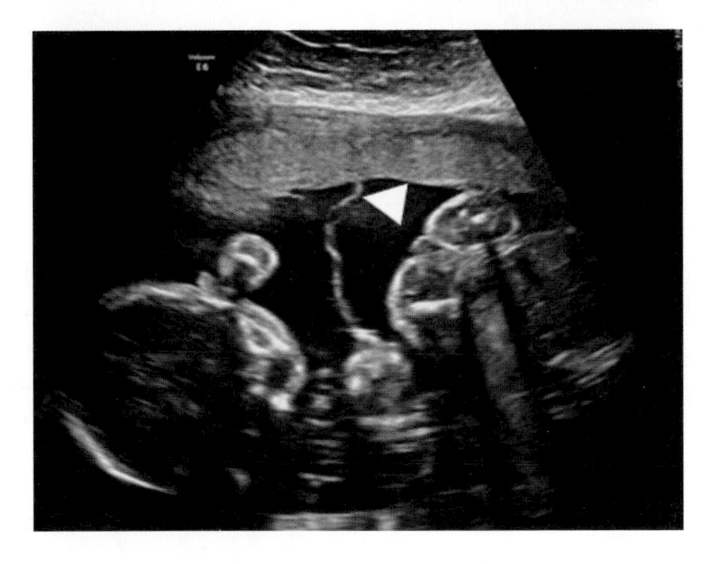

Fig. 12.3 MCDA twins showing the T sign (arrowhead).

DATING AND LABELLING

PREGNANCY DATING

- Singleton charts can be used
- Use the larger twin for dating as the smaller twin may have early growth pathology
- If twins are first seen in the second trimester, the head circumference of the larger twin should be used for dating
- Assisted conception pregnancies should be dated by adding 14 days to the oocyte retrieval date

- When frozen embryos are used, it is important to record the date of embryos replacement and their maturity when frozen
- To calculate the date of last menstrual period (LMP):
  - add 11 days to the date of embryo transfer for embryos frozen on day 3
  - add 9 days if frozen embryos were 5 days old

LABELLING FETUSES

- Fetus should be labelled in relation to the mother as maternal right/left or upper/lower
- If sex is discordant and placentas are separate, it is best to record all relevant information when labelling twins at each scan – for example, twin maternal left, female, posterior placenta
- Using the label 'Twin 1' for the fetus closest to the cervix is not advised as this may change as the pregnancy progresses

ANEUPLOIDY SCREENING

- Choice of the screening tests and counselling is more complex in twin pregnancies (see also Chapter 2)
- If a major structural anomaly is detected, invasive testing should be offered and screening tests should not be offered as an alternative

COMBINED FIRST TRIMESTER SCREENING (11^{+0} TO 13^{+6} WEEKS GA)

- Combined screening is less efficient in twins than in singleton pregnancies. This is due to the fact that when one of the twins is discordant for chromosomal abnormality, biochemical results from the affected twin/placenta may be masked by the normal twin/placenta
- For the same reason, second trimester biochemistry should no longer be considered sufficiently accurate as a screening test for aneuploidy in twin pregnancies

Procedure

- Determine chorionicity
- Determine CRL and nuchal translucency for each twin
- Some risk algorithms allow absence of the nasal bones to be used as an additional marker
- Confirm there is no obvious structural anomalies in either twin
- Twins should be clearly labelled as described above to allow possible later selective reduction with confidence
- Adjust free βhCG and PaPP-A for twin chorionicity

Interpretation for DCDA Twins

- Most likely genetically non-identical
- Calculate and quote independent aneuploidy risk for each fetus
- Risks will likely be different as CRL and nuchal translucency values typically differ

Interpretation for MCDA Twins

- If there is no structural anomaly, then these twins are likely to be genetically identical and should carry the same risk
- CRL and nuchal translucency for each twin typically vary and the risk calculated is likely to be different for each twin. The safest approach in this scenario is to offer invasive testing based on the higher risk

cffDNA PRENATAL TESTING (NIPT)

- A pre-NIPT scan should confirm viability, chorionicity and date the pregnancy.
- Screening performance is comparable to singleton pregnancies, particularly for trisomy 21, although it may be lower for trisomies 18 and 13
- Failure rates were initially reported to be higher than in singleton pregnancies, but more recent techniques have reported failure rates similar to singletons
- Screening efficacy may be affected by the methodology used. Clinicians need to be aware of whether a whole-genome sequencing or targeted SNP-based technology is used (see Chapter 2)
- NIPT for extended range of aneuploidies is increasingly commercially advertised, but there are no good-quality data to evaluate screening efficacy
- All positive screening results need to be confirmed through invasive testing

'No Call' Result

- If NIPT cannot be reported ('no call') then early recourse to combined first trimester screening is recommended

Fetal Fraction

- Most providers report fetal fraction of the cffDNA in twin pregnancy, but the proportion from the two twins may differ. There is a small risk that aneuploidy could be missed if the aneuploid placenta has particularly low fetal fraction

Vanishing Twin

- If ultrasound identifies intrauterine death of one twin ('vanishing twin') then positive NIPT test may be unreliable, that is, false positive
- If a woman accepts that somewhat higher risk of false-positive result may lead to an 'unnecessary' invasive test, NIPT remains a valid screening option

INVASIVE TESTING

- Both amniocentesis and CVS are feasible in twin pregnancy
- In MCDA pregnancies, increased nuchal translucency is also a marker for twin–twin transfusion syndrome (TTTS). It is, therefore, reasonable to delay testing until 16–18 weeks, in case a therapeutic procedure for TTTS is needed. And amniotic fluid can be obtained without additional risk to the pregnancy
- Added risk of miscarriage after invasive testing is likely to be slightly higher than in singletons (~1%)

- Counselling should include discussion regarding availability and risks associated with selective termination of pregnancy in case of an abnormal result (see Chapter 20)
- Invasive tests should be performed by individuals prepared to perform selective reduction in the same pregnancy. This is important to avoid the error in identifying the affected twin, especially as there may be a significant gap between the gestation of invasive test and planned selective reduction
- Pregnancy topography should be extensively described at the time of invasive testing
- It is good practice for a second experienced operator to confirm the description of findings during the procedure and subsequent labelling of the samples

DCDA

- As dichorionic twins are mostly dizygotic (~85%), double ('two entry') CVS or double amniocentesis should be done

MCDA

- Monochorionic twins can be assessed through a single CVS (across the whole placenta)
- The small risk of discordance for chromosomal abnormality between two twins (up to 4%) needs to be recognised
- The risk for discordance for chromosomal abnormality is much higher when monochorionic twins exhibit structural discordance (up to 10% of such cases)
- If invasive testing is indicated and zygosity is not clear (e.g. same-gender twins with single, fused placenta) both twins should be sampled
- The options and availability, including legal gestational age limits, for selective termination should be discussed

MANAGEMENT OF DCDA TWINS

WHAT TO LOOK FOR?

Pregnancy Loss

- The rate of miscarriage/fetal loss before 24 weeks is ~2%
- Loss of one twin before 24 weeks is associated with loss of the co-twin in ~3% of cases, typically within 1 week
- The rate of stillbirth is ~1%
- Stillbirth risk at 38 weeks is equivalent to risk at 42 weeks for singletons (~9 deaths/1,000 pregnancies)

Structural Anomalies

- Prevalence of structural anomalies is ~1%
- ~25% of DCDA twins with structural malformations have chromosomal abnormalities detected by microarray

Fetal Growth Restriction

- Depending on the diagnostic criteria, 12–25% of DCDA twin pregnancies will develop FGR in one twin
- Up to 10% of DCDA twin pregnancies develop FGR in both twins

Preterm Births

- The rate of preterm birth before 37 weeks is ~50%
- The rate of preterm birth before 32 weeks is ~7%
- The rate of preterm birth before 28 weeks is ~2%
- Preeclampsia leads to delivery before 34 weeks in 2.5% of DCDA pregnancies

ULTRASOUND SURVEILLANCE

20 Weeks Scan

- Biometry
- Morphology assessment
- Cervical length measurements (transvaginal assessment)
- Placentation and cord insertions

Follow-up Scans Every 4 Weeks

- Biometry
- Cervical length measurements up to 28 weeks
- Amniotic fluid – deepest vertical pocket
- Umbilical artery pulsatility index
- Fetal Doppler (ductus venosus and middle cerebral artery) – individualised according to biometry
- Last scan at 36 weeks

TIMING OF DELIVERY

- DCDA twins should be delivered no later than 37^{+6} weeks as perinatal mortality after 38^{+0} weeks is comparable to 42 weeks in singleton pregnancies

DCDA WITH SELECTIVE FETAL GROWTH RESTRICTION (SFGR)

Definition

Any of the following:

- EFW of one twin <3rd centile
- EFW of one twin <10th centile with ≥25% EFW discordance
- umbilical artery PI >95th centile

Management and Counselling

- Surveillance and assessment of FGR twin as per protocol for singleton FGR (see Chapter 4)
- Fetal demise of FGR twin is associated with:
  - ~3% risk of demise for appropriate for gestation (AGA) co-twin
  - ~2% risk of neurological damage for the surviving twin due to increased risk of very early preterm birth, rather than vascular compromise
- Elective early preterm birth to improve outcome for the affected twin carries significant risks of prematurity for the AGA co-twin

- Selective fetal reduction may be considered if an urgent delivery is needed on maternal grounds in cases of severe, early preterm preeclampsia or 'mirror' syndrome. This is to avoid the serious risk of long-term disability for a severely growth restricted twin when born at the border of viability

DCDA WITH STRUCTURAL ABNORMALITIES

- Slightly higher prevalence compared to singleton pregnancy – likely due to one in seven DC twins being monozygotic
- Indications for karyotyping and exome studies are the same as in singletons
- Counselling should include discussion regarding availability and risks associated with selective termination of pregnancy (see Chapter 20)

MANAGEMENT OF MCDA TWINS

WHAT TO LOOK FOR?

- MCDA twins have increased risk of adverse pregnancy outcome compared with DCDA twins

Pregnancy Loss

- The rate of fetal loss in MC pregnancies is highest at 16–22 weeks' gestation, corresponding to the peak incidence of acute twin–twin transfusion syndrome (TTTS)
- The rate of miscarriage/fetal loss before 24 weeks is ~8%
- The rate of perinatal death after a normal 12-week scan is ~12%
- Sudden intrauterine fetal death rate is ~5%
- The risk of stillbirth rises after 34 weeks (additional 2.5 deaths per 1,000 fetuses for each additional week)

Structural Anomalies

- Prevalence of structural anomalies ~3%
- ~15% of MCDA twins with structural malformations have chromosomal abnormalities detected by microarray
- The functional impact of the structural abnormality on the 'normal' co-twin needs to be considered, such as associated risks in case of intrauterine death of the abnormal twin, or preterm birth risk associated with polyhydramnios
- These risks need to be balanced against the risk of selective termination of pregnancy (see Chapter 20)

Fetal Growth Restriction

- ~15–20% of MCDA twin pregnancies will develop FGR in one twin
- Up to 10% of MCDA twin pregnancies develop FGR in both twins

Twin–Twin Transfusion Syndrome

- TTTS is characterised by the twin oligo-polyhydramnios sequence (TOPS) and occurs in ~10–15% MCDA twin pregnancies

Twin-Arterial Perfusion Syndrome (TAPS)

- TAPS is characterised by large inter-twin haemoglobin differences in the absence of amniotic fluid discordances
- Two-thirds of TAPS cases occur after laser treatment for TTTS
- The other cases occur spontaneously; ~1% of all monochorionic twins

Preterm Births

- Preterm birth rate before 32 weeks is ~15%
- Preterm birth rate before 28 weeks is ~3%

ULTRASOUND SURVEILLANCE

Scan every 2 weeks from 16 weeks, assessing:

- biometry
- anatomy
- bladder volumes
- amniotic fluid (deepest vertical pocket – both sacs)
- placentation
- establish cord insertion (likely possible at the first visit)
- fetal Doppler (umbilical artery, ductus venosus and middle cerebral artery from 18 weeks)
- cervical length (every 2–4 weeks until 28 weeks)

TIMING AND MODE OF DELIVERY

- All uncomplicated MCDA should be delivered by 36^{+6} weeks
- We would recommend that women carrying MCDA twin pregnancies have an elective caesarean section due to the small but not insignificant risk of acute, massive TTTS during labour

ACUTE TTTS

- TTTS should be suspected if there is a rapid increase in uterine size with tense polyhydramnios, but the diagnosis can only be made by ultrasound through recognition of polyhydramnios/oligohydramnios sequence
- Not all twins affected by TOPS will have significant weight discordance
- Ultrasound is not a good tool to evaluate the vascular patterns (e.g. number of A–A and A–V anastomoses)

Definitions and Classification

- Oligohydramnios is universally defined as maximum pool depth (MPD), also called deepest vertical pool (DVP), of less than 2 cm
- Definitions of polyhydramnios are gestation dependent. In European literature the polyhydramnios before 16 weeks is defined as MPD of >6 cm, >8 cm at 18–20 weeks and >10 cm after 20 weeks
- Five stages (Table 12.1) are of value for management planning; however, the disease does not necessarily progress serially through stages 1–5

- Other groups have produced modified scoring systems that accommodate assessment of fetal cardiac function (CHOP score, Cincinnati stage); they may be useful in planning management of Quintero Stage 1 disease

Table 12.1 Quintero's staging for TTTS.

Signs	Stage 1	Stage 2	Stage 3	Stage 4	Stage 5
Polyhydramnios / oligohydramnios	+	+	+	+	+
Absent bladder in donor		+	+	+	+
Abnormal Doppler findings in either fetus			+	+	+
Hydrops				+	+
Fetal demise					+

Quintero Stage 1

- 10–15% of stage 1 will regress spontaneously
- 50% will stay at stage 1
- 30% will progress to stage 2–4 (and then require laser)
- 5% will result to an unanticipated twin death (stage 5)
- There is no evidence to support laser treatment intervention in stage 1 TTTS. However, laser may be of benefit if:
  - there is cardiac dysfunction (AV valve regurgitation and/or diastolic dysfunction, e.g. fusion of E/A wave)
  - there is significant polyhydramnios causing clinical symptoms/short cervix

Quintero Stages 2–4

- Endoscopic laser ablation of communicating placental vessels should be offered (see Chapter 17)

Quintero Stage 5

- Management strategy is the same as for unanticipated IUFD (see below)
- Following laser treatment, TTTS can reverse, recur or become chronic (TAPS)
- Continued fortnightly surveillance is needed with two survivors
- Counselling and outcome post-laser is discussed in Chapter 17

TWIN ANAEMIA POLYCYTHAEMIA SEQUENCE (TAPS)

- TAPS occurs when there is a low volume, chronic inter-twin transfusion in the absence of TOPS
- The spontaneous form complicates ~5% of monochorionic pregnancies
- Post-laser TAPS can be as high as 15% due to the presence of minuscule residual anastomoses. This risk may be reduced somewhat with the Solomon technique (see Chapter 17 for details)

Definition

- Antenatal diagnosis of TAPS is based on MCA Doppler PSV discordance:
  - >1.5 MoM in the anaemic donor
  - <1.0 MoM in the polycythaemic recipient
  - difference between twins in MCA PSV of >0.5 MoM (ΔMoM >0.5)
- Additional ultrasound signs may be used for staging (Table 12.2 and Figs. 12.4 and 12.5):
  - echogenic/thick placenta with hydropic anaemic donor
  - hypoechoic appearance of liver in polycythaemic recipient
  - tricuspid regurgitation – only in the anaemic twin
  - abnormal fetal Doppler in either twin:
    - absent or reversed end-diastolic velocity in the umbilical artery
    - DV 'a' wave reversal
    - pulsatile flow in the umbilical vein

Management and Counselling

- Spontaneous TAPS typically occurs after 30 weeks' gestation – delivery is the safest option
- Post-laser TAPS is typically seen 1–2 weeks post-laser, more often at early gestations
- Treatment options (Table 12.3) include:
  - expectant management and early delivery
  - endoscopic laser ablation – the procedure is often technically difficult as these anastomoses are usually small; visualisation may be poor due to previous laser treatment
  - intrauterine transfusions; repeated top-up transfusions may be associated with polycythaemic morbidity in the recipient

Table 12.2 Antenatal classification of TAPS.

	Ultrasound findings		
Antenatal stage	**MCA PSV donor MoM**	**MCA PSV recipient MoM**	**Any sign of fetal compromise**
Stage 1	>1.5	<1.0	No
Stage 2	>1.7	<0.8	No
Stage 3	As stage 1 or 2	As stage 1 or 2	Abnormal fetal Doppler Tricuspid regurgitation Hypoechoic liver
Stage 4	Hydrops		Thick placenta is common in addition to signs of fetal compromise
Stage 5	Intrauterine demise of one or both fetuses		

Table 12.3 Antenatal management of TAPS depending on the disease stage and gestational age

	<28 weeks	28–30 weeks	30–32 weeks
Stage 1	Expectant	Expectant	Expectant
Stage 2	Expectant/laser*	Expectant/IUT*	IUT/delivery*
Stage 3	Laser/IUT*	IUT	Delivery

IUT, intrauterine transfusion.
* The choice depends on the local expertise and quality of neonatal facilities.

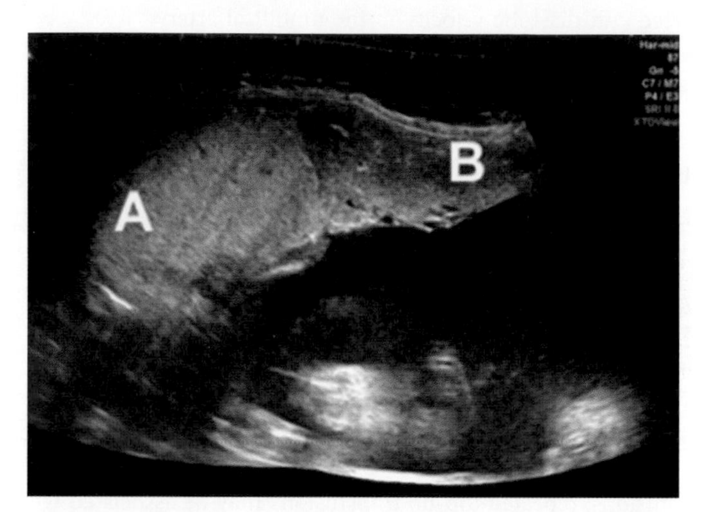

Fig. 12.4 Placenta in TAPS. Note the enlarged portion of the placenta (A) from the anaemic donor and the smaller hypoechoic area (B) from the polycytaemic recipient.

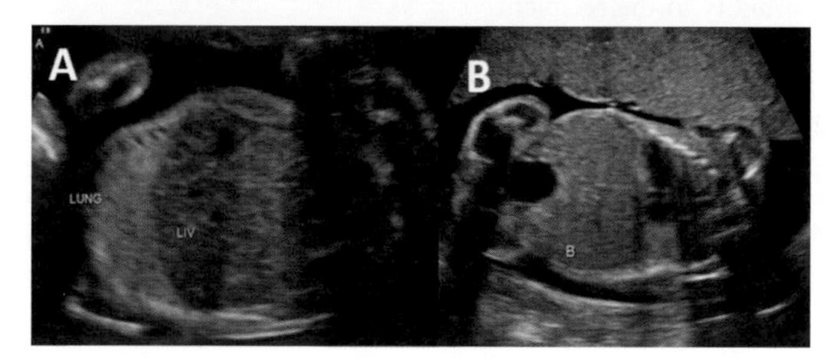

Fig. 12.5 Coronal sections of the fetal body showing the hypoechoic "starry sky" liver of the polycythaemic twin (A) and a normal liver appearance of the anaemic twin (B).

MCDA WITH SELECTIVE FETAL GROWTH RESTRICTION (SFGR)

Definition of sFGR

- EFW of one twin <3rd centile
- OR
- combination of three out of four
  - EFW <10th centile
  - AC <10th centile
  - EFW discordance of ≥25%
  - umbilical artery PI smaller twin >95th centile

sFGR type 1

Definition

Both twins have persistent end-diastolic flow (EDF) in the umbilical arteries (~80% of all cases)

Management and Counselling

- Expectant management is appropriate for most cases
- Doppler surveillance once or twice each week and, if stable, delivery by 35^{+6} weeks
- Overall, 97% intact survival and 3% risk of intrauterine demise

sFGR type 2

Definition

- Persistent absent or reversed EDF in the umbilical arteries of the smaller twin (~15% of all cases)

Management and Counselling

- If FGR baby is previable, offer selective termination/laser to protect the appropriately grown co-twin from demise and neurological damage
- If continuing, manage according to fetal Doppler findings
- If growth trajectory and/or fetal Doppler suggests that delivery will be needed before 26 weeks, offer selective reduction
- If fetal Doppler findings remain stable, plan elective delivery by 32^{+0} weeks
- Overall, ~80% survival with ~5% of neurodevelopmental disability

sFGR type 3

Definition

- Intermittently absent or reversed EDF in the umbilical arteries of the smaller twin (~5% of all cases)

Management and Counselling

- Monitoring is difficult as there is an unpredictable risk of intrauterine demise, even in the presence of stable Dopplers
- If FGR baby is previable, offer selective termination/laser to protect the appropriately grown co-twin from demise and neurological damage
- If managed expectantly, deliver by 30–32 weeks
- The actual timing of delivery will depend on the availability of neonatal cots and recent gestation-related outcomes in the local neonatal unit
- Overall, ~80% survival, but 15–30% risk of neurodevelopmental morbidity in the larger twin

MCDA TWINS WITH STRUCTURAL MALFORMATIONS

- ~90% of structural defects in MCDA twins are discordant, despite the majority being monozygotic
- Some anomalies (e.g. anencephaly) may cause morbidity to the 'normal' twin by triggering preterm labour

Management and Counselling

- Review anatomical findings for both fetuses
- Consider karyotyping both twins – each sac separately
- Provide information about prognosis for the specific anomaly in the affected twin
- Discuss the likely impact on the co-twin (e.g. polyhydramnios in the affected twin may cause preterm delivery of the unaffected twin)
- Discuss options for expectant management and/or selective reduction
- Selective reduction is complicated by the risk of co-twin demise, increased risk of preterm delivery and post-procedure exsanguination (where there is failure to close anastomoses)
- Methods of selective reduction are listed in Chapter 20

MANAGEMENT OF MCMA TWINS

WHAT TO LOOK FOR?

- MCMA twins have more adverse outcomes compared to MCDA twins, but precise quantification of this excess risk is limited by a paucity of published data

Pregnancy Loss

- The rate of pregnancy loss including terminations and selective fetocide is ~30%
- The rate of perinatal death is ~15%
- Two-thirds of fetal deaths are related to cord entanglement and/or accidents, although all cords will be tangled

Structural Anomalies

- Overall prevalence is ~30%

Fetal Growth Restriction

- FGR may occur in one or both twins, but appears less likely than the ~25% rate reported in MCDA twin pregnancies
- Recognised by serial ultrasound biometry during pregnancy

Twin–Twin Transfusion Syndrome (TTTS/TOPS)

- TTTS may occur, but appears less likely than the 10–15% described in MCDA pregnancies
- Recognised through finding of severe polyhydramnios with discrepancy in the bladder size between the donor and recipient twin

Twin-Arterial Perfusion Syndrome (TAPS)

- TAPS may occur, but appears less likely than the 5% described in MCDA twin pregnancies
- Recognised by regular MCA Doppler measurements

Preterm Births

- Preterm birth rate before 32 weeks is ~30%
- Preterm birth rate at 24–28 weeks is ~3%

ULTRASOUND SURVEILLANCE

- Ultrasound monitoring should start from the time of diagnosis
- Apart from common placental mass and no inter-twin membrane, the diagnosis can be confirmed by rolling the patient on their side and scanning again to confirm that both twins have fallen to the lowest part of the uterus
- Colour Doppler should be used to identify both umbilical cords - cord entanglement is a hallmark finding in monoamniotic pregnancy
- Counting yolk sacs to define amnionicity is a common misconception and should not be used for clinical decision-making

12–24 Weeks

- Detailed anatomy assessment
- Although TTTS is rare in this group, it is still important to look for bladder discrepancy and polyhydramnios

24–32 Weeks

- Assessments every 1–2 weeks, including fetal Doppler

MANAGEMENT AND COUNSELLING

- For monochorionic complications (sFGR, TTTS, TAPS and structural abnormalities), counsel and manage as for MCDA twins
- The risk of fetal demise of both twins at 33–34 weeks is ~2%
- Uncomplicated MCMA should be delivered by 32^{+0} weeks

TWIN REVERSED ARTERIAL PERFUSION (TRAP) SEQUENCE

Definition

- TRAP is suspected in monochorionic twin pregnancies when one fetus appears anatomically normal while the other either lacks apparent cardiac structures ('acardiac twin') or has only a rudimentary heart
- The acardiac twin gets deoxygenated blood from a healthy 'pump' twin via an arterial anastomosis
- There is usually little or no perfusion of the upper torso, resulting, most commonly, in absent head and thorax
- In some cases only the head can develop, or there could be a head with partially developed limbs or a mass with barely recognisable parts
- ~75% are MCDA and ~25% are MCMA

Ultrasound Assessment

- Beware of TRAP when the diagnosis of 'vanishing monochorionic twin' is made in early pregnancy, or when a fetus without fetal heart activity appears to be growing in size
- It is important to keep assessing the blood flow from the 'pump' twin to the secondary tissue mass at each visit (Fig. 12.6)

- At each visit calculate weight of the acardiac twin using the following formula:

  EFW(g) acardiac = $1.2 \times \text{length}^2$ (cm) – $1.66 \times$ length (cm)

Management and Counselling

- ~10% of pump twins are aneuploid; therefore, amniocentesis for chromosomal analysis is recommended
- If EFW of an acardiac twin is >50% of EFW of the pump twin, there is ~10% risk of hydrops in the pump twin. Selective reduction should be discussed as a management option
- If EFW of the acardiac twin is >70% of weight of the pump twin, there is a much higher risk of hydrops in the pump twin (~30%). Counsel for selective reduction to improve pregnancy outcome (interventions for TRAP are described in Chapter 17)

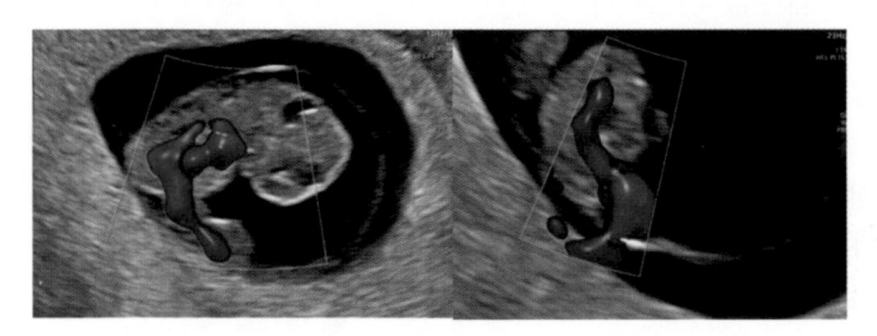

Fig. 12.6 Monochorionic twins at 9 weeks showing TRAP sequence. Sagittal view of the normal twin on the left showing normal blood flow in the umbilical artery away from the fetus (blue colour). Sagittal section of the acardiac twin on the right, showing reversed flow in the umbilical artery towards the fetus (red colour).

CONJOINED TWINS

Definition

- The term *conjoined* describes shared tissue mass between two fetuses. Conjoined twins are classified according the area of fusion (Table 12.4)

Table 12.4 Types of conjoined twins.

Type	Definition
Cephalopagus	Joined from the top of the head to the umbilicus. Two faces.
Thoracopagus	Joined from upper thorax to the upper abdomen (face-to-face). Always involves cardiac system.
Omphalopagus	Joined from lower thorax to umbilicus. No cardiac involvement.
Ischiopagus	Joined at lower abdomen with fused pelvic bones. Involves anus and external genitalia.
Parapagus	Joined laterally. Parapagus dithoracic (separated thoraces), parapagus dicephalus (separate heads) and parapagus diprosopus (two faces).
Craniopagus	Joined skulls. Typically share meninges.
Pygopagus	Joined dorsally at the sacrococcygeal area and perineum with one anus.
Rachipagus	Joined dorsally (thoracolumbar vertebrae).

Ultrasound Assessment

- Be aware of the risk of conjoined twins in MCMA pregnancies. Detailed structural survey of MCMA twins must ensure that there are no fused parts
- If fused parts are demonstrated, document the extent of fusion with respect to body compartment and organ systems
- Fetal MRI provides both panoramic accuracy and more details to ascertain the extent of organ fusion

Management and Counselling

- Management depends on fused parts and potential for separation
- If continuing the pregnancy, multidisciplinary input is essential to agree the management plan
- Delivery typically requires classic caesarean section and should be performed in a tertiary centre able to manage subsequent stabilisation and separation procedures
- If interrupting pregnancy, dilation and evacuation may provide alternative to hysterotomy at early gestations

TRIPLETS (AND HIGHER-ORDER MULTIPLES)

- The rate of spontaneous triplet pregnancies is 1/8,000 pregnancies
- Triplet pregnancies can present in varying combinations of mono-, di- or trichorionicity, as well as mono-, di- or triamnionicity
- DCTA triplets are associated with worse outcomes than TCTA triplets
- Complications related to TTTS and sFGR are likely to be responsible for the differences

Ultrasound Assessment in the First Trimester

- Early ultrasound should confirm the number of fetuses and determine chronicity and amnionicity. This information is critical for risk assessment, counselling and management
- Labelling is important for serial assessment of fetal growth later in pregnancy. The same principles are used as in twin pregnancy (see above)

Ultrasound Surveillance

- 16 weeks: DCTA should be scanned to look for early signs of TTTS
- 18–20 weeks: fetal biometry, morphological assessment, placentation, cord insertion
- 24, 28, 32 weeks: screen for FGR or growth discordance, biometry, fetal Doppler, amniotic fluid index (deepest pocket)
- Regular assessment of cervical length (e.g. 16, 20, 24 weeks) to look for significant cervical shortening/prolapsed membranes (see also Chapter 13)

Selective Reduction

- After first trimester diagnosis, the option of selective fetal reduction to twins or singleton should be discussed (Tables 12.5 and 12.6)

Aneuploidy Screening

- The risk assessment should be based on maternal age, nuchal translucency and the presence or absence of nasal bone
- Serum screening has not been validated for triplets

Management and Counselling

- Maternal complications include an increased risk of hyperemesis gravidarum, gestational diabetes (~15%), hypertensive disorders of pregnancy (~25%) and anaemia (~50%)
- There is no good-quality evidence to support 'routine' use of cerclage, pessary or vaginal progesterone
- Prophylactic antenatal corticosteroids or tocolysis are not indicated, but antenatal corticosteroids should be prescribed before planned caesarean section at 35 weeks
- The average gestational age at delivery for triplet pregnancies is 32–33 weeks; ~10% will deliver before 28 weeks

Table 12.5 Complications in trichorionic–triamniotic pregnancy (TCTA) and the impact of selective reductions.

	TCTA	Embryo reduction to twins	Embryo reduction to singleton
Miscarriage	~3%	~7%	~10%
Preterm birth <32 weeks	~35%	~13%	~8%

Table 12.6 Complications in dichorionic–triamniotic pregnancy (DCTA) and impact of selective reductions.

	DCTA	Embryo reduction to MC twins	Embryo reduction to singleton
Miscarriage	~9%	~13%	~18%
Preterm birth <32 weeks	~38%	~23%	~9%

SUGGESTED READING

PRIMARY RESEARCH

Curado J, Sileo F, Bhide A, Thilaganathan B, Khalil A. Early- and late-onset selective fetal growth restriction in monochorionic diamniotic twin pregnancy: natural history and diagnostic criteria. *Ultrasound Obstet Gynecol* 2020;55:661–666.

Glinianaia SV, Rankin J, Khalil A, et al. Prevalence, antenatal management and perinatal outcome of monochorionic monoamniotic twin pregnancy: a collaborative multicenter study in England, 2000–2013. *Ultrasound Obstet Gynecol* 2019; 53: 184–192.

Lewi L, Valencia C, Gonzalez E, et al. The outcome of twin reversed arterial perfusion sequence diagnosed in the first trimester. *Am J Obstet Gynecol* 2010;203:213.e1–4.

Sepulveda W, Sebire NJ, Hughes K, Odibo A, Nicolaides KH. The lambda sign at 10–14 weeks of gestation as a predictor of chorionicity in twin pregnancies. *Ultrasound Obstet Gynecol* 1996;7:421–423.

Syngelaki A, Cimpoca B, Litwinska E, et al. Diagnosis of fetal defects in twin pregnancies at routine 11–13 week ultrasound examination. *Ultrasound Obstet Gynecol* 2020;55:474–481.

REVIEWS AND GUIDELINES

Anthoulakis C, Dagklis T, Mamopoulos A, et al. Risks of miscarriage or preterm delivery in trichorionic and dichorionic triplet pregnancies with embryo reduction versus expectant management: a systematic review and meta-analysis. *Hum Reprod* 2017;32: 1351–1359.

Audibert F, Gagnon A. No. 262: Prenatal screening for and diagnosis of aneuploidy in twin pregnancies. *J Obstet Gynaecol Can* 2017;39:e347–e361.

Cheong-See F, Schuit E, Arroyo-Manzano D, et al. Prospective risk of stillbirth and neonatal complications in twin pregnancies: systematic review and meta-analysis. *BMJ* 2016;354:i4353.

Curado J, D'antonio F, Papageorghiou AT, et al. Perinatal mortality and morbidity in triplet pregnancy according to chorionicity: systematic review and meta-analysis. *Ultrasound Obstet Gynecol* 2019;54:589–595.

Di Mascio D, Khalil A, Rizzo G, et al. Risk of fetal loss following amniocentesis or chorionic villus sampling in twin pregnancy: systematic review and meta-analysis. *Ultrasound Obstet Gynecol* 2020;56:647–655.

Di Mascio D, Khalil A, D'Amico A, et al. Outcome of twin–twin transfusion syndrome according to Quintero stage of disease: systematic review and meta-analysis. *Ultrasound Obstet Gynecol* 2020;56:811–820.

Gil MM, Galeva S, Jani J, et al. Screening for trisomies by cfDNA testing of maternal blood in twin pregnancy: update of The Fetal Medicine Foundation results and meta-analysis. *Ultrasound Obstet Gynecol* 2019;53:734–742.

Machin G. Placentation in multiple births. *Twin Res* 2001;4:150–155.

Prefumo F, Fichera A, Pagani G, et al. The natural history of monoamniotic twin pregnancies: a case series and systematic review of the literature. *Prenat Diagn* 2015;35:274–280.

Tollenaar LS, Slaghekke F, Middeldorp JM, et al. Twin anemia polycythemia sequence: current views on pathogenesis, diagnostic criteria, perinatal management, and outcome. *Twin Res Hum Genet* 2016;19:222–233.

Townsend R, D'Antonio F, Sileo FG, et al. Perinatal outcome of monochorionic twin pregnancy complicated by selective fetal growth restriction according to management: systematic review and meta-analysis. *Ultrasound Obstet Gynecol* 2019;53:36–46.

Townsend R, Khalil A. Ultrasound surveillance in twin pregnancy: an update for practitioners. *Ultrasound* 2018;26:193–205.

CHAPTER 13

Short Cervix in Asymptomatic Women

SUMMARY BOX

INDICATIONS FOR CERVICAL LENGTH MEASUREMENT

ESTABLISHED INDICATIONS

- Previous spontaneous preterm birth (<34 weeks)
- Previous preterm prelabour rupture of membranes (PPROM) (<34 weeks)
- Knife cone biopsy
- Two or more large loop excisions (LLETZ)
- Suspected short cervix or prolapsed membranes during a transabdominal scan for other indications

RELATIVE INDICATIONS

- Extensive LLETZ (e.g. depth >10 mm)
- Known uterine anomaly
- Candidate for fetal surgery (fetoscopy, open)
- Previous full dilatation caesarean section
- Multiple pregnancy
- Routine cervical length measurement as a screening test within a preterm birth prevention programme

CORRECT TECHNIQUE

- Transvaginal scan
- Near-empty bladder
- Cervix should be as perpendicular to the vaginal probe as possible (Figs. 13.1 and 13.2)
- Avoid applying pressure on the cervix – anterior and posterior lip of the cervix should be of similar size
- Internal and external os are clearly seen
- Full length of the endocervical canal is visualised
- Still image of the cervix occupies approximately two-thirds of the ultrasound screen
- The cervix should be observed for at least 3 minutes and three separate measurements taken
- Callipers are correctly placed at the internal and external os
- The measurement is obtained by a straight line connecting the internal and external os. It is accepted that such a measurement will underestimate the true length if the cervix is curved, but this 'underestimate' is not clinically important
- The shortest measurement should be recorded for clinical decision-making

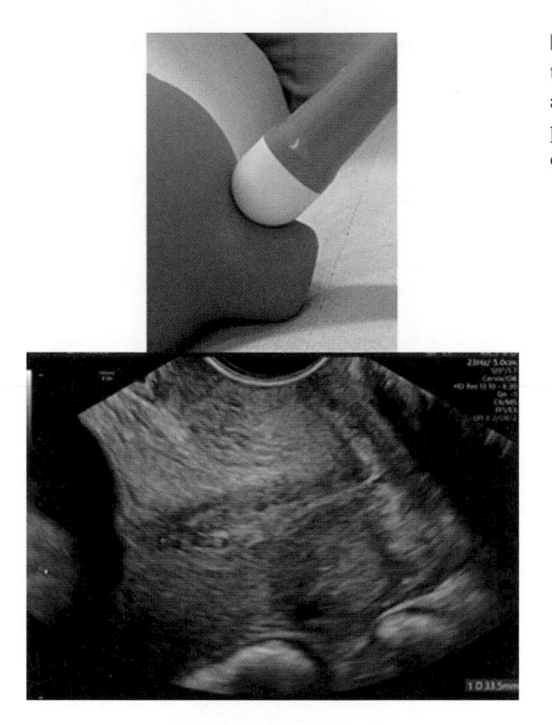

Fig. 13.1 A correctly positioned probe will allow the best visualisation of the key landmarks and accurate calliper placement. Note that the pressure applied against the anterior lip of the cervix is minimal.

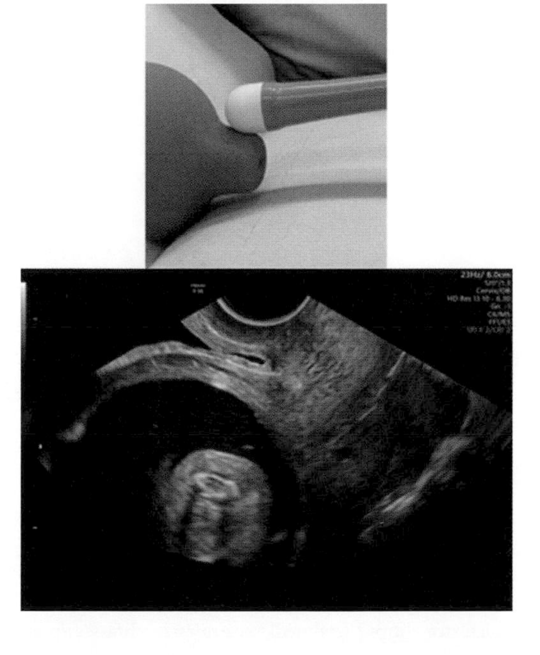

Fig. 13.2 The same cervix as in Fig. 13.1 with the vaginal probe positioned almost parallel to the cervical canal. The measurement is not attempted as it is likely to be inaccurate.

LOW-RISK SINGLETON PREGNANCY WITH SHORT CERVIX

- In otherwise low-risk pregnancy, a short cervix will be identified either within an established screening programme or suspected on a transabdominal scan and then confirmed with a transvaginal scan
- The risk of preterm birth at the time of assessment depends on cervical length (Table 13.1)

Table 13.1 Preterm birth risk for nulliparous women with singleton pregnancy with short cervix at 20–26 weeks.

Cervical length	Risk of preterm birth before 28^{+0} weeks (%)	Risk of preterm birth before 34^{+0} weeks (%)
24 mm	0.4	2.4
23 mm	0.4	2.7
22 mm	0.5	3.1
21 mm	0.6	3.5
20 mm	**0.7**	**4.1**
19 mm	0.9	4.7
18 mm	1.1	5.4
17 mm	1.3	6.2
16 mm	1.6	7.1
15 mm	**2**	**8.3**
14 mm	2.5	9.6
13 mm	3.2	11.2
12 mm	4	13.2
11 mm	5.1	15.5
10 mm	**6.6**	**18.4**
9 mm	8.6	22
8 mm	11.4	26.6
7 mm	15.3	32.6
6 mm	20.9	40.6
5 mm	**29.3**	**51.7**
4 mm	42.4	67.8
3 mm	63.6	92.5
2 mm	90	99
1 mm	90	99

Based on the Fetal Medicine Foundation risk calculator (https://fetalmedicine.org/research/assess/preterm/cervix).

MANAGEMENT

- Ask about any symptoms of threatened preterm birth or PPROM and admit for observation if clinical suspicion is high
- Ask about urinary symptoms and, if present, exclude urinary infection with urine culture
- Ask about symptoms of vaginal infection and take high vaginal swab if symptomatic

Cervical Length ≥10–24 mm

- Asymptomatic women should be prescribed vaginal progesterone 200 mg
- Advise to insert at night because of better compliance
- Weekly intramuscular injections of 17-OH progesterone caproate can be prescribed for women who cannot tolerate vaginal pessaries
- Repeat cervical length measurement 1 week later and then every 2 weeks until 28 weeks
- If follow-up scan before 26 weeks reveals cervical shortening below 10 mm, cerclage should be offered

Cervical Length <10 mm

- Perform speculum examination
- If membranes are visible and there are no contraindications, offer cervical cerclage
- If cerclage is declined, or gestation is $\geq 26^{+0}$ weeks, we offer vaginal progesterone. Cervical pessary* can be added, if available
- If cervical length is <10 mm when first measured and membranes are not visible on speculum examination, starting vaginal progesterone is a reasonable alternative to cerclage
- Irrespective of the treatment, cervical length measurement should be repeated a week later, and then every 2 weeks until 28 weeks

COUNSELLING

- Vaginal progesterone will reduce the risk of preterm birth by ~20% (e.g. 6.6.% to 5.3%; 18.4% to 14.7%)
- Progesterone treatment should be continued until 37^{+0} weeks
- Once an ultrasound-indicated cerclage is successfully placed, our advice is to continue with progesterone prophylaxis
- Removal of cerclage or cervical pessary is scheduled at ~37^{+0} weeks
- There is no good evidence to support antibiotic prophylaxis, maintenance tocolysis or continuous bed rest
- We advise to refrain for sexual intercourse with cerclage in situ

SINGLETON PREGNANCY WITH RISK FACTORS FOR PRETERM BIRTH AND SHORT CERVIX

- In women with risk factors, serial cervical length measurements usually start at 16 weeks
- Preterm birth risk at the time of diagnosis depends on the cervical length (Table 13.2)
- For women with previous preterm birth or previous cervical surgery the risk can be modified with fetal fibronectin measurement using the QUIPP calculator, available at https://quipp.org/asymptomatic.html

* A video with instructions for insertion and removal of cervical pessary can be found at: www.harris-wellbeingresearchcentre.co.uk/teaching-learning.

MANAGEMENT

- Ask about any symptoms of threatened preterm birth or PPROM and admit for observation if clinical suspicion is high
- Exclude urinary infection with urine cultures
- Ask about symptoms of acute vaginal infection and take high vaginal swab if symptomatic

Cervical Length ≥10 mm

- Asymptomatic women should be prescribed vaginal progesterone 200 mg
- Advise to insert at night because of better compliance
- Weekly intramuscular injections of 17-OH progesterone caproate can be prescribed for women who cannot tolerate vaginal pessaries
- Repeat cervical length measurement 1 week later and then every 2 weeks until 28 weeks
- If follow-up scan before 26 weeks reveals cervical shortening below 10 mm, manage accordingly

Cervical Length <10 mm

- If no contraindications, offer cervical cerclage before 26 weeks
- If cerclage is declined, as an alternative we offer a combination of vaginal progesterone and cervical pessary* if available
- Repeat cervical length measurement should be done 1 week later and then every 2 weeks until 28 weeks

COUNSELLING

- Vaginal progesterone will reduce the risk of preterm birth by ~20% (e.g. 12.3% to 9.8%; 58.4% to 46.4%)
- Progesterone treatment should be stopped at 37^{+0} weeks
- Once cerclage is successfully placed our advice is to continue with progesterone prophylaxis
- Removal of cerclage or cervical pessary is scheduled around 36–37 weeks
- To avoid repeated courses, antenatal corticosteroids should be prescribed only if preterm birth is judged to be imminent (within 72 hours)
- There is no good-quality evidence to support antibiotic prophylaxis, maintenance tocolysis or continuous bed rest
- We advise women with cervical length <15 mm to refrain from sexual intercourse

* A video with instructions for insertion and removal of cervical pessary can be found at: www.harris-wellbeingresearchcentre.co.uk/teaching-learning.

Table 13.2 Preterm birth risk for women with history of previous preterm birth <34 weeks, singleton pregnancy and short cervix at 20–26 weeks.

Cervical length	Risk of preterm birth before 28^{+0} weeks (%)	Risk of preterm birth before 34^{+0} weeks (%)
24 mm	0.7	8.5
23 mm	0.8	9.6
22 mm	1	11
21 mm	1.2	12.5
20 mm	**1.4**	**14.3**
19 mm	1.7	16.3
18 mm	2	18.6
17 mm	2.5	21.3
16 mm	3.1	24.4
15 mm	**3.8**	**28**
14 mm	4.7	32.2
13 mm	5.9	37.1
12 mm	7.5	42.9
11 mm	9.5	49.8
10 mm	**12.3**	**58.4**
9 mm	16	67.9
8 mm	21.1	80.1
7 mm	28.4	95.4
6 mm	38.9	99
5 mm	**54.6**	**99**
4 mm	78.8	99
3 mm	90	99
2 mm	90	99
1 mm	99	99

Based on the Fetal Medicine Foundation risk calculator (https://fetalmedicine.org/research/assess/preterm/cervix).

TWINS WITH SHORT CERVIX

- Preterm birth risk depends on the cervical length (Table 13.3)
- The risk can be modified with fetal fibronectin measurement using the QUIPP calculator, available at https://quipp.org/asymptomatic.html

MANAGEMENT

- Ask about any symptoms of threatened preterm birth or PPROM and admit for observation if clinical suspicion is high
- Exclude urinary infection with urine cultures
- Ask about symptoms of acute vaginal infection and take high vaginal swab if symptomatic
- If cervical length <10 mm, perform speculum examination to look for bulging membranes

Cervical Length <25 Mm with No Evidence of Dilated External Os/Bulging Membranes

- There is at present no good-quality evidence that progesterone improves perinatal outcome in this group
- If cervical pessary is available and adequate expertise is available, we offer pessary when cervix is <15 mm before 20 weeks
- If quantitative fibronectin is available and QUIPP risk is very high, cervical cerclage may be preferable to a pessary
- Cervical length measurements should be repeated every 1–2 weeks to look for prolapsed membranes

Dilated External Os/Prolapsed Membranes

- Offer cervical cerclage before 24 weeks
- If cerclage is declined, we offer cervical pessary as an alternative to cerclage
- If surgery is successful, repeat ultrasound assessment 1 week later and then every 2 weeks until 28 weeks to exclude further cervical dilatation

COUNSELLING

- Removal of cerclage or cervical pessary* is scheduled around 36^{+0} weeks
- To avoid repeated courses, antenatal corticosteroids should be prescribed only if preterm birth is judged to be imminent (within 72 hours)
- There is no good-quality evidence to support antibiotic prophylaxis, maintenance tocolysis or continuous bed rest
- We advise women with cervical length <15 mm to refrain from sexual intercourse

Table 13.3 Preterm birth risk* for women with twin pregnancy and cervical length measured at 20 weeks' gestation.

Cervical length	Risk of preterm birth within 1 week (%)	Risk of preterm birth before 30^{+0} weeks (%)
30 mm	0.3	10.5
29 mm	0.3	11.4
28 mm	0.3	12.4

* A video with instructions for insertion and removal of cervical pessary can be found at: www.harris-wellbeingresearchcentre.co.uk/teaching-learning.

Table 13.3 (*cont.*)

Cervical length	Risk of preterm birth within 1 week (%)	Risk of preterm birth before 30^{+0} weeks (%)
27 mm	0.4	13.5
26 mm	0.4	14.7
25 mm	**0.4**	**16.1**
24 mm	0.5	17.7
23 mm	0.6	19.4
22 mm	0.6	21.3
21 mm	0.7	23.5
20 mm	**0.8**	**25.9**
19 mm	0.9	28.5
18 mm	1	31.5
17 mm	1.2	34.8
16 mm	1.4	38.4
15 mm	**1.7**	**42.4**
14 mm	2	46.7
13 mm	2.4	51.3
12 mm	2.9	56.2
11 mm	3.5	61.3
10 mm	**4.4**	**66.4**
9 mm	5.5	71.5
8 mm	6.4	76.3
7 mm	8.8	80.8
6 mm	11.4	84.8
5 mm	**14.6**	**88.1**
4 mm	18.4	90.7
3 mm	22.5	92.6
2 mm	262	93.6
1 mm	28.8	94.6

* Risks are calculated using the QUIPP calculator (https://quipp.org/asymptomatic.html).

SUGGESTED READING

EPPPIC Group. Evaluating Progestogens for Preventing Preterm birth International Collaborative (EPPPIC): meta-analysis of individual participant data from randomised controlled trials. *Lancet.* 2021;397(10280):1183–1194.

Norman JE, Norrie J, MacLennan G, et al. Evaluation of the Arabin cervical pessary for prevention of preterm birth in women with a twin pregnancy and short cervix (STOPPIT-2): an open label randomised trial and updated meta-analysis. *PLoS Med* 2021;18(3):e1003506.

Roman A, Zork N, Haeri S, et al. Physical examination-indicated cerclage in twin pregnancy: a randomized controlled trial. *Am J Obstet Gynecol* 2020;223(6):902.e1–902.e11.

CHAPTER 14

Fetal Infections

SUMMARY BOX

CYTOMEGALOVIRUS

MOTHER

- ~40% of pregnant women are seronegative at booking
- Seroconversion during pregnancy occurs in ~1–2%
- Most women will remain asymptomatic
- Symptomatic women may develop fever, malaise, myalgia and lymphadenopathy

FETUS

- Fetal infection can occur after primary infection, reinfection with a different strain or reactivation of a previous infection
- Transmission rates after non-primary infections are very low (~1%)
- The transmission rate after primary infection is ~30% during the first and second trimester and 40–70% in the third trimester (Fig. 14.1)
- Although the transmission rate in the third trimester is high, any long-term problems are very rare
- The most severe complications are seen when fetal infection occurs in the embryonic period (3–8 weeks' gestation) (Figs. 14.2–14.4)

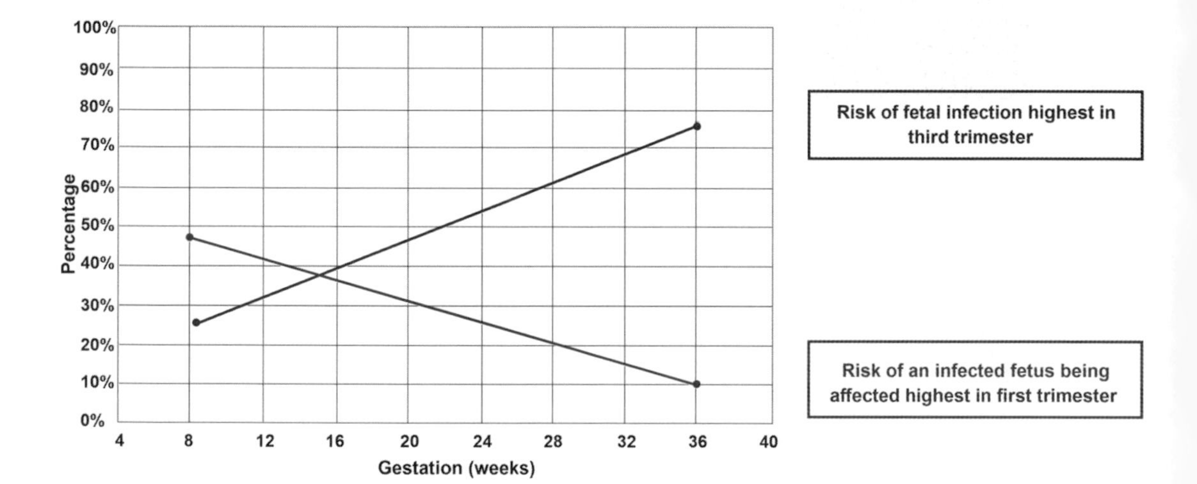

Fig. 14.1 Impact of gestational age on the risk of fetal infection and infant morbidity.

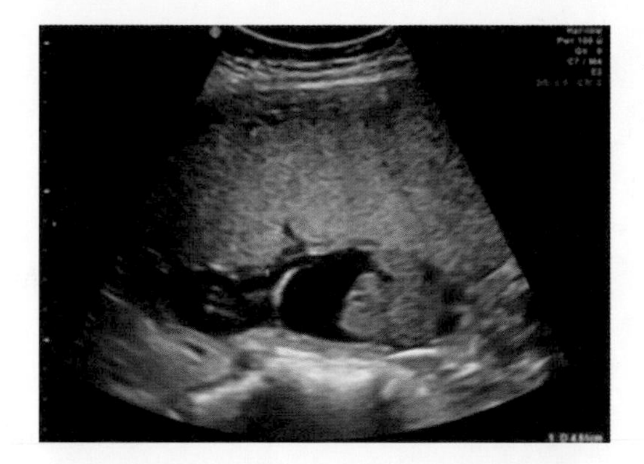

Fig. 14.2a CMV infection. Affected fetus at 25 weeks' gestation with ascites and placentomegaly.

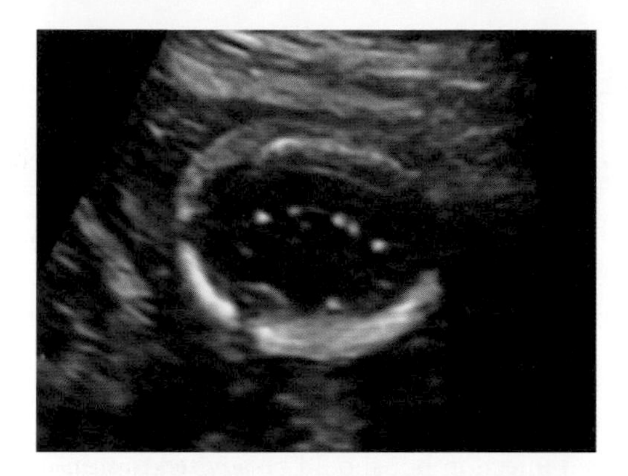

Fig. 14.2b Parasagittal view of the head showing multiple periventricular calcifications.

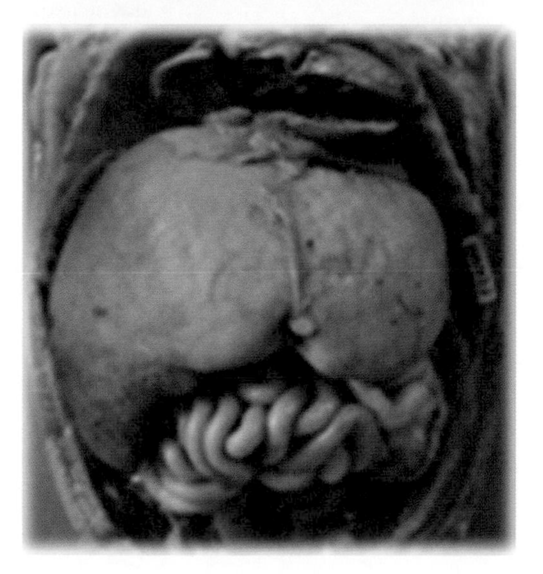

Fig. 14.3 Autopsy specimen of a fetus with CMV infection showing enlarged liver with nodular surface.

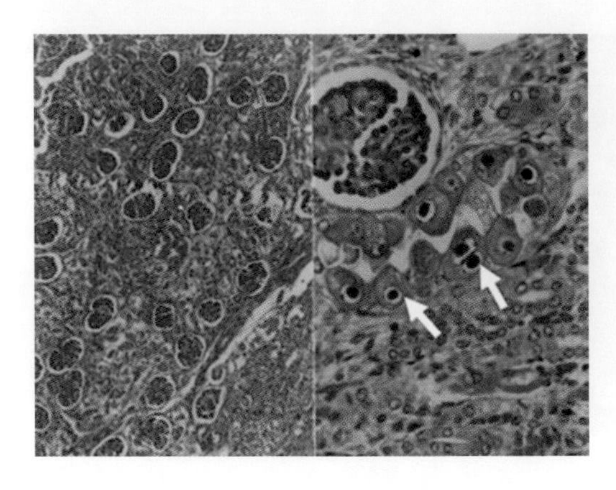

Fig. 14.4 Low- and high-power renal histology image showing cytomegaly with nucleomegaly (arrows).

INTERPRETATION OF MATERNAL SEROLOGY

IgM negative	IgG positive	**IMMUNE** • No risk to the fetus • Woman can be considered immune
IgM negative	IgG negative	**SUSCEPTIBLE** • Repeat in 2–4 weeks if the incubation period has not passed • If the incubation period has passed, the woman has not developed infection but should be advised to minimise the risk of exposure
IgM positive	IgG negative	**RECENT PRIMARY INFECTION POSSIBLE** • Repeat in 2–4 weeks and if IgG negative reassure – no recent primary infection
IgM positive	IgG positive	**INFECTION** • Test IgM and IgG in earlier sample if available • Low IgG avidity index* ≤30% – infection in the last 3 months • Intermediate IgG avidity index 30–60% – repeat in 3 weeks • High IgG avidity index >60% – infection >3 months ago

* Avidity index is the proportion of IgG bound to the antigen after exposure to denaturing agents.

CLINICAL PRESENTATION

Maternal Seroconversion Detected before 16 Weeks with a Normal Initial Scan

Management

- Offer amniocentesis for DNA PCR 8 weeks after seroconversion, but not before 18^{+0} weeks

Counselling

CMV PCR Negative (~70%)

- Reassure and return to normal antenatal care

CMV PCR Positive (~30%)

- Only ~25% of CMV PCR positive babies will become affected to some degree
- Of those who are affected:
  - ~60% will develop sensory neural hearing loss, but only a small proportion will require a cochlear implant
  - ~20% will have prenatal or postnatal symptoms, but not long-term problems
  - ~20% will have long-term problems including seizures and disabilities of mental and physical function
- Offer valacyclovir 2 g four times daily as primary therapy to mitigate the effects of viremia
- Ultrasound assessment every 2–3 weeks to look for signs of fetal infection and MRI at 28–32 weeks; if normal, offer repeat MRI in 4–6 weeks for further reassurance
- When ultrasound and MRI scan of the fetal brain remain normal, the risk of neurodisability is very low, but hearing could be affected

Maternal Seroconversion Detected after 16 Weeks with a Normal Initial Scan

Management

- Offer amniocentesis for CMV PCR

Counselling

CMV PCR Negative

- Reassure and return to the normal care pathway

CMV PCR Positive

- ~90% of babies will remain asymptomatic
- Use valacyclovir 2 g four times daily as primary therapy to mitigate the effect of viremia
- Ultrasound assessment every 2–3 weeks to look for signs of fetal infection
- MRI at 28–32 weeks; if normal, offer repeat 4–6 weeks later
- There is no good evidence to justify the risks of fetal blood sampling (cordocentesis) for monitoring of the disease
- When ultrasound and MRI scan of the fetal brain remain normal the risk of neurodisability is very low, but hearing could still be affected

Confirmed Fetal Infection with Non-severe Brain Signs or Extra Cerebral Signs

Non-severe Brain Signs on Ultrasound/MRI

- Isolated ventriculomegaly
- Parenchymal calcifications
- Isolated subependymal cysts
- Isolated intraventricular septations

Extracerebral Signs

- Fetal growth restriction (rarely isolated)
- Ascites/pleural effusion

- Cardiomegaly/pericardial effusions
- Echogenic bowel
- Hepatosplenomegaly
- Liver calcifications
- Placentomegaly, placental calcifications

Counselling

- There is no good evidence to justify the risks of fetal blood sampling in this group
- There is no good-quality evidence to suggest that valacyclovir reduces the risk of complications in this already symptomatic group
- ~40–50% will have no long-term problems
- ~10–15% will develop severe brain signs either before or after birth
- ~40–45% will have long-term problems (mainly hearing loss)

Confirmed Fetal Infection with Severe Brain Signs

Severe Brain Signs on Ultrasound/MRI

- Periventricular hyperechogenicity/cysts
- Cystic periventricular leukomalacia
- Polymicrogyria – too many small folds
- Pachygyria – too few gyri that are broad and flat
- Enlarged pericerebral spaces
- Microcephaly

Counselling

- It is too late for antiviral therapy
- All babies will have severe life-long problems (developmental delay, cognitive impairment, cerebral palsy, epilepsy, impaired vision)
- Offer termination of pregnancy if this option is legal

PARVOVIRUS B19

MOTHER

- Also known as erythema infectiosum, fifth disease or slapped cheek syndrome
- Incubation period is 7–14 days
- Majority of adults are asymptomatic
- Most common symptom in adults is arthropathy and may last several weeks
- In children, the disease usually presents as a flu-like illness, followed by a characteristic facial rash that may spread to the trunk and limbs, but is rarely extensive

FETUS

- Only primary infection can cause fetal harm
- Fetal anaemia and thrombocytopaenia are caused by a transient aplastic crisis
- Ascites/hydrops caused by anaemia, myocarditis and high-output cardiac failure is a relatively common ultrasound feature
- Hydrops is rare if infections occur after 30 weeks

- Intrauterine death before 20 weeks (~13%) most probably due to multiorgan failure
- Fetal loss after 20 weeks ≤1%

Interpretation of Maternal Serology

IgM negative	IgG positive	**IMMUNE** • No risk to the fetus • Woman can be considered immune
IgM negative	IgG negative	**SUSCEPTIBLE** • Repeat in 2–4 weeks if the incubation period has not passed • If the incubation period has passed, the woman has not developed infection but should be advised to minimise the risk of exposure
IgM positive	IgG negative	**VERY RECENT INFECTION OR FALSE-POSITIVE RESULT** • Repeat in 2–4 weeks
IgM positive	IgG positive	**SUBACUTE INFECTION** • If stored blood is available, it should be tested to confirm seroconversion • If stored blood is not available, repeat testing should confirm rising IgG titre • If IgG titre is not rising this could be an older infection (up to 6 months prior)

PCR FOR VIRAL DNA

- If maternal serology is consistent with recent infection, there is no need to perform amniocentesis to confirm or refute the diagnosis
- Viral DNA can be detected in amniotic fluid or fetal serum by PCR when amniocentesis, or fetal blood sampling, are performed as part of the hydrops workup

CLINICAL PRESENTATION

Confirmed Recent Maternal Infection *and* Normal MCA PSV (≤1.5 MoM)

- Repeat ultrasound scans with MCA Doppler every week for 12 weeks after infection
- MRI in the third trimester is not indicated as long as there is no evidence of fetal anaemia

Counselling

- If there is no evidence of anaemia 12 weeks after infection, reassure and return to normal antenatal care
- There is no good evidence to suggest that this group has higher risk of anomalies or neurological disability

Confirmed Recent Maternal Infection *and* Raised MCA PSV (>1.5 MoM) with or without Ascites/Hydrops

- Fetal intravascular transfusion should be performed within 24 hours to reduce the risk of intrauterine death
- If the first transfusion was successful (post-transfusion haemoglobin is ~14 g/dl), a second transfusion is best avoided as it will slow erythropoiesis recovery
- If MCA PSV is extremely high or the fetus is already hydropic, it is advisable to have platelets ready for possible transfusion
- Our empirical cutoff for platelet transfusion is $\leq 20 \times 10^9$/L
- When fetal haemoglobin is extremely low ($\leq$5 g/dl) and, therefore, a relatively large amount of blood needs to be transfused, our preference is to aim for fetal haemoglobin of around 10 g/dl and, if MCA PSV is still high, transfuse again 1 week later
- If there is no improvement in ascites and/or MCA Doppler after 7–10 days the prognosis is very poor
- Offer MRI of the fetal brain 4–6 weeks after 'rescue transfusion'

Counselling

- The evidence regarding the long-term risks of neurological problems (delayed psychomotor development) in this group is conflicting and ranges from no increased risk to ~30%
- Full fetal recovery after successful 'rescue transfusion' with normal follow-up ultrasound scans and normal third trimester MRI is very reassuring

CHICKENPOX (VARICELLA ZOSTER)

MOTHER

- Incubation period lasts 10–20 days; symptoms usually last 2–6 days
- Pruritic maculopapular/vesicular rash, first on the chest, back and face
- Typically, lesions are in different stages (macule, papule, vesicle, crusting)
- People are infectious 48 hours before the rash develops
- ~70% of susceptible women will be infected when exposed
- Most women will be either afebrile or have mild fever with fewer than 50 skin lesions
- Serious complications do occur in pregnancy, mainly pneumonia, leading to respiratory failure and even maternal death
- Oral acyclovir should be prescribed within 24 hours of the onset of rash
- Intravenous acyclovir should be used for severe disease and immunocompromised women
- Varicella-zoster immunoglobulin (VZIG) has no benefit and should not be prescribed for symptomatic women
- Secondary varicella zoster (shingles) poses no risk to the fetus

FETUS

- Fetal growth restriction
- Ventriculomegaly and/or microcephaly (cortical atrophy)
- Limb reduction defects (typically terminal part of digits) (Figs. 14.5 and 14.6)
- Cataracts/chorioretinitis
- Scarring skin lesions
- Prematurity

Table 14.1 Risk of congenital varicella syndrome.

Primary maternal infection	Risk of fetal disease
≤12 weeks	0.5%
12–28 weeks	1.4%
>28 weeks	No cases reported

PREVENTION FOR SUSCEPTIBLE PREGNANT WOMEN WHO HAVE HAD A HIGH-RISK EXPOSURE

- A high-risk exposure is considered to be face-to-face contact lasting ≥5 minutes, or being in the same room for ≥15 minutes with the index case
- Seronegative women should be offered treatment after a high-risk exposure up to 2 weeks after appearance of the rash in the index case
- Post-exposure treatment protocols vary, so it is best to consult a local public health team
- Currently, common advice is to give varicella-zoster immunoglobulin (VZIG) before 20 weeks; after 20 weeks valacyclovir (1 g three times daily from 7–15 days post-exposure) or acyclovir (800 mg four times daily from 7–15 days post-exposure) should be offered
- A second dose may be required if another exposure is reported more than 3 weeks after the last dose

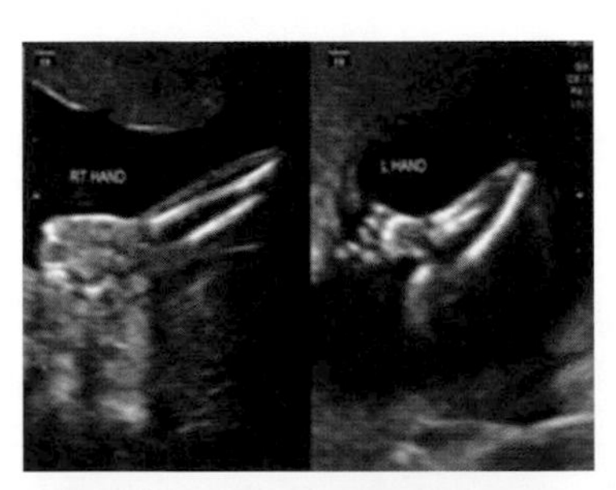

Fig. 14.5a Fetal varicella: upper limbs with contractures. Both elbow joints are flexed.

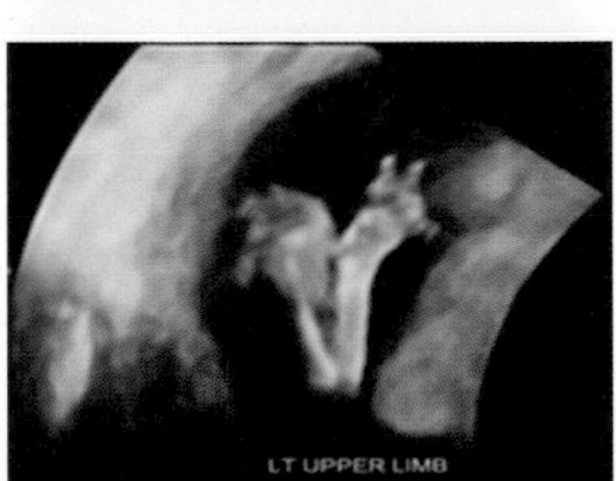

Fig. 14.5b 3D picture of the same fetus showing deformed fingers.

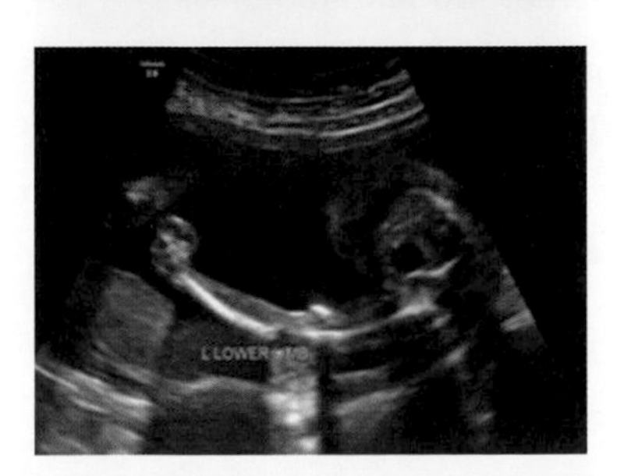

Fig. 14.5c Lower limbs showing talipes.

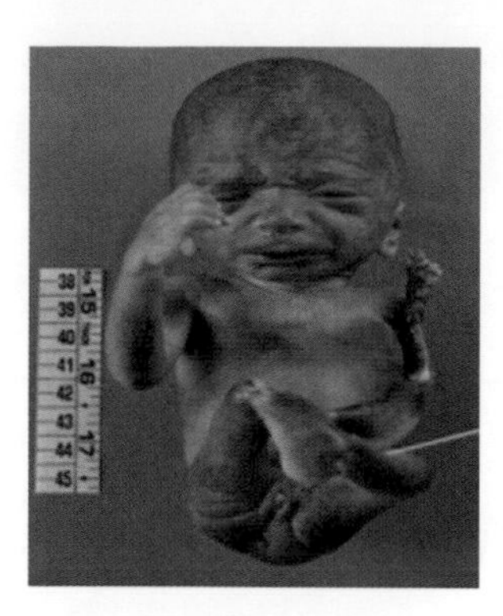

Fig. 14.6a Fetal varicella. Note the multiple contractures.

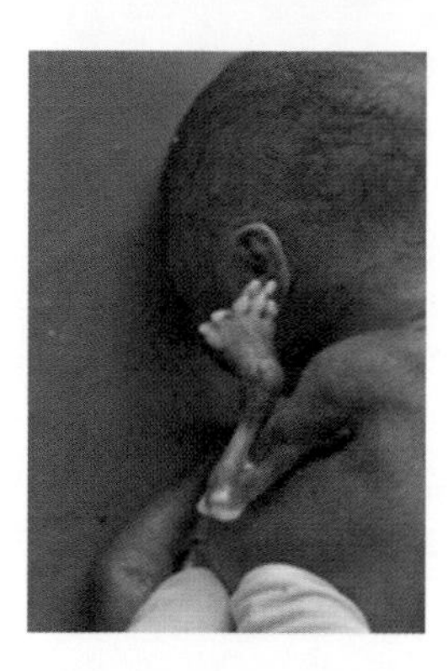

Fig. 14.6b Note the deformed hands and wasting of forearm muscles.

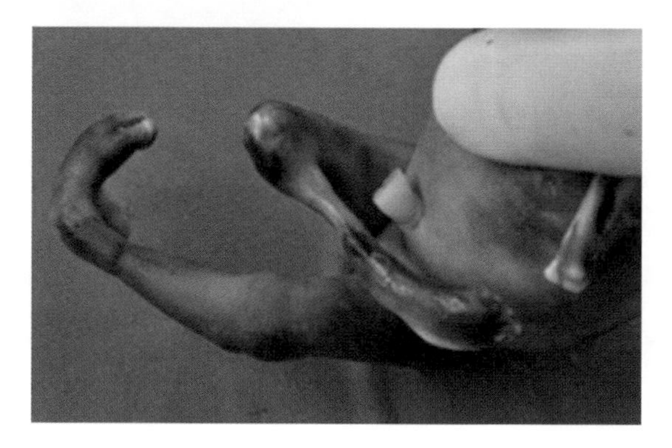

Fig. 14.6c The same fetus showing talipes, the right lower limb contractures and severe muscle wasting.

INTERPRETATION OF MATERNAL SEROLOGY

IgM negative, IgG positive	• Prior infection or immunisation
IgM negative, IgG negative	• Repeat if contact was within 3 weeks of the first test • Repeat if symptoms developed within 7 days of the first test
IgM positive, IgG negative	• Recent infection likely

- If a woman is identified as seronegative during the pregnancy and doesn't contract varicella, it is important to advise vaccination postnatally

MATERNAL INFECTION DURING PREGNANCY

Management

- Ultrasound scan at 16 weeks, or 5 weeks after infection
- Regular scans at 3–4-week intervals looking for the evidence of:
  - limb deformities/contractures
  - microcephaly
  - ventriculomegaly
  - calcifications (intracerebral, intrahepatic, myocardial)
  - fetal growth restriction
- Amniocentesis should be offered for viral PCR, but careful counselling is important (see below)
- Amniocentesis should not be performed before the skin lesions have completely healed
- MRI should be offered if cerebral lesions are suspected

Counselling

- It is important to stress that, while negative PCR is reassuring, positive PCR in amniotic fluid does not imply fetal damage
- If serial ultrasound scans are normal, the risk of clinically important neonatal disease is very small
- If maternal infection occurs in the last 4 weeks of pregnancy, there is a significant risk of clinical newborn infection (~25%)
- A planned delivery should be delayed for at least 7 days after the onset of the maternal rash to allow for the transfer of antibodies from mother to child

RUBELLA

MOTHER

- Incubation period lasts 14–21 days
- Infectious period starts 7 days before onset of symptoms and lasts ~10 days after onset of the rash
- Pruritic, fine, red maculopapular rash that usually starts behind the ears and spreads to the head, neck and body
- Symptoms include mild fever, sore throat, cough, runny nose, conjunctivitis and lymphadenopathy
- Up to 50% of adults remain asymptomatic

FETUS

- Risk of transplacental infection is highest at extremes of gestation and lowest in the late second/early third trimester (Fig. 14.7)
- Risk of fetal defect with secondary infection (low IgG on previous serology) is low
- Affected fetus may develop:
  - pulmonary stenosis

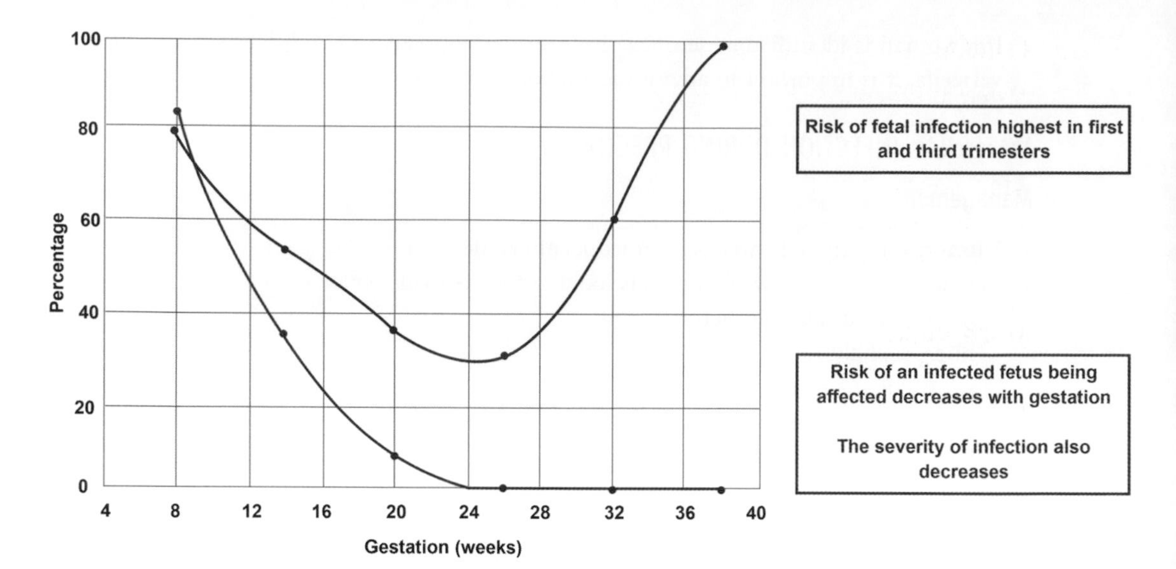

Fig. 14.7 Impact of gestational age on the risk of fetal infection and infant morbidity.

- microcephaly
- cataracts/microphthalmos
- fetal growth restriction

INTERPRETATION OF MATERNAL SEROLOGY

IgM negative	IgG positive	**PREVIOUS EXPOSURE** • IgG >10 IU/L minimal risk of reinfection • IgG ≤15 IU/L reimmunise after delivery
IgM negative	IgG negative	**SUSCEPTIBLE** • Repeat in 2–4 weeks if the incubation period has not passed
IgM positive	IgG negative	**RECENT PRIMARY INFECTION POSSIBLE** • Repeat if contact was within 3 weeks of the first test • Repeat if symptoms developed within 7 days of the first test
IgM positive	IgG positive	**SUBACUTE INFECTION** • If stored blood is available, testing of the stored sample should confirm recent seroconversion • If stored blood is not available, repeated testing should confirm rising IgG titre • If IgG titre not rising and/or avidity is high, this is likely to be an older infection (up to 6 months prior)

CLINICAL PRESENTATION

Maternal Infection <20 Weeks

Management

≤10^{+0} Weeks

- ~90% chance of multiple defects
- Offer termination of pregnancy

10–20 Weeks

- ~10–20% risk, likely single defect
- CVS can be offered for viral PCR, but the risk of maternal cross-contamination is high
- Amniocentesis should be offered, but careful counselling is important (see below)
- Amniocentesis should not be performed before the skin lesions have completely healed
- Ultrasound scan at 16 weeks, or 5 weeks after infection
- Regular scans at 3–4 weeks interval looking for the evidence of:
  - cardiac septal defects and pulmonary stenosis
  - microcephaly (Fig 14.8a,b)
  - microphthalmia
  - cataracts (Fig. 14.8c)
  - hepatosplenomegaly
  - ascites/hydrops
  - fetal growth restriction
- MRI should be offered if cerebral lesions are suspected

Counselling

- It is important to stress that, while negative PCR is reassuring, positive PCR in amniotic fluid does not imply fetal damage
- The most common long-term problem is bilateral sensory neural hearing loss (~75%), which is not detectable by ultrasound

Confirmed Maternal Infection >20 Weeks

- Reassure that there have been no confirmed cases of congenital rubella
- One third trimester scan will provide additional reassurance

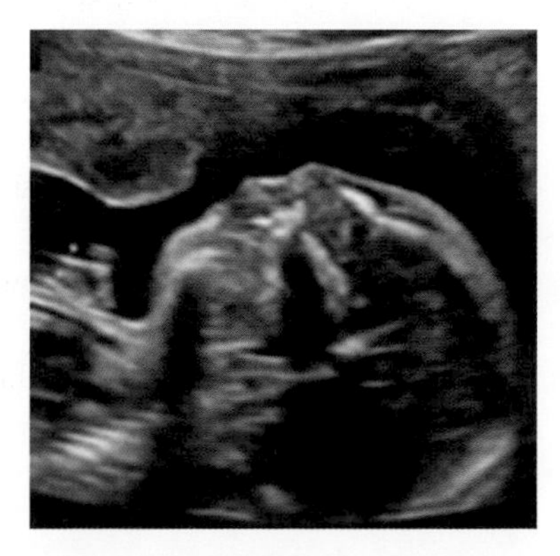

Fig. 14.8a Microcephaly in a fetus with rubella.

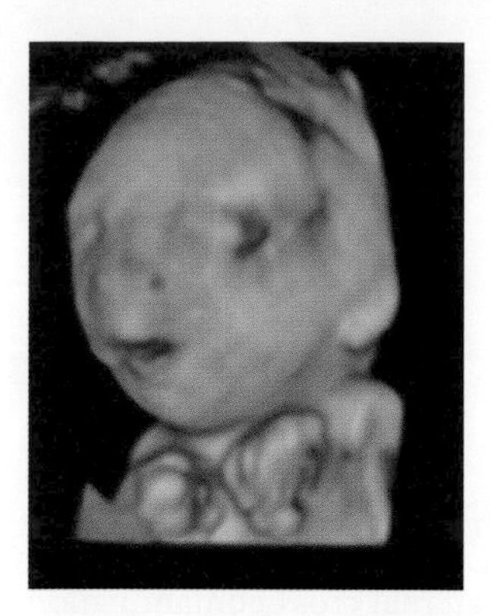

Fig. 14.8b 3D picture of the same fetus showing typical microcephaly phenotype.

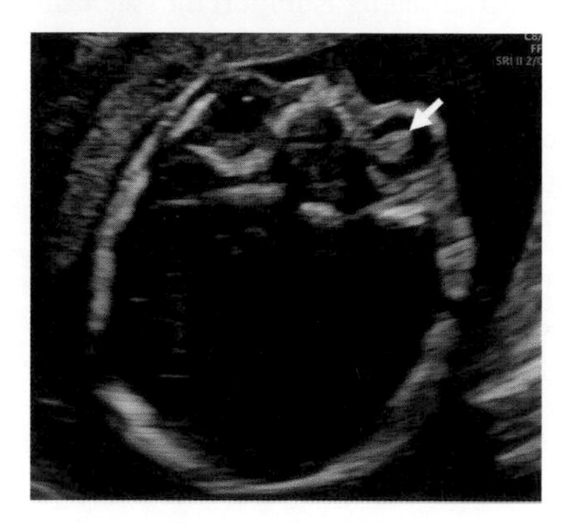

Fig. 14.8c Cataract (arrow) seen in the axial view of the orbit in a fetus with rubella infection.

MEASLES

MOTHER

- Incubation period lasts 10–14 days
- Maculopapular rash usually appears ~3 days after initial symptoms (high fever, coryza, cough, conjunctivitis)
- Hospitalisation may be required for pneumonia and encephalitis
- Severe respiratory distress may lead to death (~4%)
- Non-immune women should receive intravenous immunoglobulin within 6 days of exposure

FETUS

- Miscarriage
- Stillbirths
- Preterm birth
- No known risk of congenital malformations

INTERPRETATION OF MATERNAL SEROLOGY

IgM negative, IgG positive	• Prior infection or immunisation
IgM negative, IgG negative	• Repeat if contact was within 3 weeks of the first test • Repeat if symptoms developed within 7 days of the first test
IgM positive, IgG negative	• Recent infection likely

MATERNAL INFECTION DURING PREGNANCY

- Supportive care for the mother
- Daily CTG in the acute phase of the disease if the fetus is judged to be viable
- Reassure that there is no risk of congenital defects

ZIKA VIRUS

MOTHER

- It is important to identify a pregnant woman, or her partner, who resides in or has travelled to an area with identified mosquito-borne (*Aedes aegypti*) Zika virus transmission
- Current potential 'hot-spots' include South America, the Indian subcontinent, South East Asia and sub-Saharan Africa, although the prevalence of Zika virus infection has fallen in many of these regions since 2017
- There is no specific treatment for Zika virus
- Zika RNA persists about three times longer in a pregnant woman
- Acute symptoms include:
  - maculopapular rash (may be pruritic)
  - arthralgia
  - conjunctivitis
  - mild fever

FETUS

- ~50% of infected mothers had an affected fetus
- Unclear whether transmission and fetal disease are related to gestation of infection
- Signs of fetal infection can appear ≥20 weeks after maternal infection:
  - ventriculomegaly
  - cortical atrophy
  - microcephaly
  - intracranial calcification
  - abnormalities of cortical migration/sulcation
  - corpus callosum abnormalities
  - microphthalmia/cataracts

- talipes/arthrogryposis
- fetal growth restriction

TESTING PROTOCOL

- Definitive diagnosis is established by RNA PCR in serum and/or urine
- Negative viral PCR does not exclude infection and should be complemented with serology (IgM and plaque reduction neutralisation test (PRNT))
- There is a potential window between 7 and 15 days where infection may not be identified by either Zika RNA or IgM testing
- IgM remains positive for ~120 days post-infection, up to 240 days
- Serology is prone to false positives due to cross-reactivity with other flaviviruses such as dengue

	Recent exposure	**Ongoing exposure**
Currently asymptomatic	Laboratory testing currently not advocated	Offer testing in each trimester (Zika PCR)
Currently symptomatic	Zika PCR Zika serology (IgM/IgG)	Repeat PCR each trimester if initially negative
Fetal anomalies consistent with Zika infection	Zika PCR + serology (IgM and IgG) Test stored serum in tandem (if available)	
Placental tissue analysis	Restricted to symptomatic women or circumstances with evidence of fetal effect	

CLINICAL PRESENTATION

Positive or Inconclusive Maternal Serology *and* Normal Ultrasound Scan

Management

- Amniocentesis for viral PCR should be offered, but not before 20 weeks
- By analogy with other fetal infections, the gap between infection and amniocentesis should be at least 8 weeks
- Positive PCR result is considered diagnostic, but negative result does not exclude congenital infection
- Ultrasound every 3–4 weeks from 20 weeks to exclude developing microcephaly that may be an isolated finding

Counselling

- Confirmed maternal infection during pregnancy is associated with a significant (~50%) risk of intracranial abnormalities on a late pregnancy scan
- It may take more than 20 weeks from the infection to a visible fetal abnormality
- No therapeutic strategies have been described yet that prevent transplacental viral transmission or teratogenic effect on the fetus

- Microcephaly is associated with significant neurodevelopmental impairment
- Termination may be offered/chosen by some families based on the risk of a fetus being affected – this option will also be dependent on local law

Ultrasound Suggestive of Congenital Zika Syndrome

Management

- Offer amniocentesis as PCR is diagnostic
- If termination is not an option, antenatal assessment should follow local fetal growth restriction protocol

Counselling

- Microcephaly is associated with significant neurodevelopmental impairment
- Termination may be offered/chosen by some families based on the risk of a fetus being affected – this option will also be dependent on local law

TOXOPLASMOSIS

MOTHER

- Routine screening for toxoplasmosis is not universally recommended but is offered in some countries
- Screening for toxoplasmosis is indicated if a woman is symptomatic or with exposure to:
  - undercooked meat
  - unfiltered water
  - animal faeces/contaminated soil
- ~ 80% of women will remain asymptomatic during primary infection
- Symptoms and signs include:
  - fever
  - headache
  - myalgia
  - lethargy
  - lymphadenopathy
  - hepatosplenomegaly
  - diffuse non-pruritic maculopapular rash

FETUS

- The risk of the disease is gestation-dependent (Fig. 14.9)
- Classic CNS ultrasound signs are:
  - ventriculomegaly (Fig. 14.10)
  - intracranial calcifications
  - microcephaly
- Other ultrasound signs include:
  - intrahepatic calcifications
  - hepatosplenomegaly
  - ascites/hydrops
  - fetal growth restriction

- MRI provides added diagnostic value by identifying white matter signal change, intraparenchymal echogenic nodules, abscesses and oedema
- Chorioretinitis is a common feature but is not detectable antenatally

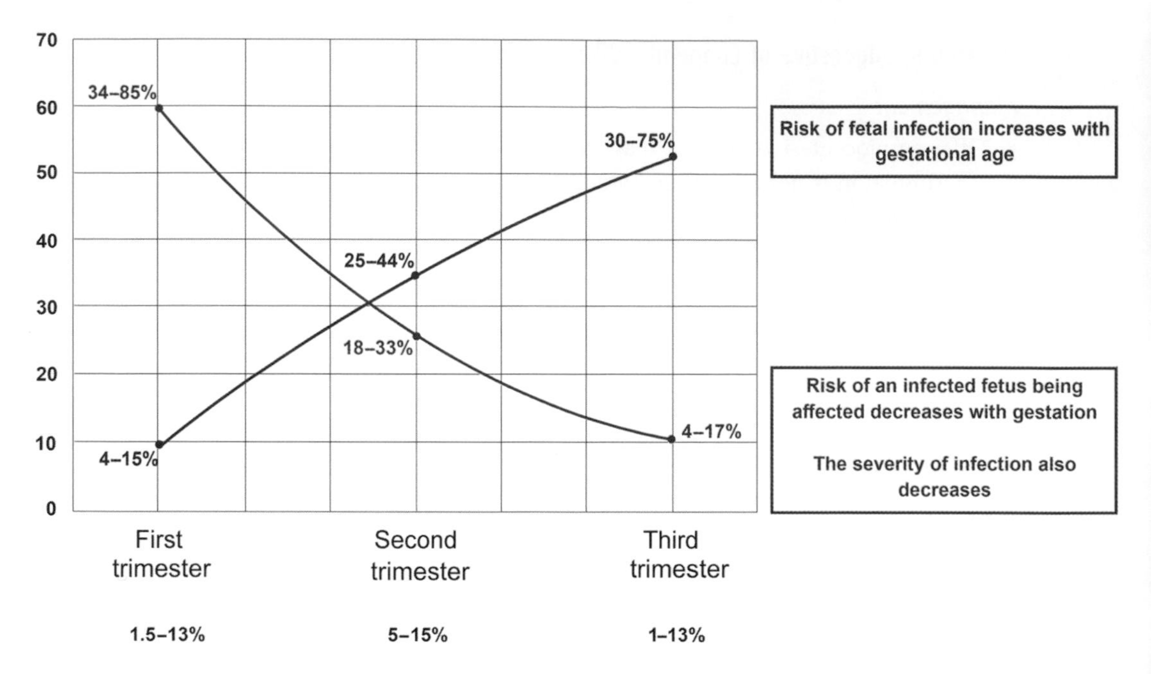

Fig. 14.9 Impact of gestational age on the risk of fetal infection and infant morbidity.

INTERPRETATION OF MATERNAL SEROLOGY

IgM negative, IgG positive	• Low risk of recent infection • High avidity within first 12 weeks rules out maternal infection during this pregnancy
IgM positive or equivocal, IgG negative	• Repeat in 2 weeks • If result unchanged likely to be a false-positive result as IgM may stay positive for years
IgM positive, IgG positive (low avidity)	• High risk of recent infection • Spiramycin may slow down the conversion from low to intermediate/high avidity.

CLINICAL PRESENTATION

Maternal Seroconversion with Normal Initial Scan

Management

- Spiramycin 1 g every 8 hours until delivery
- Amniocentesis should be offered ≥5 weeks after maternal infection, but not before 18 weeks

- The overall risk of false-negative PCR is relatively high (~17%), but decreases with advanced gestation

PCR Negative

- Continue with spiramycin until delivery
- Offer third trimester follow-up scan for reassurance to exclude a false-negative PCR result

PCR Positive

- Triple oral therapy:
  1. pyrimethanamine 50 mg once daily
  2. sulfadiazine 1.5 g once daily or 1 g three times daily
  3. folinic acid 25 mg twice a week, or 6 mg three times daily
- If spiramycin has been commenced continue only for 1 week then switch to triple therapy
- Continue until delivery and ensure weekly monitoring with a maternal full blood count
- Ultrasound scans every 3–4 weeks to look for signs of fetal infection

Counselling

- Risk of an infected fetus being affected is highest in the first trimester and decreases through pregnancy (Fig. 14.9)
- Antenatally treated fetuses have relatively good long-term prognosis (~75% will be asymptomatic, ~25% will develop chorioretinitis)
- The risk of severe neurological handicap is ~1%, but ~30% may have long-term problems (chorioretinitis which may cause blindness)
- There is no advantage in early (preterm) delivery

PCR Positive Fetus with Ultrasound/MRI Signs of Infection

- Signs of fetal infection can be visible as early as 2 weeks after maternal infection, but also as late as 14 weeks post-infection
- ~50% of affected fetuses will have only intracranial signs (ventriculomegaly, intracranial calcifications, microcephaly, white matter signal change, intraparenchymal echogenic nodules, abscesses and oedema)

Management

- Triple oral therapy:
  1. pyrimethanamine 50 mg once daily
  2. sulfadiazine 1.5 g once daily or 1 g three times daily
  3. folinic acid 25 mg twice a week, or 6 mg three times daily

Counselling

- The prognostic value of most ultrasound signs remains uncertain
- ~80% of babies with intracranial calcification (thickened echogenic ventricular walls) but no ventriculomegaly will have normal neurodevelopment
- Termination of pregnancy may be offered/chosen by some families based on the risk of a fetus being affected – this option will be dependent on local laws

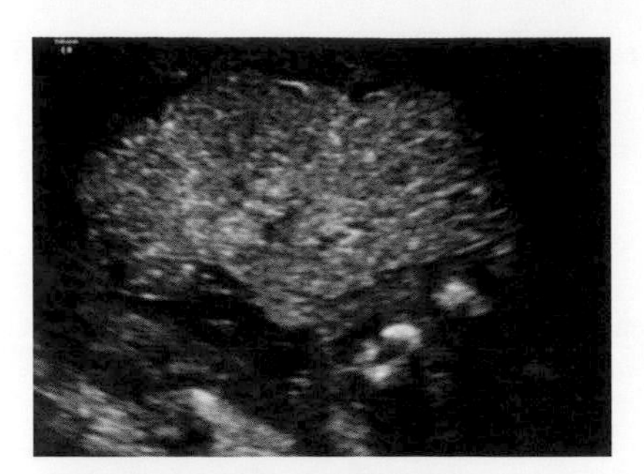

Fig. 14.10a Toxoplasmosis: placentomegaly and small calcifications.

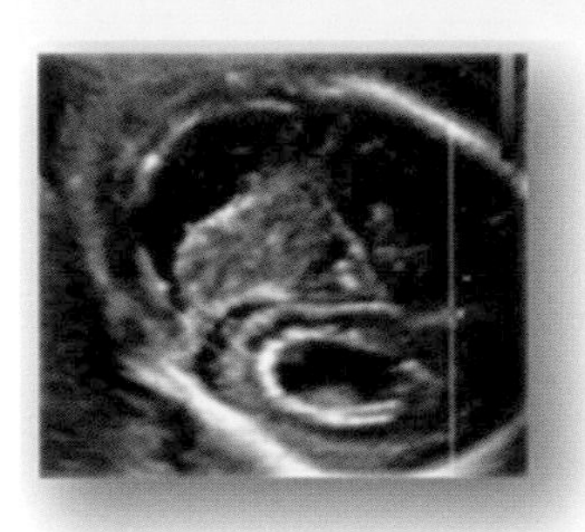

Fig. 14.10b Fetal toxoplasmosis: ventriculomegaly with diffuse periventricular echogenicity.

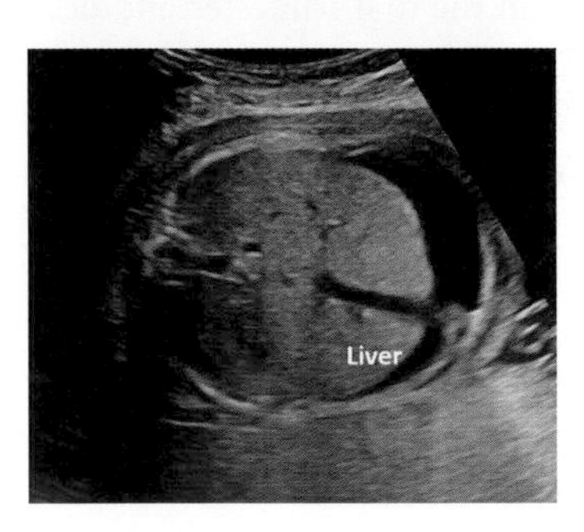

Fig. 14.10c Ascites and hepatomegaly in fetal toxoplasmosis.

SYPHILIS

MOTHER

- Rates of syphilis and congenital syphilis are rising
- Primary syphilis is characterised by a painless genital/anal ulcer (chancre)
- Secondary syphilis develops several months later, commonly with a diffuse maculopapular skin rash of the trunk and extremities (palms and soles)
- Diagnosis of primary or secondary syphilis in pregnancy through clinical presentation is rare
- More commonly a potential diagnosis is made through antenatal screening

RISK OF FETAL INFECTION

- Signs of fetal infection are the consequence of a robust inflammatory response and, therefore, unlikely to be present before 20 weeks
- Risk of fetal infection depends on maternal stage of illness:
  - maternal untreated primary infection ~80% risk
  - maternal untreated secondary infection ~50% risk

  - maternal latent infection (no visible signs of infection) ~10% risk
  - adequately treated screening positive women ~0% risk

AFFECTED FETUS

- Hepatomegaly (~80%)
- Anaemia – abnormal MCA Doppler (~30%)
- Placentomegaly (~30%)
- Polyhydramnios (~10%)
- Ascites (~10%)
- Intrauterine fetal death
- Preterm delivery
- ~30% will have more than one feature

DIAGNOSTIC TESTS FOR SYPHILIS

- Direct detection tests (e.g. dark field microscopy, PCR) may allow the diagnosis before a serologic response, but they are not commonly available and most centres must rely on serological testing and clinical manifestation
- Interpretation of serological results is complex and must be done by experts, taking into account the clinical and geographical background
- In low-prevalence populations, most initial screen positive results will be false positives
- As a precaution, a pregnant woman with positive treponemal serology should be treated as if for syphilis, unless previous treatment can be documented
- False-negative results may be seen in HIV-infected patients

Treponemal Tests

- CLIA (chemiluminescent immunoassay)
  - more sensitive than TPPA in primary syphilis, but more false positives
- EIA (enzyme immunoassay)
- TPPA (Treponema pallidum particle agglutination assay)
  - becomes reactive earlier than TPHA
- TPHA (Treponema pallidum haemagglutination assay)
- TPLA (Treponema pallidum agglutination test automated turbidimetric assay)
  - second line test; high lipid levels may cause false results
- FTA-ABS (fluorescent treponemal antibody-absorption)

Non-treponemal Tests

- Non-treponemal tests measure antilipid antibodies (IgG and IgM) released in response to lipoidal material from damaged hosts cells and to cell surface lipids from treponeme
- In pregnant women non-treponemal titres can rise non-specifically
- RPR (rapid plasma regain)
  - a titre of at least 16 is usually found in recent infection
- VDRL (Venereal Disease Research Laboratory carbon antigen test)
- TRUST (toluidine red unheated serum test)

CLINICAL PRESENTATION

Newly Diagnosed Untreated Syphilis

- Benzathine benzylpenicillin 2.4 million units IM single dose
- In the third trimester a repeated dose should be offered after 1 week to reduce risk of treatment failure
- Regular ultrasound follow-up including MCA Doppler every 2 weeks to assess the fetal response to treatment
- Fetal anaemia and ascites should resolve within 4 weeks of successful treatment
- Persistent fetal hepatomegaly does not indicate treatment failure; it may take months to resolve
- Vaginal birth is preferable unless the patient has an active genital lesion

Adequately Treated Previous Infection *and* Normal 20 Weeks Scan

- No need for additional fetal surveillance
- Reassure and refer back to antenatal care

SUGGESTED READING

Khalil A, Sotiriadis A, Chaoui R, et al. ISUOG Practice Guidelines: role of ultrasound in congenital infection. *Ultrasound Obstet Gynecol* 2020;56:128–151.

CYTOMEGALOVIRUS

Buca D, Di Mascio D, Rizzo G, et al. Outcome of fetuses with congenital cytomegalovirus infection: a systematic review and meta-analysis. *Ultrasound Obstet Gynecol* 2020;57:551–559.

RCOG. Congenital cytomegalovirus infection: update on treatment: scientific impact paper No. 56. *BJOG* 2018;125:e1–e11.

Shahar-Nissan K, Pardo J, Peled O, et al. Valaciclovir to prevent vertical transmission of cytomegalovirus after maternal primary infection during pregnancy: a randomised, double-blind, placebo-controlled trial. *Lancet* 2020;396(10253):779–785.

PARVOVIRUS B19

Bascietto F, Liberati M, Murgano D, et al. Outcome of fetuses with congenital parvovirus B19 infection: systematic review and meta-analysis. *Ultrasound Obstet Gynecol* 2018;52:569–576.

Dembinski J, Haverkamp F, Maara H, et al. Neurodevelopmental outcome after intrauterine red cell transfusion for parvovirus B19-induced fetal hydrops. *BJOG* 2002;109(11):1232–1234.

Dijkmans AC, de Jong EP, Dijkmans BAC, et al. Parvovirus B19 in pregnancy: prenatal diagnosis and management of fetal complications. *Curr Opin Obstet Gynecol* 2012;24:95–101.

Zavattoni M, Paolucci S, Sarasini A, et al. Diagnostic and prognostic value of molecular and serological investigation of human parvovirus B19 infection during pregnancy. *New Microbiologica* 2016;39:181–185.

RUBELLA

Bouthry E, Picone O, Hamdi G, et al. Rubella and pregnancy: diagnosis, management and outcomes. *Prenat Diagn* 2014;34:1246–1253.

Yazigi A, De Pecoulas AE, Vauloup-Fellous C, et al. Fetal and neonatal abnormalities due to congenital rubella syndrome: a review of literature. *J Matern Fetal Neonatal Med* 2017;30:274–278.

MEASLES

Congera P, Maraolo AE, Parente S, et al. Measles in pregnant women: a systematic review of clinical outcomes and a meta-analysis of antibodies seroprevalence. *J Infect* 2020;80(2):152–160.

ZIKA

Viens LJ, Fleck-Derderian S, Baez-Santiago MA, et al. Role of prenatal ultrasonography and amniocentesis in the diagnosis of congenital Zika syndrome. *Obstet Gynecol* 2020;135:1185–1197.

TOXOPLASMOSIS

Australasian Society for Infectious Diseases. Toxoplasmosis Gondii. In *Management of Perinatal Infections* (Palasanthiran P, Starr M, Jones C, Giles M, eds). Australasian Society for Infectious Diseases, Sydney, 2014; 69–74.

Azevedo C, Brasil P, Guida L, Moreira ME. Performance of polymerase chain reaction analysis of the amniocytic fluid of pregnant women for the diagnosis of congenital toxoplasmosis: a systematic review and meta-analysis. *PLoS One* 2016;11:e1049938.

Berrébi A, Assouline C, Bessières M-H, et al. Long-term outcome of children with congenital toxoplasmosis. *Am J Obstet Gynecol* 2010;203:552.e1–6.

CNGO. Toxoplasmosis screening during pregnancy in France: opinion of an expert panel for the CNGO. *J Gynecol Obstet Hum Reprod* 2020;49:101814.

Codaccioni C, Picone O, Lambert V et al. Ultrasound features of fetal toxoplasmosis: a contemporary survey in 88 fetuses. *Prenat Diagn* 2020;40:1741–1752.

Mandelbrot L, Keffer F, Sitta R, et al. Prenatal therapy with pyrimethamine and sulfadiazine versus spiramycin to reduce placental transmission of toxoplasmosis: a multicentre, randomised trial. *Am J Obstet Gynecol* 2018;219:386.e1–386.e9.

SYPHILIS

Adhikari EH. Syphilis in pregnancy. *Obstet Gynecol* 2020;135:1121–1135.

Lin JS, Eder ML, Bean SI. Screening for syphilis infection in pregnant women: updated evidence report and systematic review for the US Preventive Services Task Force. *JAMA* 2018;320(9):918–925.

Public Health England. (2015). *Syphilis Serology: UK Standards for Microbiology Investigations.* www.gov.uk/uk-standards-for-microbiologyinvestigations-smi-quality-and-consistency-in-clinical-laboratories

Rac MW, Bryant SN, McIntire DD, et al. Progression of ultrasound findings of fetal syphilis after maternal treatment. *Am J Obstet Gynecol* 2014;211(4):426.e1–426.e6.

CHAPTER 15

Drugs in Pregnancy and Teratogenesis

SUMMARY BOX

DEFINITIONS AND PHASES OF EXPOSURE

Teratogen Physical, chemical, drug, infectious or metabolic agents or maternal diseases which causes a structural or functional derangement of a developing fetus

Susceptibility of a Fetus to a Teratogenic Insult*

1. Depends on fetal genotype and the way the fetus reacts to the adverse agent
2. Varies according to the gestational age at the time of exposure
3. Depends on ways by which the agent acts on fetal tissues to initiate abnormal development
4. Depends on the nature of the agent, which can be physical (such as ionising radiation) or chemical, which can reach fetal tissues through the placenta
5. Results in four possible outcomes: death, malformation, impaired function or growth restriction
6. Dosage of exposure and effect can vary from nothing to lethality

PREIMPLANTATION EXPOSURE

- In the first 2 weeks from conception
- Cells are totipotent and can multiply quickly, even if there is mild damage or cell loss
- 'All or nothing effect': severe insult usually results in death of embryo or no damage
- Malformations are still possible during this time period

Example

- Excessive alcohol intake is associated with an increased risk of miscarriage

EMBRYONIC EXPOSURE

- From third to eighth week of embryo development
- Period known as organogenesis
- Exposure at this stage is most likely to cause malformations

Example

- Coumarin derivatives, such as warfarin, causing nasal bone hypoplasia, epiphyseal stippling and cardiac malformations

FETAL EXPOSURE

- From the ninth week onwards
- Growth and functional maturation of organs take place during this phase
- Organ systems have formed; therefore, exposure results in functional derangement rather than structural malformations

* Wilson JG. *Environment and Birth Defects.* New York, Academic Press, 1973.

Example

- ACE inhibitors causing increased risk of fetal growth restriction and oligohydramnios

CLASSIFICATIONS

THE US FOOD AND DRUG ADMINISTRATION (FDA)

- The FDA categorises drugs into five groups based on evidence-based risk of teratogenicity
  - **Category A:** Controlled studies in women have failed to demonstrate a risk to the fetus in the first trimester and there is no evidence of risk in later trimesters. Medications in this class are considered safe to use in pregnancy
  - **Category B:** Either animal-reproduction studies have not demonstrated a fetal risk, but there are no controlled studies in pregnant women, or animal studies have demonstrated risk to the fetus that was not confirmed in controlled studies in pregnant women in the first trimester and there is no evidence of a risk in later trimesters
  - **Category C:** Studies in animals have revealed adverse effects on the fetus and there are no controlled studies in women, or studies in women and animals are not available. Drugs from this class can be given to pregnant women if the benefit to the mother outweighs the risk to the fetus
  - **Category D:** Evidence of human fetal risk has been documented, but the benefits to the mother may be acceptable despite the risk to the fetus
  - **Category X:** Studies in animals or humans have demonstrated teratogenic effects. The risk to the fetus clearly outweighs any potential benefit to the mother. Drugs in this category are contraindicated in pregnancy
- The FDA are phasing out the use of the above categories in favour of an overview of the known risks and summary of the available data. This means some drugs now are given a 'not assigned' (NA) status

THE AUSTRALIAN THERAPEUTIC GOODS ADMINISTRATION (TGA)

The TGA categorises drugs into the following groups based on evidence-based risk of teratogenicity

- **Category A:** Drugs which have been taken by a large number of pregnant women without any proven increase in the frequency of malformations, or other direct or indirect harmful effects on the fetus having been observed
- **Category B:** Drugs which have been taken by only a limited number of pregnant women, without an increase in the frequency of malformation or other direct or indirect harmful effects on the human fetus having been observed. Subcategorisations are based on animal data only as human data are lacking
  - **B1:** Studies in animals have not shown evidence of an increased occurrence of fetal damage
  - **B2:** Studies in animals are inadequate or may be lacking, but available data show no evidence of an increased occurrence of fetal damage
  - **B3:** Studies in animals have shown evidence of an increased occurrence of fetal damage, the significance of which is considered uncertain in humans
- **Category C:** Drugs which, due to their pharmacological effects, have caused or may be suspected of causing harmful effects on the human fetus or neonate without causing malformations. These effects may be reversible

- **Category D:** Drugs which have caused, are suspected to have caused or may be expected to cause an increased incidence of human fetal malformations or irreversible damage
- **Category X**: Drugs which have such a high risk of causing permanent damage to the fetus that they should not be used in pregnancy

COUNSELLING REGARDING DRUG USE IN PREGNANCY AND TERATOGENIC POTENTIAL

- Ideally, counselling should be arranged preconception
- Some drugs, such as sodium valproate, warfarin and isotretinoin, should not be commenced in women of childbearing potential without appropriate counselling and ideally should be avoided. If they need to be prescribed then specialist counselling regarding the risks and appropriate contraceptive advice and provisions are imperative
- Any teratogenic drug should be stopped or replaced by a less teratogenic drug or reduced to its lowest effective dose in conjunction with the woman's medical specialist or GP
- Good control of the maternal disease is the priority. The effects of poorly controlled maternal disease have the potential for poor pregnancy outcomes, often worse than many of the potential risks of drug treatments
- An early pregnancy scan is essential in order to elucidate the timing of any exposure and therefore the potential risks
- Reassurance should be given for FDA and TGA category A, B and C drugs
- Specialist fetal medicine ultrasound assessment may be needed for Class D or X drugs

TERATOGENS

ANTIBIOTICS

Name	FDA/TGA category	Risk of congenital malformations
Aminoglycosides *e.g. gentamicin*	D/D	No evidence of increased risk (but known association with ototoxicity and nephrotoxicity)
Cefalosporins *e.g. cefalexin*	B/A	Evidence shows no increased risk
Clindamycin	B/A	No evidence of increased risk in first trimester Evidence shows no increased risk in second and third trimesters or with topical/gel preparations
Macrolides *e.g. azithromycin* *e.g. erythromycin* *e.g. clarithromycin*	 B/B1 NA/A C/B2	No strong evidence of increased risk
Metronidazole	NA/B2	No strong evidence of increased risk
Penicillins *e.g. amoxicillin*	B/A	Evidence shows no increased risk

(*cont.*)

Name	FDA/TGA category	Risk of congenital malformations
Quinolones *e.g. ciprofloxacin*	C/B3	No strong evidence of increased risk
TB treatment: isoniazid and rifampicin	C/C	No evidence of increased risk
Tetracyclines *e.g. doxycycline*	D/D	No strong evidence of increased risk (but known association with teeth and bone discoloration with use from 18 weeks)
Trimethoprim	NA/B3	Possible increased risk of neural tube defects, cardiac defects and orofacial clefts with use in first trimester No evidence of increased risk in second and third trimesters

ANTICOAGULANTS

Name	FDA/TGA category	Risk of congenital malformations*
Clopidogrel	NA/B1	Evidence shows no increased risk
Heparin and low molecular weight heparin	B/C	Evidence shows no increased risk
Novel oral anticoagulants (NOACs) *e.g. rivaroxaban* *apixaban* *dabigatran*	 NA/C NA/C NA/C	No evidence of increased risk
Warfarin	**NA/D**	• **Fetal warfarin syndrome** (Fig. 15.1): – **Nasal hypoplasia** – **Epiphyseal calcification of long bones and vertebrae** – **Cardiac defects (thin atrial septum, coarctation)** • **Situs inversus** • **Risk could be as high as 30%** • **Doses above 5 mg pose the highest risk** • **Should be stopped at least 1 month prior to conception**

* Those highlighted in bold require specialist fetal medicine referral and targeted ultrasound assessment.

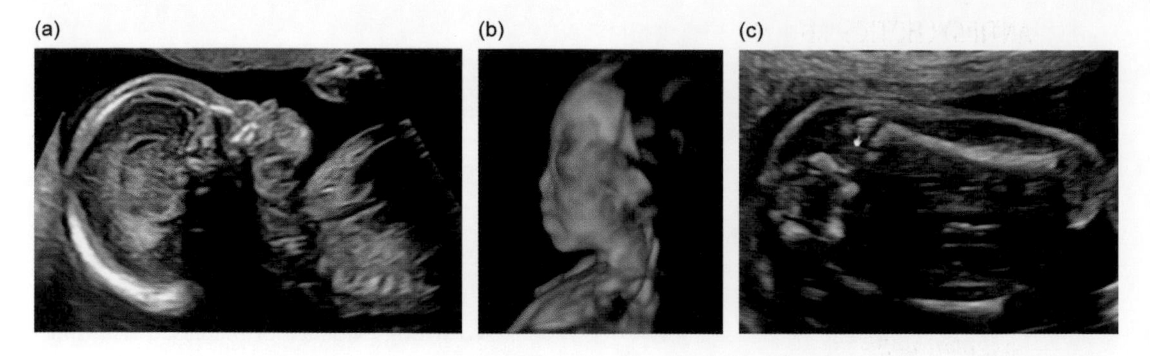

Fig. 15.1 Warfarin embryopathy: (a) mid-sagittal view of the face showing midfacial hypoplasia, hypoplastic nasal bone and depressed nasal bridge; (b) 3D image of the fetal face showing the typical facial phenotype; (c) typical focal bone calcifications (stippling).

ANTIDEPRESSANTS

Name	FDA/TGA category	Risk of congenital malformations
Selective serotonin reuptake inhibitors (SSRIs) *e.g. citalopram* *e.g. fluoxetine* *e.g. sertraline* *e.g. paroxetine*	 C/C C/C NA/C D/D	No strong evidence of increased risk
Serotonin and norepinephrine reuptake inhibitors (SNRIs) *e.g. duloxetine* *e.g. venlafaxine*	 NA/B3 C/B2	Evidence suggests no increased risk
Tricyclics *e.g. amitriptyline*	C/C	No strong evidence of increased risk

ANTIPSYCHOTICS AND MOOD STABILISERS[§]

Name	FDA/TGA category	Risk of congenital malformations*
First generation		No evidence of increased risk
e.g. haloperidol	C/C	
e.g. chlorpromazine	NA/C	
Second generation		
e.g. olanzapine	C/C	Evidence shows no increased risk
e.g. clozapine	B/C	No evidence of increased risk
e.g. quetiapine	C/C	Evidence shows no increased risk
e.g. risperidone	C/C	No strong evidence of increased risk
e.g. aripiprazole	NA/C	Evidence shows no increased risk
Lithium*	**NA/D**	• **Cardiac defects (Ebstein's anomaly)** (Fig. 15.2)

[§] See Antiepileptics for more commonly used mood stabilisers.
* Those highlighted in bold require specialist fetal medicine referral and targeted ultrasound assessment.

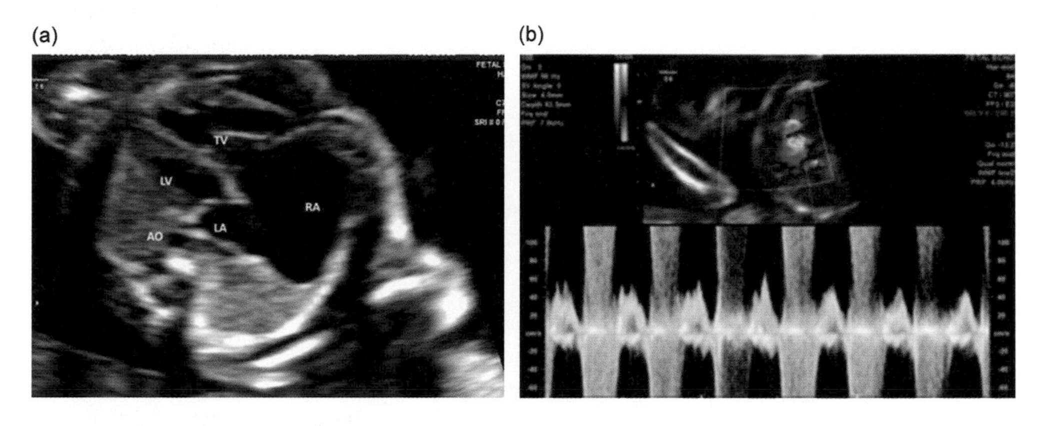

Fig. 15.2 Ebstein's anomaly.(a) Four chamber view of the heart showing a dilated right atrium (RA), apically placed tricuspid valve (TV). AO, aorta; LA: left atrium; LV, left ventricle. (b) Colour and pulsed Doppler of the same fetus showing severe tricuspid regurgitation. Note the significant aliasing on the pulsed Doppler.

ANTIEPILEPTICS

- Women on antiepileptic drugs (AEDs) planning pregnancy need to undergo pre-pregnancy counselling with an experienced clinician to discuss options around switching over to less teratogenic drugs or lowering the dose to reduce any risk of fetal malformations while balancing good seizure control
- All should be commenced on 5 mg folic acid once daily from 3 months preconception until at least 12 weeks of pregnancy

- Women on AEDs are at increased risk of a small for gestational age fetus and therefore should have ultrasound surveillance of fetal growth
- The background risk of congenital malformations in women with epilepsy is ~3%, which is similar to the general population risk
- The lowest risk seems to be with lamotrigine <300 mg/day; risk is similar to background risk
- Risk for valproate ~11%
- Polytherapy is also high-risk, but the data are too variable to suggest any accurate risk values. The risk will depend on the combination and dosages prescribed.

Name	FDA/TGA category	Risk of congenital malformations*
Carbamazepine	**D/D**	**Evidence suggests possible increased risk with doses >1,000 mg/day:** • **orofacial clefts** • **facial: hypertelorism, nose hypoplasia** • **neural tube defects** • **cardiac defects**
Clonazepam	NA/B3	No evidence of increased risk
Gabapentin	NA/B3	No evidence of increased risk
Lamotrigine	NA/D	Evidence shows no increased risk
Levetiracetam	C/B3	Evidence shows no increased risk
Lorazepam	NA/C	No evidence of increased risk
Phenobarbital	**D/D**	• **Cardiac malformations** • **Facial clefts**
Phenytoin	**D/D**	• **Orofacial clefts** • **Cardiac defects** • **Microcephaly** • **Digit hypoplasia**
Pregabalin	NA/B3	Evidence shows no increased risk
Primidone	**NA/D**	• **Neural tube defects** • **Orofacial clefts** • **Cardiac defects**
Sodium valproate	**NA/D**	• **Neural tube defects** • **Craniofacial defects (flat nasal bridge, orofacial clefts, craniosynostosis)** • **Cardiac defects (ASD)** • **Limb abnormalities** • **Genitourinary defects**
Tiagabine	C/B3	No evidence of increased risk

(*cont.*)

Name	FDA/TGA category	Risk of congenital malformations*
Topiramate	**NA/D**	• **Orofacial clefts**
Trimethadione	**NA/–**	• **Orofacial clefts** • **Cardiac defects** • **Genitourinary defects** • **Limb abnormalities**
Zonisamide	C/D	No evidence of increased risk

* Those highlighted in bold require specialist fetal medicine referral and targeted ultrasound assessment.

ANTIHYPERTENSIVES

Name	FDA/TGA category	Risk of congenital malformations*
Alpha-blockers *e.g. doxazosin*	NA/B3	No evidence of increased risk
Angiotensin-converting enzyme (ACE) inhibitors *e.g. ramipril*	**D/D**	• First trimester: evidence shows no increased risk • **Second and third trimester: risk of oligohydramnios, fetal growth restriction and stillbirth**
Angiotensin II receptor blockers (ARBs) *e.g. candesartan*	**D/D**	• First trimester: evidence shows no increased risk • **Second and third trimester: risk of oligohydramnios and resulting joint contractures, incompletely formed skull bones, pulmonary hypoplasia**
Beta blockers *e.g. bisoprolol*	C/C	Evidence shows no increased risk of malformations but increased risk of fetal growth restriction – should have ultrasound surveillance of fetal growth
Calcium channel blockers *e.g. nifedipine*	C/C	No strong evidence of increased risk
Clonidine	C/B3	No evidence of increased risk
Methyldopa	B/A	Evidence shows no increased risk
Thiazides *e.g. indapamide*	C/C	No strong evidence of increased risk

* Those highlighted in bold require specialist fetal medicine referral and targeted ultrasound assessment.

AUTOIMMUNE DISEASE DRUGS

Name	FDA/TGA category	Risk of congenital malformations*
Anti-TNF agents *e.g. infliximab*	NA/C	No strong evidence of increased risk
Azathioprine	D/D	Evidence shows no increased risk
B-cell depleting agents *e.g. rituximab*	NA/C	No evidence of increased risk
Calcineurin inhibitors *e.g. tacrolimus* *e.g. ciclosporin*	 NA/C C/C	Evidence shows no increased risk Should have ultrasound surveillance of fetal growth
Corticosteroids	C/A	Topical, inhaled, intranasal: evidence shows no increased risk Oral: no strong evidence of increased risk High-dose prolonged courses require ultrasound surveillance of fetal growth
Hydroxychloroquine	NA/D	Evidence shows no increased risk
Leflunomide	**X/X**	**No specific malformations in the literature, but pregnancy should be avoided for at least 2 years after treatment** **If conception occurs while taking medication, advise a cholestyramine drug elimination procedure**
Methotrexate	**X/D**	**Risk of fetal methotrexate syndrome with high doses ≥ 50 mg/m^2** • **Craniofacial defects (microcephaly, craniosynostosis)** • **Cardiac defects (tetralogy of Fallot)** • **Renal defects** • **Limb and digit abnormalities** • **Skeletal abnormalities (spine and ribs)** • **Pregnancy should be avoided for at least 3 months after treatment**

(cont.)

Name	FDA/TGA category	Risk of congenital malformations*
Mycophenolate mofetil	D/D	• **Orofacial clefts** • **Cardiac defect** • **Craniofacial defects: microtia, microcephaly, micrognathia, microphthalmia** • **Oesophageal atresia** • **Congenital diaphragmatic hernia** • **Skeletal abnormalities** **Risk ~25%** **Should be stopped at least 3 months prior to conception**
Non-steroidal anti-inflammatory drugs (NSAIDs)	NA/C	• First and second trimester: no strong evidence of increased risk • **Third Trimester: evidence suggests increased risk of oligohydramnios and premature closure of the ductus arteriosus with prolonged use**
Penicillamine	D/D	No strong evidence of increased risk
Sulfasalazine	B/A	Evidence shows no increased risk

* Those highlighted in bold require specialist fetal medicine referral and targeted ultrasound assessment.

CHEMOTHERAPY AGENTS

- Chemotherapy should be avoided in the first trimester of pregnancy, but it is crucial that there are minimal delays to any treatment for any women diagnosed with cancer
- Many chemotherapy agents are considered safe in the second trimester (from 14 weeks) and third trimester of pregnancy
- Women on chemotherapy should have ultrasound monitoring in view of the risk of fetal growth restriction and preterm birth

Breast Cancer

Name	FDA/TGA category	Risk of congenital malformations*
Cyclophosphamide	NA/D	• **Skeletal abnormalities** • **Limb abnormalities** • **Orofacial clefts** • **Ocular abnormalities** **Pregnancy should be avoided for 12 months after treatment**

(*cont.*)

Name	FDA/TGA category	Risk of congenital malformations*
Docetaxel	D/D	No strong evidence of increased risk
Doxorubicin	D/D	No strong evidence of increased risk Pregnancy should be avoided for 6 months after treatment
Epirubicin	**NA/D**	**No strong evidence of increased risk when used in the second or third trimester but cardiotoxicity has been reported** **Pregnancy should be avoided for 6 months after treatment**
Fluorouracil	D/D	No strong evidence of increased risk Pregnancy should be avoided for 6 months after treatment
Idarubicin	**D/D**	**One reported case of use in pregnancy which resulted in stillbirth**
Tamoxifen	**D/B3**	• **Goldenhar syndrome (oculoauriculovertebral dysplasia)** • **Genital abnormalities** **Pregnancy should be avoided for 2 months after treatment**
Trastuzumab (Herceptin)	**NA/D**	**Risk of reversible oligo/anhydramnios causing pulmonary hypoplasia and/or skeletal abnormalities** **Pregnancy should be avoided for 7 months after treatment**

* Those highlighted in bold require specialist fetal medicine referral and targeted ultrasound assessment.

Ovarian Cancer

Name	FDA/TGA category	Risk of congenital malformations
Bevacizumab	NA/D	No strong evidence of increased risk
Carboplatin	D/D	No strong evidence of increased risk
Paclitaxel	NA/D	No strong evidence of increased risk Pregnancy should be avoided for 6 months after treatment

Cervical Cancer

Name	FDA/TGA category	Risk of congenital malformations
Cisplatin	NA/D	No strong evidence of increased risk but some reports of oligohydramnios Pregnancy should be avoided for 14 months after treatment

Haematological Cancers

Name	FDA/TGA category	Risk of congenital malformations
Cytarabine	D/D	Evidence suggests no increased risk
Vincristine	D/D	No strong evidence of increased risk

Skin Cancer

Name	FDA/TGA category	Risk of congenital malformations
Dacarbazine	C/D	No strong evidence of increased risk

ABORTIFACIENTS[§]

Name	FDA/TGA category	Risk of congenital malformations*
Mifepristone	X/–	Evidence shows no increased risk
Misoprostol	**NA/X**	• **Limb abnormalities** • **Arthrogryposis** • **Facial defects**

§ See Autoimmune Disease Drugs for methotrexate.

* Those highlighted in bold require specialist fetal medicine referral and targeted ultrasound assessment.

SUBSTANCE MISUSE

Name	Risk of congenital malformations*
Alcohol	**Teratogenic effects seen in pregnant women who are chronic, heavy drinkers (>5 units/day)** **Fetal alcohol syndrome:** • **maxillary hypoplasia** • **macrophthalmia** • **cardiac defects** • **fetal growth restriction**
Amphetamine	No strong evidence of increased risk, but regular use during pregnancy requires ultrasound surveillance of fetal growth
Cannabis/marijuana	No strong evidence of increased risk, but some cases of neural tube defects, gastroschisis and ventricular septal defects have been reported Regular use during pregnancy requires ultrasound surveillance of fetal growth
Cocaine	**Teratogenic effects have been seen in pregnant women using cocaine:** • **limb abnormalities** • **gastrointestinal tract defects** • **urinary tract defects** • **skeletal abnormalities** • **cardiac defects** • **fetal growth restriction**
Heroin	No strong evidence of increased risk Requires ultrasound surveillance of fetal growth
LSD	**Teratogenic effects may be seen with frequent or high-dose usage:** • **limb abnormalities** • **ocular defects** • **central nervous system defects**
MDMA/ecstasy	**No conclusive evidence of increased, risk but possible association with gastroschisis reported. Consider fetal medicine review with frequent or high-dose usage.**

* Those highlighted in bold require specialist fetal medicine referral and targeted ultrasound assessment.

VITAMINS

Name	FDA/TGA category	Risk of congenital malformations*
Vitamin isotretinoin	**X/X**	• **Craniofacial defects (small/abnormal/absent ears, micrognathia, cleft palate, ocular hypertelorism)** • **Thymic abnormalities (hypoplasia, aplasia, ectopia)** **>10,000 IU/day:** • **Cardiac defects (Fallot's tetralogy, AVSDs, TGA, aortic arch hypoplasia)** • **CNS abnormalities (microcephaly, hydrocephalus, cortical and cerebellar defects)** • **Has a very long half-life; therefore, has to be discontinued at least 1 month before pregnancy** • **Risk ~20%**
Vitamin B/ C/D/E/K		No strong evidence of increased risk with excess or deficiency General malnutrition is a risk factor for fetal growth restriction

* Those highlighted in bold require specialist fetal medicine referral and targeted ultrasound assessment.

IONISING RADIATION

- Ionising radiation due to exposure to X-rays and CT scans is calculated in terms of the dosage that is delivered during the examination
- The dosage is expressed as rads or, currently preferred, milligray (mGy); 1 rad = 10 mGy
- Most diagnostic imaging modalities deliver <50 mGy to the fetus
- Fetal exposure to <50 mGy is considered to be of minimal teratogenic risk
- Exposure between the second and fifteenth week of gestation is considered 'high risk' – doses exceeding 150 mGy should be considered as a potential indication for therapeutic abortion.

	Radiation dose	Comment
X-ray		
A single radiograph	0.001–10 mGy	Well below the risk threshold Lumbar spine radiograph is the highest radiation dose at 10 mGy

(*cont.*)

	Radiation dose	Comment
Computed tomography		
CT abdomen and pelvis	Dose varies depending on type of CT performed Highest dose is with a CT pelvis at ~50 mGy	To be avoided during pregnancy if possible
CT that does not involve the abdomen and pelvis, e.g. CTPA (CT pulmonary angiogram)	Minimal scattered radiation to the fetus but this needs to be weighed up against high-dose to maternal breast tissue	Can be performed as per institutional protocol An ultrasound to first rule out DVT is advisable

Nuclear medicine	Exposure	Comment
VQ (ventilation/perfusion) scan	Slightly higher radiation dose to fetus than CTPA but still considered minimal and lower radiation to maternal breast tissue	• Can be performed as per institutional protocol • Lowest risk is with low-dose perfusion scan only • An ultrasound to first rule out DVT is advisable
Other radiopharmaceutical imaging with or without CT	Exposure depends on several conditions: • maternal uptake • the dose and half-life of the radiotracer • urinary excretion • placental permeability • if CT also performed	• Best avoided unless for very compelling reasons • Alternative modalities like ultrasound and MRI should be considered first
Thyroid radioactive iodine scan	Iodine 121 and 131 cross the placenta and are taken up by the fetal thyroid	Contraindicated in pregnancy

MRI	Exposure	Comment
Standard MRI	Not associated with risk for the fetus	Considered safe at any trimester
MRI with gadolinium	Increased risk of: • inflammatory or infiltrative skin conditions • perinatal deaths	Contraindicated at any stage of pregnancy

Angiography and fluoroscopy	Best avoided and should be used only in emergency situations

SUGGESTED READING

Australian Government, Department of Health, Therapeutic Goods Administration: www.tga.gov.au
FDA categories and summaries: www.drugs.com
Kumar R, De Jesus O. Radiation effects on the fetus. 2021. www.ncbi.nlm.nih.gov/books/NBK564358
RCOG. Green-Top Guideline No. 68: Epilepsy in Pregnancy. 2016. www.rcog.org.uk/guidance/browse-all-guidance/green-top-guidelines/epilepsy-in-pregnancy-green-top-guideline-no-68.
UK Teratology Information Service: www.uktis.org

CHAPTER 16

Ultrasound Guided Invasive Diagnostic and Therapeutic Procedures

SUMMARY BOX

GENERAL PRINCIPLES

COUNSELLING

- Individual counselling should cover the indication, intended benefits, procedure-related risks and potential consequences of not performing the procedure
- Availability, advantages and disadvantages of different diagnostic tests should be discussed (PCR, conventional karyotype, microarray, exome)
- Written patient information should be provided, if available
- All invasive procedures should be subject to informed written consent
- Clear records should be maintained, including details of the information provided and options for communicating results

ANTISEPTIC PROCEDURES

- Use sterile gloves
- In most centres sterile gowns are used only for longer procedures (transfusions, shunts, amniodrainage)
- Cleaning the skin is done with an antiseptic-based solution
- Use of a sterile cover for ultrasound probe and sterile gel, although not universal, is recommended
- Prophylactic antibiotics, most commonly single IV dose of cephalosporins, are used for more complex procedures, but not for CVS or amniocentesis

TECHNIQUE

- Continuous ultrasound guidance is achieved either by using a free-hand technique or a needle guide
- The puncture site is infiltrated with a local anaesthetic (e.g. 10 ml lidocaine 1%)
- Local infiltration is also helpful to map the needle path when a free-hand technique is used

POST-PROCEDURE MANAGEMENT

- Provide anti-D prophylaxis if Rhesus-negative and non-sensitised; the dose used varies between 500 and 750 IU (200–300 μg)
- Ensure that the timeline and method of communicating results is shared with the woman
- There is no good evidence for use of prophylactic tocolysis, hospital admission or bed rest
- Women can go home as soon as they feel able post-procedure
- Routine prescription of analgesia is not required, paracetamol can be taken at home if required
- We advise that strenuous activity is avoided for 48 hours
- Women are advised to seek medical advice if pain is not relieved by paracetamol, or there are any other concerns
- Provide emergency contact details

CHORIONIC VILLUS SAMPLING

Indications

- Genetic testing in early pregnancy

Gestational Age

- 11^{+0} to 14^{+6} weeks

Procedure-Related Risk

- Miscarriage risk is less than 1 in 200 (<0.5%) in the hands of experienced operators (with at least 30 ultrasound guided procedures per annum)
- Women with multiple pregnancies should be informed that the additional risk of miscarriage for twin pregnancy may be slightly higher (~1%).

Transabdominal or Transvaginal Approach?

- There is no good evidence to prove that, in experienced hands, one approach is safer than the other (Figs. 16.1 and 16.2)
- In our centres, transvaginal CVS is performed rarely, only in cases of low-lying posterior placenta
- For most cases where the placenta cannot be accessed safely by the transabdominal route, this should be feasible 7–10 days later (Fig. 16.2)

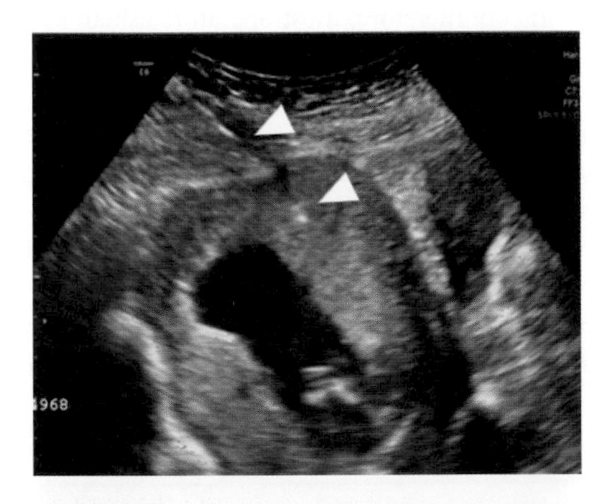

Fig. 16.1 Transabdominal CVS. An 18G needle is inserted through the abdominal wall into the anterior placenta (arrowheads).

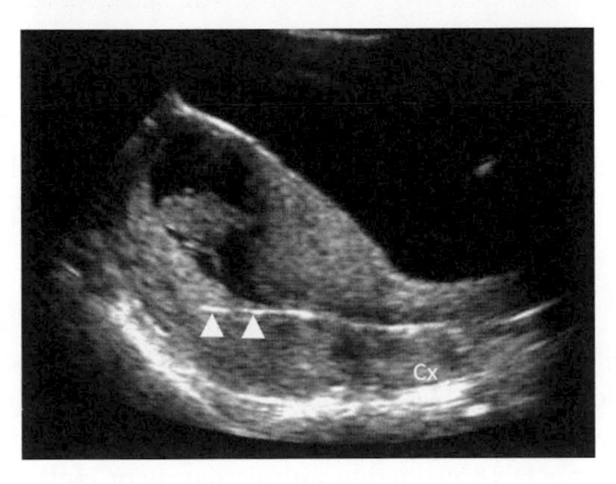

Fig. 16.2 Transcervical CVS. Note the canula (arrowheads) introduced trough the cervix into the posterior placenta. Cx, cervix.

TRANSABDOMINAL TECHNIQUE

- Draw up 3–4 ml culture medium in the suction syringe to prime the needle and syringe (and three-way tap if using) to facilitate aspiration of the villi
- Two aspiration methods are commonly used; there is no good evidence than one method is superior to the other:
  - single needle (usually 18G (1.27 mm))
  - double needle (usually 18G outer; 21G (0.82 mm) inner)
- In order to ensure optimal positioning of the needle, the ultrasound probe and the needle should be handled by the same operator. In some centres a needle guide is used to facilitate correct placement of the needle
- Once the needle is positioned within the placenta, a 10 ml or 20 ml syringe is attached to the needle, either directly or via ~20 cm plastic tube
- The sample is obtained by moving the needle back and forth 3–4 times in a fan-shaped target area
- The best samples are obtained when the needle path is parallel with the chorionic plate in the middle of placenta above cord insertion
- Some operators will choose to aspirate themselves, holding a probe with one hand and a syringe attached to the needle with the other hand. Generating adequate negative pressure using this technique may be quite difficult; therefore, most operators ask an assistant to generate negative pressure
- If an assistant is used, good communication and coordination is needed to ensure that adequate negative pressure is generated at the right time, without pulling on the needle
- The negative pressure must be maintained until the needle is fully withdrawn from the skin, allowing air to enter in the syringe
- The aspirate is transferred to a sterile container and inspected visually before transport to the lab, to ensure adequacy of the sample
- In twin pregnancies it is important to sample each fetus and to label samples appropriately in order that the results of the tests can be attributed to the appropriate fetus
- Our technique is demonstrated in the video that can be accessed at www.rcog.org.uk/en/guidelines-research-services/guidelines/gtg8

MULTIPLE PREGNANCY

- As dichorionic twins are mostly dizygotic (~85%), double ('two-entry') CVS or double amniocentesis should be done
- Monochorionic twins can be assessed through a single CVS (across the whole placenta)
- For more details, see Chapter 12

WHAT IS AN ADEQUATE SAMPLE?

- Inspection can be done with the naked eye (Fig. 16.3) or under a microscope
- 1–5 mg: limited testing may be possible (e.g. QF-PCR only). The need for additional testing is reviewed on a case-by-case basis, depending upon the reasons for referral
- 5–9 mg: will require cultured cells for DNA extraction for microarray or molecular testing. Results will take longer in view of additional time needed to grow culture material
- ≥10 mg: usually adequate for testing uncultured material

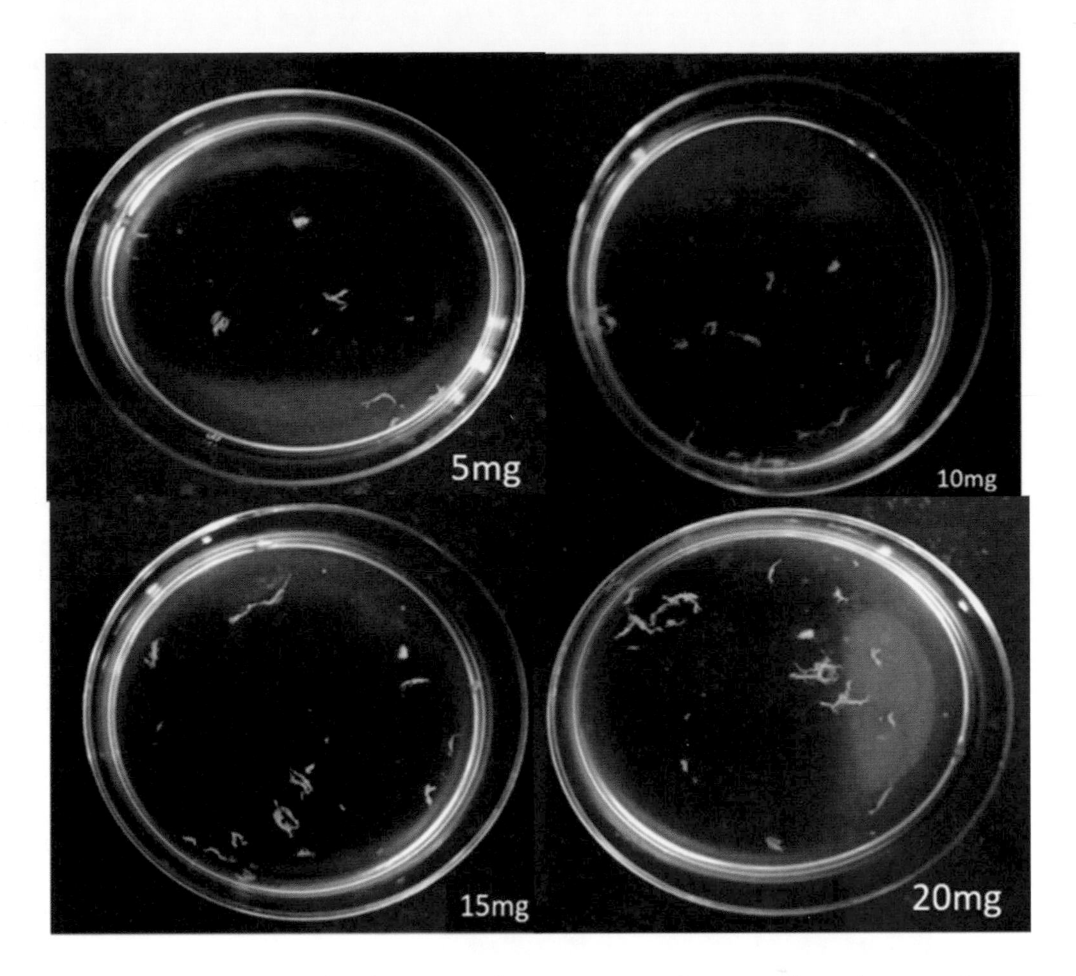

Fig. 16.3 Chorionic villi samples of 5, 10, 15 and 20 mg; 5 mg samples are usually inadequate and 10 mg are borderline. Most laboratories may ask for a second sample.

AMNIOCENTESIS

Indications

- Testing for genetic conditions, fetal infections, identification of blood group/platelet type. Testing of amniotic fluid for suspected neural tube defects or for fetal lung maturity is rarely offered

Gestational Age

- After 15^{+0} weeks
- The procedure should be delayed if amnion and chorion are not fused

Procedure-Related Risk

- In the hands of experienced operators (with at least 30 ultrasound guided procedures per annum) the risk of pregnancy loss before 24^{+0} weeks is less than 1 in 200 (<0.5%), with equivalent risk of preterm birth after 24^{+0} weeks

- Women with multiple pregnancies should be informed that the additional risk of miscarriage for twin pregnancy may be slightly higher (~1%)

TECHNIQUE

- Local anaesthesia is not used for this procedure
- A pool of liquor that is clear of fetal parts and umbilical cord is targeted (Fig. 16.4)
- Transplacental passage, avoiding placental cord insertion with the help of colour Doppler, is a reasonable alternative if this provides the safest route. There is no evidence of increased risk of procedure-related complications (Fig. 16.5)
- Using a 21 or 22G needle, a ~20 ml sample should be obtained for analysis (Fig. 16.6)
- Sample volumes <20 ml and samples and obtained before 16^{+0} weeks are at higher risk of low quantities of DNA from direct extraction, with potential for longer turnaround time for results
- Our technique is demonstrated in the video that can be accessed at www.rcog.org.uk/en/guidelines-research-services/guidelines/gtg8

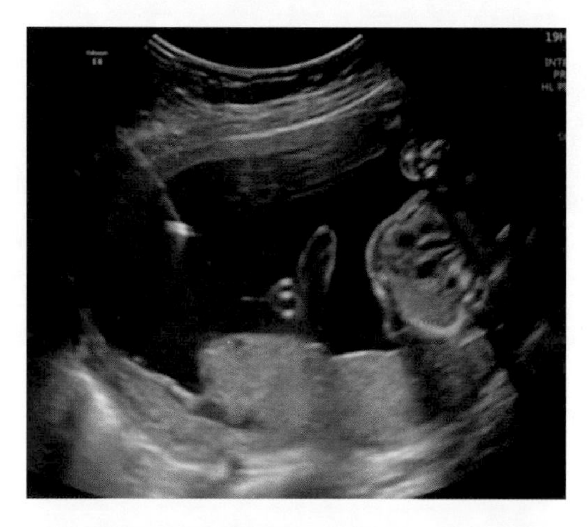

Fig. 16.4 Amniocentesis. The needle is introduced through a placenta-free window into a pool of amniotic fluid.

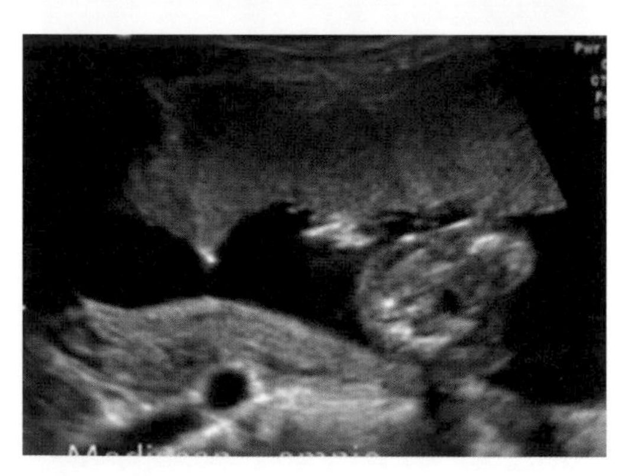

Fig. 16.5 Amniocentesis through the placenta. When unavoidable, the needle can be inserted through the placenta. A quick jab is needed to enter the amniotic cavity. A 'tenting' of the membrane is seen due to slow introduction of the needle.

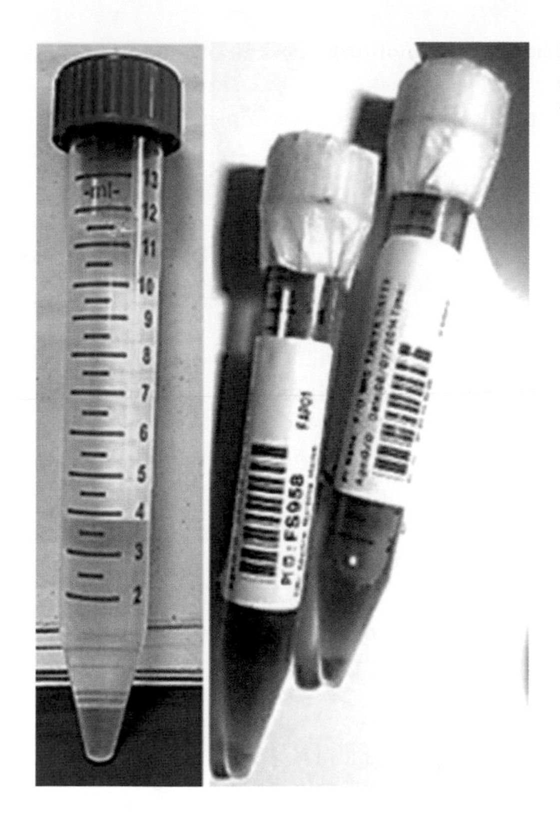

Fig. 16.6 Amniotic fluid samples. The first tube shows clear amniotic fluid. The second and third tubes are blood-stained.

FETAL BLOOD SAMPLING

Indications

- Full blood count analysis for suspected anaemia and thrombocytopenia
- Liver function tests in fetal infections (some centres)
- Genetic studies (rarely needed)

Procedure-Related Risks

- ~1–2 in 100 (1–2%) procedure-related risk of pregnancy loss before 24^{+0} weeks, with equivalent risk of preterm birth after 24^{+0} weeks
- Overall risk of pregnancy loss or preterm birth is likely to be higher due to underlying pathology

Gestational Age

- Feasible from 16 weeks, but technically very challenging before 20 weeks

TECHNIQUE

- Consider using vecuronium or pancuronium (0.1 mg/kg) for fetal paralysis, particularly where fetal blood sampling may be followed by an in utero transfusion
- If the fetus is judged to be viable, it is good practice to liaise with the delivery suite to discuss the most appropriate time when an emergency theatre can be made available in

case of persistent fetal bradycardia (≥3 min, not responsive to cessation of procedure and change to left lateral position)
- Liaise with the onsite laboratory to alert them to expect samples for immediate processing
- At least two assistants are required, one to remain in the procedure room and receive blood samples, and the other to take fetal blood samples to the laboratory if fetal transfusion is planned
- As a rule, placental cord insertion or intrahepatic umbilical vein can be sampled to obtain blood (Figs. 16.7 and 16.8)
- We avoid free loops of cord as a target because mobility increases the challenge of sighting the needle. Dislodging of the needle during infusion is also much more likely
- Cardiocentesis is only used in cases of early ascites (<20 weeks) when access to fetal vessels is not possible and the risk of imminent fetal demise is high (Fig. 16.9)
- Using a 20G needle, the target vessel is approached and the needle tip placed next to the vessel wall. The needle is then advanced swiftly to puncture the vessel wall
- If the needle is positioned correctly, the blood should be flowing freely into the needle
- 1 ml sample volume is usually sufficient for haemoglobin estimation; more will be needed if additional tests are necessary (e.g. direct Coomb's test)

POST-PROCEDURE MANAGEMENT: PROCEDURE-SPECIFIC POINTS

- Fetal heart rate should be checked after the procedure. If there is no transient bradycardia and no signs of bleeding from the puncture site, there is no need for further fetal monitoring
- If transient fetal bradycardia is observed in a viable fetus for more than 30 seconds, or there is bleeding from the puncture site (≥1 min), a CTG should be arranged within 1 hour of the procedure, lasting at least 30 minutes
- An individualised plan should be made regarding hospital admission, but most uncomplicated fetal blood sampling cases (+/– transfusions) can be discharged home post-procedure

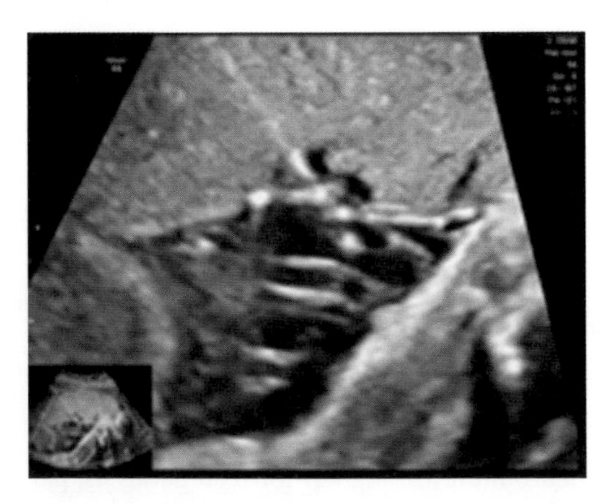

Fig. 16.7 Fetal blood sampling. The needle is inserted through the base of the cord.

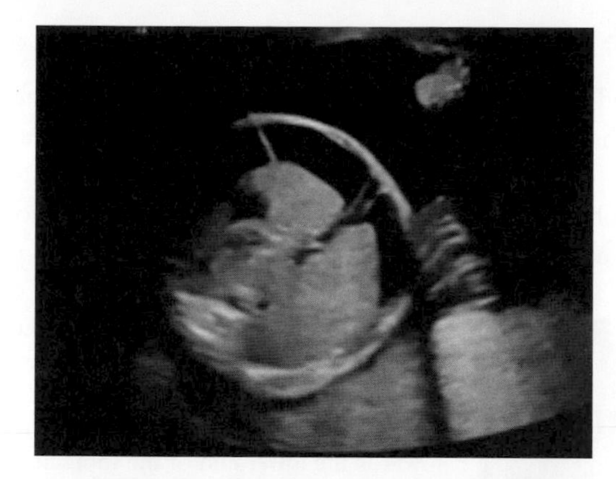

Fig.16.8 Intrahepatic fetal blood sampling. The needle is introduced into the intrahepatic portion of the umbilical vein.

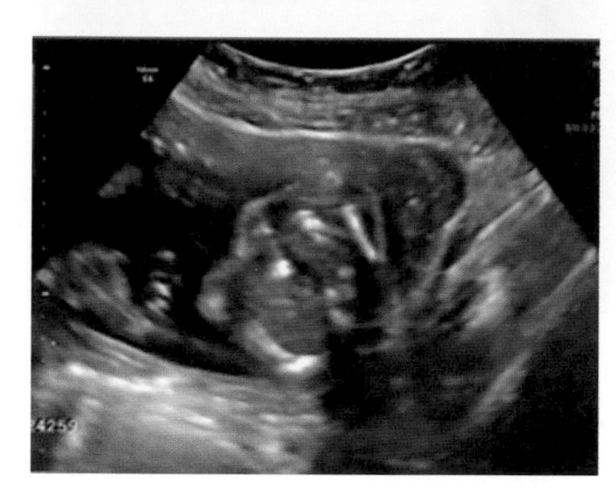

Fig.16.9 Fetal cardiac sampling. Sampling of fetal blood can be done directly from the fetal heart when there is no other access.

FETAL TAPS

Indications

- Fluid-filled fetal body cavities (bladder, ascites, chest, cysts) may be aspirated for diagnostic purposes, such as to analyse fluid constituents (biochemistry, cytology) and to assess the rate for reaccumulation (Fig. 16.10)
- These procedures may also be therapeutic to facilitate neonatal resuscitation (ventilation) and prevent soft tissue dystocia during vaginal delivery

Gestational Age

- 18 weeks onwards

Procedure-Related Risks

- ~1–2 in 100 (1–2%) procedure-related risk of pregnancy loss before 24^{+0} weeks, with equivalent risk of preterm birth after 24^{+0} weeks
- Overall risk of pregnancy loss or preterm birth is likely to be higher due to underlying pathology

POST-PROCEDURE MANAGEMENT: PROCEDURE-SPECIFIC POINTS

- Fetal heart rate should be checked after the procedure – if there is no transient bradycardia and no signs of bleeding from the puncture site, there is no need for further fetal monitoring post-procedure
- If transient fetal bradycardia is observed in a viable fetus, or there is bleeding from the puncture site, a CTG should be arranged within 1 hour of the procedure

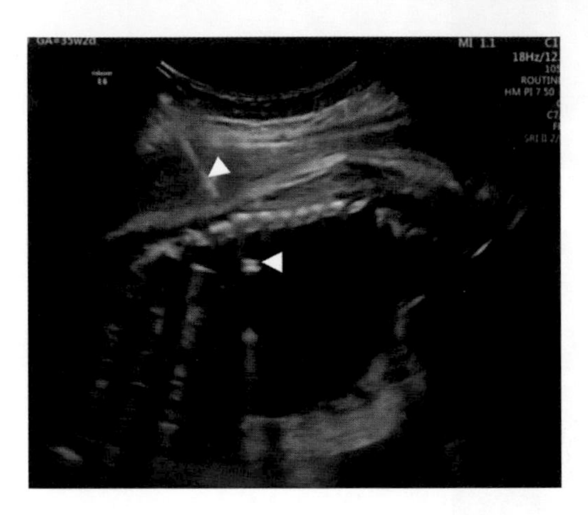

Fig. 16.10 Thoracocentesis. Percutaneous aspiration of a large hydrothorax. The needle (arrowheads) is inserted through the intercostal space, preferably along the mid-clavicular line, towards the lower end of the thoracic cavity.

AMNIODRAINAGE AND AMNIOINFUSION

Indications

Amniodrainage

- Clinically symptomatic polyhydramnios (breathlessness, pain)

Amnioinfusion

- May be used to improve visualisation of fetal anatomy in anhydramnios
- There is no good evidence to support its use to improve lung development in oligo/anhydramnios caused by PPROM or renal disease

Procedure-Related Risks

- ~1–2 in 100 (1–2%) risk of pregnancy loss before 24^{+0} weeks with equivalent risk of preterm birth after 24^{+0}, but overall risk of pregnancy loss or preterm birth is likely to be significantly higher due to underlying pathology

TECHNIQUE

- When performing amnioinfusion, a three-way tap should be connected to the needle on one side and on the other side to a giving set connected to a 1 L bag of 0.9% normal saline, which can be manually squeezed or infused using a pressure bag
- Sufficient volume should be infused to normalise maximum pool depth

FETAL BLOOD TRANSFUSION

Indications

- Fetal anaemia
- Severe fetal thrombocytopenia ($<20 \times 10^9$/L)

Gestational Age

- Feasible from 16 weeks, but more technically challenging before 20 weeks

Procedure-Related Risks

- ~1–2 in 100 (1–2%) risk of pregnancy loss with equivalent risk of preterm birth after 24 weeks, attributable to the procedure
- Overall risk of pregnancy loss will be significantly higher in hydropic fetuses and fetuses with severe thrombocytopenia

BLOOD PRODUCTS FOR TRANSFUSION

- A local blood transfusion team should be contacted to prepare O-negative haemoconcentrated blood (haematocrit 70–85%)
- Red cells should be irradiated (24-hour shelf life) to prevent graft-versus-host disease
- Additional notice is required to prepare blood if maternal antibodies other than anti-D, -c, -C, -E or -K are present
- A non-irradiated alternative, or neonatal exchange blood units, are acceptable in an emergency because these components have been leucodepleted
- Maternal blood should not be used as there is a significant risk of graft-versus-host disease for the fetus
- Platelets for transfusion should be obtained from a single donor, irradiated and hyper-concentrated to $\geq 2{,}000 \times 10^9$/L

PREPARATION

- Prescribe steroids for fetal lung maturation where the fetus is considered viable. We prescribe a maximum of two courses during pregnancy
- There is no good evidence to support use of antibiotics or tocolytics
- It is good practice to estimate transfusion volumes needed to normalise fetal haemoglobin for a range of fetal haemoglobins before the procedure starts
- The calculations take account of donor haematocrit/haemoglobin, expected range of fetal haemoglobin (usually 5–10 g/dl) and fetoplacental volume for gestational age (Table 16.1)
- Liaise with obstetric theatre to agree the time for the procedure for when an emergency caesarean section can be performed in case of persistent fetal bradycardia
- Liaise with onsite laboratory to alert them to expect samples for immediate processing
- It is a good practice to heparinise syringes used for aspiration and infusion to minimise the risk of clotting
- An assistant is required to infuse blood. Two other assistants are required to receive samples; one should remain in the procedure room and receive samples for point-of-care testing (e.g. HemoCue) and the other is to take fetal blood samples to the laboratory for more detailed, confirmatory analysis

TECHNIQUE

- Continuous ultrasound guidance is achieved using a free-hand technique
- The puncture site is infiltrated with 10 ml of local anaesthetic (lidocaine 1%) – this is also helpful to map the initial needle path
- Consider vecuronium or pancuronium (0.1–0.2 mg/kg) for fetal paralysis if an intrahepatic approach is planned
- Ideally, an intravascular target (placental cord insertion or intrahepatic umbilical vein) should be used
- Free loops of cord are best avoided
- Intraperitoneal transfusions (~20 ml) are a reasonable alternative before 20 weeks when an attempt to perform intravascular transfusion has failed or is judged not to be feasible
- Using a 20G needle, the target vessel is approached and the needle tip placed next to the vessel wall and then advanced swiftly to puncture the vessel
- The stylet is removed to confirm that blood is flowing freely into the needle
- Two separate 1 ml syringes are filled for point-of-care testing and laboratory estimation prior to beginning the transfusion
- It is good practice to send additional fetal blood samples for fetal blood grouping, Rh typing and direct Coombs test
- Start transfusion when point-of-care testing has confirmed significant fetal anaemia
- Intracardiac transfusion should be considered as a last resort, mainly for an already severely hydropic fetus before 20 weeks when an attempt to perform intravascular transfusion has failed
- The assistant uses the three-way tap to draw down donor blood into a 10 ml syringe and then inject slowly 10 ml volumes into the fetal circulation (Fig. 16.11)
- The assistant should communicate with the operator and keep track of the volume infused
- When drawing down, it is advisable to avoid injecting the full syringe to prevent air entering the fetal circulation
- The operator should keep track of the fetal heart rate during the procedure
- When the planned volume (according to calculation) has been transfused, samples should be obtained for point-of-care and laboratory estimation
- Our practice is to aspirate/inject back and forth three times before the sample is obtained to ensure a thoroughly mixed representative sample. A saline flush can also be used
- If required, additional volume can be transfused based on the fetal haemoglobin, followed by repeat testing before completion of the procedure

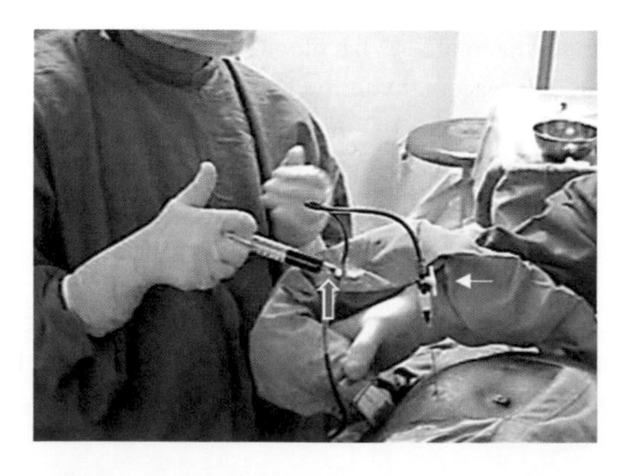

Fig. 16.11 Intrauterine transfusion. The O-negative, haemoconcentrated donor blood is drawn using a 10 ml syringe using a three-way (large arrow) and pushed through an extender tube which has a three-way attaching to the needle (arrow). The second three-way helps to sample the fetal blood to check haemoglobin.

Table 16.1 Estimated volume of transfused blood needed to reach fetal haemoglobin of around 14 g/dl.

Gestation (donor Hct %)	Fetal haemoglobin pre-transfusion					
	5 g/dl	6 g/dl	7 g/dl	8 g/dl	9 g/dl	10 g/dl
18 weeks						
60%	37	33	29	25	21	17
65%	29	26	23	19	16	13
70%	24	21	19	16	13	11
75%	20	18	16	14	11	9
80%	18	16	14	12	10	8
19 weeks						
60%	41	37	32	27	23	18
65%	32	28	25	21	18	14
70%	26	24	21	18	15	12
75%	22	20	17	15	12	10
80%	21	18	16	14	11	9
20 weeks						
60%	47	41	36	31	26	21
65%	36	32	28	24	20	16
70%	30	27	23	20	17	13
75%	25	23	20	17	14	11
80%	22	20	17	15	12	10
21 weeks						
60%	54	48	42	36	30	24
65%	42	37	33	28	23	19
70%	35	31	27	23	19	15
75%	29	26	23	20	16	13
80%	26	23	20	17	14	11
22 weeks						
60%	63	56	49	42	35	28
65%	49	43	38	33	27	22

Table 16.1 (*cont.*)

Gestation (donor Hct %)	Fetal haemoglobin pre-transfusion					
	5 g/dl	6 g/dl	7 g/dl	8 g/dl	9 g/dl	10 g/dl
70%	40	36	31	27	22	18
75%	34	30	27	23	19	15
80%	30	26	23	20	17	13
23 weeks						
60%	73	65	57	49	41	33
65%	57	51	44	38	32	25
70%	47	42	37	31	26	21
75%	40	36	31	27	22	18
80%	35	31	27	23	19	15
24 weeks						
60%	86	76	67	57	48	38
65%	67	59	52	44	37	30
70%	55	49	43	37	31	25
75%	47	42	36	31	26	21
80%	41	36	32	27	23	18
25 weeks						
60%	100	89	78	66	55	44
65%	78	69	60	52	43	35
70%	64	57	50	43	36	29
75%	54	48	42	36	30	24
80%	47	42	37	32	26	21
26 weeks						
60%	116	103	90	77	64	51
65%	90	80	70	60	50	40
70%	75	66	58	50	41	33
75%	63	56	49	42	35	28
80%	55	49	43	37	31	24

Table 16.1 (*cont.*)

Gestation (donor Hct %)	Fetal haemoglobin pre-transfusion					
	5 g/dl	6 g/dl	7 g/dl	8 g/dl	9 g/dl	10 g/dl
27 weeks						
60%	133	118	104	89	74	59
65%	104	92	81	69	58	46
70%	86	76	67	57	48	38
75%	73	65	57	48	40	32
80%	63	56	49	42	35	28
28 weeks						
60%	153	136	119	102	85	68
65%	119	106	92	79	66	53
70%	98	88	77	66	55	44
75%	83	74	65	55	46	37
80%	73	65	57	48	40	32
29 weeks						
60%	174	154	135	116	96	77
65%	135	120	105	90	75	60
70%	112	100	87	75	62	50
75%	95	84	74	63	53	42
80%	83	74	64	55	46	37
30 weeks						
60%	197	175	153	131	109	87
65%	153	136	119	102	85	68
70%	127	113	99	85	70	56
75%	107	95	83	71	60	48
80%	94	83	73	62	52	42
31 weeks						
60%	221	197	172	147	123	110
65%	172	153	134	115	96	77
70%	143	127	111	95	79	63

Table 16.1 *(cont.)*

Gestation (donor Hct %)	Fetal haemoglobin pre-transfusion					
	5 g/dl	6 g/dl	7 g/dl	8 g/dl	9 g/dl	10 g/dl
75%	121	107	94	80	67	54
80%	105	94	82	70	58	47
32 weeks						
60%	247	220	192	165	137	110
65%	193	171	150	129	107	86
70%	160	142	124	106	89	71
75%	135	120	105	90	75	60
80%	118	105	92	79	65	52
33 weeks						
60%	275	245	214	184	153	122
65%	215	191	167	143	119	95
70%	178	158	138	118	99	79
75%	150	134	117	100	83	67
80%	131	117	102	87	73	58

Values are calculated using The Fetal Medicine Foundation calculator available at https://fetalmedicine.org/research/assess/anemia.

FETAL MONITORING DURING PROCEDURE

- Transient bradycardias (<30 seconds) are relatively common
- When they occur, an infusion should be temporarily stopped without removing the needle, and restarted as soon as the fetal heart rate returns to normal
- On occasions, when the needle has been dislodged from the umbilical vein, fetal blood can be seen jetting into the amniotic fluid. Although this looks dramatic, the bleeding will stop spontaneously within 1–2 minutes and no action is needed as long as the fetal heart rate remains normal
- If fetal bradycardia persists for more than ~1 minute, the patient should be put in the left lateral position and fetal heart rate observed for another 1 minute
- If bradycardia persists, the needle should be removed and the fetal heart rate observed for another 30–60 seconds
- If the fetal heart rate has not fully recovered after ~3 minutes and the baby is judged to be viable, the patient should be moved to an obstetric theatre for immediate caesarean section
- Once the patient is on the operating table, the fetal heart rate should be checked once more, ideally with an ultrasound machine rather than a handheld Doppler device. If persistent asystole is confirmed the operation should be abandoned

FETAL MONITORING AFTER PROCEDURE

- If the fetal heart rate remained normal throughout the procedure and there was no evidence of fetal blood loss ('jetting'), there is no need for post-procedure CTG
- If there were episodes of transient fetal bradycardia, or bleeding from the cord was seen, fetal CTG should be performed 30–60 minutes after the procedure for at least 30 minutes
- If CTG is normal, the patient can be discharged home
- Interpretation of a suboptimal CTG trace can be quite difficult, particularly if the fetus was paralysed for the procedure
- Paralysis and hypervolaemia post-transfusion result in loss of accelerations and reduced variability
- Our advice is that any post-procedure CTG should be interpreted by the fetal medicine specialists who have performed the procedure
- As a rule, any interpretation of a suboptimal CTG should be complemented by detailed ultrasound scan, including MCA PSV measurements

POST-PROCEDURE MANAGEMENT: PROCEDURE-SPECIFIC POINTS

- An individualised plan should be made regarding hospital stay; in most cases women are discharged within 1–2 hours (i.e. as soon as they feel comfortable enough)

VESICO-AMNIOTIC SHUNT

Potential candidates should fulfil the following criteria:

- no obvious significant structural abnormality
- longitudinal bladder diameter ≥15 mm
- no umbilical cord cysts
- gestation between 16 and 24 weeks

INVESTIGATIONS

- There is no clear diagnostic benefit of (repeated) bladder taps to measure urinary electrolytes (calcium, sodium, β2-microglobulin) before the procedure
- If shunting is performed, urine can be sent for chromosomal analysis
- Fetal urine can be tested for gamma-glutamyl transferase (GGT) if a uro-digestive fistula is suspected
- Fetal cystoscopy has been proposed as a method to improve diagnostic accuracy by attempting to visualise the obstruction of the posterior urethra. Even in the most experienced hands the technical difficulties (~30%) and preterm rupture of membranes are common (~20%) (see Chapter 17)

COUNSELLING

Arguments in Favour of Vesico-amniotic Shunt

- Improved perinatal survival from 39% to 57%
- Higher chance of good renal function for infants age 6 months to 2 years (from 48% to 68%)
- There is no benefit of repeated bladder taps as urine will reaccumulate quickly unless significant fetal anuria is already present

Arguments Against Vesico-amniotic Shunt

- No difference in survival at the age of 2
- Lack of good-quality evidence of improved long-term renal function
- Complications are common, including pregnancy loss following shunt insertion (up to 10%), dislodgment and/or blockage of the shunt (up to 30%), bladder rupture and chorioamnionitis
- Very rare risks include maternal sepsis and maternal vascular injury

TECHNIQUE

- Continuous ultrasound guidance is achieved using a free-hand technique
- The most commonly used shunts are larger Rocket KCH Fetal Bladder Drain (Rocket Medical, Hingham, MA) and Harrison Fetal Bladder Stent Set (Cook Medical Inc., Bloomington, IN). The size (diameter) of the Harrison stent and the Rocket double pigtail catheter are 1.7 mm and 2.1 mm, respectively (Fig. 16.12)
- It has been our preference to use the Rocket device despite the larger trocar (3 mm outer diameter) (Fig. 16.13). Anecdotally, we have experienced less migration and 'blockages' than with the Harrison device

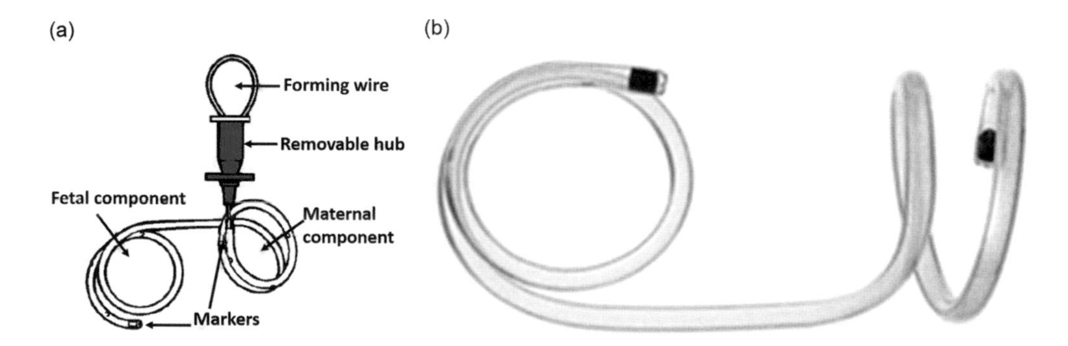

Fig. 16.12 (a) Schematic diagram of the Rocket double pigtail catheter; (b) real-life image of the catheter with the fetal end to the left and the amniotic cavity end on the right (images courtesy of Rocket Medical).

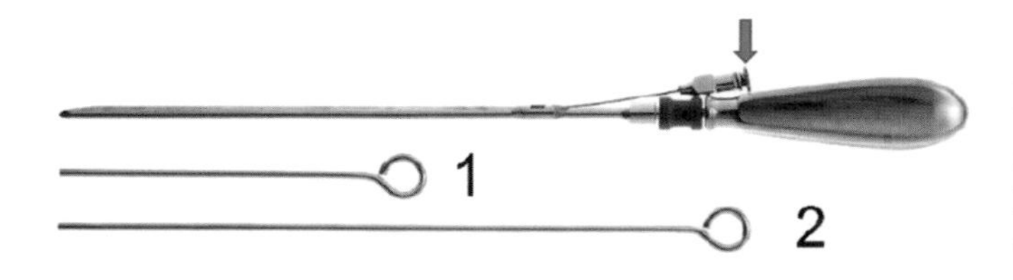

Fig. 16.13 Rocket trocar with a port for amnioinfusion (arrow) and two 'pushers' – the short one (1) is used to insert the catheter into the bladder and long one (2) for the insertion in the amniotic cavity (images courtesy of Rocket Medical).

PREPARATION

- The procedure can be performed either in an obstetric theatre or in an outpatient setting, providing full sterile precautions are taken
- We offer oral sedation with 2 mg lorazepam; we don't use intravenous sedation

- Prophylactic antibiotics are given before the procedure (most commonly a single IV dose of a cephalosporine)
- Corticosteroids are prescribed for fetal lung maturation after 24 weeks
- We do not use prophylactic tocolysis
- Fetal paralysis with vecuronium or pancuronium (100–200 μg/kg) is rarely needed
- If anhydramnios is present, it is advisable to perform amnioinfusion to ensure safe placement of the proximal end of the shunt within the amniotic cavity
- The trocar puncture site should be infiltrated with local anaesthetic (e.g. 10 ml of lidocaine 1%)
- A trocar and cannula are inserted under direct ultrasound guidance into the amniotic cavity, aiming for the infra-umbilical part of the anterior abdominal wall
- The placenta should be avoided if at all possible
- Once the full length of the trocar and the distended bladder are aligned, the trocar is introduced. The tip of the trocar has to be clearly visible in the middle of the bladder (Fig. 16.14)
- When the trocar is removed, fetal urine will start jetting from the canula – samples for genetic analysis could be taken if needed, but the shunt should be introduced without delay
- Good coordination between the main operator and the assistant is essential at this point. The main operator holds the probe and the cannula while the assistant introduces the shunt through the cannula
- Every effort should be made to avoid kinking of the silicone shunt – the kinking can make the advancement through the cannula very difficult and sometimes impossible
- Once the shunt is placed within the cannula, a shorter pusher rod is used to advance the distal part of the shunt into the bladder
- Once the distal part of the shunt is clearly visible protruding through the cannula, the cannula is withdrawn into the amniotic cavity
- The most critical part of the procedure is to ensure that as soon as the main operator has withdrawn the cannula from the fetal skin, the assistant uses the long pusher to deposit the shunt into the amniotic cavity. If the long pusher is pushed through the whole cannula too early, the whole shunt will end up within the bladder/abdomen. If pushed too late, the cannula may have already pulled the whole shunt into the amniotic cavity, or even the uterine wall
- The most commonly used shunts are the Rocket KCH Fetal Bladder Drain (Rocket Medical, Hingham, MA) and Harrison Fetal Bladder Stent Set (Cook Medical Inc., Bloomington, IN)
- The outer diameter of the Harrison and the Rocket stents are 1.7 mm and 2.1 mm, respectively; therefore, a smaller trocar can be used for the insertion of the Harrison stent
- There is no good-quality evidence for superiority of either in terms of outcomes and complications

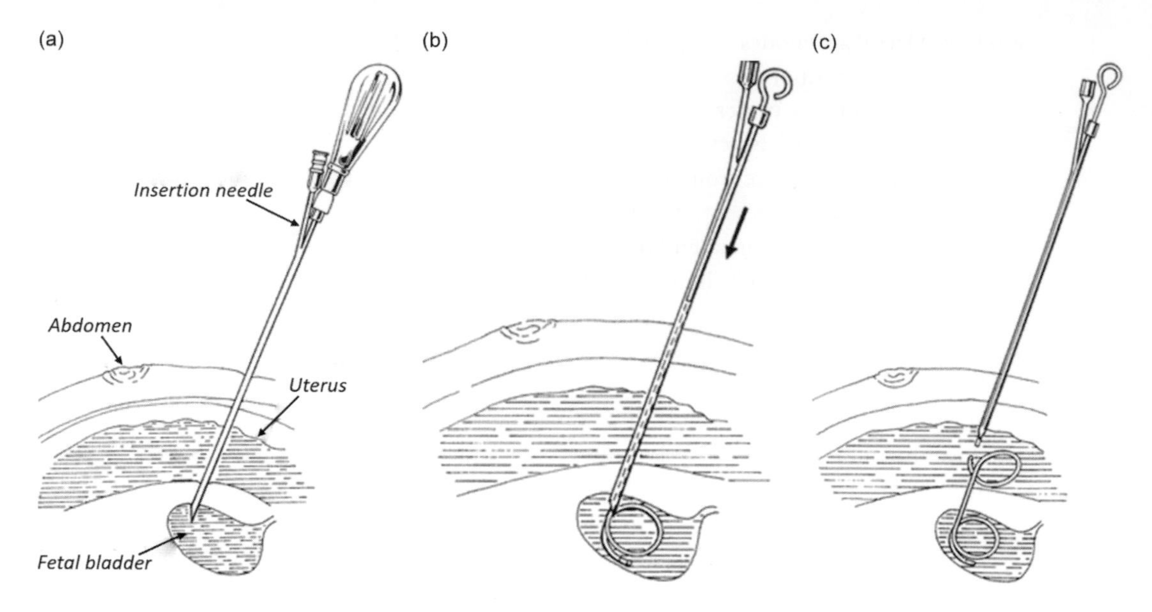

Fig. 16.14 Three key steps during the shunt placement. (a) trocar placement; (b) the shunt is pushed with the short pusher into the bladder; (c) once the trocar has been withdrawn into the amniotic cavity the long pusher is used to place the proximal end of the shunt in the amniotic cavity (images courtesy of Rocket Medical).

POST-PROCEDURE MANAGEMENT: PROCEDURE-SPECIFIC POINTS

- An individualised plan should be made regarding hospital admission
- After uncomplicated shunt placements, the patient can be discharged from hospital on the same day
- We advise women that strenuous activity should be avoided for 48 hours and ask them to seek medical advice if pain is not relieved by paracetamol, if they experience any vaginal loss, fever or flu-like symptoms or have any concerns with fetal movements
- Emergency contact details should be provided
- Plan the follow-up interval (usually 1 week) to assess the effectiveness of the shunt

PLEURO-AMNIOTIC SHUNTS

- Potential candidates should fulfil the following criteria:
  - bilateral hydrothorax associated with ascites and/or skin oedema
  - no evidence of structural abnormalities
  - normal fetal echocardiography
  - no evidence of fetal anaemia or congenital infections
- Some centres offer shunting for apparently isolated large, rapidly accumulating pleural effusions without evidence of hydrops, particularly if mediastinal shift is present
- Some centres offer shunting in large congenital cystic pulmonary airway (adenomatoid) malformation (CPAM/CCAM)

INVESTIGATIONS

- Aneuploidy testing (mainly trisomy 21 and Turner syndrome)
- Chromosomal microarray and testing for Noonan syndrome is recommended in such cases, but is not a prerequisite for offering the shunt insertion
- Exome testing is increasingly carried out in the presence of skin hydrops or structural abnormalities
- Diagnostic/therapeutic thoracocentesis is sometimes offered, particularly if amniocentesis is being performed as part of the diagnostic work-up, but its role remains controversial
- High lymphocyte count (≥80%) is not diagnostic for chylothorax – it is common irrespective of the underlying pathology

COUNSELLING

Arguments in Favour of Shunting

- There are no clear therapeutic benefits of pleural taps other than, possibly, just before birth to assist in neonatal resuscitation
- Although dramatic improvement may be seen immediately after the pleural tap, the fluid will reaccumulate within hours
- There have been case reports when reaccumulation after tapping does not happen, but one has to question whether in such cases the fluid would resorb spontaneously anyway
- Prolonged thoracic decompression with shunting is likely to reduce the risk of pulmonary hypoplasia
- Improvement in venous return may improve hydrops/ascites
- Reduction of oesophageal compression may improve polyhydramnios and, by doing so, reduce the risk of preterm birth
- Hydrops will resolve in ~50% of cases
- Overall, perinatal survival for hydropic fetuses is increased to ~50%

Arguments Against Shunting

- Preterm birth after shunting, with or without PPROM, is common (~80%)
- Risk of chorioamnionitis is ~10%
- Fetal deaths are rare, but have been described due to fetal haemorrhage or traumatic cord accidents
- Catheter migration is relatively common (~20%)
- The catheter may end up inside the fetal thorax and even in the maternal peritoneal cavity
- Up to 25% of cases may need a repeated procedure
- Long-term data are very limited; ~15% of infants will be using home oxygen and ~35% will be readmitted in early childhood for respiratory complications
- Sclerotherapy should be discussed as an alternative for fetuses with primary hydrothorax, particularly at early gestations

TECHNIQUE

- The procedure is almost identical to the placement of a vesico-amniotic shunt, shown in Figs. 16.12–16.14

- Once the full length of the trocar and the intrathoracic target (large pocket of pleural effusion in the mid-axillary line) are aligned, the trocar is introduced with reasonable force to penetrate the chest wall
- The movement is best described as 'jerky' – initially fast, with a sudden stop
- Once the chest wall has been penetrated, the tip of the trocar has to be clearly visible in the middle of the pleural effusion at least 1–2 cm from the chest wall
- Bilateral effusions can be treated in one sitting. The baby can be safely manipulated with the distal end of the cannula that has to be kept 'closed' with a pusher to avoid excessive drainage of amniotic fluid
- Amnioreduction may be performed at the end of the procedure, if needed

POST-PROCEDURE MANAGEMENT

- This is the same as for vesico-amniotic shunting

SUGGESTED READING

PRIMARY RESEARCH

Vinit N, Gueneuc A, Bessières B, et al. Fetal cystoscopy and vesicoamniotic shunting in lower urinary tract obstruction: long-term outcome and current technical limitations. *Fetal Diagn Ther* 2020;47(1):74–83.

REVIEWS AND GUIDELINES

Carson E, Devaseelan P, Ong S. Systematic review of pleural-amniotic shunt insertion vs. conservative management in isolated bilateral fetal hydrothorax without hydrops. *Ir J Med Sci* 2020;189:595–601.

Morris RK, Quinlan-Jones E, Kilby MD, et al. Systematic review of accuracy of fetal urine analysis to predict poor postnatal renal function in cases of congenital urinary tract obstruction. *Prenat Diagn* 2007;27:900–911.

Nassr AA, Shazly SAM, Abdelmagied AM, et al. Effectiveness of vesicoamniotic shunt in fetuses with congenital lower urinary tract obstruction: an updated systematic review and meta-analysis. *Ultrasound Obstet Gynecol* 2017;49:696–703

Navaratnam K, Alfirevic Z on behalf of the Royal College of Obstetricians and Gynaecologists. Amniocentesis and chorionic villus sampling. Green-top Guideline No. 8. *BJOG* 2021;129:e1–e15.

New HV, Berryman J, Bolton-Maggs PHB, et al. on behalf of the British Committee for Standards in Haematology. Guidelines on transfusion for fetuses, neonates and older children. https://b-s-h.org.uk/media/2884/2016-neonates-final-v2.pdf.

Nimrah A, Ryan, G. Fetal primary pleural effusions: prenatal diagnosis and management. *Best Pract Res Clin Obstet Gynaecol* 2019;58:66–77.

CHAPTER 17

Fetoscopy and Ultrasound Guided Thermal Therapeutic Procedures

SUMMARY BOX

INTRODUCTION

- Fetoscopy is a surgical technique for accessing the placenta and the fetus using a semi-rigid fetoscope connected to a light source and camera
- Fetoscopes have side channels to introduce a laser fibre, catheter with a balloon or instruments to facilitate specific procedures such as photocoagulation of vessels, tracheal occlusion or spina bifida surgery
- Radio frequency ablation (RFA) is a percutaneous technique which uses electromagnetic energy to induce thermal injury and coagulation of the tissue. It is used mainly for selective fetal reduction in monochorionic twins
- Bipolar cord coagulation is used for selective fetal reduction in complicated monochorionic twins. A bipolar forceps is used to coagulate the whole of the umbilical cord, using standard surgical diathermy equipment
- Interstitial laser uses laser energy directly delivered in the tissue to occlude vessels inside the fetus

INDICATIONS

LASER FETOSCOPY

Monochorionic Twins

- Twin–twin transfusion syndrome (16–26 weeks)
  - Quintero's stages 2–4
  - In stage 1, fetoscopic surgery is done if the cervical length is <25 mm and there is maternal discomfort due to significant polyhydramnios in the recipient
- Twin anaemia polycythaemia sequence (18–28 weeks in most centres)
- Selective fetal growth restriction (type 2 and 3) in monochorionic twins (18–26 weeks in most centres)
- Cord coagulation in selective fetal growth restriction or TRAP sequence (after 18 weeks)

Singletons

- Release of amniotic bands (after 17 weeks)
- Laser coagulation of the placental or fetal tumour feeding vessels (timing depends on the clinical presentation, but usually in the third trimester)
- Tracheal occlusion devices – insertion (27–32 weeks), removal (34 weeks)
- Fetal cystoscopy (18–22 weeks)
- Myelomeningocele repair (usually 24–26 weeks)

RADIOFREQUENCY ABLATION

- Can be performed between 16–26 weeks
- Twin reversed arterial perfusion (TRAP) sequence
- Selective fetal growth restriction (sFGR) type II/III
- Twin–twin transfusion syndrome (TTTS) with severe selective fetal growth restriction
- Discordant anomalies in MC twins

BIPOLAR CORD COAGULATION

- Always done after 18 weeks as risk of PPROM is doubled prior to 18 weeks
- Indications are similar to RFA
- Selective reduction of the hydropic recipient twin in stage 4 TTTS

INTERSTITIAL LASER

- TRAP after 14 weeks.
- Ablation of the aberrant arterial supply in bronchopulmonary sequestration. Usually late second or early third trimester
- Intra-tumoural vessels in chorioangiomas. Usually late second or early third trimester

PRE- AND POST-PROCEDURE MANAGEMENT

GENERAL PRINCIPLES

- A detailed ultrasound is essential to evaluate the fetal condition and assess the need for and the type of procedure to be performed
- Individual counselling should cover the indication, intended benefits, procedure-related risks and potential consequences of not performing the procedure
- Written patient information should be provided, if available
- Obstetric history-taking should focus on any risk factors that may influence the overall management of the pregnancy, in particular issues related to increased risk of preterm birth/PPROM
- Booking blood tests including blood group and type, serology, full blood count and hemoglobinopathy screen should be reviewed, and treated and/or repeated, if necessary
- Maternal comorbidities should be noted and any compliance issues with treatment resolved
- Anticoagulation including aspirin should be stopped 24 hours before the procedure
- All invasive procedures should be subject to informed written consent
- Contemporaneous records should be maintained, including details of the information provided and options for communicating results

MATERNAL PREPARATION

- It is preferable to have the patient fasting at least 4 hours before the procedure
- Tocolysis is achieved by oral (25 or 50 mg) or rectal indomethacin (100 mg once only), or nifedipine (10–20 mg orally) 30 min prior to the procedure
- Oral prescriptions may be continued post operatively for 24–48 hours, if deemed necessary
- Cefazolin 2 g IV is given preoperatively. If the patient is allergic to penicillin or cephalosporins, clindamycin 900 mg IV can be given
- The mother should lie supine or in a lateral decubitus position, depending on the choice of the entry site

POST-PROCEDURE MANAGEMENT

- Provide anti-D prophylaxis if Rhesus negative and non-sensitised; the dose used varies between 200 and 600 μg (500–1,500 IU)

- Following fetoscopy, the patient can be discharged home on the same day or admitted overnight (longer if clinically indicated)
- If nifedipine is used for tocolysis it can cause headache, palpitation or hypotension – the dose can be reduced to 10 mg or stopped
- Strenuous activity should be avoided for 48 hours
- Medical advice should be sought if pain is not relieved by paracetamol or there are any other concerns
- The patient is rescanned after 6–12 hours
- In cases of TTTS the donor bladder is usually visible 24–48 hours after the procedure and liquor normalisation is expected within 1–2 weeks
- Subsequently, 2-weekly follow-up should be arranged depending on the growth, liquor volume and fetal Doppler
- Emergency contact details are provided to the patient, who is advised to report to the hospital if there are signs of contractions, leaking, bleeding or fever

INSTRUMENTS AND TECHNIQUE

LASER FETOSCOPY

Standard Instruments

- Straight or curved sheath with an obturator; these instruments can have either sharp or blunt tip (Fig. 17.1)
- The sharp-tip instrument can be directly introduced through the skin after a local anaesthetic
- When a blunt instrument is used, a cannula (10 or 12 Fr) has to be introduced first, with the help of the Seldinger technique (described below)

Integrated Scopes

- Integrated scopes have a light source, telescope and channels for laser fibre, all moulded as a single unit
- They can only be introduced into the uterine cavity through a cannula (introducer set) with the help of the Seldinger technique (Fig. 17.2)

Optics

- A standard laparoscopic setup (light source, camera and monitor) can be used to connect with the fetoscope

Laser

- An Nd–YAG laser machine with power output of 60–100 watts or a diode laser capable of delivering up to 60 watts can be used
- An 'end firing' laser fibre of 400–600 nm diameter that can pass through the side channel of the fetoscope is used (Fig. 17.3)

The Theatre Setup

- Prior to the procedure it is important to ensure that all the instruments are functioning well
- The positioning of the equipment, including the ultrasound machine, the tower with the light source, camera and the laser machine, is arranged to allow a clear line of sight for the surgeon (Fig. 17.4)
- The theatre technician should have easy access to the tower and ultrasound machine
- The type of scope (i.e. straight, curved or 30 degree) is selected prior to the procedure. In some cases more than one type may be needed and should be kept ready
- Fetoscopic procedures are mostly done under local anaesthesia, but when regional anaesthesia is planned (spinal, epidural or combined), the anaesthetic team must be involved in the theatre setup

Technique

- The patient is positioned, and draped in a sterile fashion
- An ultrasound transducer is placed in a sterile cover and used to map the placental location and cord insertion sites, and to ensure the absence of any vascularity along the planned access route
- The fetoscope entry site is then selected to ensure that the target (e.g. the placental surface between the two cords in TTTS) can be visualised well
- The fetoscope should be directed perpendicular to the axis of the donor twin. This will ensure that the collapsed membrane is visualised at 90 degrees to the fetoscope
- If blunt instruments or an integrated fetoscope are used, the first step is to introduce a guide wire into the amniotic space through the 18G needle under direct ultrasound guidance
- Once the 18G needle is removed, a 10/12 Fr cannula (also called an introducer set) is introduced over the guide wire in the amniotic cavity (the Seldinger technique is shown in Fig. 17.5)
- The fetoscope is then introduced through the cannula to visualise the placental surface/fetal parts as needed
- If at any point during the procedure local anaesthesia appears inadequate, supplementation with midazolam or remifentanil may be needed

Limitations for Fetoscopic Laser Surgery

- After 27 weeks laser is technically challenging due to vernix in the liquor limiting visibility
- A very short distance between the two umbilical cord insertions may pose an unacceptably high risk as the communicating vessels will be very large and close to the base of the two cords. In this scenario, selective fetal reduction with RFA of bipolar coagulation may be a safer alternative
- In women with severe preeclampsia the risk of pulmonary oedema from excess intrauterine fluid infusion may be unacceptably high
- With prolapsed membranes the increased intra-amniotic pressure from fluid infusion may cause perioperative PPROM

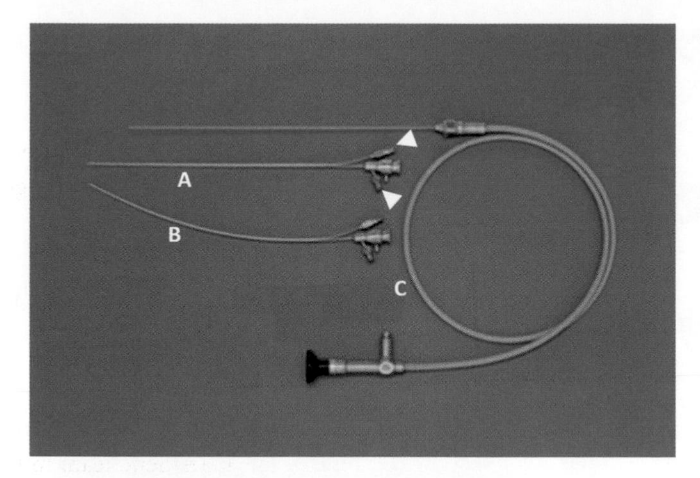

Fig. 17.1 Standard straight fetoscope for posterior placentas with 2 mm straight sharp-tip sheath that has a removable obturator (A). The side channels (arrowheads) are used to introduce the laser fibre and for saline infusion.
A curved fetoscope is used for anterior placentas (B). A semi-rigid scope (C) goes into the straight or curved sheath after removing the obturator (A).

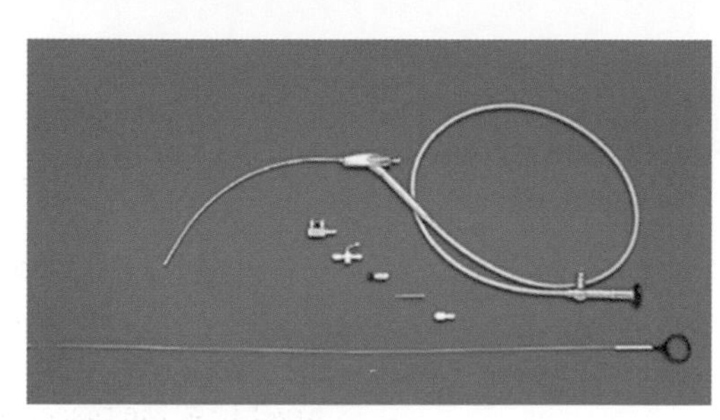

Fig. 17.2 Integrated curved fetoscope for anterior placentas that is introduced through a separate 10/12 Fr cannula (not shown). The cable for the light source, the camera interface and the scope form a single unit. The cleaning brush is also shown.

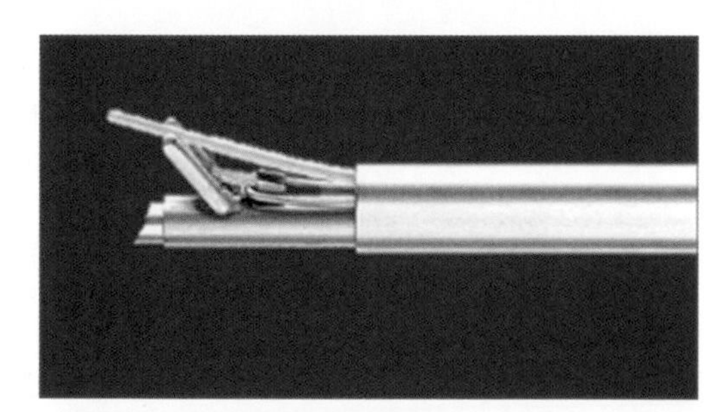

Fig. 17.3 Straight scope with a 30° viewing angle for anterior placentas. Note the laser fibre can be tilted upwards to help obtain a better angle of the laser beam to the vessel.

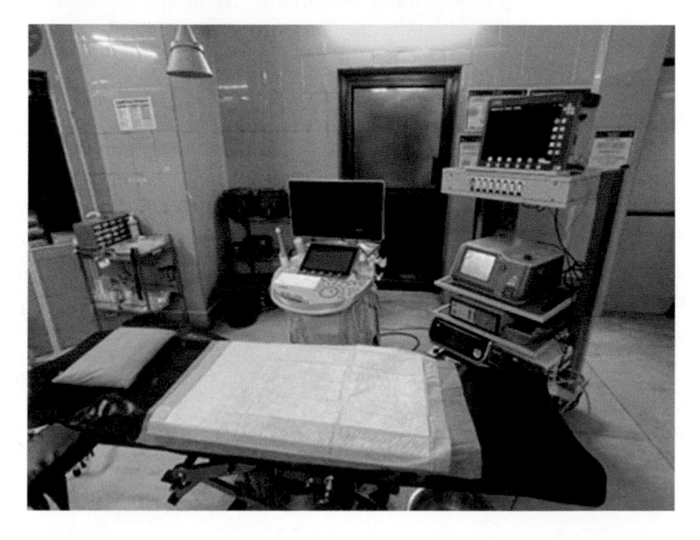

Fig 17.4 An example of a fetoscopy suite setup.

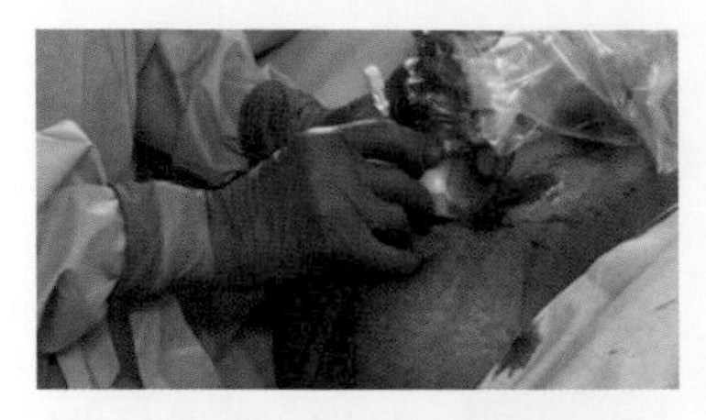

Fig. 17.5a Seldinger technique step 1: introduction of an 18G needle under ultrasound guidance.

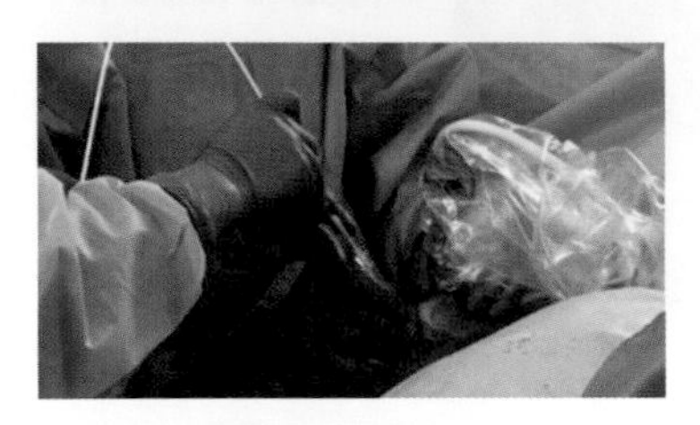

Fig. 17.5b Seldinger technique step 2: guidewire threaded through the 18G needle into the amniotic cavity.

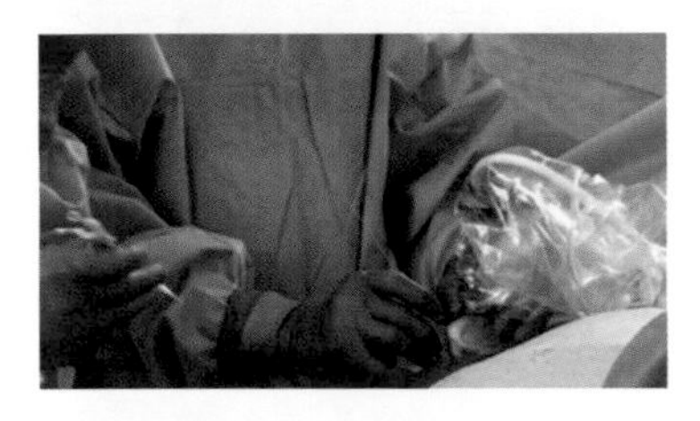

Fig. 17.5c Seldinger technique step 3: the needle is removed, leaving the guidewire in place.

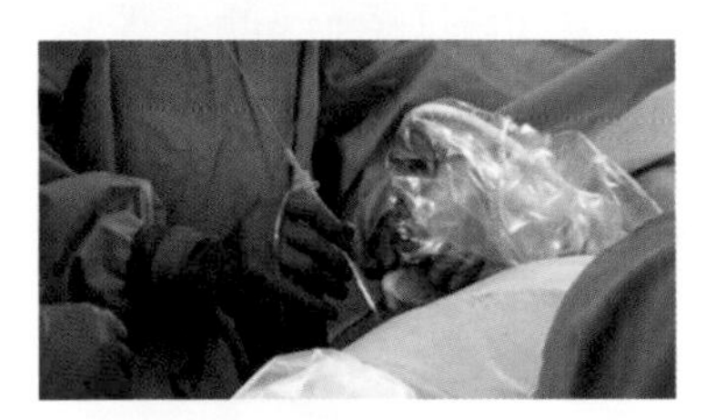

Fig. 17.5d Seldinger technique step 4: a 10 Fr flexible cannula with a dilator is introduced through the guidewire till the cannula reaches the amniotic cavity.

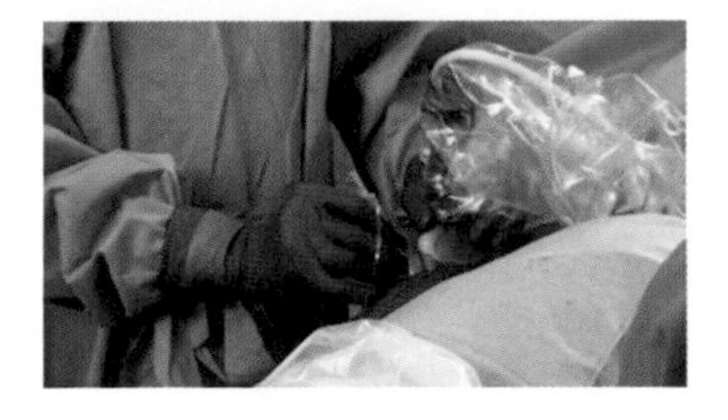

Fig. 17.5e Seldinger technique step 5: The guidewire is removed, followed by the dilator, leaving the flexible cannula in the amniotic cavity.

RADIOFREQUENCY ABLATION

Instruments

- The equipment for RFA consists of an RF generator, a needle connected to the generator by a cable and grounding pads (Fig. 17.6)

Temperature-Controlled System

The needle electrodes are of two types:

1. Multiple expanding tines with tips that contain a thermocouple to read the temperature of the tissue
2. Internally cooled electrodes in which internal cooling is achieved by chilled saline, thus preventing the overheating of tissue near the electrode

Impedance-Controlled System

- The impedance-based systems come with a 14G needle with retractable curved electrodes (Fig. 17.7)
- The generator is switched on when electrodes are opened in the fetal abdomen at the level of the umbilical cord insertion
- As the tissue is ablated, the ability to conduct heat decreases, leading to an increase in impedance
- When the tissue is completely ablated, the generator shuts off automatically ('roll off'). When this happens, it is assumed that the tissue is fully ablated

Technique

- Prior to the procedure, the needle should be checked for temperature increase by grasping the tip of the needle or each of the tines – the instrument should show an increase in temperature from the body heat by 1–2 °C
- Under local anaesthesia, the RFA needle is introduced into the fetal abdomen and the tines are opened to about 2 cm
- The RFA generator is set for 150 watts and 110 °C, timed at 3 minutes per cycle
- The generator is then switched on and the gradual increase of temperature is noted on the display, depicting each of the tines
- If one of the tines is not heating, then the needle is gently rotated to ensure that the temperature is increasing
- Once the target of 150 watts is achieved in all tines, as indicated on the display, the ablation starts and should continue for 3 minutes, followed by a 10 second cooling time
- A fetal heart rate of <50 bpm, with absence of colour Doppler flow in the cord, can be considered as the completion of the procedure
- If ablation is not complete after the first attempt, the tines may need to be repositioned. However, visibility of the tines will become difficult since they will become brightly echogenic after the first cycle

Limitations

- If the sac of the affected fetus is below the healthy co-twin, the needle may need to be introduced through the co-twin's sac. This can potentially cause a tear in the membrane and leak of amniotic fluid from the co-twin
- Intrauterine death of the co-twin can happen in ~20% of cases
- If repeated attempts are needed, the risk of losing the healthy twin increases with each additional attempt

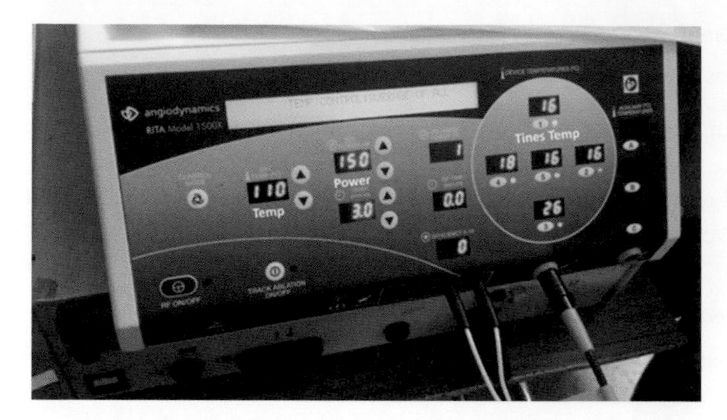

Fig. 17.6 RFA generator. The displays shows the temperature set at 110 °C. Power is set at 150 W and the cycle time is 3 min. The temperatures of the five tines are individually displayed ('Tines Temp'). The lower display shows a higher temperature as the surgeon touches the tine to test.

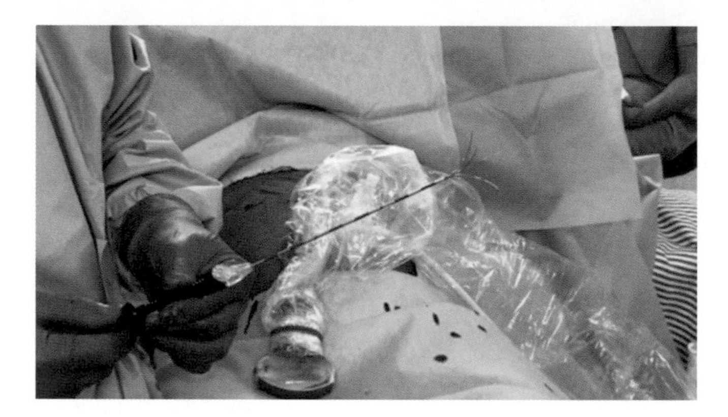

Fig. 17.7 Impedance-controlled RFA needle with the tines open.

BIPOLAR COAGULATION

Instruments

- Bipolar cord coagulation is done using a bipolar forceps connected to standard surgical diathermy equipment (Fig. 17.8)
- A grounding pad with good contact with the patient's leg is necessary to complete the circuit
- The bipolar forceps has a long handle and two blades which are used to grasp the umbilical cord of the affected twin
- Once the cable is connected between the forceps and the machine, a test coagulation is done on a wet gauze to check whether adequate heat is generated as evidenced by the vapour that should arise from the gauze between the blades
- The settings required can vary with the equipment used; usually 25–40 watts

Technique

- Bipolar cord occlusion is usually done only after 18 weeks since the risk of PPROM is much higher if done prior to 18 weeks
- The fetus and sac are scanned to ensure there is a placenta-free window for introducing either a flexible trocar with the Seldinger technique or a rigid trocar directly as described above

- If there is oligohydramnios, amnioinfusion will be required to create a window for entry of the trocar
- The bipolar forceps is connected to a diathermy machine with the coagulation setting switched on
- Ultrasound is used to visualise a straight segment of the umbilical cord close to the fetal end
- The forceps is then introduced through a trocar and the umbilical cord is fully grasped
- A gentle movement of the forceps is done to ensure that the cord is held firmly by the forceps
- The machine is set at 25 watts and can be increased up to 40 watts if required. These settings may vary depending on the type of machine used
- As coagulation occurs, first there is bubbling, followed by steam rise seen as bright echoes rising through the amniotic cavity
- The process should be repeated in two or three locations in the umbilical cord to ensure complete occlusion (Fig. 17.9)
- Fetal bradycardia <50 bpm and absence of colour Doppler signal in the cord is considered as completion of the procedure

Limitations

- If there is an anterior placenta with no significant window to introduce the trocar, RFA may be a safer alternative
- If there is severe oligohydramnios, amnioinfusion may be technically very difficult and will prolong the procedure time considerably

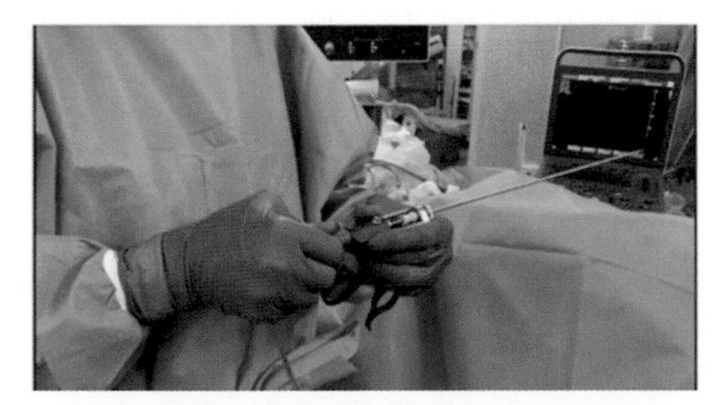

Fig. 17.8a Bipolar forceps: attaching the cable to the forceps.

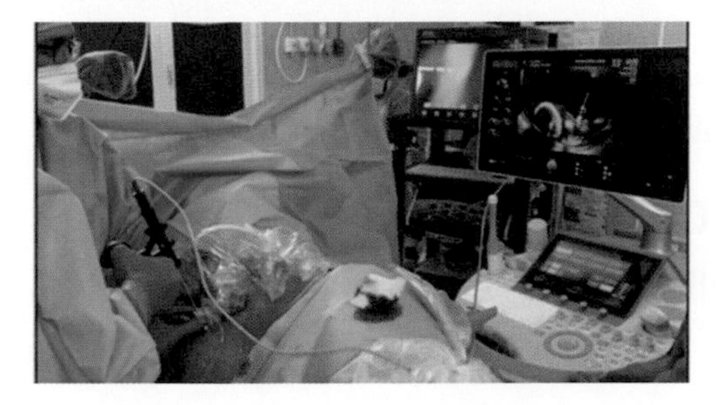

Fig. 17.8b Bipolar cord coagulation under ultrasound guidance.

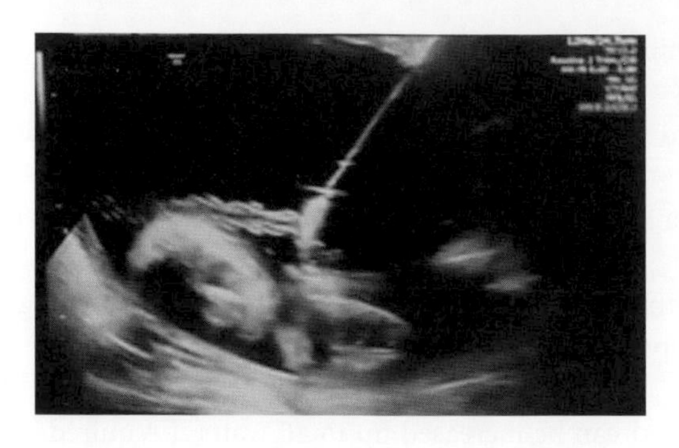

Fig. 17.9 Ultrasound image of bipolar forceps grasping the full thickness of the cord.

INTERSTITIAL LASER

Instruments

- The equipment needed includes an ultrasound machine, a 40 watt diode or Nd–YAG laser and an 18G 13–15 cm needle

Technique

- The vessels for ablation are identified by ultrasound and colour Doppler
- A needle path is chosen such that the tip of the needle once introduced into the fetus will be perpendicular to the vessels to be ablated
- An 18G needle is passed under ultrasound guidance into the tissue and the tip is positioned 1 cm away from the vessels
- A 400 or 600 nm diameter laser fibre is introduced through the needle until the tip of the fibre is seen projecting out of the needle in close contact with the vessel wall
- The fibre can be marked with tape to the correct length before starting the procedure
- Laser energy is applied in short bursts until the vessels are coagulated, as evidenced by the absence of colour Doppler signal

Limitations

- As gestational age increases, the vessel diameter increases, making the coagulation more difficult
- After the initial laser energy has been applied, it may be difficult to locate the laser tip by ultrasound because the surrounding tissue will become hyperechogenic
- Inadvertent withdrawal of the laser fibre into the needle may cause the needle to be charred and it may have to be replaced with a new needle

INTERVENTIONS FOR COMPLICATED TWINS

LASER FETOSCOPY FOR TWIN–TWIN TRANSFUSION SYNDROME

Technique: Specific Considerations

- Best performed between 16^{+0} and 26^{+0} weeks
- Before 16^{+0} weeks there may be a separation of amnion and chorion

- After 26 weeks, the liquor turbidity makes visualisation difficult
- A straight scope is used for a posterior placenta
- For anterior placentas, a placenta-free window is chosen and a curved scope is introduced through it
- In some centres a 30° telescope is used with a 'deflecting mechanism' for the laser fibre to help obtain the optimal angle of the laser beam
- The patient may need to be repositioned to get good access
- Once the scope is in the amniotic cavity, the membrane is identified and traced until the avascular area in the edge of the placenta is seen at both ends (Fig. 17.10)
- The vascular anastomoses are then identified by following each of the vessels from the membrane as they course towards the donor
- The anastomotic sites are identified when the vessel from the donor and a corresponding vessel from the recipient 'dip down' into the placenta close to each other
- The communicating vessels may be small, medium or large in diameter
- The anastomotic sites form the 'vascular equator' which is usually in a line
- After mapping the anastomoses, the larger vessels are chosen first for 'selective laser photocoagulation'
- The laser beam is directed towards the donor vessel at an angle close to 90°
- An energy of 40 watts is applied till 'blanching' of the vessel is achieved. The same is repeated for the vessel on the recipient's side
- The process is continued till all the anastomoses, large and small, are coagulated. The sites are inspected again to ensure completeness of the coagulation
- Some centres prefer 'joining the dots' by drawing a line with the laser which connects all the areas previously coagulated. This is also called the 'Solomon technique' and may reduce the incidence of post-procedure TAPS
- Once the procedure is done, the fetoscope is removed and the excess amniotic fluid is drained, aiming for the single deepest vertical pool of less than 8 cm
- The cannula is then removed and pressure is kept on the site of entry with a gauze for a few minutes to stop the leakage of amniotic fluid
- The fetal cardiac activity is confirmed and shown to the patient before transfer to the ward

Counselling

It is important to describe several clinical scenarios that may follow the procedure:

- 1 in 3 TTTS pregnancies that require laser will end up with two healthy survivors
- In ~20% of cases both babies will die within one week of the procedure
- One of the babies may die in ~40% of cases
- If one or both babies survive there could be serious antenatal complications in ~10% of cases (very early PPROM, TAPS) that may have important long-term health consequences for survivors (e.g. neurodevelopmental delay)

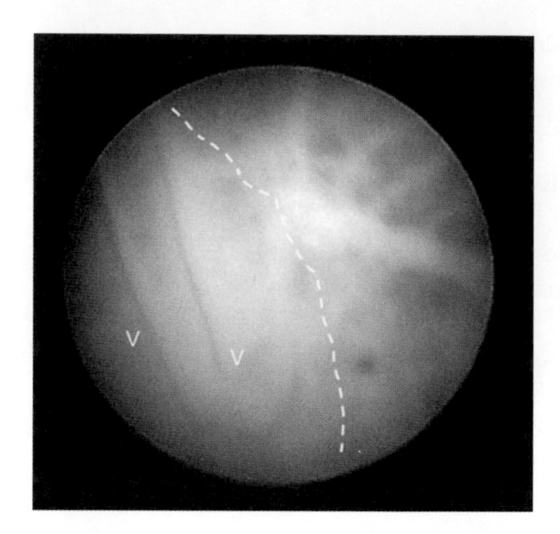

Fig. 17.10 Fetoscopic view of the placental edge (dotted line). Placental vessels are seen to the left of the dotted line (V, V) The bare area of the placenta is seen to the right of the dotted line.

SELECTIVE FETAL GROWTH RESTRICTION

Isolated sFGR – No TTTS (Type 2/3)

- If a decision is taken to intervene, then selective reduction is done either by bipolar cord coagulation after 18 weeks or RFA after 16 weeks

Technique: Specific Considerations

- The fetus for selective reduction is identified and a cross section of the abdomen is visualised at the level of the umbilical cord entry
- The RFA needle is introduced into the abdomen so that the tip of the needle goes beyond 50% of the abdominal diameter
- When the tines are advanced caution is needed to ensure that they do not perforate the whole fetal abdomen and come into contact with the uterine wall
- The needle can be inserted through the placenta, although there will be some self-limiting bleeding when the needle is removed

Counselling

- Both RFA and bipolar cord occlusions have a livebirth rate of ~85% for the surviving twin
- RFA is a technically simpler procedure to perform
- Higher rates of PPROM have been reported for bipolar cord occlusion, and amnioinfusion is usually required when there is oligohydramnios

sFGR with TTTS

- Management of sFGR with coexisting TTTS would depend on the severity of the discordancy and the Doppler assessment
- Selective fetal reduction may be a better choice when there is a significant discordance (≥35%), phenotype type II/III or a stuck twin before 24 weeks
- Selective laser photocoagulation of anastomotic vessels may be offered when there is type 1 sFGR with TTTS

Technique: Specific Considerations

- In severe sFGR a non-selective laser along the membrane can be performed, but carries a high risk of demise of the smaller twin
- Even if selective laser photocoagulation is done, there is a risk of vascular compromise for the smaller twin as it may draw its supply from the recipient's territory

Counselling

- Post-laser survival does not depend on whether coexisting TTTS is present or not
- Overall survival rate for both twins is ~50%
- At least one survivor is seen in ~70%
- Only ~12% of the smaller twins survive if the ductus venosus is abnormal prior to the procedure

TWIN ANAEMIA POLYCYTHAEMIA SEQUENCE (TAPS)

Technique

- Fetoscopic laser is the only definitive treatment for TAPS
- Absence of oligo/polyhydramnios sequence, the small size of the anastomoses and the large donor size of the placenta make the treatment challenging as these conditions limit the accessibility to the residual vascular anastomoses
- The procedure is even more difficult when the placenta is anterior
- Since the residual anastomoses are usually miniscule, the use of the Solomon technique is recommended

Counselling

- Perinatal mortality occurs in 9% of spontaneous TAPS and in 18% of TAPS cases that occur after laser fetoscopy
- The rate of PPROM after laser for TAPS is ~35%
- Post-laser TAPS donors have a ~25% mortality as compared with ~10% in recipient (polycythaemic) twins
- Perinatal mortality increases with increasing severity of the TAPS and lower gestational age at birth
- Significant neonatal morbidity is present in ~30–40% of either donor or recipient survivors
- After birth, in addition to anaemia, TAPS donors may show short-term renal dysfunction, low albumin and neutropenia due to decreased erythropoiesis
- The polycythaemic (recipient) twin may have reduced splenic perfusion and tissue hypoxia causing neonatal thrombocytopenia

FETOSCOPIC TRACHEAL OCCLUSION FOR CONGENITAL DIAPHRAGMATIC HERNIA (FETO)

Indication

- Compression of the lung by the herniated organs is causing efflux of lung liquid, leading to collapse of the lung and impaired lung development

- The aim of FETO is to prevent efflux by blocking the trachea, thereby allowing expansion of the lung and lung growth that will reduce the risk of bronchopulmonary dysplasia
- The observed to expected lung area/head circumference ratio (O/E LHR) has been used to predict the severity of congenital diaphragmatic hernia
- O/E LHR of <25% irrespective of the liver position is considered severe and FETO is usually scheduled at 27–29 weeks' gestation
- O/E LHR of 25–34.9% irrespective of the liver position and 35–44.9% with intrathoracic liver herniation is considered moderately severe; in this group FETO is performed up to 30^{+6} weeks

Balloon Insertion Technique

- Using the Seldinger technique as described above, a flexible cannula is introduced in the direction of the fetal mouth (Fig. 17.11)
- A 3.3 mm fetoscope with side channels for the occlusive device, puncture needle and fluid infusion is introduced through the cannula into the fetal mouth
- Lactated Ringer's solution, warmed to body temperature, is infused in the fetal mouth to help visualisation and dilatation of the vocal cords
- The scope is advanced through the fetal mouth into the trachea, ensuring that the tongue, epiglottis, vocal cords and carina are identified (Fig. 17.12)
- The catheter with a detachable balloon is introduced through the scope. The balloon is then inserted to lie between the carina and the vocal cord
- The balloon is inflated with 0.6 ml of isotonic fluid. When fully inflated the balloon is 20 mm long and 7 mm wide
- If the liquor is reduced due to leakage, amnioinfusion is performed prior to removal of the instruments

Balloon Removal

- Centres planning to deliver babies after FETO must be equipped with personnel skilled in balloon removal techniques, which may be required under emergency circumstances if the patient reports with iatrogenic PPROM or preterm labour
- Elective balloon removal is performed between 34^{+0} and 34^{+6} weeks, either fetoscopically or by ultrasound guided puncture
- In case of an unplanned preterm birth, the balloon should be removed before the cord is clamped. Alternatively, direct puncture of the balloon can be done immediately after delivery

Counselling

- Iatrogenic preterm prelabour rupture of membranes <37 weeks can occur in about 40–50% of cases
- Neonatal complications in survivors include bronchopulmonary dysplasia (~65%), pulmonary hypertension (~75%), sepsis (~30%) and neonatal death (~30%)
- Survival to discharge after FETO in the severe group is ~40% compared with ~15% in the expectant management group
- Survival to discharge after FETO in the moderate group is ~60% compared with ~50% in the expectant management group

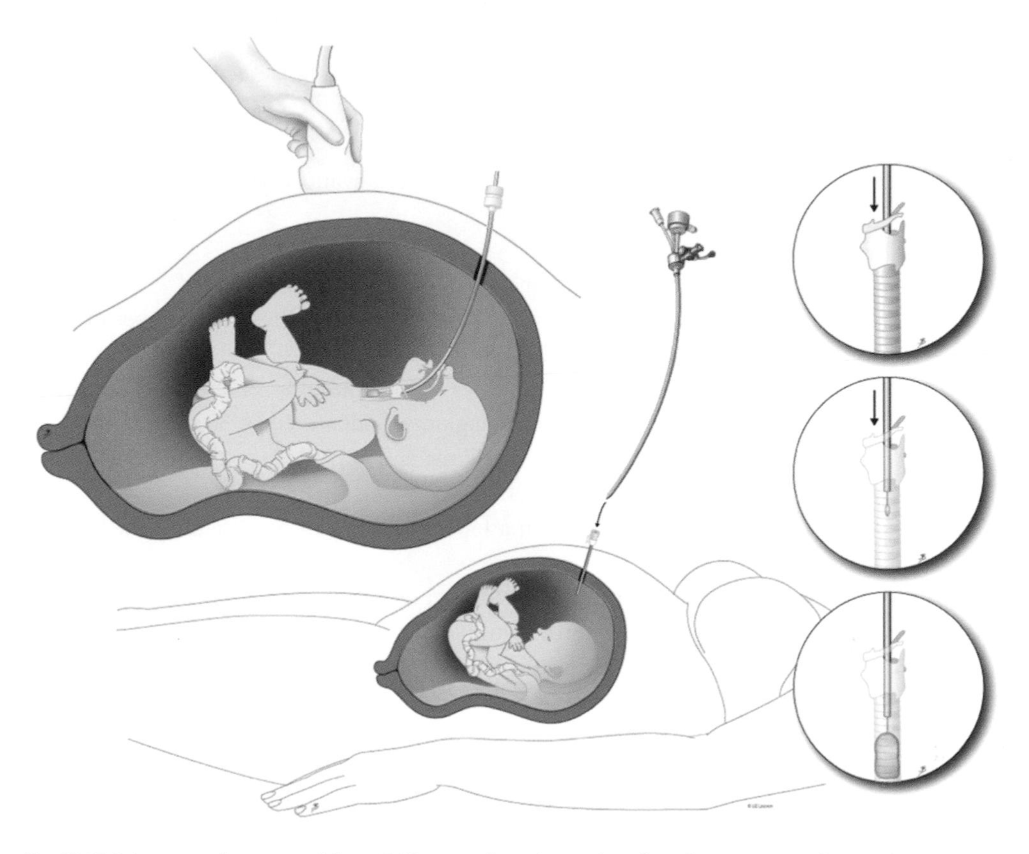

Fig. 17.11 Schematic drawing of the FETO procedure (reproduced with permission from UZ Leuven, Belgium).

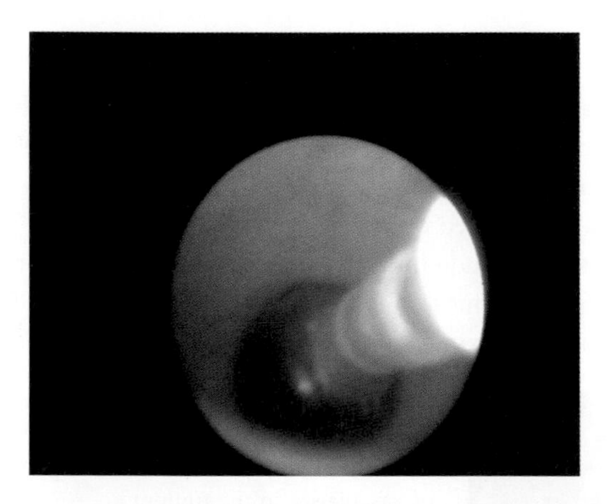

Fig. 17.12 Fetoscopic view of the fetal trachea with a balloon in situ (reproduced with permission from UZ Leuven, Belgium).

INTERVENTIONS FOR CHORIOANGIOMA

Indications

- In utero treatment should be discussed when large chorioangioma is associated with:
  - polyhydramnios
  - increased MCA PSV (fetal anaemia)
  - fetal cardiac failure and hydrops

Technique

- Therapeutic methods targeting the tumour itself include:
  - fetoscopic laser ablation of the feeding vessel
  - interstitial laser (Fig. 17.13)
  - injection of embolisation agents (Histoacryl, cyanoacrylates mixed with Lipiodol) (Fig. 17.14)
  - radiofrequency ablation
  - embolisation coils and bipolar occlusion
- Choice of the procedure is operator-dependant, since the total number of published case series is small and no randomised controlled trials exist.
- If *fetoscopy* is chosen, a 2 mm fetoscope is introduced as described earlier in this chapter and the feeding artery to the chorioangioma is identified. A 30 watt diode laser is used to ablate the vessel. If the vessel is very large and very close to the placental cord insertion site, laser may not be feasible
- *Interstitial laser* has been tried in a few cases, but can be difficult if the tumour is highly vascular
- *Radiofrequency ablation* can be performed (as described elsewhere in this chapter) but has the risk of thermal injury to the fetus
- *Embolisation agents* can be injected slowly into the feeding vessel within the tumour and immediate cessation of blood flow in the tumour can be achieved. The target vessel should be the feeding artery and not the vein
- If treatment is successful, complete cessation of flow in the tumour is expected
- Intrauterine transfusion may have to be performed when necessary, along with any of the treatment options described above
- If there is polyhydramnios, amnioreduction is done at the end of the procedure
- MCA Doppler should be done post-procedure to exclude fetal anaemia

Counselling and Management

- In large untreated chorioangiomas (>10 cm) perinatal mortality is ~30–50%, while in treated cases series the reported perinatal mortality is ~30%
- Treatment can help in the resolution of hydrops in ~60% of cases
- Preterm delivery occurs in 50–60% of treated cases
- Other, less invasive treatment options include intrauterine transfusion when there is fetal anaemia, amnioreduction for polyhydramnios and, if there is cardiac failure, transplacental therapy with maternal digoxin

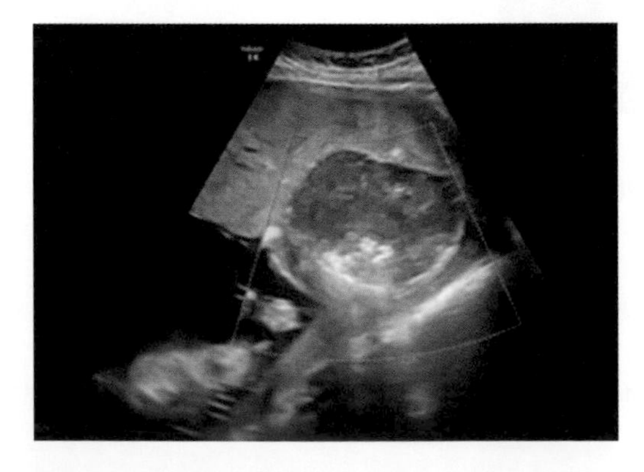

Fig. 17.13 Large chorioangioma after treatment with interstitial laser in a 25-week pregnancy. Note the echogenic areas and complete absence of vascularity in the tumour.

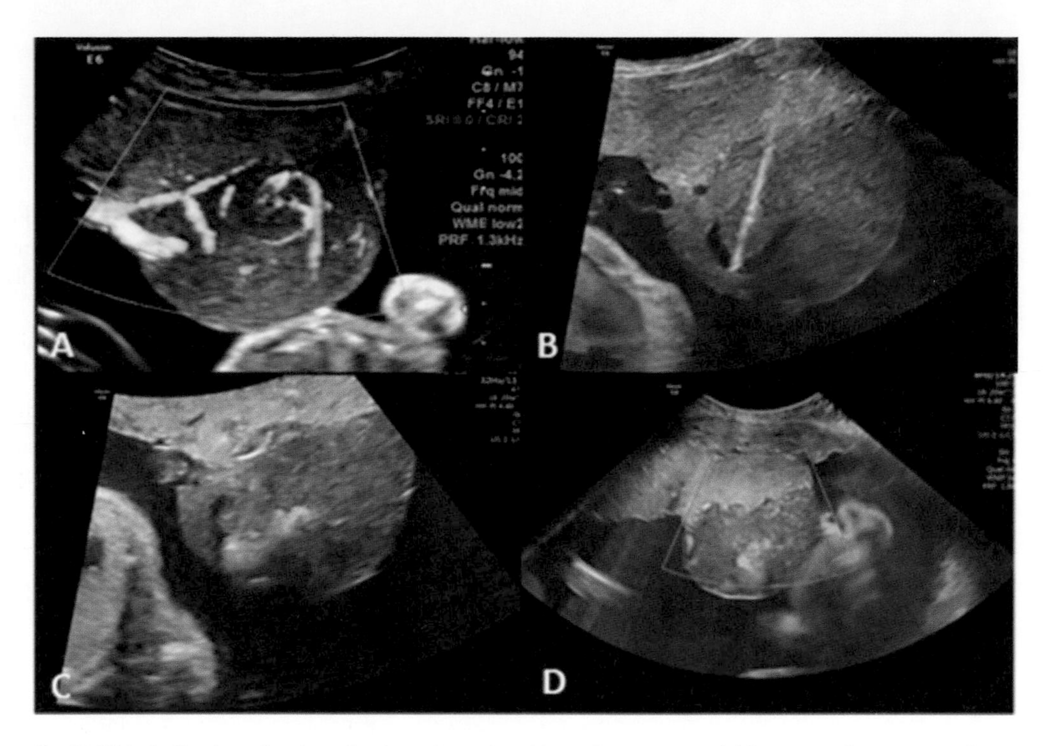

Fig. 17.14 Embolisation of a giant chorioangioma in a 28-week pregnancy. (a) Pre-procedure picture shows significant vascularity. (b) A 20G needle was placed within the large feeding vessel. (c) A slow injection of 5 ml of a mixture of cyanoacrylate glue and Lipiodol resulted in an echogenic vessel indicating occlusion. (d) Post-procedure scan shows significant reduction in the colour Doppler flow within the tumour.

FETAL CYSTOSCOPY

Indication

- Fetal cystoscopy is an experimental alternative to vesico-amniotic shunting; this method may also serve as a diagnostic tool for urethral atresia
- Optimal gestational age is 18–22 weeks

Technique

- A 1 mm curved fetoscope is used to enter the fetal bladder percutaneously through the superior surface of the bladder
- Once in the bladder, the scope is passed through the posterior urethra and the valve is identified (Fig. 17.15)
- A 400 or 600 nm laser fibre is introduced through the side channel and a 30 watt laser is used to create holes in the valve
- Sudden decompression of the bladder and passage of fluid through the urethra into the amniotic fluid is considered as success of the procedure

Counselling

- The theoretical advantage of fetal cystoscopy is that it attempts to ‘restore’ normal anatomy, thus enabling physiological bladder function as opposed to shunting, wherein the bladder remains collapsed for several weeks till delivery

- However, the currently available instrumentation is not ideally suited for fetal cystoscopy and the procedure remains largely experimental and limited to a few centres
- Even in the most experienced hands technical difficulties (~30%) and preterm rupture of membranes are common (~20%)

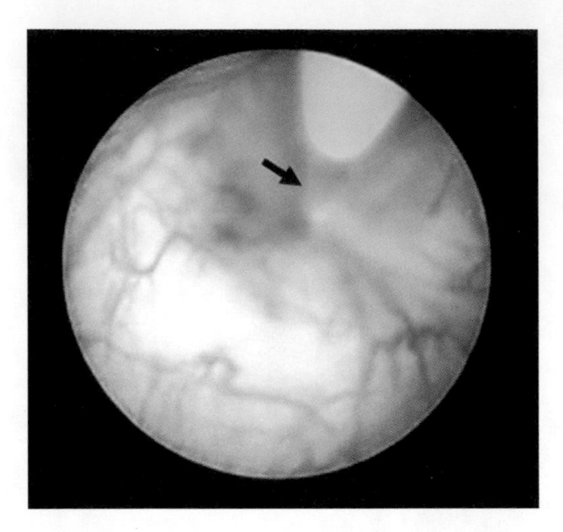

Fig. 17.15 Fetal cystoscopy for lower urinary tract obstruction. The 1 mm curved fetoscope is in the posterior urethra and the laser fibre (black arrow) is just touching the valve.

SUGGESTED READING

PRIMARY RESEARCH

Deprest JA, Nicolaides KH, Benachi A, et al. TOTAL Trial for Severe Hypoplasia Investigators: randomized trial of fetal surgery for severe left diaphragmatic hernia. *N Engl J Med* 2021;385(2):107–118.

Ruano R, Sananes N, Sangi-Haghpeykar H, et al. Fetal intervention for severe lower urinary tract obstruction: a multicenter case–control study comparing fetal cystoscopy with vesicoamniotic shunting. *Ultrasound Obstet Gynecol* 2015;45(4):452–458.

Senat MV, Deprest J, Boulvain M, et al.. Endoscopic laser surgery versus serial amnioreduction for severe twin-to-twin transfusion syndrome. *N Engl J Med* 2004;351(2):136–144.

Vinit N, Gueneuc A, Bessières B, et al. Fetal cystoscopy and vesicoamniotic shunting in lower urinary tract obstruction: long-term outcome and current technical limitations. *Fetal Diagn Ther* 2020;47:74–83.

REVIEWS AND GUIDELINES

Akkermans J, Peeters SHP, Klumper F, et al. Twenty-five years of fetoscopic laser coagulation in twin-twin transfusion syndrome: a systematic review. *Fetal Diagn Ther* 2015;38:241–253.

Buca D, Pagani G, Rizzo G, et al. Outcome of monochorionic twin pregnancy with selective intrauterine growth restriction according to umbilical artery Doppler flow pattern of smaller twin: systematic review and meta-analysis. *Ultrasound Obstet Gynecol* 2017;50(5):559–568.

Buca D, Iacovella C, Khalil A, et al. Perinatal outcome of pregnancies complicated by placental chorioangioma: systematic review and meta-analysis. *Ultrasound Obstet Gynecol* 2020;55:441–449.

Khalil A, Cooper E, Townsend R, Thilaganathan B. Evolution of stage 1 twin-to-twin transfusion syndrome (TTTS): systematic review and meta-analysis. *Twin Res Hum Genet* 2016;19(3):207–216.

CHAPTER 18

Fetal Surgery for Spina Bifida

SUMMARY BOX

RATIONALE

- Long-term morbidity related to spina bifida stems from the primary spinal lesion and secondary intracranial effects
  - More than 90% of infants with spina bifida will have hindbrain herniation (Arnold Chiari malformation)
  - ~80% will develop hydrocephalus requiring cerebral spinal fluid diversion
  - While children with spina bifida will typically have a normal IQ, the requirement of a ventriculo-peritoneal (VP) shunt with possible complications (e.g. shunt revision, obstruction, infection) can be associated with neurodevelopmental delay
  - Impaired neurodevelopment affects lower limb mobility; adults with lesions above L4 are unlikely to be fully ambulant
  - Children with spina bifida may need orthopaedic intervention for talipes and/or other spinal problems such as kyphosis, scoliosis and spinal cord tethering
  - Impairment of bladder and/or bowel function is a common feature, irrespective of the lesion severity
  - Adults with spina bifida may experience sexual dysfunction
- In utero repair of spina bifida may:
  - prevent ongoing spinal nerve injury through protection against mechanical and chemical (amniotic fluid) injury
  - reduce the chance of severe hindbrain herniation and progressive hydrocephalus

COUNSELLING

POTENTIAL BENEFITS OF IN UTERO SURGERY*

- ~50% reduction in VP shunt placement
- ~30% reduction in hindbrain herniation
- ~50% increase in independent walking at 30 months of age

RISKS OF FETAL SURGERY*

- Increased risk of preterm birth (13% of preterm births before 30 weeks in the prenatal surgery group compared with 0% in the postnatal surgery group)
- Increased risk of spontaneous membranes rupture (46% in prenatal vs 8% in postnatal surgery group)
- Increased maternal risk of pulmonary oedema and placental abruption (~6%)
- Increased risk of uterine dehiscence (~10%)
- Need for blood transfusion at delivery (~9%)
- Need to deliver by caesarean section, including all future pregnancies
- Future pregnancies at risk of placenta accreta and uterine rupture/dehiscence
- Surgery performed in a limited number of centres, which may have socio-economic implications for the family

* Estimates based on the data from the MOMS Trial.

INCLUSION CRITERIA

Fetal

- Meningomyelocele (including myeloschisis) at level T1 through to S1
- Normal chromosomes
- Gestational age between 19^{+0} and 25^{+6} weeks

Maternal

- Age $\geq$18 years
- Able to provide informed consent
- Meets psychosocial criteria, including appropriate support at home

EXCLUSION CRITERIA

Maternal

- Poorly controlled pregestational diabetes
- Other relevant maternal medical condition, e.g. chronic hypertension
- BMI >35 kg/m^2
- Previous history of spontaneous preterm delivery or cervical incompetence
- Short cervix (<20 mm) measured by transvaginal scan
- Placenta praevia
- Alloimmune disease (anti-red cell or anti-platelet antibodies)
- Hepatitis B or C, or HIV positive
- Uterine anomaly – Mullerian duct abnormality or multiple fibroids
- Previous uterine surgery (except previous lower uterine segment caesarean section)

Fetal

- Multiple pregnancy
- Other structural anomalies
- Fetal growth restriction
- Fetal kyphosis >30°
- Ventriculomegaly >15 mm

PREOPERATIVE ASSESSMENT

ULTRASOUND

- Assess level of lesion
- Look for evidence of kyphosis or scoliosis
- Assess cranial features, including head shape, lateral cerebral ventricles, cerebellum and posterior fossa
- Exclude other fetal structural malformations
- Measure fetal biometry and amniotic fluid volume, and estimate fetal weight
- Assess lower limbs for function and talipes
- Determine placental site and measure cervical length by transvaginal ultrasound

MRI

- Assess intracranial anatomy to look for features associated with spina bifida and to exclude other fetal brain anomalies
- Assess the fetal spine and measure the level and size of spina bifida defect

GENETIC TESTING

- Amniocentesis for chromosomal microarray, unless CVS was already done earlier in pregnancy

TECHNIQUE

OPEN SURGERY VIA HYSTEROTOMY

- Involves maternal laparotomy and hysterotomy under general anaesthesia and antibiotic cover
- The hysterotomy is usually undertaken using a uterine stapling device which secures the membranes, myometrium and serosa all in one layer (Fig. 18.1)
- The procedure is done under general anaesthesia, which will also reach the fetus
- The fetus will also receive an intramuscular injection of a muscle relaxant (e.g. pancuronium 0.2 mg/kg) and fentanyl, with the dose calculated based on the estimated fetal weight
- The fetal spina bifida defect is exposed at the maternal hysterotomy site and the spina bifida defect repair is undertaken while the fetus remains in utero
- The spina bifida repair includes:
  - release of the neural placode (Fig. 18.2)
  - closure of the dura
  - skin closure
- Warmed Hartmann's solution is delivered into the amniotic sac by controlled infusion during the procedure
- Ongoing ultrasound monitoring of cardiac function (heart rate, contractility) and amniotic fluid volume with a sterile probe in direct contact with the uterus
- Once the amniotic fluid volume is restored, the hysterotomy incision is repaired (Fig. 18.3)
- Delivery by caesarean section is scheduled for 37 weeks, although the majority will be delivered preterm for obstetric indications (PPROM, abruption, chorioamnionitis) (Fig. 18.4)

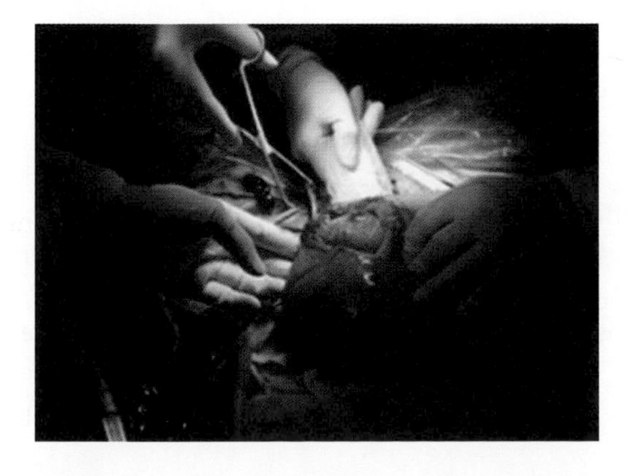

Fig. 18.1 The uterus is exposed and opened, securing the myometrium, serosa and membranes in a single layer. Stay sutures are used to keep the hysterotomy incision under tension while the fetus is manipulated into the wound.

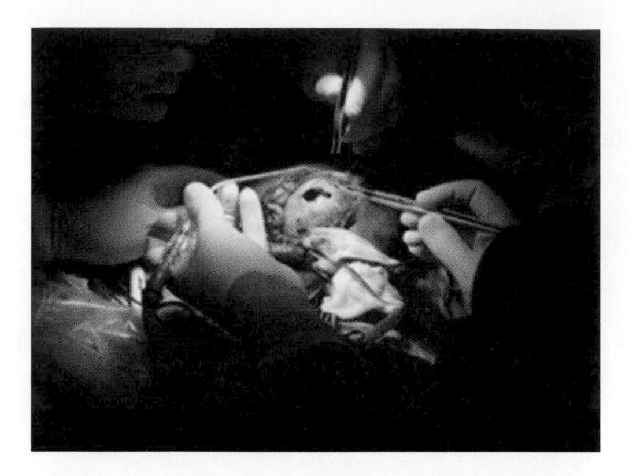

Fig. 18.2 The neural placode is released and the dura and skin are then closed in layers. A catheter runs into the uterus to maintain amniotic fluid volume with warmed Hartmann's solution.

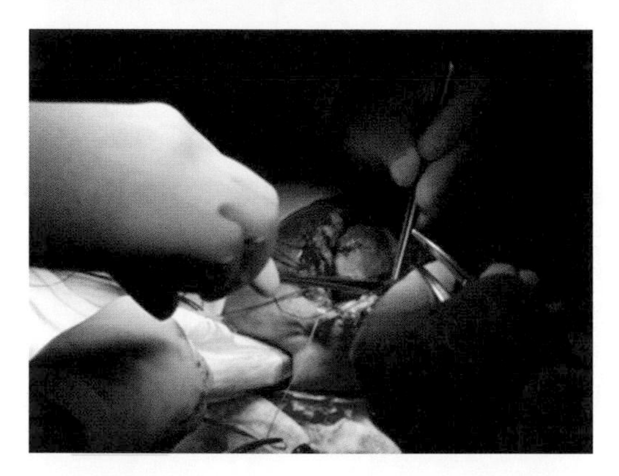

Fig. 18.3 The hysterotomy incision is repaired and amniotic fluid volume normalised. Caesarean section is indicated for future obstetric deliveries.

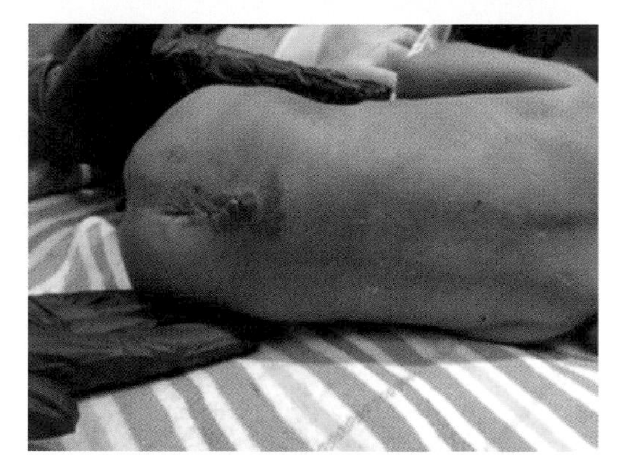

Fig. 18.4 The neonatal scar at delivery.

LAPAROSCOPIC APPROACH

- An increasing number of groups are offering an endoscopic approach to the spine bifida repair
- CO_2 is commonly used for insufflation
- The learning curve is likely to be longer than with open surgery – initial case series have reported higher rates of PPROM and preterm births
- The technique is being continuously modified and improved in order to minimise the risk of associated complications

SUGGESTED READING

Adzick NS, Thom EA, Spong CY, et al. A randomized trial of prenatal versus postnatal repair of myelomeningocele. *N Engl J Med* 2011;364:993–1004.

Lapa DA. Endoscopic fetal surgery for neural tube defects. *Best Pract Res Clin Obstet Gynaecol* 2019;58:133–141.

Moldenhauer JS, Flake AW. Open fetal surgery for neural tube defects. *Best Pract Res Clin Obstet Gynaecol* 2019;58:121–132.

Nagaraj UD, Kline-Fath BM. Imaging of open spinal dysraphisms in the era of prenatal surgery. *Pediatr Radiol* 2020;50:1988–1998.

Ravindra VM, Aldave G, Weiner HL, et al. Prenatal counseling for myelomeningocele in the era of fetal surgery: a shared decision-making approach. *J Neurosurg Pediatr* 2020;28:1–8.

Sanz Cortes M, Chmait RH, Lapa DA, et al. Experience of 300 cases of prenatal fetoscopic open spina bifida repair: report of the International Fetoscopic Neural Tube Defect Repair Consortium. *Am J Obstet Gynecol* 2021;225:678.e1–678.e11.

Sherrod BA, Ho WS, Hedlund A, et al. A comparison of the accuracy of fetal MRI and prenatal ultrasonography at predicting lesion level and perinatal motor outcome in patients with myelomeningocele. *Neurosurg Focus* 2019;47(4):E4.

CHAPTER 19
Genetic Syndromes

SUMMARY BOX

DEFINITIONS

Syndrome

- A group of features frequently occurring together which may have a single unifying cause or presumed cause
- *Example:* Down syndrome

Association

- An association is a group of signs and symptoms occurring together more frequently than would be expected by chance alone, but the underlying genetic cause is unknown
- *Example:* VACTERL association

Sequence

- In a sequence, one anomaly or event leads to the other abnormalities
- *Example:* Amniotic band leading to ring-like constriction or amputation limb defects

PRENATAL PHENOTYPING

- When a genetic syndrome is suspected, detailed phenotyping should be done by experts in ultrasound
- Standard ultrasound evaluation should be complemented with 3D/4D ultrasound, targeted echocardiography and fetal neurosonography including MRI
- Fetal phenotyping is increasingly informed by exome sequencing and vice versa. Genetic testing limited to only karyotyping and/or microarray testing should be considered suboptimal for difficult cases
- Clinical geneticists should be an integral part of the diagnostic process, but their availability may be limited
- If genetic specialists are not available, fetal medicine specialists should be transparent regarding their limitation in the interpretation of complex results (e.g. variants of unknown significance)
- For complex cases, fetal phenotyping and counselling performed jointly by experienced fetal medicine specialists and clinical geneticists should be considered the gold standard

Useful Resources

- OMIM: www.ncbi.nlm.nih.gov/omim
- GeneReviews: www.ncbi.nlm.nih.gov/books/NBK1116/
- Orphanet: www.orpha.net/consor/cgi-bin/index.php

ACROCALLOSAL SYNDROME

Characteristics

Three of the four criteria are needed for diagnosis:

- Agenesis of corpus callosum and/or Dandy–Walker malformation
- Craniofacial anomalies: macrocephaly, hypertelorism
- Limb abnormalities: pre- or post-polydactyly, polysyndactyly
- Moderate to severe intellectual disability and hypotonia

Inheritance

- Autosomal recessive: *KIF7* and *GLI3*

Ultrasound/MRI Detectable Features in Affected Fetuses

- Agenesis of corpus callosum
- Dandy–Walker malformation
- Polydactyly

AICARDI SYNDROME

Characteristics

- Severe neurodevelopmental delay with infantile spasms, low muscle tone and retinal defects
- Almost exclusively in females

Inheritance

- Likely X-linked
- Genetic cause currently unknown

Ultrasound/MRI Detectable Features in Affected Fetuses

- Agenesis of corpus callosum, asymmetry of cerebral hemispheres, ventriculomegaly
- Polymicrogyria, periventricular heterotopia, cerebellar hypoplasia
- Microphthalmia

AICARDI GOUTIERES SYNDROME (AGS)

Characteristics

- Early-onset encephalopathy
- Acquired microcephaly
- Intermittent sterile pyrexias
- Chilblain lesions
- Intracranial basal ganglia calcifications, white matter changes with temporal cyst-like formation
- Subgroup will present at birth with features mimicking congenital infection

Inheritance

- Autosomal recessive: *ADAR*, *RNASEH2A*, *RNASEH2B*, *RNASEH2C*, *SAMHD1* and *TREX1*
- Autosomal dominant: *IFIH1*

Ultrasound/MRI Detectable Features in Affected Fetuses

- Mimics fetal infection
- Growth restriction
- Cerebral changes (parenchymal calcification, gyral abnormalities)
- Hyperechogenic bowel

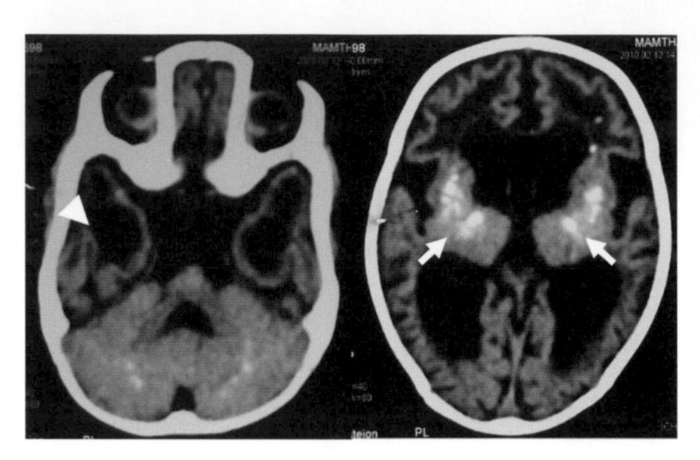

Fig. 19.1 Aicardi Goutieres syndrome. Postnatal CT showing basal ganglia calcifications (arrows) and white matter changes including temporal cyst (arrowhead). These changes are likely due to mutations in the *RNASEH2C* gene

APERT SYNDROME

Characteristics

- Craniosynostosis and syndactyly

Inheritance

- Autosomal dominant
- Variants in *FGFR2* in most cases

Ultrasound/MRI Detectable Features in Affected Fetuses

- Craniosynostosis, hypertelorism
- Complex syndactyly of hands and feet (mitten appearance)

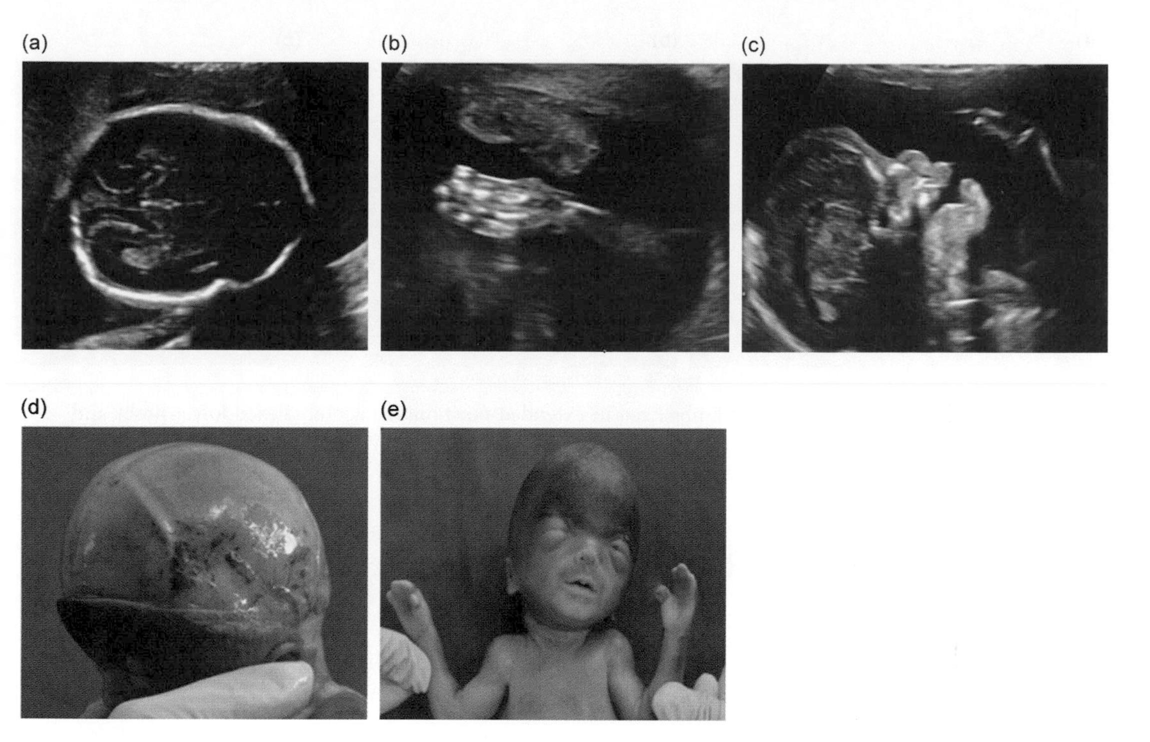

Fig. 19.2 Apert syndrome. (a) Fetal head at 20 weeks showing an abnormal shape and absence of cranial sutures due to craniosynostosis; (b) syndactyly ('mitten hands'); (c) depressed nasal bridge and midface hypoplasia; (d) craniosynostosis with fused coronal and lambdoid sutures; (e) midfacial hypoplasia with depressed nasal bridge and syndactyly.

ARTHROGRYPOSIS MULTIPLEX CONGENITA (AMC)

Characteristics

- Multiple joint contractures affecting two or more areas of the body
- Muscle atrophy

Inheritance

- AMC is not a specific diagnosis, but rather a manifestation of many different conditions (syndromes, genetic, neurological, connective tissue or muscle disorders) – inheritance depends on the underlying condition

Ultrasound/MRI Detectable Features in Affected Fetuses

- Fixed joints
- Reduced fetal movements

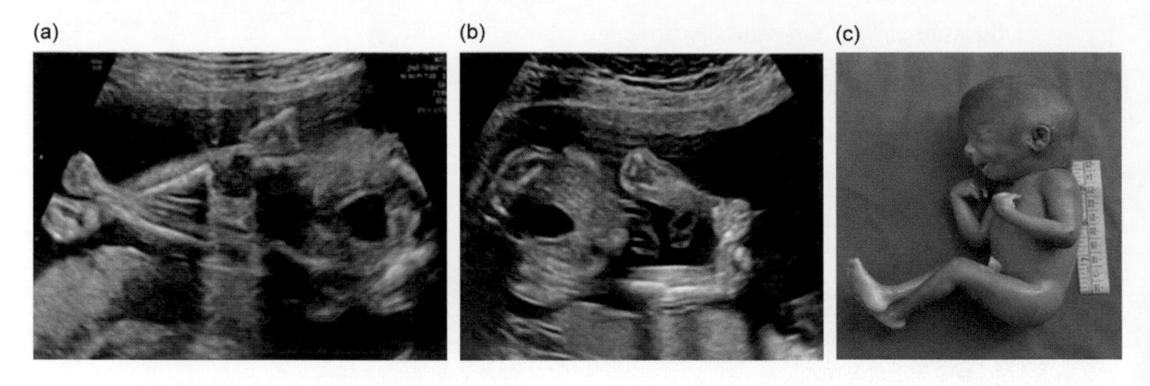

Fig. 19.3 Arthrogryposis: (a) fetal lower limbs fixed in extended position; (b) acutely flexed lower limbs and clenched hands; (c) same fetus after birth.

BANNAYAN–RILEY–RUVALCABA SYNDROME

Characteristics

- Large head size, multiple benign tumours and tumour-like growths, mostly in skin and digestive system (hamartomas, haemangiomas, lipomas)
- Can have intellectual disability or delayed development, hypotonia, seizures, autism
- Can have skeletal abnormalities (scoliosis, kyphosis, pectus excavatum) and joint hyperextensibility

Inheritance

- Autosomal dominant: *PTEN* mutations

Ultrasound/MRI Detectable Features in Affected Fetuses

- Macrocephaly, macrosomia
- Tumours unlikely to be seen prenatally

BARTSOCAS–PAPAS SYNDROME

Characteristics

- Microcephaly
- Craniofacial anomaly – short palpebral fissures, fused eyelids, hypoplastic nose, orofacial clefting, filiform bands between the jaws
- Severe popliteal webbing
- Renal anomalies
- Oligosyndactyly
- Ectodermal abnormalities

Inheritance

- Autosomal recessive
- Variants in *RIPK4* have been found in some cases

Ultrasound/MRI Detectable Features in Affected Fetuses

- Dysmorphic face, hypoplastic nose, facial clefts
- Microcephaly
- Characteristic popliteal webbing (pterygium)
- Renal anomalies

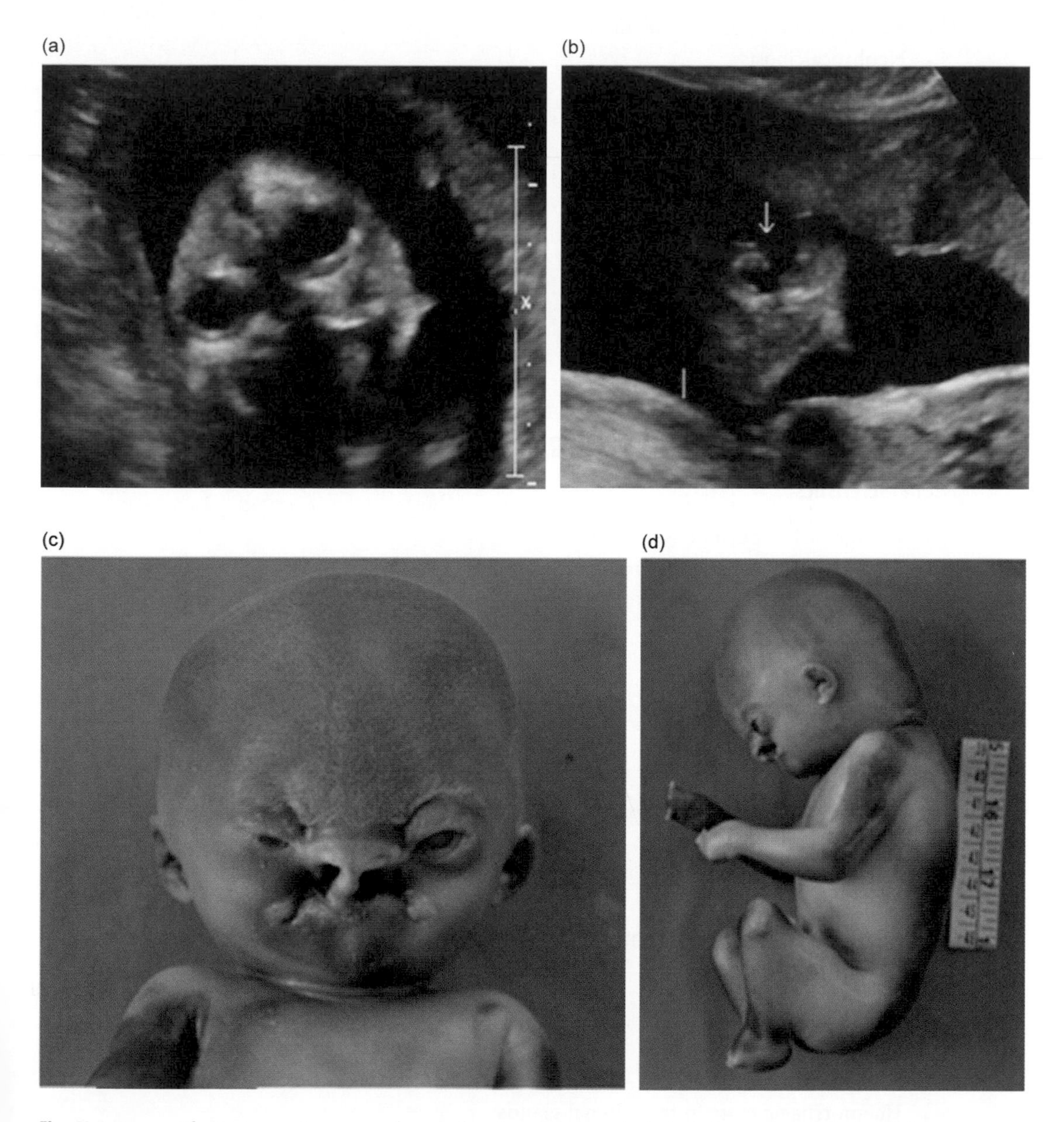

Fig. 19.4 Fetus with Bartsocas–Papas syndrome showing the characteristic facies and popliteal webbing. (a) Hypertelorism; (b,c) facial cleft; (d) popliteal webbing.

BARTTER SYNDROME

Characteristics

- Renal tubular salt wasting disorder
- Electrolyte abnormalities – hypokalaemia metabolic acidosis, hypomagnesaemia and hypocalcaemia
- Severe failure to thrive, polyuria
- Nephrocalcinosis

Inheritance

- Autosomal recessive: types I, II, III, IV caused by variants in *SLC12A1, KCNJ1, CLCNKB, BSND, CLCNKA*
- Autosomal dominant: type V caused by variants in *CASR*
- Types I, II, III present antenatally

Ultrasound/MRI Detectable Features in Affected Fetuses

- Severe polyhydramnios

BECKWITH–WIEDEMANN SYNDROME

Characteristics

- Overgrowth syndrome – macrosomia
- Macroglossia (most common finding)
- Hemi-hypertrophy, organomegaly (liver, spleen, kidneys)
- Omphalocele
- Ear creases/pits
- Increased risk of childhood cancers (i.e. Wilm's tumour, hepatoblastoma, rhabdomyosarcoma)
- Rarely structural congenital heart disease or cardiac hypertrophy

Inheritance

- 75% of patients will have a methylation abnormality or uniparental disomy of 11p15

Ultrasound/MRI Detectable Features in Affected Fetuses

- Macrosomia, macroglossia
- Hepatomegaly
- Omphalocele
- Echogenic kidneys
- Haemorrhagic cysts in the adrenal glands
- Embryonal tumours
- Placentomegaly, polyhydramnios

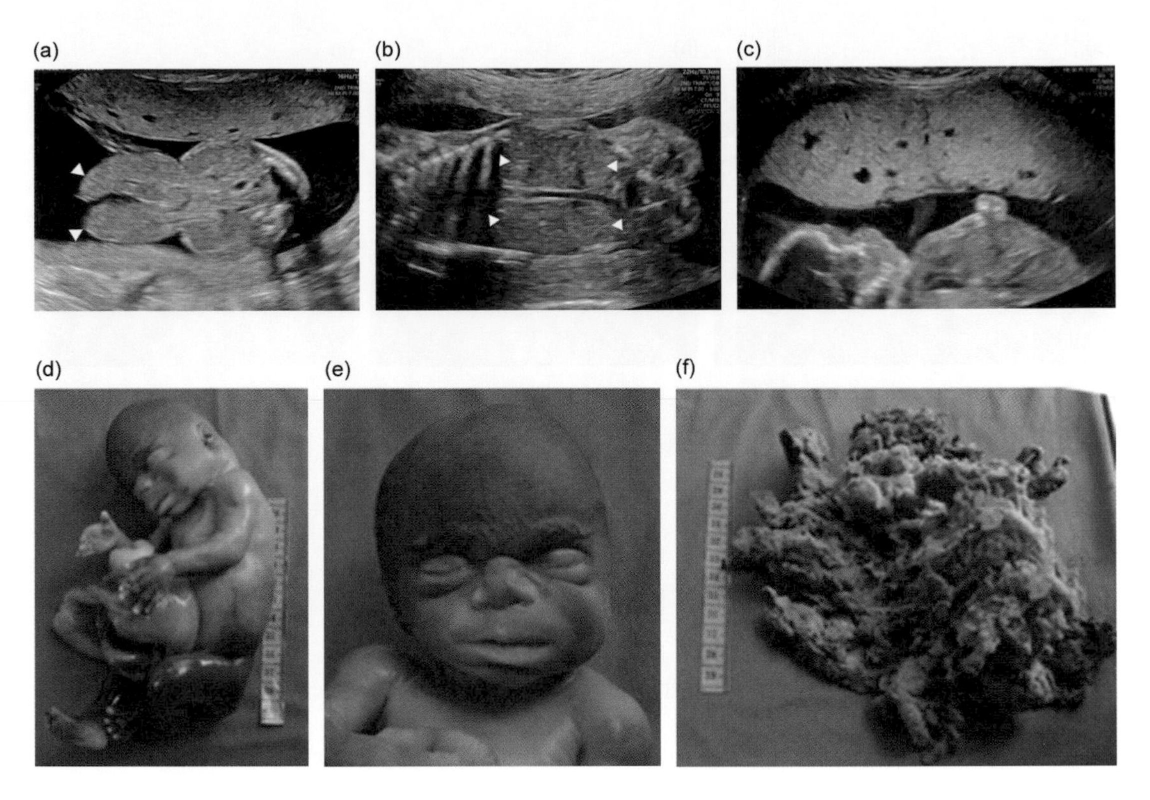

Fig. 19.5 Beckwith–Wiedemann syndrome. (a) Omphalocele (arrowheads); (b) coronal view of the abdomen showing bilateral nephromegaly (arrowheads); (c) placentomegaly with cystic spaces suggestive of mesenchymal dysplasia. (d) Same fetus after birth with omphalocele and (e) facial asymmetry which is difficult to diagnose antenatally. (f) Placenta after expulsion showing mesenchymal dysplasia confirmed on histology.

BINDER PHENOTYPE OR SYNDROME

Characteristics

- Maxillo-nasal dysplasia
- Short nose with flat nasal bridge, short columella and an acute naso-labial angle
- Heterogeneous aetiology
  - *Familial* where several members of the same family have a similar facial profile and are otherwise normal
  - *Secondary* to maternal autoimmune disorders, vitamin K deficiency, mothers on warfarin or phenytoin
  - Seen in *chondrodysplasia punctate* – associated with stippling of epiphyses and sometimes shortening of bones

Inheritance

- Variable – depends on underlying aetiology

Ultrasound/MRI Detectable Features in Affected Fetuses

- Nasal hypoplasia with reduced frontonasal angle

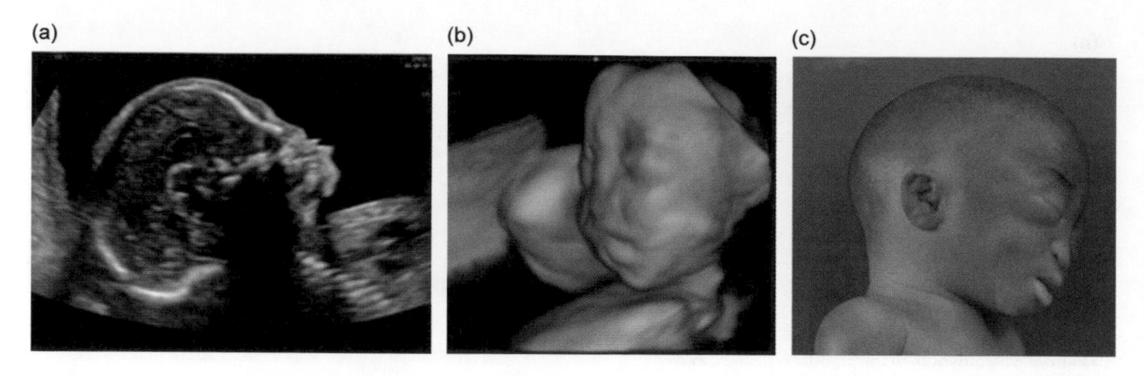

Fig. 19.6 Binder phenotype: (a) sagittal view of a fetus at 21 weeks showing flat facial profile; (b) 3D image of the same fetus; (c) fetus after birth with characteristic flat nose.

BLOOM SYNDROME

Characteristics

- Short stature
- Skin rash after sun exposure (butterfly-shaped patch of reddened skin across the nose and cheeks)
- Increased risk of cancer and subsequent reduced life expectancy
- Reduced fertility in women, infertility in men
- Moderate immunodeficiency and endocrine disorders

Inheritance

- Autosomal recessive – *BLM* mutations

Ultrasound/MRI Detectable Features in Affected Fetuses

- Reduced growth – symmetric
- Possibly micrognathia and dolichocephaly

CAUDAL REGRESSION SYNDROME

Characteristics

- Sacral hypoplasia or agenesis, can involve lumbar part of the spine and pelvic bones
- Usually able to walk but bowel and bladder control usually affected

Inheritance

- Mostly sporadic
- Association with maternal diabetes

Ultrasound/MRI Detectable Features in Affected Fetuses

- Absent/hypoplastic sacrum
- Abnormal lumbar spine/pelvis
- Abnormal lower limbs

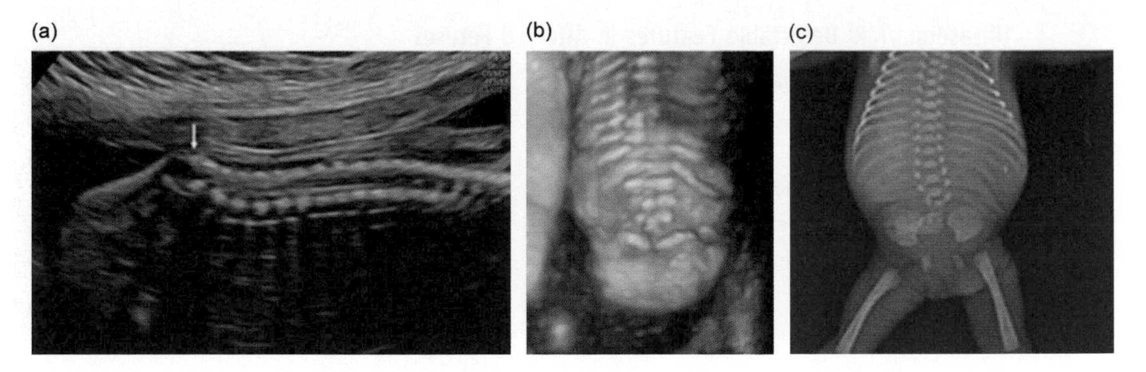

Fig. 19.7 Caudal regression syndrome. (a) Sagittal view of the spine showing lower lumbar and sacral agenesis (arrow); (b) 3D coronal view and (c) postnatal X-ray of the same fetus showing absence of lower lumbar and sacral vertebrae.

CEREBRO-OCULO-FACIO-SKELETAL SYNDROME

Characteristics

- Neurodegenerative disorder with antenatal onset
- Pre- and postnatal growth failure
- Microcephaly, cataract, microphthalmia, micrognathia
- Brain dysmyelination and calcium deposits
- Flexion contractures, camptodactyly (bent fingers), rocker-bottom feet
- Considered to overlap with a severe form of Cockayne syndrome

Inheritance

- Autosomal recessive – *ERCC6*, *ERCC8* and *ERCC2* genes

Ultrasound/MRI Detectable Features in Affected Fetuses

- Growth restriction
- Microphthalmia, cataract
- Micrognathia
- Multiple joint contractures
- Rocker-bottom feet

CHARGE SYNDROME

Characteristics

- Coloboma, choanal atresia, ear abnormalities
- Heart defects
- Growth restriction
- Genital abnormalities

Inheritance

- Autosomal dominant
- Changes in *CHD7* – single variants (98%) or copy number changes (2%)
- Usually *de novo*

Ultrasound/MRI Detectable Features in Affected Fetuses

- Difficult to diagnose prenatally as features are non-specific
- Ventriculomegaly
- Cardiac defects
- Fetal growth restriction
- Abnormal genitalia
- Fetal growth restriction, polyhydramnios

CILIOPATHIES

- Ciliopathies are associated with genetic mutations encoding defective proteins leading to abnormal formation or function of primary or motile cellular cilia
- Ciliary dysfunction is genetically very heterogeneous and phenotypically very diverse – ~100 single-gene causes have been already described

BARDET–BIEDL SYNDROME

Characteristics

- Intellectual disability
- Progressive visual impairment due to retinal degeneration
- Truncal obesity
- Postaxial polydactyly
- Kidney abnormalities, hypogonadism

Inheritance

- Autosomal recessive
- At least 26 causative genes identified

Ultrasound/MRI Detectable Features in Affected Fetuses

- Polydactyly
- Polycystic kidneys
- Difficult to diagnose clinically as there is significant overlap with other ciliopathies

ELLIS–VAN CREVELD SYNDROME

Characteristics

- Short limbs (mesomelia)/short stature, short ribs/narrow chest, polydactyly
- Abnormal fingernails
- Over half have congenital heart defects
- Cleft palate, dental abnormalities

Inheritance

- Autosomal recessive
- Variants in *EVC* and *EVC2*

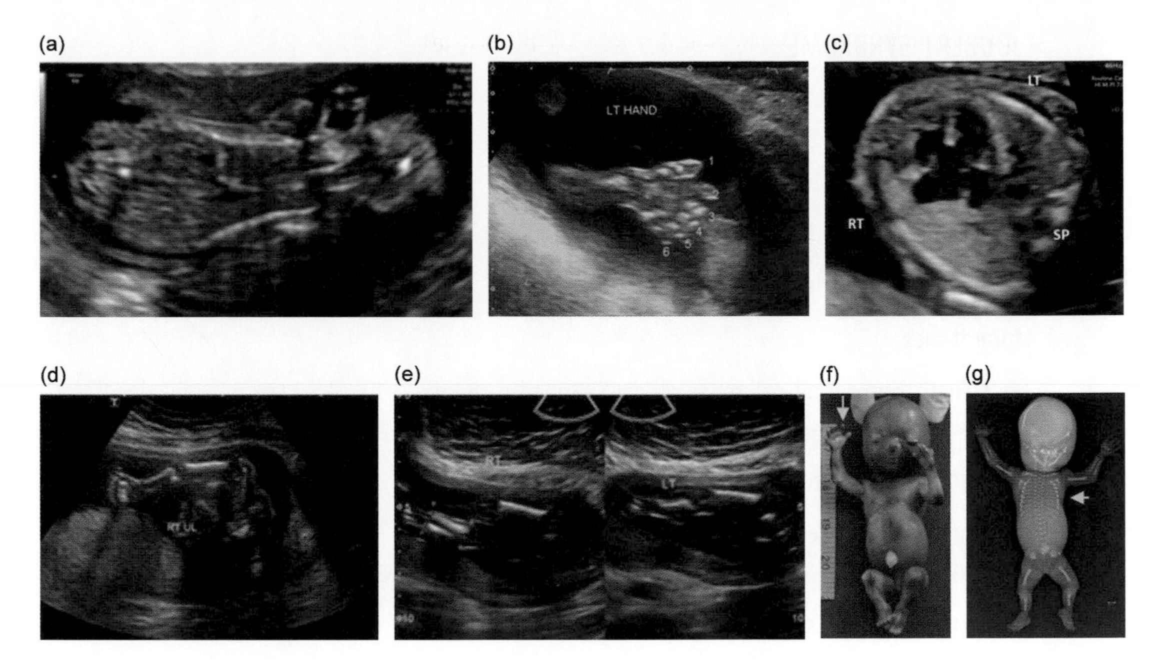

Fig. 19.8 Ellis–van Creveld syndrome. (a) Coronal section of the body showing narrow thorax; (b) mesoaxial polydactyly; (c) AVSD with common AV valve; (d,e) bilateral mesomelic shortening of the upper and lower limbs. (f) The same fetus after birth – note mesoaxial polydactyly (arrow) and narrow thorax. (g) X-ray shows short ribs and short tibia, fibula, radius and ulna.

Ultrasound/MRI Detectable Features in Affected Fetuses

- Narrow thorax, short ribs, short long bones
- Cardiac defects (ASD, VSD, single atrium, patent ductus, hypoplastic left heart syndrome, abnormal AV valves)
- One of very few disorders presenting with a central cleft lip

JEUNE SYNDROME (ASPHYXIATING THORACIC DYSPLASIA)

Characteristics

- Small chest/short ribs, restricted lung development, life-threatening breathing difficulties
- Short long bones, abnormal pelvis
- Polydactyly
- Kidney problems

Inheritance

- Autosomal recessive
- At least four causative genes identified

Ultrasound/MRI Detectable Features in Affected Fetuses

- Short ribs, small thorax, short long bones
- Polydactyly

JOUBERT SYNDROME

Characteristics

- Intellectual disability
- Hypotonia, ataxia, abnormal eye movements
- Distinctive facial features (broad forehead, arched eyebrows, ptosis, hypertelorism, low-set ears, triangle-shaped mouth)
- Abnormal breathing patterns

Inheritance

- Usually autosomal recessive, rarely X-linked recessive
- Multiple causative genes

Ultrasound/MRI Detectable Features in Affected Fetuses

- Abnormal cerebellar peduncles (molar tooth sign)
- Hypoplasia or absence of the cerebellar vermis with cleft between cerebellar hemispheres

MECKEL–GRUBER SYNDROME

Characteristics

- Occipital encephalocele
- Polycystic kidneys
- Facial deformities (micrognathia, cleft lip/palate)
- Pulmonary hypoplasia due to oligohydramnios
- Lethal disorder

Inheritance

- Autosomal recessive
- At least 13 causative genes identified

Ultrasound/MRI Detectable Features in Affected Fetuses

- Classic triad: polydactyly, polycystic kidney and occipital encephalocele (at least two needed for diagnosis)

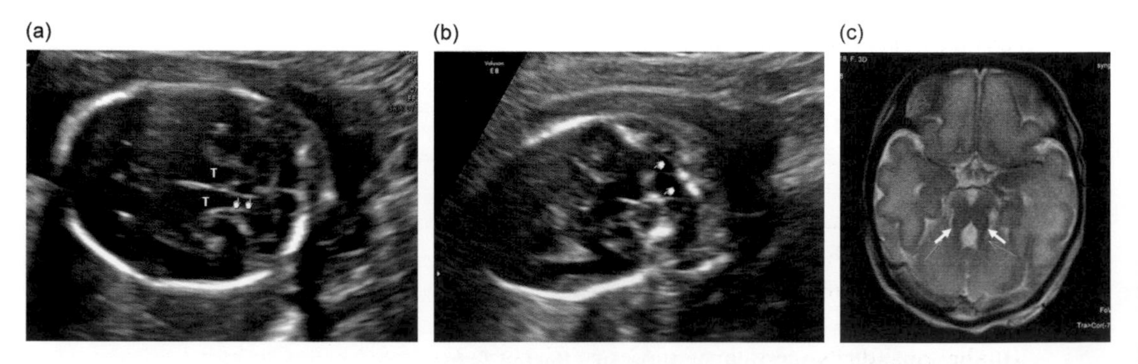

Fig. 19.9 Joubert syndrome. (a) Transverse section of the fetal head showing the molar tooth sign of the thalami (T) and elongated fourth ventricle (pointed fingers). (b) Transversal view of the posterior fossa showing absence of cerebellar vermis and a cleft between cerebellar hemispheres (pointed fingers). (c) Typical molar tooth sign seen on the MRI (arrows).

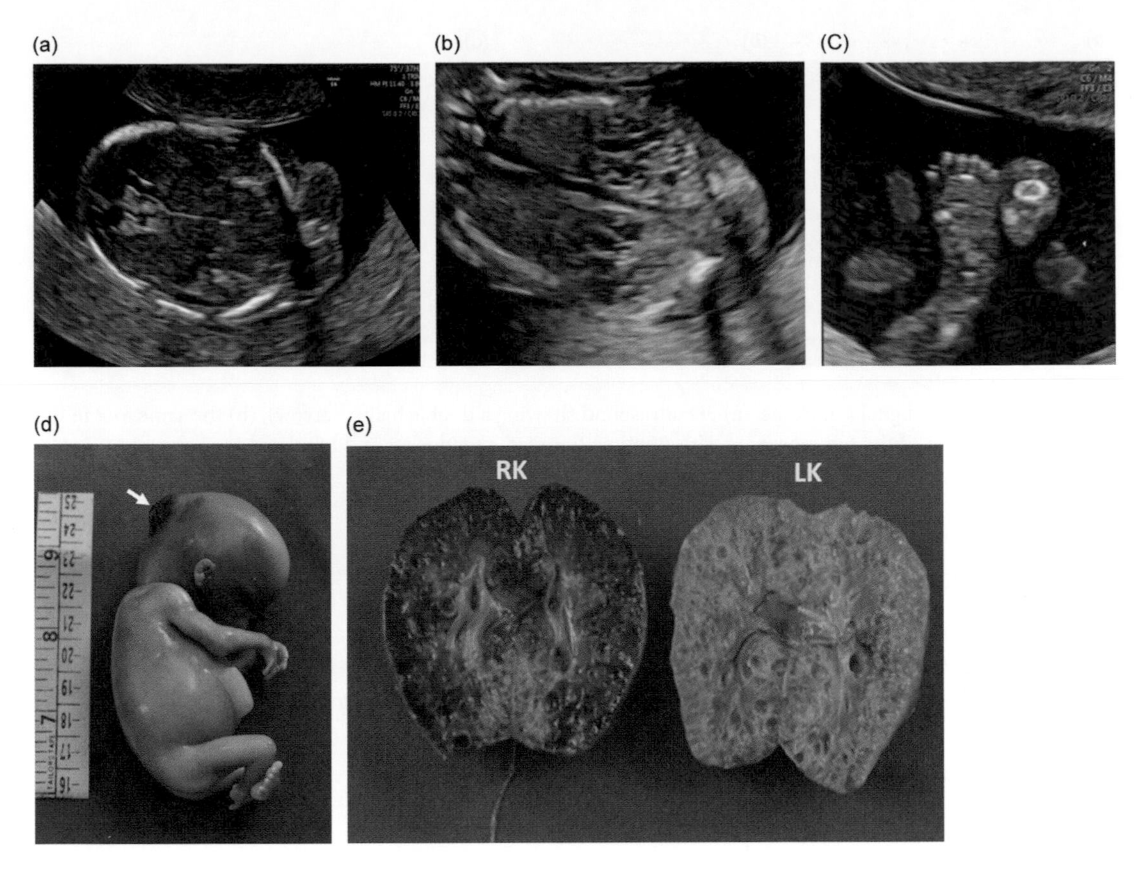

Fig. 19.10 (a) Meckel–Gruber syndrome: transverse view of the head with occipital encephalocele. (b) Coronal section of the abdomen showing bilateral polycystic kidneys. (c) Fetal foot with polydactyly. (d) Post mortem picture of the same fetus with occipital encephalocele (arrow) and (e) autopsy specimen showing enlarged cystic kidneys.

- Ventriculomegaly
- Facial abnormalities
- Oligohydramnios

ORO-FACIAL-DIGITAL SYNDROME (OFDS)

Characteristics

- Heterogenous group of 16 disorders characterised by facial dysmorphism, abnormalities of oral cavity and digits
- Central nervous system, renal cystic disease and cardiac involvement may be seen
- Many types overlap with ciliopathy spectrum
- Oral manifestations – lobed tongue, tongue hamartomas, lipomas, median cleft or pseudocleft, cleft palate, multiple frenulae
- Abnormal digits – pre- or postaxial polydactyly, duplicated hallux or broad thumb, syndactyly

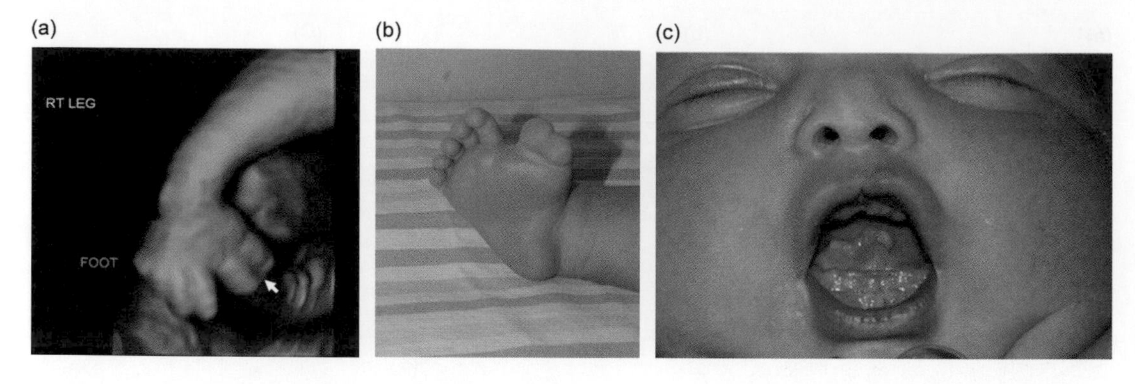

Fig. 19.11 Oro-facial-digital syndrome: (a) 3D ultrasound showing a double hallux (arrow); (b) the same foot in the neonate; (c) mouth of the same neonate with multiple frenulae, pseudocleft and lobulated tongue.

Inheritance

- OFDS I is inherited in an X-linked dominant manner with male lethality due to variants in *OFD1*
- Most of the others are autosomal recessive or currently unknown

Ultrasound/MRI Detectable Features in Affected Fetuses

- Polydactyly – pre- or postaxial, duplicated hallux
- Cleft lip and palate
- Echogenic kidneys

SHORT RIB POLYDACTYLY SYNDROMES

Characteristics

- Short ribs, hypoplastic thorax, polydactyly, micromelia
- Multiple types with significant clinical overlap with EVC and Jeune syndrome
- This is a lethal skeletal dysplasia due to severe lung hypoplasia

Inheritance

- Autosomal recessive
- Multiple causative genes

Ultrasound/MRI Detectable Features in Affected Fetuses

- Short ribs, hypoplastic thorax, polydactyly, micromelia
- Most common associated congenital abnormalities are cardiac and renal
- Difficult to diagnose clinically prenatally due to features overlapping with other ciliopathies

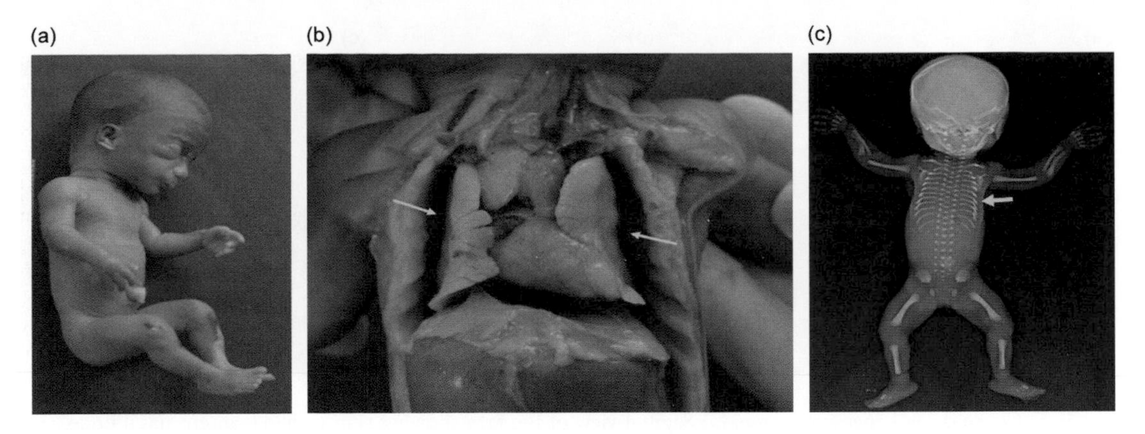

Fig. 19.12 Short rib polydactyly syndrome. (a) Bilateral shortening of both upper and lower limbs, with postaxial polydactyly of hands and feet; (b) narrow thorax with hypoplastic lungs and (c) very short horizontal ribs.

CORNELIA DE LANGE SYNDROME

Characteristics

- Developmental delay
- Distinctive facial features with hypertrichosis (small nose, downturned mouth, thin upper lip, long and smooth philtrum, thick eyebrows)
- Congenital diaphragmatic hernia
- Small stature, missing toes/fingers
- Microcephaly

Inheritance

- Linked to multiple genes (60% of variants in *NIPBL*) – mostly *de novo*
- Can be inherited as X-linked or autosomal dominant

Ultrasound/MRI Detectable Features in Affected Fetuses

- Abnormal facial profile
- Limb abnormalities (mostly asymmetrical defects in upper limbs – ulnar aplasia and a flexed elbow are typical, but can be more subtle)
- Fetal growth restriction
- Diaphragmatic hernia

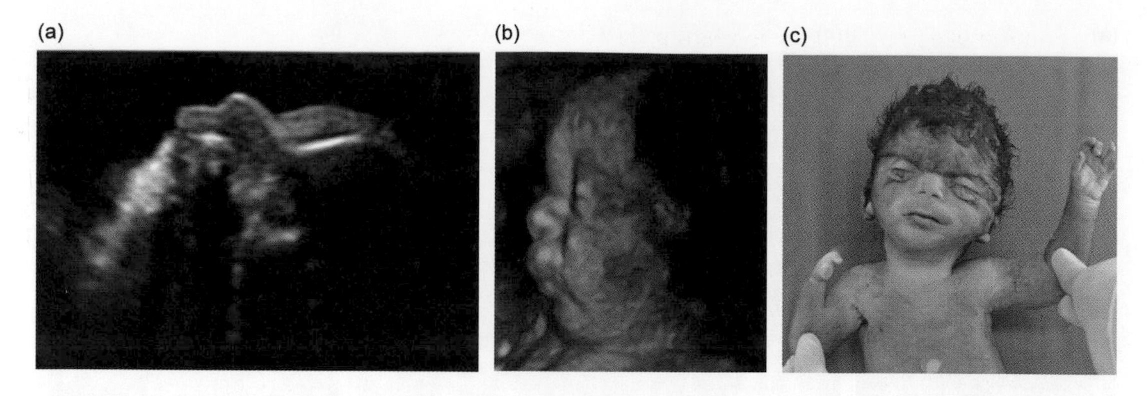

Fig. 19.13 Cornelia De Lange syndrome. (a) Sagittal view of the face showing skin oedema, absent nasal bone, an overlapping upper lip and micrognathia; (b) 3D facial profile of the same fetus. (c) Fetus after birth showing hypertrichosis, fusion of the eyebrows above the bridge of nose (synophrys), long eyelashes and abnormal left upper limb.

CROUZON SYNDROME

Characteristics

- Craniosynostosis
- Hypertelorism, psittichorhina (beak-like nose), strabismus, hypoplastic maxilla
- Can develop Chiari malformation and hydrocephalus
- Exomphalos
- Most patients have normal intelligence
- May have vision and hearing problems

Inheritance

- Autosomal dominant
- Variants in *FGFR2*

Ultrasound/MRI Detectable Features in Affected Fetuses

- Abnormal shape of the skull (i.e. brachycephaly)
- Midface hypoplasia, beaked nose, mandibular prognathism

DIGEORGE SYNDROME

Characteristics

- Heart defects
- Cleft lip/palate
- Learning difficulties, behavioural problems
- Speech and hearing problems
- Hyperparathyroidism
- Frequent infections

Inheritance

- Autosomal dominant deletion of 22q11.2
- 90% *de novo* mutations

Ultrasound/MRI Detectable Features in Affected Fetuses

- Heart defects (commonly tetralogy of Fallot, interrupted aortic arch, truncus arteriosus)
- Cleft lip/palate
- Thymic hypoplasia or aplasia
- Fetal growth restriction

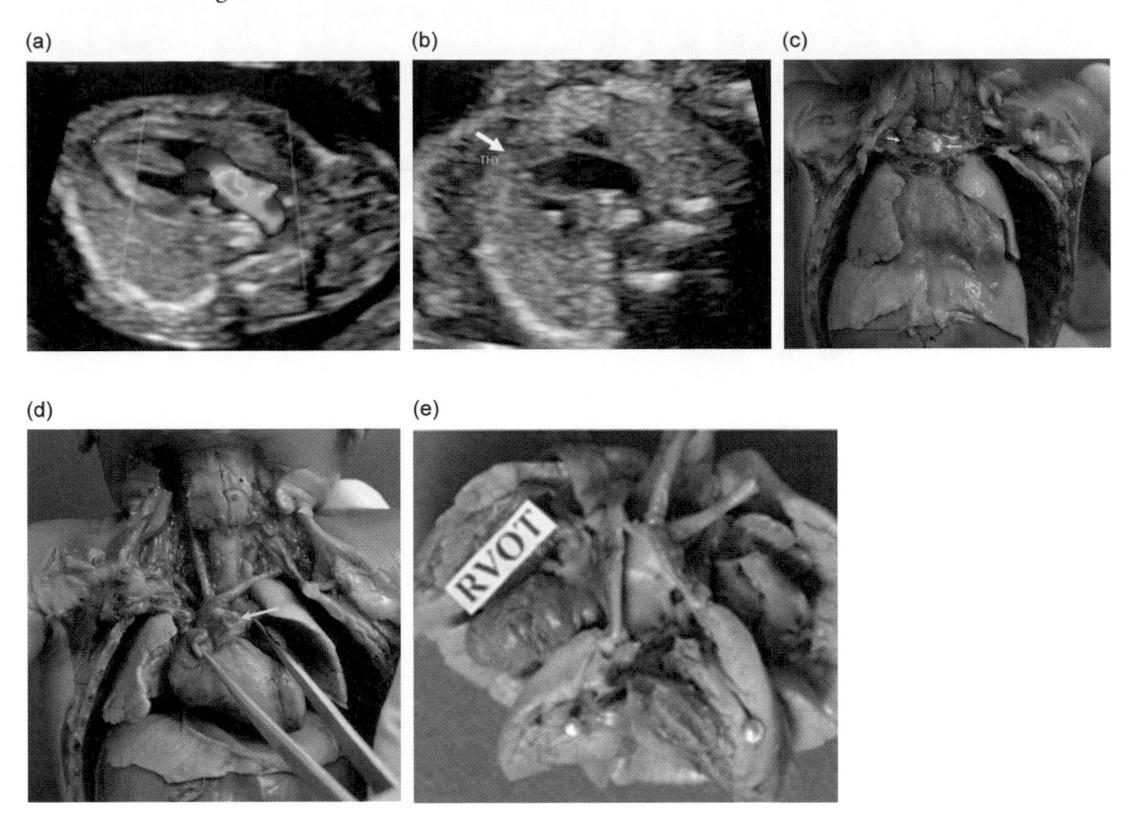

Fig. 19.14 DiGeorge syndrome. (a) Ultrasound images of the truncus arteriosus arising from right ventricle and (b) hypoplastic thymus (arrow). (c) Autopsy images of the hypoplastic thymus (d) a single outflow tract and (e) common trunk arising from the right ventricle.

ECTRODACTYLY-ECTODERMAL DYSPLASIA-CLEFT (EEC) SYNDROME

Characteristics

- Facial clefts
- Ecterodactyly (cleft hand)
- Ectodermal dysplasia (abnormal teeth, skin, sweat glands, nails)

Inheritance

- Autosomal dominant
- *TP63* genetic variants

Ultrasound/MRI Detectable Features in Affected Fetuses

- Cleft lip/palate, abnormal hand (cleft hand, syndactyly, polydactyly)
- Ectrodactyly, but significant overlap with other ectrodactyly disorders

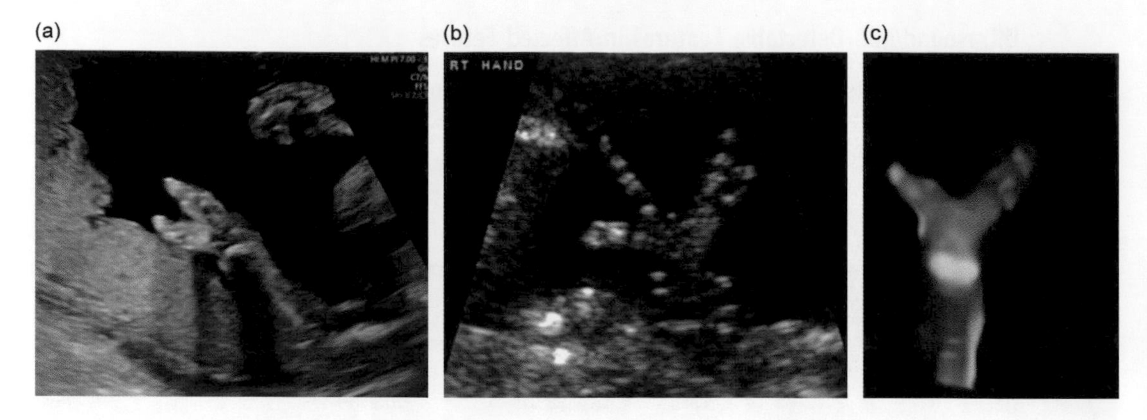

Fig. 19.15 EEC syndrome. Ectrodactyly (split hand) seen on (a,b) 2D and (c) 3D scan images.

FANCONI ANAEMIA

Characteristics

- Prenatal and postnatal growth failure
- Abnormal skin pigmentation
- Progressive bone marrow failure
- Skeletal malformations (radial ray defect)
- CNS – microcephaly, corpus callosum defects and ventriculomegaly
- Ophthalmic and genitourinary anomalies
- The diagnosis is confirmed by increased chromosomal breakage in the lymphocytes induced with mitomycin C (MMC) or diepoxybutane (DEB) via DEB/MMC stress test

Inheritance

- Autosomal recessive – 19 genes: *FANCA*, *FANCC*, *FANCG*, etc.
- Autosomal dominant – *RAD51*
- X-linked – *FANCB*

Ultrasound/MRI Detectable Features in Affected Fetuses

- Fetal growth restriction
- Radial ray defects ranging from partial to completely absent radius, with or without abnormal bones
- Microcephaly, rarely corpus callosal defects and ventriculomegaly have been reported
- Horseshoe kidney
- Vertebral abnormalities

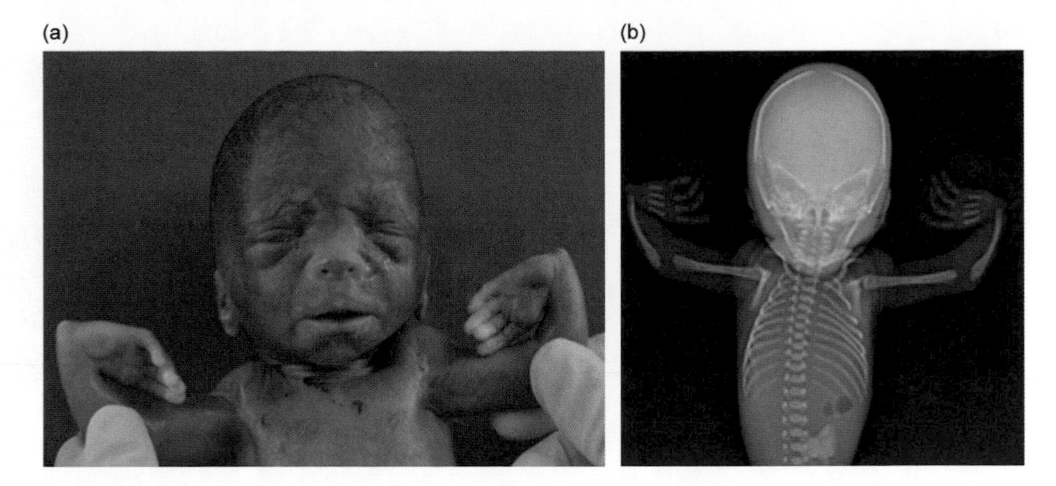

Fig. 19.16 Fanconi anaemia. (a) Bilateral radial ray defect. (b) X-ray of the same fetus showing absence of radius on both sides.

FEMORAL–FACIAL SYNDROME (FEMORAL HYPOPLASIA–UNUSUAL FACIES SYNDROME)

Characteristics

- Bilateral femoral hypoplasia
- Characteristic facial features (short nose with broad tip, long philtrum, thin upper lip, micrognathia, cleft palate, upward-slanting eyes)

Inheritance

- Sporadic occurrence
- Association with maternal diabetes

Ultrasound/MRI Detectable Features in Affected Fetuses

- Short, often bowed femur
- Micrognathia, facial clefts

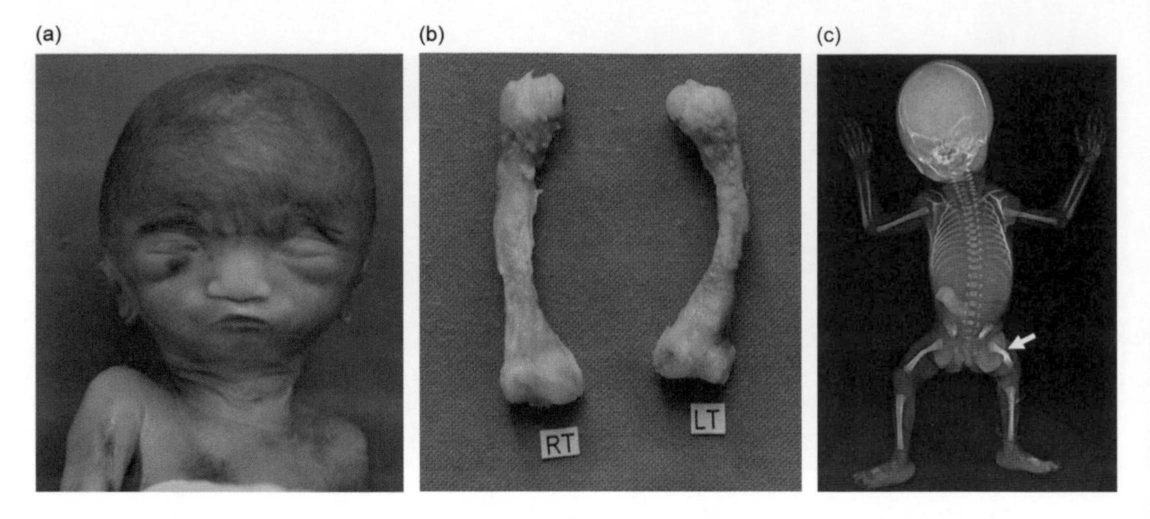

Fig. 19.17 Femoral–facial syndrome. (a) Dysmorphic face with depressed nasal bridge, flattened nose, micrognathia. (b) Bilateral shortened and bowed femora and (c) fetogram of the same fetus.

FRASER SYNDROME

Characteristics

- Intellectual disability
- Fused eyelids (cryptophthalmos), malformations of nose and ears
- Syndactyly
- Laryngeal/tracheal atresia
- Abnormal or missing kidneys, ambiguous genitalia
- Autosomal recessive
- *FRAS1*, *GRIP1*, *FREM1* and *FREM2* genetic variants

Ultrasound/MRI Detectable Features in Affected Fetuses

- Fused eyelids and syndactyly are key features
- Microphthalmia
- Enlarged echogenic lungs
- Abnormal kidneys
- Ambiguous genitalia or abnormal male genitalia

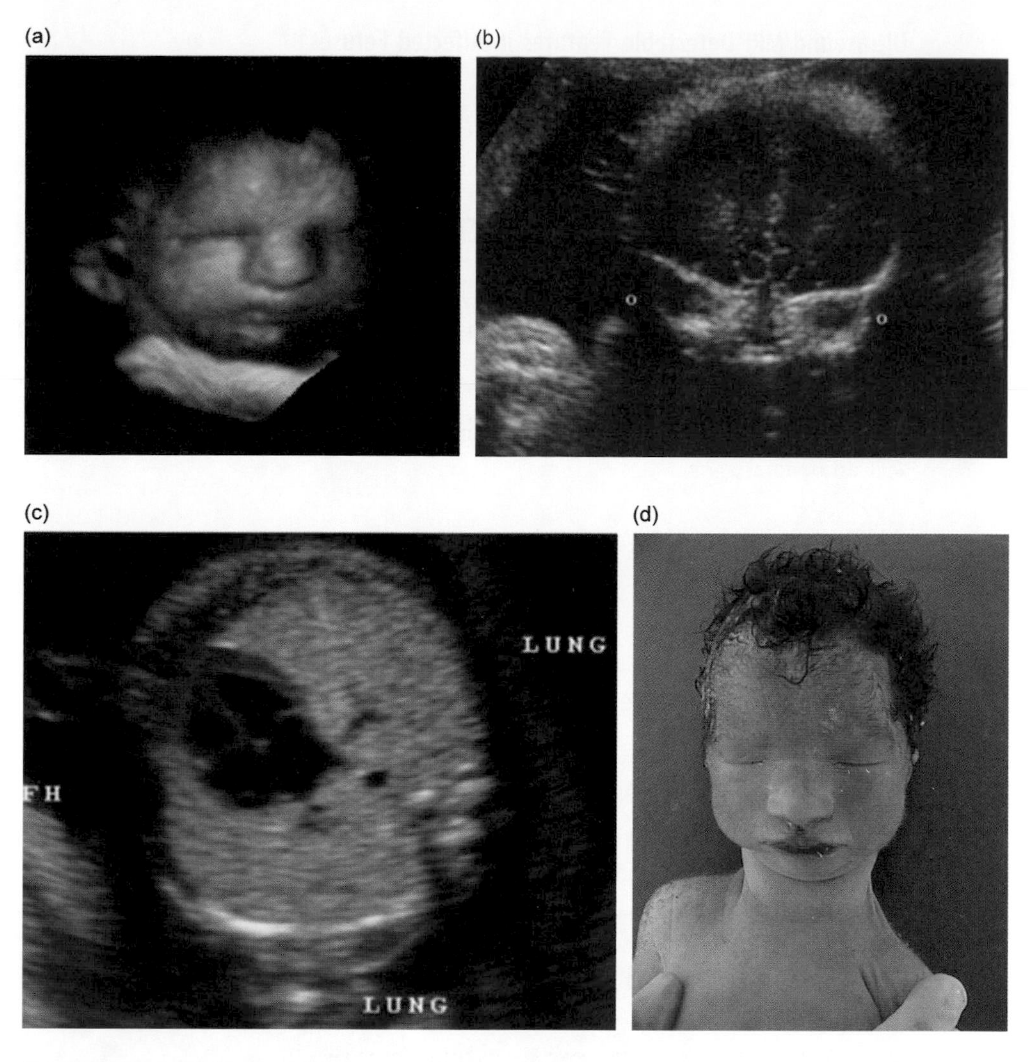

Fig. 19.18 Fraser syndrome. (a) Left cryptophthalmos (skin passing continuously from the forehead to the cheek); (b) microphthalmia; (c) enlarged echogenic lungs. (d) Same fetus after birth with microphthalmia.

FRYNS SYNDROME

Characteristics

- Congenital diaphragmatic hernia (90%), lung hypoplasia
- Distinctive facial features (coarse face, hypertelorism, cloudy cornea, broad and flat nasal bridge, anteverted nostrils, dysplastic and low-set ears, wide mouth and micrognathia)
- Cleft lip/palate
- Abnormalities of toes and fingers and multiple other organs
- Mostly fatal in early infancy due to lung hypoplasia

Inheritance

- Thought to be autosomal recessive
- No specific genes identified

Ultrasound/MRI Detectable Features in Affected Fetuses

- Microphthalmia, micrognathia
- Diaphragmatic hernia
- Polyhydramnios

GENERALISED ARTERIAL CALCIFICATION OF INFANCY (GACI)

Characteristics

- Abnormal accumulation of calcium in the walls of blood vessels, aorta and pulmonary artery in particular, leading to stenosis and stiffness of the vessels (heart failure may develop)
- Deposits of calcium in other organs and tissues (e.g. joints)
- Can be fatal

Inheritance

- Autosomal recessive
- *ENPP1*, *ABCC6* genetic variants

Ultrasound/MRI Detectable Features in Affected Fetuses

- Echogenic great arteries, abnormal cardiac contractility, cardiomegaly, pericardial effusion
- Hydrops, polyhydramnios
- Hyperechoic kidneys

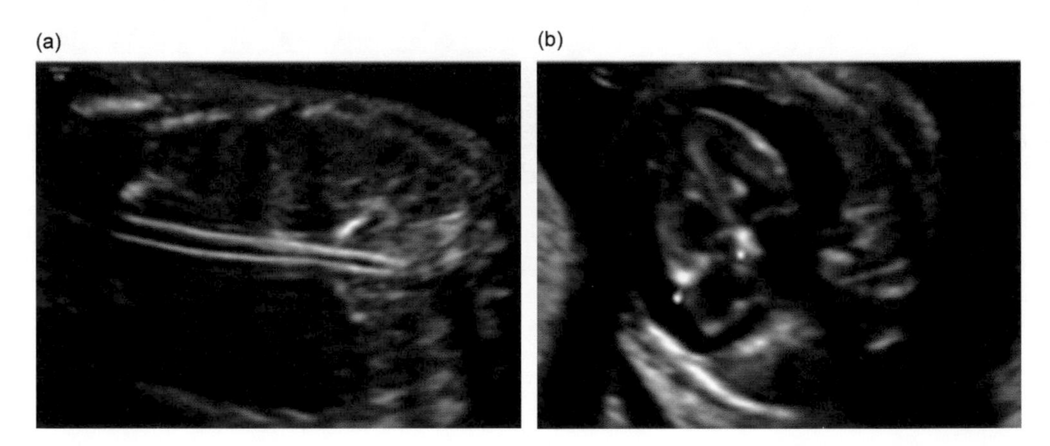

Fig. 19.19 Generalised arterial calcification of infancy. (a) Coronal view of the fetal abdomen with calcified abdominal aorta and (b) four chamber view with echogenic, calcified valves.

GOLDENHAR SYNDROME

Characteristics

- Facial asymmetry, abnormal or absent ears, periaurical tags, benign tumours of the eye (ocular dermoid cysts), cleft lip/palate
- Spinal abnormalities
- May also affect the heart, lungs, kidneys and brain

Inheritance

- Sporadic occurrence, but does have considerable overlap with other genetic disorders

Ultrasound/MRI Detectable Features in Affected Fetuses

- Facial asymmetry (hemifacial hypoplasia), ear abnormalities, orbital anomalies, retrognathia/micrognathia
- Difficult to diagnose prenatally as need to exclude other genetic conditions such as Treacher Collins syndrome

GOLTZ–GORLIN SYNDROME (FOCAL DERMAL HYPOPLASIA)

Characteristics

- Genodermatosis
- Skin involvement – areas of thin and atrophic skin following Blaschko's lines
- Asymmetry of face, small or absent eyes, intraocular abnormalities
- Fat nodules and herniation
- Dystrophic nails, sparse hair
- Limb abnormalities – oligodactyly, syndactyly, ectrodactyly, limb shortening
- Dental anomalies, renal anomalies, diaphragmatic hernia

Inheritance

- X-linked dominant –*PORCN*; females are affected and usually lethal in male

Ultrasound/MRI Detectable Features in Affected Fetuses

- Growth restriction in some fetuses
- Variable limb anomalies – ectrodactyly, syndactyly, oligodactyly, limb shortening
- Occasionally diaphragmatic hernia, renal anomalies

HOLT–ORAM SYNDROME

Characteristics

- Upper limb malformations (different presentations, i.e. abnormal wrist bones, thumb that looks like a finger)
- Congenital heart defects (ASD, VSD most common) and cardiac conduction defects (heart block)

Inheritance

- Autosomal dominant with very variable penetrance; may find a mildly affected parent
- *TBX5* genetic variants

Ultrasound/MRI Detectable Features in Affected Fetuses

- Upper limb defects, cardiac defects

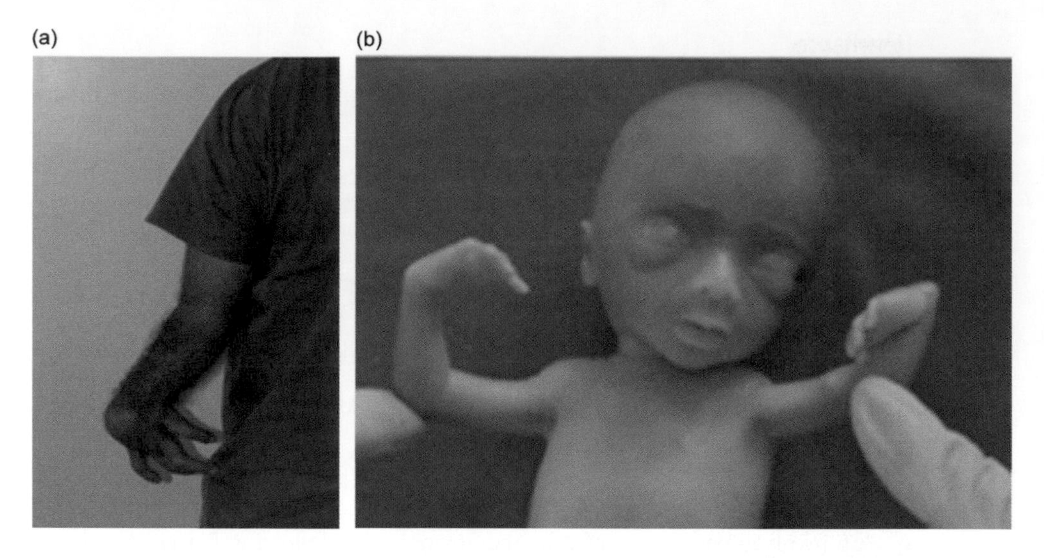

Fig. 19.20 Holt–Oram syndrome. (a) Father with radial ray defect. (b) Post mortem picture of his baby. The fetus also had large VSD. Both harboured heterozygous pathogenic variants of the *TBX5* gene.

HYDROLETHALUS SYNDROME

Characteristics

- Lethal malformation syndrome
- Hydrocephalus, absence of upper midline structures of the brain (corpus callosum, cerebellar vermis, septum pellucidum)
- Postaxial polydactyly in hands and preaxial polydactyly in feet and micrognathia
- Other associated anomalies include talipes, cardiac defects, cleft lip and palate, keyhole-shaped defect in occipital bone, abnormal genitalia and abnormal airways

Inheritance

- Autosomal recessive – *HYLS1* and *KIF7*

Ultrasound/MRI Detectable Features in Affected Fetuses

- Severe ventriculomegaly, agenesis of corpus callosum and other intracranial midline structures
- Cleft lip and palate
- Cardiac defects
- Characteristic polydactyly (postaxial in hands but preaxial in feet)

JARCHO–LEVIN SYNDROME (SPONDYLOCOSTAL DYSPLASIA)

Characteristics

- Defects of the vertebrae and the ribs (abnormal, fused or missing in chaotic patterns), scoliosis, kyphosis, short neck, small thorax, hypoplastic lungs
- Can be fatal due to lung hypoplasia

Inheritance

- Autosomal recessive
- Multiple genes

Ultrasound/MRI Detectable Features in Affected Fetuses

- Abnormal vertebrae/spine and ribs, small thorax

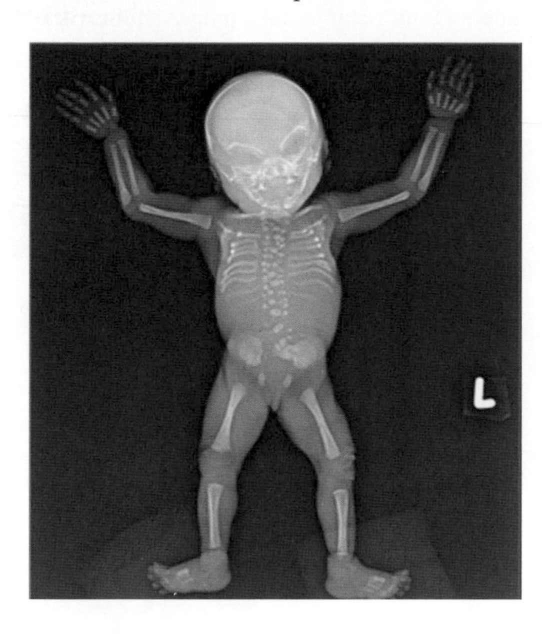

Fig. 19.21 Jarcho–Levin syndrome. Short spine with abnormal vertebrae showing multiple missing or abnormal vertebrae – 'pebble beach' sign.

KLIPPEL–FEIL SYNDROME

Characteristics

- Abnormal fusion of two or more cervical vertebrae +/− narrowing of spinal canal/cord compression
- Three classic signs: (1) short neck; (2) low hairline at the back of the head and (3) a limited range of motion in the neck
- Can have associated abnormalities (cardiac, intracranial, spinal)

Inheritance

- Autosomal dominant or autosomal recessive
- Diagnostic genetic testing often not available

Ultrasound/MRI Detectable Features in Affected Fetuses

- Hyperextended neck, fused cervical vertebrae

LARSEN SYNDROME

Characteristics

- Dysmorphic facial profile (hypertelorism, frontal bossing, depressed nasal bridge)
- Ligamentous hyperlaxity, multiple joint dislocation
- Talipes equinovarus

Inheritance

- Autosomal dominant – *FLNB* (common)
- Autosomal recessive – *CHST3* (rare)

Ultrasound/MRI Detectable Features in Affected Fetuses

- Dysmorphic facial profile
- Joint dislocations, hyperextended knees (genu recurvatum), talipes equinovarus
- Polyhydramnios

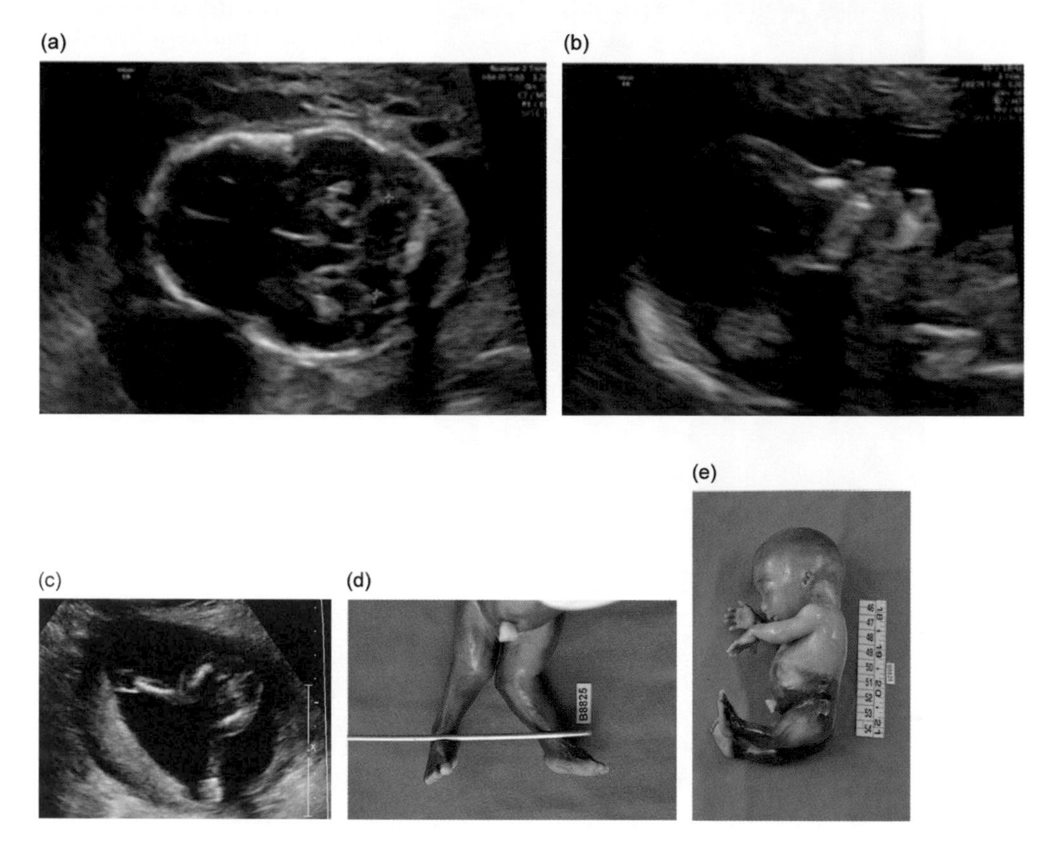

Fig. 19.22 Larsen syndrome. (a) Ultrasound images showing abnormal head shape due to craniosynostosis; (b) profile with flattened nasal bridge and dysmorphic face and (c) bilateral genu recurvatum. (d,e) Post mortem picture of the same fetus showing extended legs with bilateral genu recurvatum.

MICROCEPHALIC OSTEODYSPLASTIC PRIMORDIAL DWARFISM TYPES I/III, II

Characteristics

- Severe intrauterine and postnatal growth restriction
- Intellectual deficit and seizures, microcephaly
- Variable dislocation of hips and elbows, flexion contractures, short limbs, skeletal anomalies
- Corpus callosal abnormalities and gyral pattern abnormalities reported with type I
- Skeletal dysplasia with progressive scoliosis, radial head dislocation and abnormal skin involvement is seen in type II

Inheritance

- MOPD I/III: autosomal recessive – *RNU4ATAC*
- MOPD II: autosomal recessive – *PCNT*

Ultrasound/MRI Detectable Features in Affected Fetuses

- Microcephaly
- Severe fetal growth restriction

MILLER–DIEKER SYNDROME

Characteristics

- Lissencephaly causing severe intellectual disability, seizures, swallowing difficulties, hypotonia
- Distinctive facial features – prominent forehead, upturned nose, midface hypoplasia, low-set abnormal ears, micrognathia, thick upper lip
- Short life span

Inheritance

- Most cases sporadic
- Can be caused by 17p13.3 deletions

Ultrasound/MRI Detectable Features in Affected Fetuses

- Abnormal gyration, lissencephaly
- Can have other intracranial abnormalities (ventriculomegaly, agenesis of corpus callosum)
- Fetal growth restriction
- Polyhydramnios

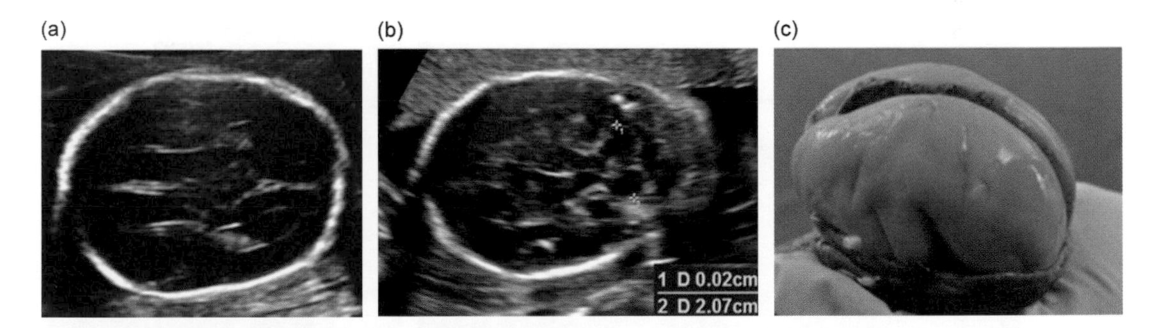

Fig. 19.23 Miller–Dieker syndrome. Fetal head at 26 weeks showing (a) smooth brain and (b) cerebellar hypoplasia. (c) Post mortem of the same fetus brain showing obvious lissencephaly.

NEU–LAXOVA SYNDROME

Characteristics

- Microcephaly, brain abnormalities
- Facial abnormalities (sloping forehead, hypertelorism, exophthalmos, micrognathia, abnormal ears)

- Generalised oedema (especially hands and feet)
- Skin abnormalities (ichthyosis, hyperkeratosis)
- Lethal condition

Inheritance

- Autosomal recessive
- *PHGDH*, *PSAT1*, *PSPH* genetic variants

Ultrasound/MRI Detectable Features in Affected Fetuses

- Exophthalmos (bulging eyeballs) is a key feature, but is also seen in other genetic conditions
- Microcephaly, intracranial abnormalities (lissencephaly, cerebellar hypoplasia)
- Severe fetal growth restriction
- Skin oedema, joint contractures, digit deformities
- Polyhydramnios

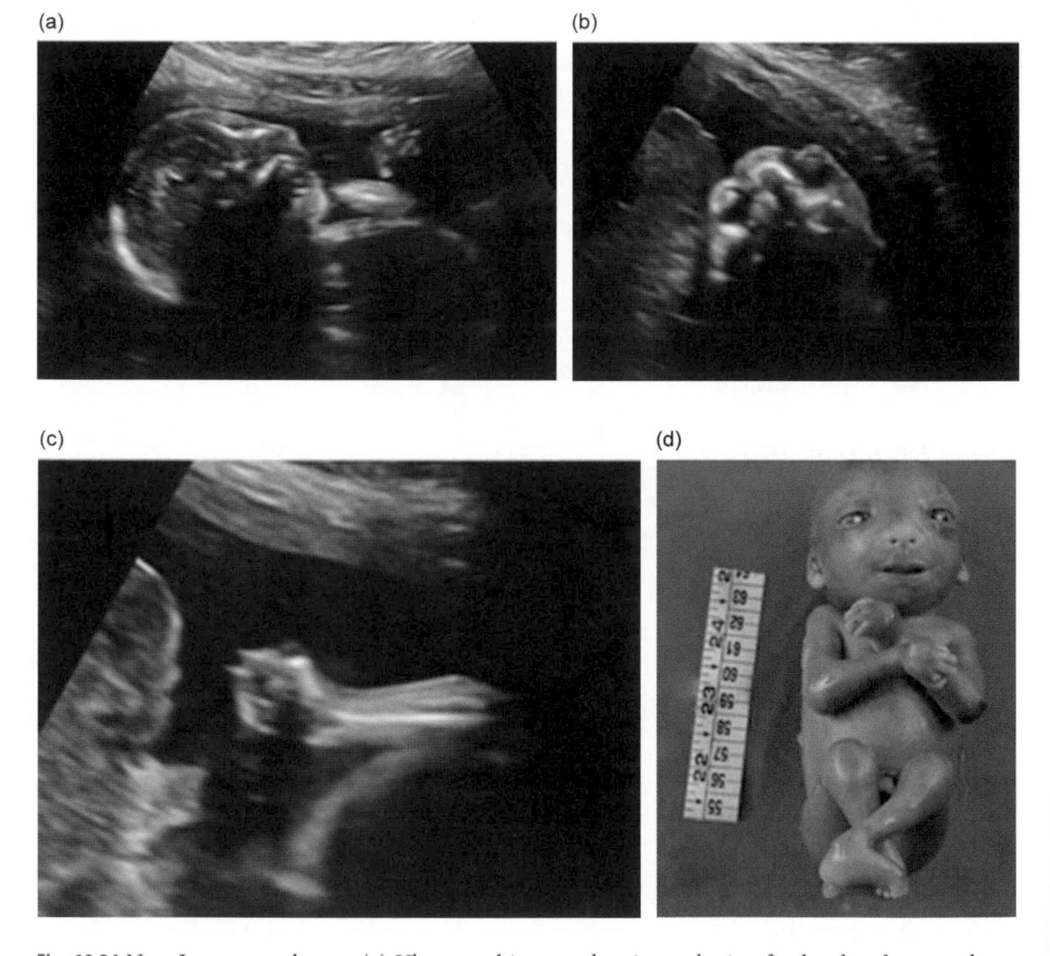

Fig. 19.24 Neu–Laxova syndrome. (a) Ultrasound images showing a sloping forehead and prenasal oedema; (b) hypertelorism and cataract and (c) abnormal posture with clenched fingers. (d) Post mortem findings confirmed microcephaly, thickened and stretched skin contractures and clenched hands. The fetus also had lissencephaly and agenesis of corpus callosum.

PFEIFFER SYNDROME

Characteristics

- Craniosynostosis, midfacial hypoplasia, broad thumbs and toes, variable intellectual disability
- Type I – mildest form, normal intelligence
- Type II – most severe; cloverleaf skull, maxillary hypoplasia, severe proptosis, elbow ankylosis, broad thumbs and big toe
- Type III – similar to type II except for absence of cloverleaf skull

Inheritance

- Autosomal dominant
- Type I: *FGFR1* and *FGFR2*
- Types II and III: *FGFR2*

Ultrasound/MRI Detectable Features in Affected Fetuses

- Craniosynostosis
- Abnormal eye protrusion (exophthalmos)
- Elbow ankylosis, broad thumbs and great toes

PIERRE–ROBIN SEQUENCE

Characteristics

- Micrognathia, retraction of the tongue, cleft palate, upper airway obstruction, feeding difficulties
- Can be isolated or part of a syndrome

Inheritance

- At least 50% have an underlying genetic basis
- Most commonly seen as part of Stickler syndrome

Ultrasound/MRI Detectable Features in Affected Fetuses

- Severe micrognathia
- Polyhydramnios (due to impaired swallowing)

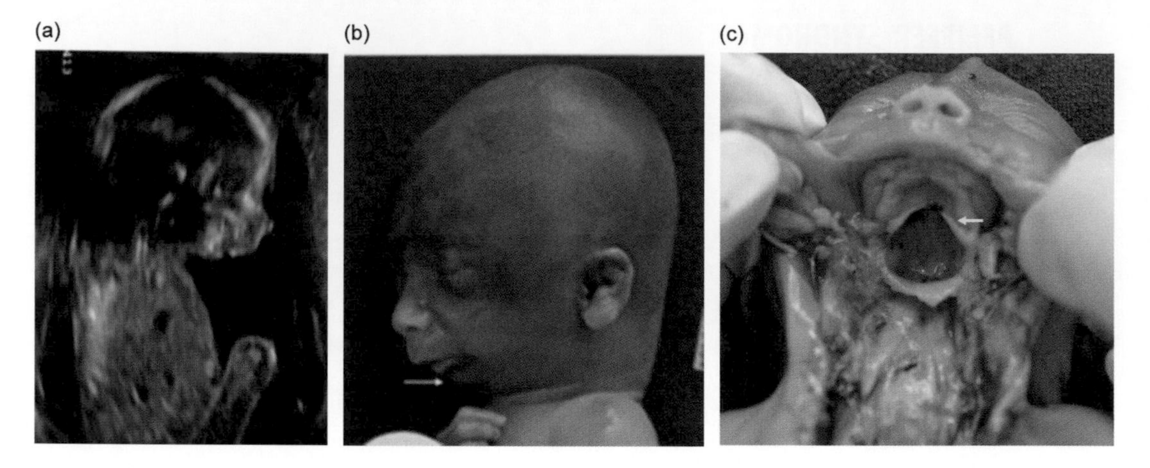

Fig. 19.25 Pierre–Robin sequence. (a) Fetal profile with severe micrognathia. (b) Post mortem pictures of the same fetus showing micrognathia (arrow) and (c) the roof of the mouth with posterior cleft palate.

PROTEUS SYNDROME

Characteristics

- Progressive disorder of tissue overgrowth (skin, bones, muscles, fatty tissues, blood and lymphatic vessels); usually asymmetric
- Increased risk of deep vein thrombosis and pulmonary embolism
- Increased risk of embryonic tumours

Inheritance

- Sporadic occurrence – *AKT1* mutations
- Mosaic condition

Ultrasound/MRI Detectable Features in Affected Fetuses

- Difficult diagnosis as features of the syndrome might not be obvious in prenatal life
- Megalencephaly
- Brain and eye malformations
- Focal soft tissue enlargement and ambiguous genitalia reported in the literature

PSEUDO-TORCH SYNDROME

Characteristics

- Mimics intrauterine infection
- Severe intellectual disability
- Intrauterine growth restriction
- Microcephaly, gyral abnormalities, spasticity
- Intracranial calcifications
- Cataract
- Seizures
- Neonatal hyperbilirubinemia, hepatosplenomegaly, thrombocytopenia

Inheritance

- Autosomal recessive: *OCLN, USP18, STAT2*

Ultrasound/MRI Detectable Features in Affected Fetuses

- Fetal growth restrictions
- Microcephaly and intracranial calcification
- Cataracts

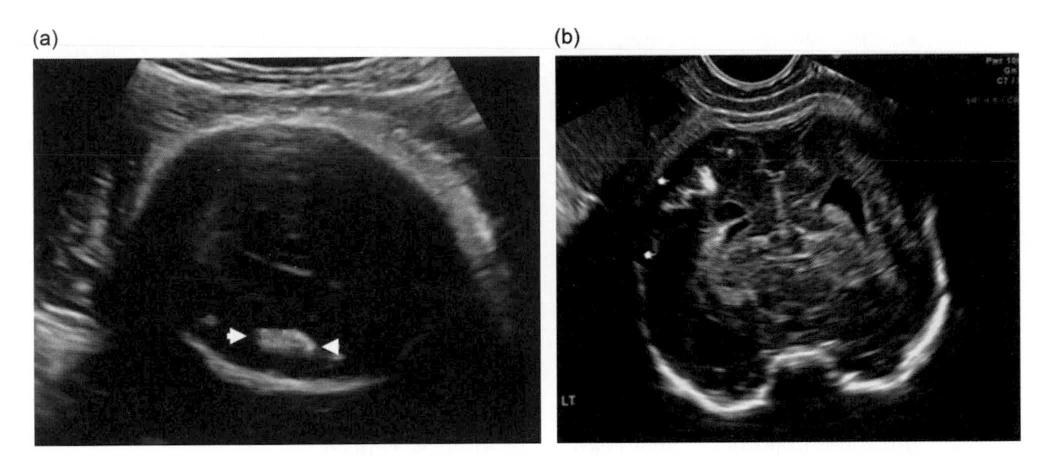

Fig. 19.26 Pseudo-TORCH syndrome. (a) Intracranial calcification (arrows). (b) Transvaginal scan of the same fetus confirmed cortical calcifications (finger arrows). Note the presence of a band in the ventricle. Maternal infection screen was negative.

RASopathies

- The RASopathies are caused by germ-line mutations in genes that encode components, or regulators, of the RAS/mitogen-activated protein kinase (MAPK) pathway – a chain of proteins that communicate signals from receptors on the cell surface to the nuclear DNA
- Most RASopathies have overlapping clinical features and clinical diagnosis is not always possible

COSTELLO SYNDROME

Characteristics

- Short stature, intellectual disability
- Loose skin folds (especially around hands and feet), abnormally flexible joints
- Congenital heart defects, arrythmia

Inheritance

- Autosomal dominant
- *HRAS* genetic variants, usually *de novo*

Ultrasound/MRI Detectable Features in Affected Fetuses

- Ventriculomegaly, macrocephaly
- Fetal atrial tachycardia
- Short long bones
- Polyhydramnios, hydrops

NOONAN SYNDROME

Characteristics

- Short stature
- Congenital heart defects
- Characteristic facial features (hypertelorism, down-slanting eyes, ptosis, low-set ears, bulbous nose tip and depressed root, prominent forehead, low hairline in the back)
- Skeletal malformations
- Lymphoedema

Inheritance

- Autosomal dominant and can have a very mildly affected parent
- 50% will have a variant in *PTPN11*

Ultrasound/MRI Detectable Features in Affected Fetuses

- Cystic hygroma
- Cardiac defects (pulmonary valve stenosis, ASD, VSD, hypertrophic cardiomyopathy)
- Pleural effusions
- Polyhydramnios

ROBERTS SYNDROME

Characteristics

- Severe pre- and postnatal growth restriction
- Symmetrical limb defects ranging from tetraphocomelia to absence of a few bones (upper limbs are more severely affected)
- Dysmorphic face, cleft lip and palate and microbrachycephaly, dysplastic ears
- Cardiac anomalies
- Genitourinary anomalies

Inheritance

- Autosomal recessive: *ESCO2*

Ultrasound/MRI Detectable Features in Affected Fetuses

- Severe fetal growth restriction
- Limb abnormalities (arms usually more affected than legs)
- Cleft lip and palate
- Cardiac and kidney anomalies may be present

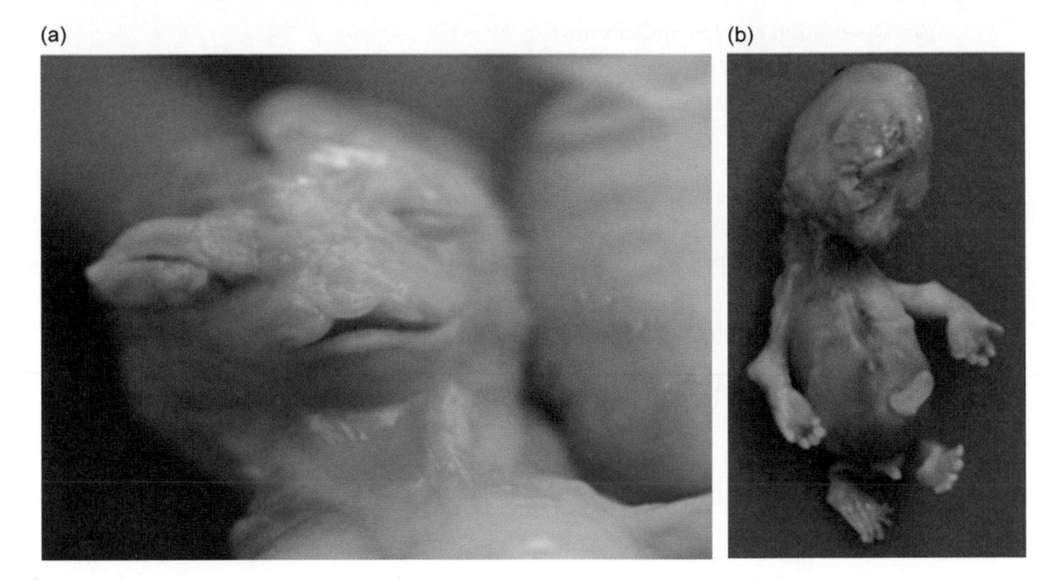

Fig. 19.27 Roberts syndrome. (a) Severely dysmorphic fetal face with bilateral cleft lip and severe micrognathia; (b) all limbs are severely shortened and the lower limbs are attached to the hip by a pedicle.

ROBINOW SYNDROME

Characteristics

- Short stature, mesomelic limb shortening predominantly of the upper limbs and brachydactyly
- Dysmorphic facies, dental abnormalities
- Cleft lip and palate, cardiac, renal and vertebral anomalies (hemivertebrae and vertebral fusion) are occasionally seen

Inheritance

- Autosomal dominant: *DVL1*, *DVL3* and *WNT5A*
- Autosomal recessive – *ROR2* (the limb shortening and brachydactyly is much more severe in the recessive type)

Ultrasound/MRI Detectable Features in Affected Fetuses

- Short long bones – mesomelic shortening of upper limbs
- Narrow thorax
- Dysmorphic facies or cleft lip/palate

SECKEL SYNDROME

Characteristics

- Low birth weight, short stature, microcephaly
- Micrognathia, large eyes/hypotelorism, low-set ears, beak-like nose
- Intellectual disability

- Dislocation of hips and elbows
- Cryptorchidism/clitoromegaly
- Haematological disorders (pancytopaenia)

Inheritance

- Autosomal recessive
- At least nine genes identified

Ultrasound/MRI Detectable Features in Affected Fetuses

- Severe fetal growth restriction
- Microcephaly, micrognathia, low-set ears

SOTOS SYNDROME

Characteristics

- Overgrowth, acromegaly
- Characteristic facial appearance – long and narrow face, flushed cheeks, prominent forehead with frontotemporal hair scarcity, down-slanting palpebral fissures, hypertelorism, a high arched palate and pointed chin
- Learning disabilities and delayed development

Inheritance

- Autosomal dominant – *NSD1* mutations but ~95% is *de novo*

Ultrasound/MRI Detectable Features in Affected Fetuses

- Overgrowth, macrocephaly, dolichocephaly
- Brain abnormalities (non-specific)
- Possible polyhydramnios, renal abnormalities, raised nuchal translucency

RUSSELL–SILVER SYNDROME

Characteristics

- Poor growth, short stature
- Triangular face, large head in relation to body size
- Body asymmetry (arms and legs of different length)
- Clinodactyly
- Feeding problems, hypoglycaemia

Inheritance

- 40–60% of patients have a detectable methylation defect at 11p15
- Some of them have uniparental disomy (UPD) of chromosome 7, or rarely UPD of chromosome 11
- Some have intragenic variants in *CDKN1C, IGF2, PLAG2* or *HMGA2*
- The genetic mechanism is still unknown in 40% of children with Russell–Silver syndrome

Ultrasound/MRI Detectable Features in Affected Fetuses

- Early fetal growth restriction with normal liquor and Doppler
- Relative macrocephaly, short long bones
- Fifth-digit clinodactyly

RAINE SYNDROME (OSTEOSCLEROTIC BONE DYSPLASIA)

Characteristics

- Generalised increase in bone density, increased ossification in the skull in particular
- Craniofacial features (exophthalmos with everted lower eyelids, gum hyperplasia, prominent forehead, small nose with depressed nasal bridge, choanal atresia, low-set ears and midface hypoplasia, wide anterior fontanelle) and cerebral calcifications
- Lethal in most cases, although surviving children are increasingly reported

Inheritance

- Autosomal recessive: *FAM20C*

Ultrasound/MRI Detectable Features in Affected Fetuses

- 'Fish-like' facies: craniofacial dysplasia, including exophthalmos, hypoplastic nose and midface, and triangular-shaped mouth
- Intracranial calcifications (periventricular, around corpus callosum)
- Microcephaly

SIRENOMELIA

Characteristics

- Partial or complete fusion of the legs
- Lethal condition

Inheritance

- Sporadic occurrence
- Association with maternal diabetes

Ultrasound/MRI Detectable Features in Affected Fetuses

- Fused lower limbs
- Associated abnormalities: renal agenesis, oligohydramnios, cardiac abnormalities, abdominal wall defects, spinal abnormalities, imperforate anus

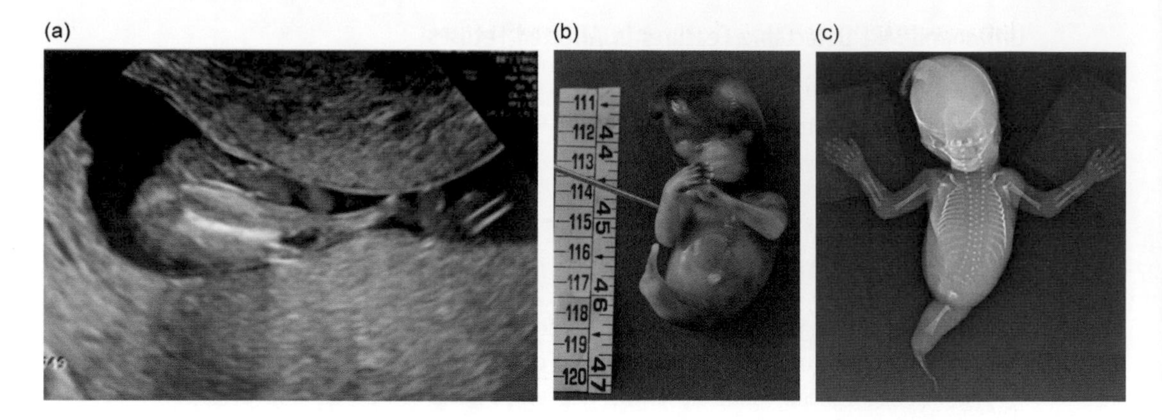

Fig. 19.28 Sirenomelia. (a) Ultrasound image showing fused lower limbs; (b) post mortem image of the same fetus with (c) an X-ray showing a single bone in the lower limb and no bones in the distal segment. The mother had uncontrolled diabetes.

SMITH–LEMLI–OPITZ SYNDROME (SLO)

Characteristics

- Growth restriction, microcephaly, mild to moderate intellectual disability
- Multiple birth defects (brain, cleft palate, heart, fused second and third toes, ambiguous genitalia)

Inheritance

- Autosomal recessive
- *DHCR7* genetic variants

Ultrasound/MRI Detectable Features in Affected Fetuses

- Fetal growth restriction
- Microcephaly, agenesis or hypoplasia of the corpus callosum, cerebellar hypoplasia, ventriculomegaly
- Cleft palate
- Polydactyly
- Cardiac defects
- Renal agenesis
- Ambiguous genitalia

TAR (THROMBOCYTOPENIA AND ABSENT RADIUS) SYNDROME

Characteristics

- Absent radius, preserved thumb
- Thrombocytopaenia (risk of life-threatening bleeding and intracranial haemorrhage)

Inheritance

- Autosomal recessive
- *RBM8A* genetic changes – usually one allele has a deletion and one a single nucleotide variant

Ultrasound/MRI Detectable Features in Affected Fetuses

- Absent radius with preserved thumb

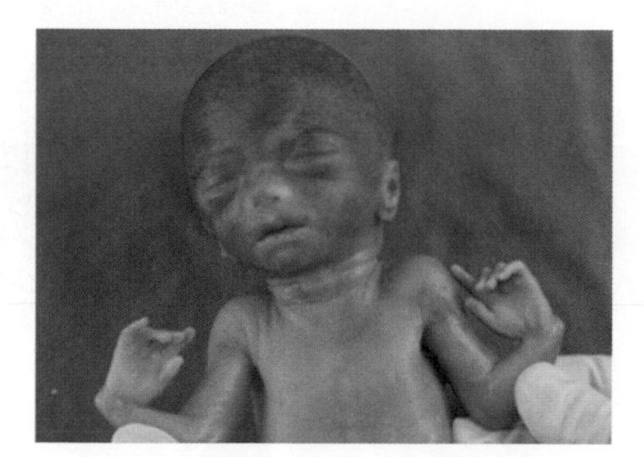

Fig. 19.29 TAR syndrome. Note the radial ray defect with preserved thumb.

TREACHER COLLINS SYNDROME

Characteristics

- Affects the development of bones and other tissues of the face – facial dysmorphia (underdeveloped zygomatic bone, micrognathia, eyes slanted downwards, eyelid coloboma, absent/small/dysmorphic ears, cleft palate)

Inheritance

- Autosomal dominant
- *TCOF1* genetic variants most common
- 40% inherited, 60% *de novo* mutation

Ultrasound/MRI Detectable Features in Affected Fetuses

- Abnormal facial profile, abnormal face 3D/4D, abnormal or absent ears
- Significant clinical overlap with other genetic disorders

TUBEROUS SCLEROSIS

Characteristics

- Neurocutaneous syndrome (phakomatosis) where benign hamartomas develop in multiple organ systems
- Angiofibromas, forehead plaque, periungual fibromas, hypomelanotic macules, shagreen patches, retinal nodular hamartomas, cortical tubers, subependymal nodules, cardiac rhabdomyomas
- Variable intellectual impairment, seizures

Inheritance

- Autosomal dominant:*TSC1* and *TSC2*
- Tremendous variability in organs involved and extent of severity

Ultrasound/MRI Detectable Features in Affected Fetuses

- Cardiac rhabdomyomas
- Echogenic/cystic kidneys
- MRI may pick up subependymal nodules and/or cortical tubers

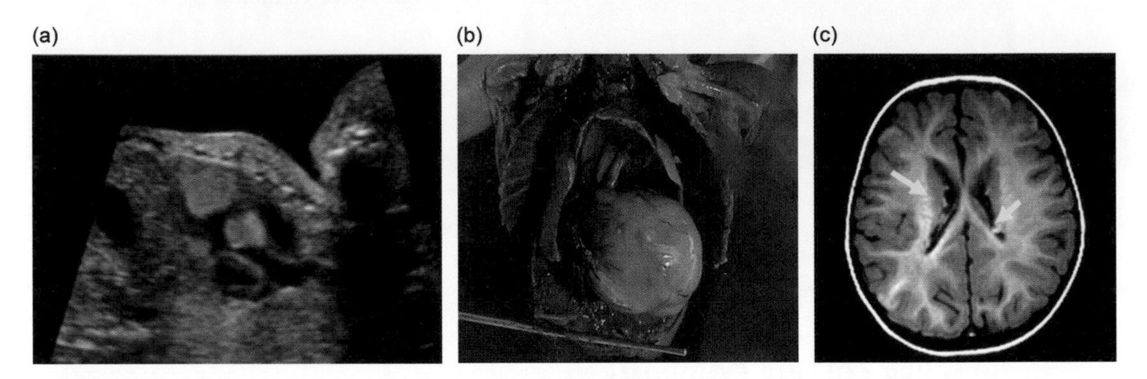

Fig. 19.30 Tuberous sclerosis. (a) Parasagittal view of the fetal heart showing multiple rhabdomyomas. (b) Post mortem picture of the heart with rhabdomyoma; (c) brain CT showing subependymal nodules (arrows).

VACTERL ASSOCIATION

Characteristics

- At least three to make diagnosis: **v**ertebral anomalies (60–80%), **a**norectal malformations (60–90%), **c**ardiovascular anomalies (40–80%), **t**racheoesophageal fistula (50–80%), o**e**sophageal atresia, **r**enal abnormalities (50–80%) and **l**imb defects (50%)

Inheritance

- No consistent genetic abnormality identified, probably sporadic

Ultrasound/MRI Detectable Features in Affected Fetuses

- Hemivertebrae
- Anal atresia/imperforate anus
- Cardiac defects (VSD, ASD and tetralogy of Fallot most common)
- Signs of oesophageal atresia/tracheoesophageal fistula (absent or small stomach and polyhydramnios)
- Abnormal kidneys
- Limb defects (displaced or hypoplastic thumb, poly/syndactyly, radial aplasia)

VAN DER WOUDE SYNDROME

Characteristics

- Cleft lip, cleft palate or both
- Pits (depressions) near the centre of the lower lip
- Other features: hypodontia, congenital heart defects, syndactyly

Inheritance

- Autosomal dominant – parent can be very mildly affected
- *IRF6* genetic variants

Ultrasound/MRI Detectable Features in Affected Fetuses

- Facial clefts of all types

VICI SYNDROME

Characteristics

- Multi-system disorder with profound developmental delay, acquired microcephaly and failure to thrive
- Five principal diagnostic features (1) agenesis of corpus callosum, (2) cataracts, (3) cardiomyopathy, (4) hypopigmentation and (5) combined immunodeficiency

Inheritance

- Autosomal recessive: *EPG5*

Ultrasound/MRI Detectable Features in Affected Fetuses

- Agenesis of corpus callosum
- Abnormal gyral pattern

WALKER–WARBURG SYNDROME

Characteristics

- Congenital muscular dystrophy associated with brain and eye abnormalities (microphthalmia, retinal abnormalities)
- Hypotonia, developmental delay, intellectual disability, seizures
- Reduced life expectancy

Inheritance

- Autosomal recessive
- At least 14 genes identified

Ultrasound/MRI Detectable Features in Affected Fetuses

- Lissencephaly, encephalocele, ventriculomegaly, Dandy–Walker
- Distinctive dorsal ‘kink’ at the mesencephalic–pontine junction

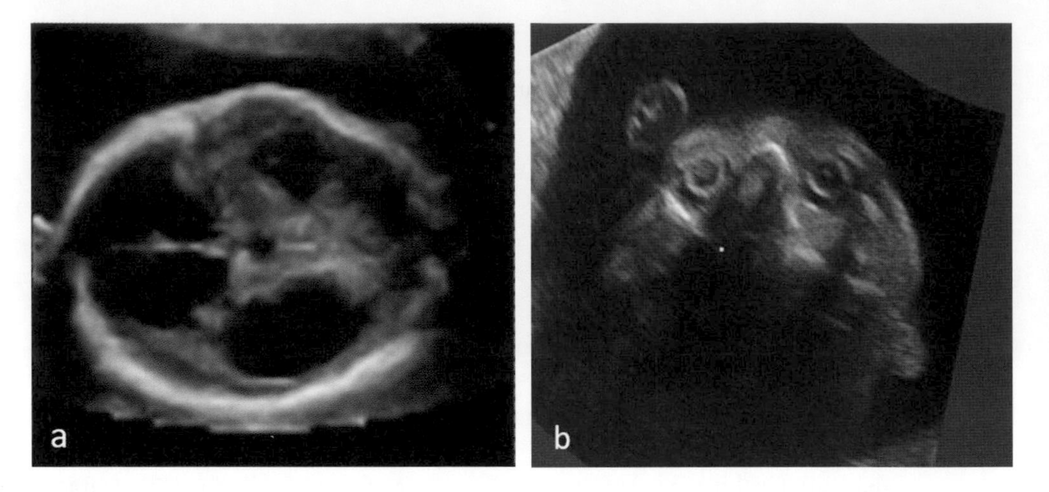

Fig. 19.31 Walker–Warburg syndrome. (a) Scan images showing ventriculomegaly and (b) the orbits with retinal detachment.

WEAVER SYNDROME

Characteristics

- Tall stature with or without macrocephaly, rapid growth
- Variable degree of intellectual disability (usually mild)
- Facial features: broad forehead, hypertelorism, large, low-set ears, micrognathia
- Contractures of joints (toes and fingers in particular), advanced bone age

Inheritance

- Autosomal dominant: *EZH2* mutations but most cases are *de novo*

Ultrasound/MRI Detectable Features in Affected Fetuses

- Overgrowth
- Macrocephaly
- Abnormal hands and feet – flexion deformities, in particular camptodactyly and talipes

WOLF–HIRSCHHORN SYNDROME

Characteristics

- Distinctive facial features (microcephaly, high forehead, hypertelorism, broad flat nasal bridge, micrognathia, dysplastic ears, downturned mouth, cleft lip/palate)
- Intellectual disability, seizures
- Congenital heart defects
- Scoliosis/kyphosis

Inheritance

- Mostly *de novo* microdeletion of the short arm of chromosome 4
- Can be inherited from a parent with a balanced translocation

Ultrasound/MRI Detectable Features in Affected Fetuses

- Fetal growth restriction
- Microcephaly, abnormal facial profile (flat nose)
- Cardiac defects (ASD)
- Scoliosis/kyphosis

X-LINKED HYDROCEPHALUS

Characteristics

- Most severe clinical subtype of L1 syndrome involving Sylvian aqueduct stenosis and severe hydrocephalus as a consequence
- Apart from hydrocephalus, clinical features include corpus callosum hypoplasia, severe intellectual disability, adducted thumbs, spasticity

Inheritance

- Can be X-linked and caused by variants in *L1CAM*

Ultrasound/MRI Detectable Features in Affected Fetuses

- Hydrocephalus, male fetus
- Adducted thumbs is a significant clue to *L1CAM*

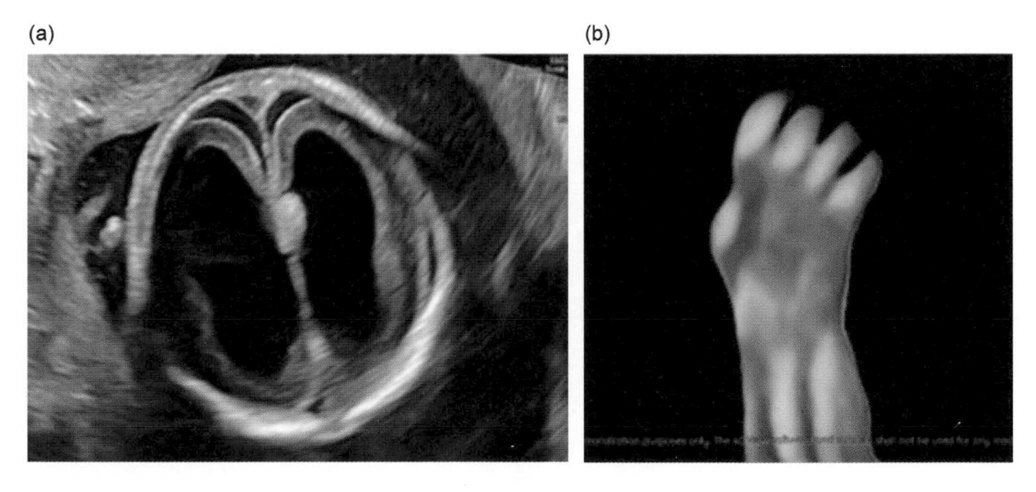

Fig. 19.32 X-linked hydrocephalus. (a) Coronal view of the head showing dilated lateral ventricles in a male fetus; (b) 3D picture of the hand of the same fetus showing characteristic palmar thumb adduction with the thumb folded under the other fingers.

ZELLWEGER SYNDROME

Characteristics

- Cerebro-hepato-renal syndrome
- Most severe form of peroxisomal biogenesis disorders
- Dysmorphism with large fontanelle, cataracts, neurological impairment, severe hypotonia, punctate calcification of patella, cystic renal impairment and hepatic disorder

Inheritance

- Autosomal recessive
- 13 genes are currently known to be associated, with *PEX1* accounting for ~60%
- Prenatal diagnosis is feasible by molecular testing and biochemically by assays of peroxisomal metabolites

Ultrasound/MRI Detectable Features in Affected Fetuses

- Increased nuchal translucency and fetal hypokinesia in the first trimester
- In later gestation, fetuses present with cerebral ventriculomegaly, hyperechogenic kidneys and hepatomegaly
- MRI in third trimester may reveal cerebral ventricular enlargement, abnormal cortical gyral patterns, impaired myelination, cerebral periventricular microcysts, renal microcysts and hepatosplenomegaly

CHAPTER 20

Termination of Pregnancy for Fetal Abnormality

SUMMARY BOX

INDICATIONS

- Structural abnormalities ~50%, mainly CNS abnormalities
- Chromosomal abnormalities ~40%; mainly due to trisomy 21
- PPROM ~5%
- Multiple factors ~5%

- In countries where late termination is legal, ~10% of terminations of pregnancy (TOPs) for fetal abnormalities are performed after 24 weeks' gestation

LEGAL FRAMEWORK

UNITED KINGDOM

- The Abortion Act 1967, amended in 1990, sets out the framework in which TOP for fetal abnormality is lawful when two registered medical practitioners are of the opinion, formed in good faith, that grounds for TOP are satisfied
- Out of seven statutory grounds for TOP, clause E is the most relevant for fetal medicine specialists: *There is a substantial risk that if the child were born it would suffer from such physical or mental abnormalities as to be seriously handicapped*

AUSTRALIA AND NEW ZEALAND

- There is considerable variation in abortion legislation across states and territories of Australia and between Australia and New Zealand
- In most territories, late termination is legal for anomalies detected or apparent >20 weeks, including discordant anomalies in multiple pregnancies
- In most territories, once a gestation threshold for late termination is reached (varies from 14 to 20 weeks), two doctors must agree that the grounds for TOP are met
- In the Northern Territory TOP >23 weeks is permitted only if the woman's life is at risk, while in Western Australia TOP is heavily restricted after 20 weeks

INDIA

- The Medical Termination of Pregnancy Act 1971 stipulates that TOP is permissible when there is substantial risk that the child, if born, would be seriously handicapped due to physical or mental abnormalities
- The Act was amended in 2021 to raise the cutoff gestational age from 20 to 24 weeks

MEDICAL MANAGEMENT

- Combination of mifepristone and misoprostol
- Mifepristone is an oral progesterone receptor antagonist
- Misoprostol is a synthetic prostaglandin E1 analogue; it can be administered orally, sublingually vaginally or rectally

GESTATIONAL AGE

- The mifepristone/misoprostol combination can be used at any gestation

PROCEDURE-RELATED RISKS

- Failure ~2%
- Infection is unlikely, but can occur, particularly if there is a subclinical pre-existing infection
- Haemorrhage ~0.1% during the first trimester rising to 0.4% at 20 weeks
- Retained tissue and need for operative intervention ~5%
- Uterine rupture is rare <0.1%
- Misoprostol induced side effects are relatively common, mainly shivering and diarrhoea
- Misoprostol induced maternal hyperpyrexia may occur, but it will be short-lasting and self-limiting. When it occurs standard supporting measures (cooling, paracetamol) should suffice

PROCEDURE

- In selected cases, early first trimester TOP (<10 weeks) may be completed at home
- If home TOP is arranged, we advise a follow-up scan to ensure that the process is complete
- Wherever possible, women should be cared for in a private room, away from other expectant mothers
- Women should receive supportive, non-judgemental one-to-one nursing/midwifery care
- Best practice is to allow a birth partner to remain with the woman throughout
- Adequate analgesia is important. For most women undergoing first and early second trimester TOP this is achieved with oral paracetamol and codeine
- Access to parenteral opiates and/or epidural analgesia should be available, if needed, mainly during late TOP in primiparous women

MIFEPRISTONE

- 200 mg orally is adequate; there is no good evidence to support higher doses
- Mifepristone can be administered in an outpatient setting; there is no minimum required observation period
- The *standard protocol* requires 48–72 hours gap between mifepristone and the first misoprostol dose
- The *short protocol* (<24 hours gap between mifepristone and misoprostol) is also acceptable, particularly for women who may find the delay unacceptable
- Standard protocol will require fewer doses of misoprostol with more women delivering within 12 hours of the first misoprostol dose
- The average mifepristone–delivery interval of the standard protocol is longer compared with the short protocol

MISOPROSTOL

Intact Uterus (No Previous Uterine Scar)

- $\leq 23^{+6}$ weeks, misoprostol 800 µg vaginally, then up to four oral doses of 400 µg
- 24^{+0} to 31^{+6} weeks, misoprostol 400 µg vaginally, then up to four oral doses of 200 µg
- 32^{+0} to term, misoprostol 50 µg vaginally, repeat every 6 hours to a maximum of four doses

Placenta Praevia

- Placenta praevia is not a contraindication to vaginal delivery before 24 weeks
- In cases of complete placenta praevia after 24 weeks, a hysterotomy is a safer option

Scarred Uterus

- $\leq 23^{+6}$ weeks, misoprostol 400 µg vaginally, then up to four oral doses of 400 µg
- 24^{+0} to 31^{+6} weeks, misoprostol 200 µg vaginally, then up to four oral doses of 100 µg
- 32^{+0} to term, misoprostol 25 µg vaginally, repeat every 6 hours to a maximum of four doses

No Significant Progress after 24 Hours

- Arrange detailed clinical review by senior obstetrician
- Be alert to the possibility of uterine rupture
- Be alert to the possibility of an abdominal pregnancy
- It is advisable to perform another ultrasound scan, transvaginal if necessary, to confirm that the fetus is still within the uterine cavity, in close proximity to the internal cervical os with intact myometrium
- If clinically stable, the medical management protocols can be safely repeated after a 12-hour rest period
- If mifepristone/misoprostol protocol has failed, intramuscular carboprost (250 µg) should be tried before contemplating hysterotomy
- Carboprost injections can be repeated every 1.5–2 hours up to eight doses
- There is no good evidence to support routine curettage after medical TOP

SURGICAL MANAGEMENT

GESTATIONAL AGE

- Can be performed at any gestational age, but the approach and techniques must be adapted according to fetal size and maternal factors
- It is important to mention to patients that it will not be possible to see the baby after the procedure – this can only be arranged after medical TOP

PROCEDURE-RELATED RISKS

- Overall risks increase with gestational age, but the risks are comparable to the risks of medical management
- Retained tissue ~2%
- Haemorrhage ~0.1% during the first trimester, 0.4% at 20 weeks
- Cervical trauma $\leq 1\%$
- Uterine perforation 0.1–0.4%
- Infection is unlikely, but can occur, particularly if there is a pre-existing subclinical infection
- A significant proportion of risks can be mitigated by adhering to good practice where appropriate (e.g. antibiotics, cervical ripening, perioperative ultrasound)

TECHNIQUE

First Trimester

- Cervical ripening with 400 μg vaginal misoprostol ~3 hours pre-op is advised for cases with a higher chance of uterine perforation, including those with cervical scarring or stenosed endocervical canal following previous treatment
- Pre-op misoprostol can be safely self-administered at home
- Antimicrobial prophylaxis is advised with a single dose of oral doxycycline 200 mg or azithromycin 500 mg
- Procedures should be performed in theatre, with aseptic technique
- Effective anaesthesia/analgesia is required
- Conscious sedation +/− paracervical block and NSAIDs can be used effectively for procedures before 14 weeks
- Suction evacuation can be safely performed without cervical dilatation up to 12 weeks
- Good practice is to avoid suction catheters that are too small as this increases the risk of uterine perforation
- Sharp curettage can be used to remove retained tissue, but should not be routinely used for every surgical TOP due to increased risk of uterine perforation

Second Trimester

- Cervical ripening with 400 μg vaginal misoprostol 3 hours pre-op, or laminaria (Dilapam) is advised for all cases >14 weeks
- After 16 weeks, we give 400 μg of misoprostol 4 hours before scheduled surgery, followed by 200 μg 3 hours later
- Antimicrobial prophylaxis is advised with a single dose of oral doxycycline 200 mg or azithromycin 500 mg
- Procedures should be performed in theatre, with aseptic technique
- Performing a perioperative scan is important to:
  - confirm appropriate path of dilatation
  - reduce the risk of perforation
  - confirm that evacuation is complete
- Due to the need for greater instrumentation in the second trimester, general or regional anaesthesia are generally used. However, deep sedation combined with NSAIDs and local anaesthesia may be an acceptable alternative, after appraising individual factors, with the informed consent of the woman
- After 14 weeks, cervical dilatation is required to allow passage of larger fetal parts (Fig. 20.1)
- As the second trimester progresses, destructive procedures using instruments may also be required to allow delivery through the cervix
- Cervical dilatation before the procedure reduces the risk of cervical injury from instruments
- Sharp curettage can be used to remove retained tissue, but should not be routinely used for every surgical TOP due to increased risk of uterine perforation

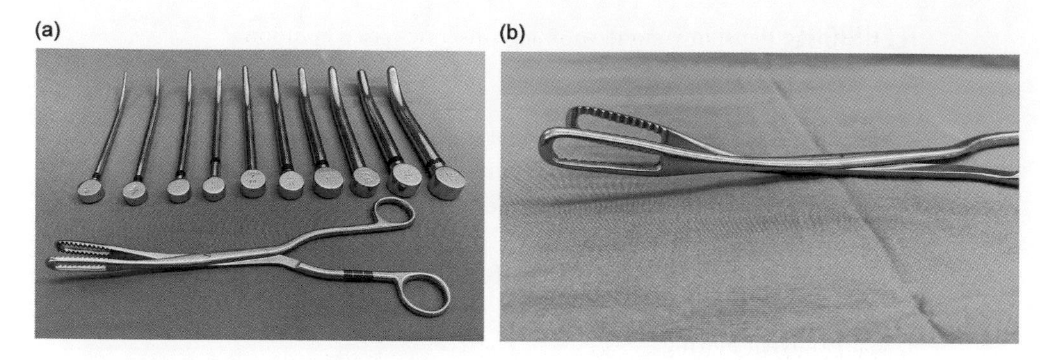

Fig. 20.1 (a) Amber Hawkin tapered dilators used for mechanical dilatation of the cervix before surgical TOP. (b) Fink forceps are used to grasp products of conception; the profile of the jaws facilitates easy insertion in the uterine cavity, minimising risk of perforation. Continuous ultrasound guidance of the procedure further minimises the risk of complications.

TERMINATION AFTER TRANSABDOMINAL CERCLAGE

- Medical TOP is generally contraindicated, because the risk of cervical tears and even uterine rupture is considered to be too high
- Early surgical procedures usually require only minimal manual dilatation with dilators, in order to accommodate suction cannulas
- In skilled hands, ultrasound guided surgical procedures may be performed safely even after 20 weeks' gestation
- Laminaria, rather than misoprostol, tends to be used for cervical preparation for procedures at later gestations
- If adequate skill is not available for a transvaginal procedure, hysterotomy has to be performed
- Several successful pregnancies following TOP with TAC in situ have been reported

FETOCIDE IN SINGLETONS

GESTATIONAL AGE

- Offered from 21^{+0} weeks to prevent a possibility of a livebirth with related legal and ethical implications
- Advised beyond 21^{+6} weeks to avoid fetus being born with signs of life
- Ensure that relevant consent and notification forms have been signed according to local laws

PROCEDURE-RELATED RISKS

- Maternal discomfort
- <1:1,000 risk of severe maternal infection
- Visceral or vascular injuries are extremely rare

ANTISEPTIC PROCEDURES

- Use sterile gloves
- In most centres sterile gowns are used only for longer procedures (transfusions, shunts, amniodrainage)

- Cleaning the skin is done with an antiseptic-based solution
- Use of a sterile cover for ultrasound probe and sterile gel, although not universal, is recommended
- There is no good evidence to support use of antibiotics or tocolytics

TECHNIQUE

- The puncture site is infiltrated with 10 ml of local anaesthetic (lidocaine 1%) – this is also helpful to map the needle path
- Fetal heart or umbilical vein at the site of placental cord insertion are targeted with 20G needle
- Free loops of cord are best avoided as additional mobility increases the challenge of siting the needle and risk of dislodging
- A fetal blood sample can be obtained for diagnostic purposes, if required
- For intracardiac injection, up to 10 ml of 15% potassium chloride can be used. A higher dose is rarely required
- Potassium should be injected only when the needle tip is clearly visible and a flush-back of fetal blood is obtained to avoid injecting into the pericardium
- Alternatively, a bolus of 10–20 ml of 1% lidocaine can be injected to induce fetal asystole, particularly when placental insertion of the umbilical vein is used to access the fetal circulation
- Leave the needle in place until asystole has been sustained for at least 5 minutes
- We advise that fetal asystole is confirmed after a period of 20–30 minutes

FETOCIDE IN MULTIPLE PREGNANCIES

DICHORIONIC PREGNANCY

- Dichorionic twins, and some higher-order multiples, have individual placentas with no shared vascular connections. Therefore, intravascular agents (potassium chloride or lidocaine) can be used safely for selective termination of an affected twin

GESTATIONAL AGE

- Safest between 11^{+0} and 14^{+0} weeks
- If legally permissible, procedures carried out after 32^{+0} weeks reduce the risk of procedure-related miscarriage of the whole pregnancy, or extreme preterm birth of the healthy twin

PROCEDURE-RELATED RISKS

- Pregnancy loss and preterm birth rates are gestation dependent (see Table 20.1)
- Discomfort/pain is relatively common
- Maternal visceral/vascular injury are very rare
- Infection (<1/1,000)
- Inadvertent termination of a healthy twin is very rare

Table 20.1 Pregnancy loss and preterm birth rates: fetocide in multiple pregnancies

	Timing of the procedure		
	First trimester	Second trimester	Third trimester
Loss of a healthy twin	~5%	~15%	Rare
Preterm birth/PPROM	~5%	~15%	~15%

TECHNIQUE

- Following review of any cytogenetic results, accurate mapping should be performed jointly by two operators
- As a rule, the procedure is performed as an outpatient procedure with local anaesthetic
- The procedure is carried out with continuous ultrasound guidance using a free-hand technique
- The rest of the fetocide technique is the same as described for singletons
- The intracardiac route is preferable to avoid the risk of misidentification
- There is no risk of hypoperfusion injury to the healthy twin following demise of the affected twin

SELECTIVE TERMINATION WITH SHARED CHORIONICITY

MONOCHORIONIC PREGNANCY

- Monochorionic twins (and some higher multiples) have placentas with shared vascular connections and for this reason vaso-occlusive techniques must be used (see Chapter 17)
- Intravascular agents (potassium chloride and lidocaine) cannot be used as they are likely to enter the circulation of the unaffected twin
- There is a risk of hypoperfusion injury to the healthy twin following demise of the affected twin

GESTATIONAL AGE

- Safest between 11^{+0} and 14^{+0} weeks
- If legally permissible, the procedure carried out after 32^{+0} weeks reduces the risk of procedure-related miscarriage of the whole pregnancy, or extreme preterm birth of the healthy twin

PROCEDURE-RELATED RISKS

- Pregnancy loss and preterm birth rates are gestation dependent (see Table 20.2)
- Discomfort/pain is relatively common
- Maternal visceral or vascular injuries are very rare
- Infection rate is <1/1,000
- Inadvertent termination of healthy twin is very rare

Table 20.2 Pregnancy loss and preterm birth rates: selective termination with shared chorionicity

	Timing of the procedure		
	First trimester	**Second trimester**	**Third trimester**
Loss of a healthy twin	~15%	~15%	~15%
Preterm birth/PPROM	~15%	~15%	~15%

TECHNIQUE

Bipolar coagulation, radiofrequency ablation and interstitial laser are described in Chapter 17

POST-PROCEDURE MANAGEMENT

- If delivery is uncomplicated and the woman is well, there is no need to remain in hospital for a set period, but women should be afforded as much time to stay as they wish
- Ideally, they should recover in a private hospital room, in the presence of their birth partner and stillborn baby, if they so wish
- Information on post-abortion support (locally available and/or online) should be provided
- Rhesus negative, non-sensitised women should receive anti-D prophylaxis
- An individualised plan should be made regarding follow-up and timing of delivery of a healthy twin, taking account of the woman's wishes
- Ensure that all relevant tests, including genetic tests, have been offered and the plan for investigations is communicated to the obstetric team
- Debrief should be offered once all investigation results are available and complete information can be shared with the woman
- For twin pregnancies, the registration of a stillborn baby can be complex and needs to be carefully communicated in advance

SUGGESTED READING

Beriwal S, Impey L, Ioannou C. Multifetal pregnancy reduction and selective termination. *TOG* 2020; 22(4):284–292.

Dethier D, Lassey SC, Pilliod R, et al. Uterine evacuation in the setting of transabdominal cerclage. *Contraception*. 2020;101(3):174–177.

RCOG. Best practice in abortion care (Best Practice Paper No.2). 2015. www.rcog.org.uk/en/guidelines-research-services/guidelines/bpp2.

Sharp A, Navaratnam K, Abreu P, Alfirevic Z. Short versus standard mifepristone and misoprostol regimen for second- and third-trimester termination of pregnancy for fetal anomaly. *Fetal Diagn Ther* 2016;39:140–146.

Index